CANINE and FELINE CYTOLOGY

A Color Atlas and Interpretation Guide

SECOND EDITION

CANINE and FELINE CYTOLOGY

A Color Atlas and Interpretation Guide

Rose E. Raskin, DVM, PhD, DACVP
Director of Continuing Education and
Professor of Veterinary Clinical Pathology
Department of Comparative Pathobiology
School of Veterinary Medicine
Purdue University
West Lafayette, Indiana;
Courtesy Professor
Department of Physiological Sciences
College of Veterinary Medicine
University of Florida
Gainesville, Florida

Denny J. Meyer, DVM, DACVIM, DACVP
Chief Scientific Officer
Charles River Preclinical Services
Reno, Nevada

with more than 1,200 illustrations

SAUNDERS

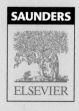

ELSEVIER

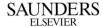

SAUNDERS
ELSEVIER

11830 Westline Industrial Drive
St. Louis, Missouri 63146

CANINE AND FELINE CYTOLOGY: A COLOR ATLAS AND INTERPRETATION
GUIDE, SECOND EDITION   ISBN: 978-1-4160-4985-2
Copyright © 2010, 2001 by Saunders, an imprint of Elsevier Inc.

Notice

ISBN: 978-1-4160-4985-2

Vice President and Publisher: Linda Duncan
Senior Acquisitions Editor: Anthony Winkel
Developmental Editor: Maureen Slaten
Publishing Services Manager: Julie Eddy
Senior Project Manager: Andrea Campbell
Designer: Margaret Reid

Printed in China

Last digit is the print number: 9   8   7   6   5   4   3   2

Contributors

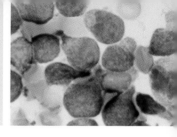

**A. Rick Alleman, DVM, PhD, DABVP, DACVP
(Companion Animal Practice)**
Professor, Clinical Pathology
Department of Physiological Sciences
College of Veterinary Medicine
University of Florida
Gainesville, Florida
Chapter 16: Endocrine System

Claire B. Andreasen, DVM, PhD, DACVP
Professor and Chair
Department of Veterinary Pathology
College of Veterinary Medicine
Iowa State University
Ames, Iowa
*Chapter 7: Oral Cavity, Gastrointestinal Tract, and
Associated Structures*

Anne C. Avery, VMD, PhD
Associate Professor
Department of Microbiology, Immunology and
Pathology
College of Veterinary Medicine & Biomedical Sciences
Colorado State University
Fort Collins, Colorado
Chapter 17: Advanced Diagnostic Techniques

Paul R. Avery, VMD, PhD, DACVP
Assistant Professor
Department of Microbiology, Immunology and
Pathology
College of Veterinary Medicine & Biomedical Sciences
Colorado State University
Fort Collins, Colorado
Chapter 17: Advanced Diagnostic Techniques

Anne M. Barger, DVM, MS, DACVP
Clinical Associate Professor, Pathobiology
Clinical Associate Professor, Veterinary Diagnostic
Laboratory
College of Veterinary Medicine
University of Illinois at Urbana-Champaign
Urbana, Illinois
Chapter 13: Musculoskeletal System

Dori L. Borjesson, DVM, PhD, DACVP
Associate Professor
Department of Pathology, Microbiology &
Immunology
School of Veterinary Medicine
University of California, Davis
Davis, California
Chapter 10: Urinary Tract

Mary Jo Burkhard, DVM, PhD, DACVP
Associate Professor
Department of Veterinary Biosciences
College of Veterinary Medicine
The Ohio State University
Columbus, Ohio
Chapter 5: Respiratory Tract

Ul Soo Choi, DVM, PhD
Instructor
Department of Veterinary Clinical Pathology
College of Veterinary Medicine
Chonbuck National University
Jeonju, Korea
Chapter 16: Endocrine System

Sara L. Connolly, DVM
Department of Comparative Pathobiology
School of Veterinary Medicine
Purdue University
West Lafayette, Indiana
*Chapter 1: The Acquisition and Management of
Cytology Specimens*

Keith DeJong, DVM
Department of Pathology, Microbiology & Immunology
School of Veterinary Medicine
University of California, Davis
Davis, California
Chapter 10: Urinary Tract

Davide De Lorenzi, DVM, DECVP
Specialist, Clinic and Pathology of Companion Animals
San Marco Veterinary Clinic
Padua, Italy
Chapter 14: The Central Nervous System

Hock Gan Heng, DVM, MVS, MS, DACVR, DECVDI
Clinical Assistant Professor
Department of Veterinary Clinical Sciences
School of Veterinary Medicine
Purdue University
West Lafayette, Indiana
*Chapter 1: The Acquisition and Management of
Cytology Specimens*

Albert E. Jergens, DVM, MS, PhD, DACVIM
Associate Professor and Section Head
Professor, Small Animal Medicine
Department of Veterinary Clinical Sciences
College of Veterinary Medicine
Iowa State University
Ames, Iowa
*Chapter 7: Oral Cavity, Gastrointestinal Tract, and
Associated Structures*

Maria Teresa Mandara, DVM
Associate Professor, Neuropathology Laboratory
Department of Biopathological Science and Hygiene
    of Animal and Food Production
School of Veterinary Medicine
University of Perugia
Perugia, Italy
Chapter 14: The Central Nervous System

Laurie M. Millward, DVM
Goss Laboratory
Department of Veterinary Biosciences
College of Veterinary Medicine
The Ohio State University
Columbus, Ohio
Chapter 5: Respiratory Tract

José A. Ramos-Vara, DVM, PhD, DECVP
Associate Professor of Veterinary Pathology
Animal Disease Diagnostic Laboratory
School of Veterinary Medicine
Purdue University
West Lafayette, Indiana
Chapter 17: Advanced Diagnostic Techniques

Alan H. Rebar, DVM, PhD, DACVP
Executive Director of Discovery Park
Senior Associate Vice President for Research
Professor of Veterinary Clinical Pathology
School of Veterinary Medicine
Purdue University
West Lafayette, Indiana
Chapter 6: Body Cavity Fluids

Laia Solano-Gallego, DVM, PhD, DECVCP
Lecturer, Veterinary Clinical Pathology
Department of Pathology and Infectious Diseases
The Royal Veterinary College
North Mymms
Hatfield, Hertfordshire, United Kingdom
Chapter 12: Reproductive System

Craig A. Thompson, DVM, DACVP
Clinical Assistant Professor of Clinical Pathology
Department of Comparative Pathobiology
School of Veterinary Medicine
Purdue University
West Lafayette, Indiana
Chapter 6: Body Cavity Fluids

Heather L. Wamsley, DVM, DACVP
Assistant Professor, Clinical Pathology
Department of Physiological Sciences
College of Veterinary Medicine
University of Florida
Gainesville, Florida
Chapter 8: Dry-Mount Fecal Cytology

Preface

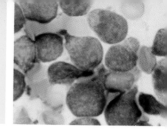

"Another source of fallacy is the vicious circle of illusions which consists on the one hand of believing what we see and, on the other, seeing what we believe."
– Sir Clifford Allbutt, M.D. (1836-1925). He introduced the diagnostic use of the microscope to the hospital ward.

The objective of the first edition of the Atlas was to compile a practical guide to cytopathology that focused primarily on the types of lesions that clinicians faced in routine practice, yet be a user-friendly teaching tool for the soon-to-be practitioner. We used tables, brief descriptions, and carefully selected photomicrographs accumulated over decades of diagnostic cytology with concise, informative figure legends to support the microscopic examination of the cytology specimen. We attempted to organize the presentations into logical and uniform approaches, thereby facilitating readability, comprehension, and learning. Based on the robust positive feedback we received, we are pleased to surmise that we have generally achieved that objective.

Constructive suggestions indicated that the cytopathologist desired additional lesions be covered, including those less commonly encountered, more histopathology correlates, and a broader use of stains and immunocytochemistry for differential cytologic characterization. The encouragement incentivized us, in this new edition, to expand the photomicrograph portfolio, including more comparative histology, and the attendant text and references. This was accomplished by adding new authors who injected their pragmatic microscopic expertise into expanded existing chapters, and adding a new chapter on fecal cytology. The enhanced portfolio of images has also been made possible by the helpful assistance of other benevolent cytopathologists, who generously contributed photomicrographs from their collections.

A significant expansion involved the chapter on advanced techniques to include more methodology and application of some current tools such as immunochemistry, electron microscopy, flow cytometry, and molecular testing. The challenge was to accommodate the recommended changes without obfuscation of the Atlas' intended objective of a practical, user-friendly cytologic compilation, which was the successful foundation of the first edition. It is our hope that, by careful editing to ensure a clear and concise narrative, seamless integration of new and updated information into the existing text, judicious selection of new and enhanced photomicrographs, and the use of lists that highlight criteria for differential diagnosis, we have produced a second edition that will continue to find preferred residence beside the microscope because of its usefulness.

We present the second edition with considerable excitement and hope that we have succeeded in transmitting to the user the beauty of the expanded application of diagnostic cytology. We share in the exhilaration of the microscopist when the unknown cytologic specimen is translated into a cytologic diagnosis, i.e., *"believe in what they see,"* with the guidance of this Atlas.

Rose & Denny

Acknowledgments

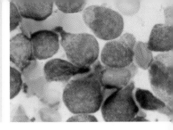

<u>Teamwork</u> = *Cooperative effort by the members of a group or team to achieve a common goal.*
<u>Achievement</u> = *Something accomplished successfully, especially by means of exertion, skill, practice, or perseverance.*
     —American Heritage Dictionary, 4th edition

An Atlas that successfully covers the broad scope of cytologic findings described and illustrated in the second edition cannot be completed without the assistance of many individuals, most of whom are transparent to us. You know who you are and thanks and gratitude are owed to all of you for help in various ways. Noteworthy recognition of folks at Elsevier is extended to Dr. Anthony Winkel for believing in us one more time, and Maureen Slaten, who exhibited remarkable patience as we missed timelines, and administered respectful, tenacious encouragement and prodding to keep the process in motion. Lastly, Andrea Campbell, who in the final stages of the project was technically terrific, conscientious, attentive to details, and responsive.

We wish to salute the authors who contributed to the first edition but were not involved in the second edition. Their cytologic expertise contributed to its success and provided a healthy foundation for the expansion of the second edition. The authors, a list that reads like recommended inductees into a Cytology Hall of Fame, include:

- Drs. Amy Valenciano and Anne Barger – Respiratory System
- Dr. Sonjia Shelly – Body Cavity Fluids
- Dr. Kristin Henson – Reproductive System
- Dr. Kathleen Freeman – Central Nervous System
- Drs. Janice Andrews and David Malarkey – Advanced Diagnostic Techniques

We also wish to extend our appreciation to those cytologists who selflessly contributed photomicrographs and are acknowledged in the figure legends. Notably, Denny thanks his longtime friend and colleague, Dr. Dave Edwards, for his impressive contributions to the liver chapter. Denny also takes the opportunity to acknowledge Rose. She was clearly the indefatigable driving force of the second edition and her passionate commitment to exhaustive completeness, accuracy, and detail translated into differentiating excellence of the second edition.

Lastly, we wish to express our sincere appreciation to the contributing authors of the second edition. They altruistically added one more burden to their primary professional duties to share their cytologic expertise for betterment of veterinary patient care. They are represented both by the seasoned and the newer, most promising purveyors of cytology today. Their collective expertise has markedly extended the range of information that is embedded in the second edition. We could not have worked with a better group of professionals. Thanks for successfully partnering with us; we hope you share in our pride with the final product.

           Rose & Denny

Contents

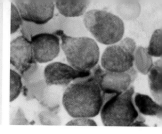

CANINE and FELINE CYTOLOGY

A Color Atlas and Interpretation Guide

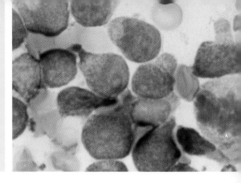

CHAPTER 1

The Acquisition and Management of Cytology Specimens

Denny J. Meyer, Sara L. Connolly, and Hock Gan Heng

The classification of events that depend on the accuracy of observation is limited by the ability of the observer to describe and of the interpreter to decipher.

—Michael Podell, M.Sc., D.V.M.

For the microscopic examination of tissue, one important factor that affects the accuracy of observation is specimen management. The successful use of aspiration cytology depends on several interrelated procedures: acquisition of a representative specimen, proper application to a glass side, adequate staining, and examination with a high-quality microscope. A deficiency in one or more of these steps will adversely affect the yield of diagnostic information. The objective of this chapter is to provide general recommendations for managing samples in a way that ensures they are diagnosed accurately.

GENERAL SAMPLING GUIDELINES

Before executing any sampling procedure, a cytology kit should be prepared and dedicated for that purpose. An inexpensive plastic tool caddie works well. Suggested contents are listed in Box 1-1. Six or more slides are placed on a firm, flat surface such as a surgical tray immediately before initiating the sampling procedure. The surface of the glass slide should be routinely wiped with a paper towel, or at least on a shirtsleeve, to remove "invisible" glass particles that interfere with the spreading procedure.

Box 1-2 lists suggested indications for the application of diagnostic cytology. The collection of specimens for cytologic evaluation from cutaneous and subcutaneous tissues and abdominal organs and masses in smaller animals is generally accomplished with a 20- or 22-gauge, 1- to 1½-inch needle firmly attached to a 6- or 12-cc syringe. For more difficult to reach internal organs, a 2½- to 3½-inch spinal needle is used. The added length amplifies the area for cell collection and enhances the diagnostic yield. Literally, cores of hepatic tissue can be obtained with the use of a longer needle. The stylet can be left in place as the cavity is entered to avoid contamination

during the "searching" process of locating the tissue of sampling interest. Coating the needle and syringe hub with sterile 4% disodium EDTA before aspiration biopsy sampling of vascular tissues, notably bone marrow, reduces the risk of clot formation that will compromise the quality of the cytologic specimen. For the relatively inexperienced, this may be a practice to consider routinely when sampling any tissue. Clotted specimens are a frequent cause of cytologic preps of poor quality.

The general steps for obtaining a cytologic specimen are illustrated in Figure 1-1A. The tip of the needle is inserted into the tissue of interest, the plunger is retracted slightly (½ to 1 cc of vacuum), the needle advanced and retracted in several different directions, the plunger released, the needle withdrawn, and the specimen placed on a glass slide or in an EDTA (purple-topped) tube as appropriate. Commercial aspiration guns (Fig. 1-1B) are available that can be loaded with various size syringes (Fig. 1-1B). The syringe plunger sits within the trigger, which allows for easier and more stable retraction. If fluid is obtained from a mass lesion, the site is completely drained, the needle withdrawn, the fluid placed in an EDTA tube, and the procedure repeated with a new needle directed at firm tissue. Both specimens are examined microscopically. To enhance operator flexibility, intravenous extension tubing (Extension Set, Abbott Laboratories) can be used to attach the needle and syringe. Positioning and redirection of the needle is easier and accommodates patient movement (Fig. 1-1C).

Aspiration is not a prerequisite for obtaining a cytologic specimen. A technique based on the principle of capillarity, referred to as "fine-needle capillary sampling," can be performed by placing a needle into the lesion with or without a syringe attached (Mair et al., 1989; Yue and Zheng, 1989). The technique has been shown to have diagnostic sensitivity similar

---

BOX 1-1   Contents of the Cytology Kit

Syringes: 6 to 12 cc
Needles: 1- and 1½-inch—20- to 22-gauge; 2½- or 3½-inch
    spinal needle with stylet
Scalpel blades: #10 and #11
Box of precleaned glass slides with frosted end
Tubes: EDTA (purple top) and serum (red top without
    separator)
Rigid, flat surface on which 6 to 10 slides can be spread out
Butterfly catheters 21- to 23-gauge and intravenous
    extension tubing
Pencil, permanent black marker (Sharpie), or slide-specific
    marker
4% sterile EDTA
Hair dryer

**BOX 1-2   General Indications for the Use
            of Diagnostic Cytology**

Effusions—thoracic, abdominal, and pericardial
Urine sediments, urinary bladder washing
Prostate—direct aspirate, washing
Lymphadenopathy—focal, generalized
Examination for metastatic disease
Diffuse organomegaly—liver, kidney, spleen
Cutaneous/subcutaneous mass, ulcerative lesion
Conjunctival/vitreous/aqueous cytology
Pulmonary/nasal aspirates/brushings, bronchoalveolar/
    nasal washing/lavage
Unidentified abdominal mass
Evaluation of a mass or lesion discovered intraoperatively

---

to that of aspiration biopsy when used to sample a variety of tissues. Its major advantage is to reduce blood contamination from vascular tissues such as liver, spleen, kidney, and thyroid. Cells are displaced into the cylinder of the needle by capillary action as the needle is incompletely retracted and redirected into the tissue three to six times. Personal preference is justified when deciding between aspiration and nonaspiration sampling for collection of the specimen. Through trial and error the operator may determine that each has value for sampling different tissues.

KEY POINT Acquisition of the cytology specimen is an art that can be honed only by practice. Selecting an appropriate mode of sampling enhances the probability of obtaining accurate diagnostic information.

KEY POINT Routinely dry-wipe the surface of the glass slide to remove "invisible" glass particles that cause spreading deficiencies. Never reuse washed glass slides.

DIAGNOSTIC IMAGING GUIDED SAMPLE COLLECTION

Cytology sample collection can be performed via the guidance of fluoroscopy, ultrasound, and computed tomography. Ultrasound guidance is the preferred method of sampling collection because of its widespread availability and portability. In addition, ultrasound provides real-time monitoring of precise needle placement. The technique and indications are detailed elsewhere (Nyland et al., 2002a). Ultrasound-guided fine-needle aspiration biopsy (FNAB) is indicated for cytologic evaluation of nodules and masses detected on ultrasound and to evaluate organomegaly when a diffuse cellular infiltrate such as lymphoma and mast cell tumor is suspected. Most sarcomas exfoliate sparsely or not at all. A surgical or ultrasound-guided cutting needle biopsy is recommended if the FNAB sample is not diagnostic. Ultrasound-guided FNAB can be performed in most patients without chemical restraint or local anesthesia. If chemical restraint is needed, agents that promote panting should be avoided because this will lead to excessive movement and gas ingestion (Nyland et al., 2002a).

Biopsy Guidance

Ultrasound-guided FNAB can be performed by freehand technique or with the aid of a biopsy guide fastened to the transducer. Freehand technique consists of holding the transducer in one hand and inserting the needle with the other at an oblique angle to the long axis of the transducer but still within the scan plane (Fig. 1-1D). This technique requires more skill but allows greater flexibility. If the needle cannot be seen during the procedure, slightly moving the transducer into the path of the needle and gently agitating the needle or injecting microbubbles in saline solution through needle will usually allow the needle's position to be determined. Better visualization of the needle can be achieved by ensuring needle placement within the focal zone of the transducer. The biopsy guide holds the needle firmly and directs the needle along a predetermined course within the scan plane of the ultrasound transducer (Fig. 1-1E). This may be easier for the beginner as the lesion is more easily and reliably sampled; however, the biopsy guide limits transducer movement.

Equipment and Technique

Sterility is maintained during the procedure. The transducer can be sterilized with transducer-compatible disinfectant and sterilizing solutions (a list of which can be found in the user manual of the ultrasound machine). Following the diagnostic ultrasound evaluation of the site of interest, the coupling gel is wiped off and alcohol or sterile water is used as the coupling media during the FNAB procedure. The use of a coupling gel is avoided because it can introduce potentially misleading artifact into the cytologic specimen. Routine skin preparation should be performed before the needle puncture through the skin.

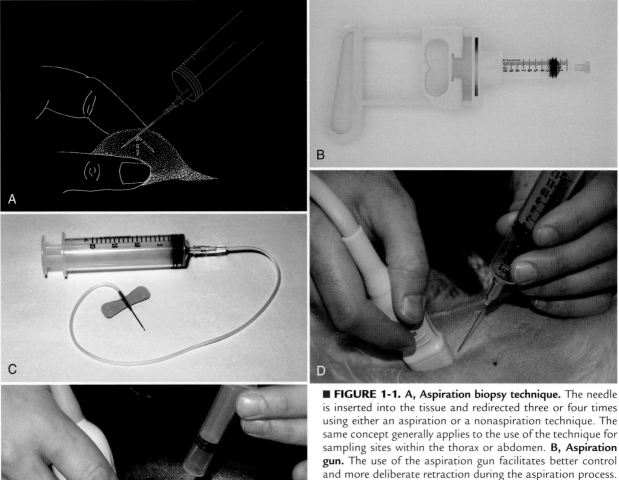

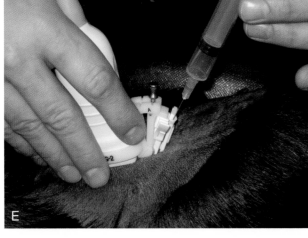

■ **FIGURE 1-1. A, Aspiration biopsy technique.** The needle is inserted into the tissue and redirected three or four times using either an aspiration or a nonaspiration technique. The same concept generally applies to the use of the technique for sampling sites within the thorax or abdomen. **B, Aspiration gun.** The use of the aspiration gun facilitates better control and more deliberate retraction during the aspiration process. **C, Butterfly needle.** Using a butterfly needle attached to the syringe will allow more flexibility with fractious patients when removing fluid. A three-way stop-cock can be placed between the butterfly tubing and syringe to facilitate removal of large amounts of fluid. **D, Ultrasound guidance.** Free-hand technique for ultrasound-guided fine needle aspiration biopsy. **E, Ultrasound guidance.** Biopsy guide is attached to a linear transducer that holds a needle firmly for ultrasound-guided fine needle aspiration biopsy. (A from Meyer DJ: The management of cytology specimens, *Compend Contin Educ Pract Vet* 9:10-17, 1987. B, Courtesy of Delasco.)

The most commonly used needles are 20- to 23-gauge hypodermic and spinal needles. These are inexpensive and long enough to pass through the biopsy guide and still reach most lesions. Larger-bore needles are easier to visualize, and they generally increase the reliability of sample collection but increase the risk of hemorrhage. A larger-bore needle is used when aspirating viscous fluids. Once the needle is in placed in the lesion, the stylet is removed and the needle is moved up and down within the lesion until a small amount of fluid is seen within the hub of the needle (Fagelman and Chess, 1990). This method generally produces a sample with less blood contamination. Alternatively, a syringe can be attached to the needle for better handling—a few milliliters of negative pressure can be applied while moving the needle up and down. The negative pressure should be released before removing the needle from the lesion. When possible, two or three samples should be obtained from each biopsy site; a new needle is used for each sample taken. A large lesion may have a necrotic center; therefore samples should also be collected from the margins.

Complications

Complications associated with ultrasound-guided FNAB are uncommon and depend on the experience of the operator, size of needle, and type of lesion aspirated (Léveillé et al., 1993). Patients should be evaluated for bleeding disorders before FNAB, especially when highly vascular tissues are sampled. Occasional needle tract tumor implantation has been reported in animals (Nyland et al., 2002b; Liu et al., 2007). In humans, implantation is associated with the used of large-bore needles but is rare with 22-gauge or smaller aspiration needles. Because pneumothorax can develop following FNAB of the thoracic structures, the patient should frequently be observed for 12 to 24 hours after the procedure. Hypertension and paradoxical hypotension has been reported in dogs following ultrasound-guided FNAB of pheochromocytoma of the adrenal glands (Gilson et al., 1994). Therefore FNAB of the adrenal gland must be performed cautiously when that tumor is suspected.

MANAGING THE CYTOLOGIC SPECIMEN

Compression (Squash) Preparation

The compression (squash) technique is an important and adaptable procedure for the management of cytology specimens that are semisolid, mucus-like, or pelleted by centrifugation. A small amount of material is placed on a clean glass slide approximately ½ inch (1 cm) from the frosted end (Fig. 1-2A). A second clean glass slide is placed over the specimen at right angles. The specimen is gently but firmly compressed between the two glass slides and in the same continuous motion the top slide is pulled along the surface of the bottom slide, directing the material away from the frosted end (Fig. 1-2B). The objective is to redistribute the material, turning a multicellular mass into a thin monolayer ideal for maximal flattening of individual cells and even stain penetration. The compression preparation thus optimizes the specimen for microscopic examination of cell morphology. A properly prepared glass slide is characterized by a feather-shaped (oblong) area with a monolayer end referred to as the "sweet spot" (Fig. 1-2C). A common mistake is the initial placement of excess sample on the glass slide, resulting in a thick preparation that is not possible to adequately examine microscopically.

> **KEY POINT** Compression and spread of the specimen is a continuum; there should be no momentary pause as the upper slide contacts the specimen. Keep the flat surfaces of the two slides parallel. A common mistake is to slightly angle the upper slide near the end of the gliding motion by allowing a slight counterclockwise rotation of the wrist (clockwise if left handed) to occur, causing cell lysis or uneven spread of the specimen. A scraping sound of glass on glass can be heard when this occurs. Again, wiping slides before the procedure will help ensure a uniform spread of the cytologic specimen.

> **KEY POINT** The term *sweet spot* refers to that area around the center mass of a baseball bat, tennis racket, or golf club that is the most effective part with which to make a successful hit. The same concept applies to the location of the cytologic specimen if it is to make a successful diagnostic hit. Cellular material too close to the ends or edges of the slide cannot be properly examined. When slides go through an automated stainer, its guiding tracks can scrape off diagnostic material

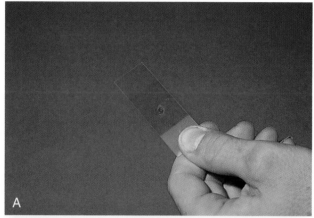

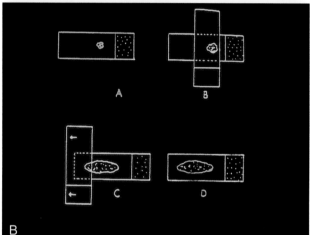

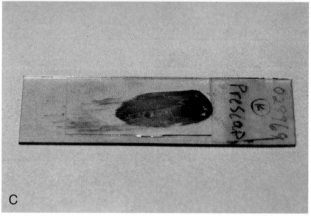

■ **FIGURE 1-2. Slide preparation. A,** The application of only a small drop or portion of the specimen on the glass slide near the frosted end is an important initial step for making a quality cytologic preparation. Placing too much material on the slide results in a preparation that is too thick and/or spreads too close to the slide edges for diagnostic purposes. **B,** The specimen is gently but firmly compressed between the two glass slides *(B)* and in the same continuous motion *(C)* the top slide is glided along the surface of the slide with the material directed away from the frosted end, resulting in a featherlike spread of the specimen *(D)* referred to as the "sweet spot." **C,** The location of the "sweet spot" is illustrated by this properly labeled and stained compression preparation of a lymph node specimen. (B from Meyer DJ, Franks PT: Clinical cytology: Part I: Management of tissue specimens, *Mod Vet Pract* 67:255-59, 1986. C from Meyer DJ: The management of cytology specimens, *Compend Contin Educ Pract Vet* 9:10-17, 1987.)

that is too close to the end of the slide (Fig. 1-3). Material placed too far from the end the specimen may not be exposed adequately to the stain. The ends and longitudinal edges of the slide cannot be adequately examined because of the inability of the 40× dry and 50× and 100× oil objectives to properly focus at those extremes.

KEY POINT If the compression preparation appears too thick, it probably is. Make another one. If the cytology specimen appears to be too close to the end or edge of the slide, it probably is. Make another one. If you have doubts regarding the quality of the preparation, make additional preparations.

Management of Fluids

A fluid specimen should be immediately placed in an EDTA tube to prevent clot formation. Fluid with a plasma-like consistency can be handled in a fashion similar to the preparation of a blood smear. A small drop of fluid is placed approximately ½ inch (1 cm) from the frosted end. The angled edge of a second glass slide, acute angle facing the operator, is backed into the specimen and drawn away from the frosted end as the fluid begins to spread along its edge (Fig. 1-4A–C). The speed at which the slide is moved depends on the viscosity of the sample—the thinner the specimen, the faster the slide should be moved to distribute the specimen evenly and thinly. For a viscous fluid specimen such as synovial fluid, the spreader slide is moved with a slow and even movement.

All fluid initially applied to the slide must remain on the slide (Fig. 1-4D&E). It is tempting to go off the end of the slide with excess fluid, referred to as the "edge-of-the-cliff syndrome," but the result is the potential loss of diagnostic material, which is thrown into the garbage with the spreader slide (Fig. 1-4D). The "edge-of-the-cliff syndrome" poses a notable threat to pleural and peritoneal fluids that contain clumps of neoplastic cells.

These cellular clumps often follow the spreader slide, finally sticking to the surface when the fluid dissipates (Fig. 1-5A&B). To avoid this cytologic disaster when excess fluid remains, simply stop ½ inch from the end of the specimen slide and apply the spreader slide to another clean glass slide and repeat the spreading procedure. When minimal excess fluid remains, the fluid can be permitted to slowly flow back on itself for a short distance. The thin part of the stained cytology slide preparation can be used to estimate cell numbers and the relatively thick, concentrated part (where the excess fluid is dried) can be evaluated for types of cells and/or infectious agents (Fig. 1-4E). Although not an optimal preparation, this "poor man's centrifuge" technique is useful in emergency settings for the initial, rapid triage of a fluid specimen.

Sedimentation preparations can also be used to concentrate cells in bloody or cloudy fluids. The sample can be centrifuged in the same tube in which it was collected after direct preparations have been made. After centrifugation, the majority of supernatant is removed with a pipette and the cell pellet resuspended in the remaining fluid. A smear and/or compression preparation can be made from the concentrated cell specimen. It is important to remember that estimates of cell counts cannot be made on concentrated samples, only from the direct smear.

The diagnostic yield of a predominantly bloody fluid specimen is enhanced with the buffy-coat concentration technique. A microhematocrit tube is prepared as if to measure a hematocrit. The tube is broken at the cell-plasma interface and the cellular concentrate (buffy coat) is applied to two or three slides and a direct smear technique is used to spread the specimen. The technique is valuable for hemorrhagic pericardial, peritoneal, and pleural samples (Fig. 1-6A&B). It is also useful for the examination of peripheral blood for neoplastic cells and cell-associated infectious organisms.

Transudates and cerebrospinal fluids are low in protein and cell numbers. The use of a cytocentrifuge (cytospin) is recommended for the capture of all the cells (Fig. 1-7A&B). For cerebrospinal fluids, a cytologic preparation should be made—ideally within 2 to 3 hours since the low specific gravity predisposes to cellular lysis. However, it appears that when inflammatory and neoplastic cells and infectious agents are present, their diagnostic cellular integrity is usually maintained for up to 12 hours with refrigeration.

KEY POINT For the management of fluid samples, routinely make direct, centrifuged (or buffy coat), and cytospin (if possible) preparations and assess each for the best diagnostic yield.

KEY POINT The refractometer-determined total solute (protein) concentration should be measured for all pleural and peritoneal fluids to facilitate classification as transudate or modified transudate when that information has diagnostic importance (Meyer and Harvey, 2004).

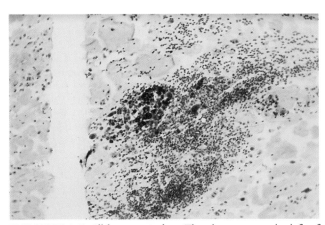

■ **FIGURE 1-3. Slide preparation.** The clear area to the left of center represents the guide track of the automated stainer that has partially scraped off the only cytologic material present on the slide because it was located too close to the slide's end.

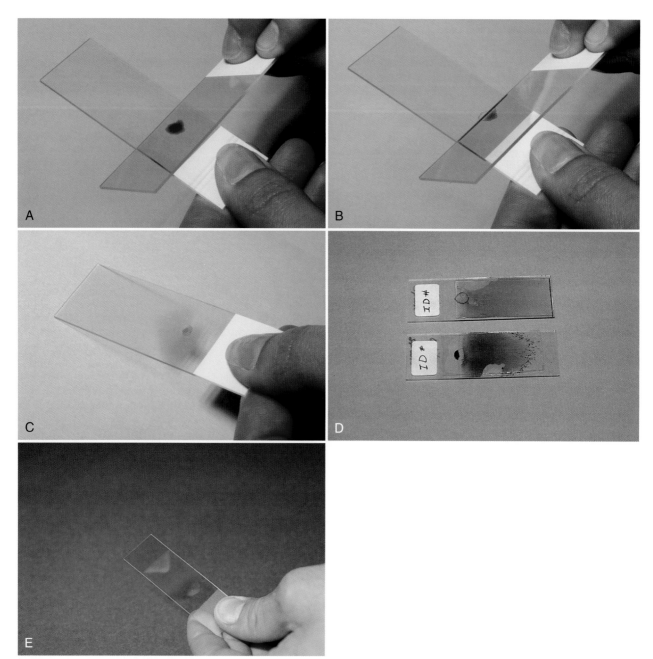

■ **FIGURE 1-4. Fluid material preparation. A,** The procedure for making a cytologic preparation from a fluid specimen is illustrated. A *small* drop of the specimen is placed approximately ½ inch (1 cm) from the frosted end of the slide. **B,** The spreader slide is slowly backed into the drop. **C,** Just as the fluid begins to spread along its edge, the spreader slide is glided away from the frosted end. **D,** All of the original fluid drop should remain on the slide and the temptation to go off the end of the slide with excess fluid must be avoided. The lower slide illustrates a properly feathered fluid specimen with the entire specimen remaining on the slide. The upper slide demonstrates the "edge-of-the-cliff syndrome" in which the excess fluid was drawn off the slide's end. **E,** Excess fluid that remains is allowed to partially flow back and is air-dried as illustrated by the small opaque dried fluid triangle near the nonfrosted end of the slide. Alternatively, the edge of the spreader slide with the excess fluid adhering is transferred to another clean slide and another smear made.

KEY POINT For low-protein fluids such as urinary sediments, cerebrospinal fluids, and transudates, the cells can be washed off during the staining process. The use of premade serum-coated slides facilitates the adhesion of the cells, which can make a diagnostic world of difference. Several drops of the excess serum not used for clinical chemistries are applied to the entire surface of a glass slide and the film of serum is air-dried. Ten to 20 slide preparations are made. Once dry (not sticky to the touch), the slides can be stacked together in an empty slide box and placed in the freezer to prevent bacterial growth. Prior to use, several slides are brought to room temperature. It is critical that no condensation develops on the surface since it causes severe cell lysis.

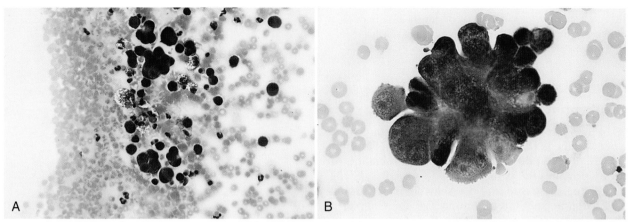

■ **FIGURE 1-5. Slide examination. A,** Examination of the feathered edge of the lower slide pictured in Figure 1-4D demonstrates clumps of cells located along the point where the fluid feathers out, emphasizing the need to leave excess fluid. The area to the right of the cell clumps consisted of only erythrocytes. (Wright; IP.) **B,** A diagnosis of a neoplastic effusion (adenocarcinoma) was made by examining the cell clumps. (Wright; HP oil.) The upper slide pictured in Figure 1-4D of the same specimen contained only erythrocytes and a few mesothelial cells but no cell clumps, precluding a cytologic diagnosis.

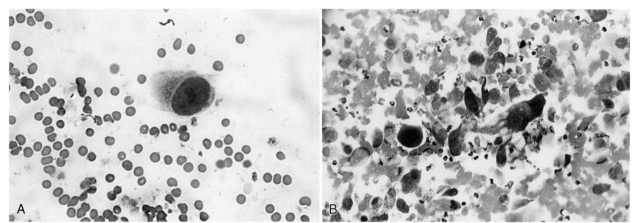

■ **FIGURE 1-6. Slide examination. A,** This bloody aspirate was obtained by pericardiocentesis. A rare large, atypical spindle-shaped cell suggestive of a sarcoma was observed among the many erythrocytes and a small number of reactive mesothelial cells. (Wright; HP oil.) **B,** After making a smear from a buffy-coat preparation of the same bloody specimen, numerous spindle-shaped cells that show malignant characteristics are observed, affording a cytologic diagnosis of a neoplastic effusion consistent with a sarcoma. (Wright; HP oil.)

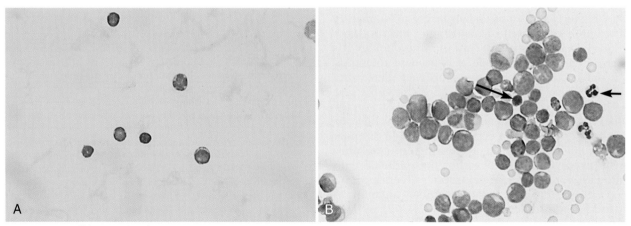

■ **FIGURE 1-7. Slide examination. A,** This is a direct smear of a pleural fluid specimen from a cat with a thoracic effusion. A small number of small, medium, and large lymphocytes were observed. (Wright; HP oil.) The triglyceride concentration of the fluid approximated the serum value, making the diagnosis of a chylous effusion less likely. (Wright; HP oil.) **B,** A cytospin preparation of the specimen easily demonstrates that most of the cells are medium to large immature lymphocytes indicative of malignant lymphoma. A normal small lymphocyte *(long arrow)* and a neutrophil *(short arrow)* are useful size comparators. (Wright; HP oil.) (A from Meyer DJ, Franks PT: Effusion: classification and cytologic examination, *Compend Contin Educ Pract Vet* 9:123-28, 1987. B fromMeyer DJ, Franks PT: Effusion: classification and cytologic examination, *Compend Contin Educ Pract Vet* 9:123-28, 1987.)

> **HELPFUL HINT** A hair dryer set on low heat enhances the even drying of fluid specimens. It can also be used to remove condensation from the serum-covered slides taken from the freezer.

Touch Imprint

Cells will often exfoliate from excised tissue when the cut surface is touched to a glass slide. This type of cytologic preparation permits immediate evaluation of a biopsy, provides the pathologist with a second means of evaluating the tissue, and is a valuable instructional tool. The clinician's interpretation can be compared with the histopathologic findings. The cut surface of the excised tissue is aggressively blotted on a paper towel to remove blood and tissue fluid. The specimen is dry enough to exfoliate cells without excessive blood contamination when the paper towel is observed to stick to it. The surface will have a dull, dry, tacky appearance. It is touched firmly to the surface of a clean glass slide in several places about the "sweet spot" (Fig. 1-8A). Properly prepared tissue is perceived to stick to the surface of the glass momentarily. If excess blood or tissue fluid is noted, the tissue is blotted again and a new touch imprint made. Imprint areas that appear too thick can be finessed to a monolayer by the gentle use of the compression technique. Touch imprints should be made of each area of tissue specimen that appears grossly different.

Tissues with a fibrous texture, such as fibromas, fibrosarcomas, and cicatricial inflammation, may not exfoliate adequately with this technique. The surface of these firm, often pale-appearing tissues needs to be roughened with a scalpel and then touched to the surface of a glass slide. In addition, the tissue on the edge of the scalpel can be used to make touch imprints and/or compression preparations (Fig. 1-8B). This technique works well on ulcerated cutaneous lesions when neoplasia or mycotic infection is suspected. Frequently, the surface is contaminated with debris, bacteria, and an attendant mixed inflammatory cell reaction composed of neutrophils, macrophages, and fibroplasia that can obscure the true etiology if a direct touch imprint is made. It is prudent to aggressively débride the area by using moistened gauze and/or by aggressive, deep scraping of the area with a scalpel. The exfoliated material, including the tissue on the scalpel blade, is used to make touch imprints and compression preparations. In certain bullous skin diseases, touching a glass slide to a freshly ruptured bulla can be used to identify acantholytic epithelial cells along with nondegenerate neutrophils (Tzanck preparation), supporting a tentative diagnosis of an immune-mediated skin disorder.

Small tissue samples such as those obtained with an endoscopic biopsy instrument or cutting biopsy needle can be rolled on a slide using a 22- or 25-gauge needle (Fig. 1-8C), or a compression preparation can be made if there is extra tissue not needed for histologic examination.

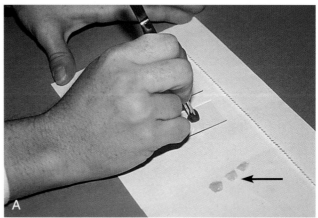

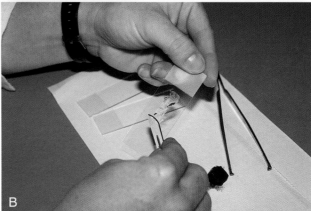

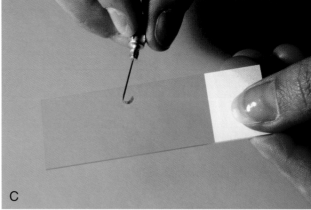

■ **FIGURE 1-8. A, Impression smear.** The touch imprint technique is illustrated. The cut surface of the specimen is firmly blotted on a paper towel (*note wet spots arrow*) until tacky and then firmly touched multiple times to the surface of a clean glass slide. **B, Tissue scraping.** If the tissue does not adequately exfoliate, a scalpel blade is used to scrape or roughen up the surface of the tissue. The tissue can be touched to a glass surface and/or the material on the edge of the blade, dragged along the surface of a slide, air-dried, and stained or, if thick, a compression preparation made. **C, Tissue rolling.** Small pieces of tissue that cannot be grasped with a forceps for imprinting can be gently rolled on a slide using a 25-gauge needle. This will allow for exfoliation of a thin layer of cells. If the tissue is not friable, multiple slides can be made. (B from Meyer DJ: The management of cytology specimens, *Compend Contin Educ Pract Vet* 9: 10-17, 1987.)

STAINING THE SPECIMEN

Romanowsky, Romanowsky-type, and new methylene blue stains are used in veterinary medicine to identify nucleated cells.

Papanicolaou Stain

The Papanicolaou (Pap) stain is used routinely in the medical profession for cytologic specimens. The stain accentuates nuclear detail and is valuable in detecting early morphologic aberrations indicative of dysplasia and neoplasia. It is not used commonly in veterinary medicine because of the multistep staining procedure and its limitations in evaluating inflammatory reactions. A rapid Papanicolaou staining procedure has recently been described in veterinary medicine that may be advantageous for enhancing the nuclear abnormalities of cancer cells (Jorundsson et al., 1999).

New Methylene Blue Stain

New methylene blue (New Methylene Blue, Fisher Scientific) is a basic dye that stains nuclei, most infectious agents, platelets, and the granules of mast cells. Eosinophil granules do not stain nor do erythrocytes, which appear microscopically as translucent circular areas. Because there is no alcohol fixation, the lipids associated with lipomas and follicular infundibular cysts can be easily recognized. The cholesterol crystals associated with the latter are highlighted (see Fig. 2-23). The staining solution consists of 0.5 g of new methylene blue dissolved in 100 ml of 0.9% saline. Full-strength formalin (1 ml) is added as a preservative. The stock solution is kept refrigerated. For clinical use, a small stoppered bottle is replenished from the stock solution; the stain is passed through filter paper first, to remove all precipitate. A small drop of stain is applied directly to an air-dried cytology preparation. A dust-free coverslip (wipe it with a paper towel or a shirtsleeve) is placed on the drop of stain, which spreads by capillary movement. Larger coverslips, 20 mm × 40 or 50 mm, allow more of the specimen to be examined. The specimen should be immediately examined since the water-based stain will evaporate. A new methylene blue-stained cytologic specimen is useful for the detection of nucleated cells, bacteria (both gram-positive and gram-negative bacteria stain dark blue), fungi, and yeast. When applied to a blood smear, leukocyte and platelet numbers can be estimated and polychromatophils (as reticulocytes) recognized. This makes it a valuable triage stain for blood and fluid specimens examined on an emergency basis. When religiously filtered, it is an ideal stain to detect hemobartonellosis since the erythrocyte is essentially "invisible," accentuating the surface silhouette of the dark blue organism.

> **HELPFUL HINT** This is a valuable, cost-effective stain for examining cytologic preparations, blood smears, and urine sediments in veterinary practice. The added responsibility of replenishing the stain with filtered stock stain weekly is well worth the time invested.

Romanowsky-Type Stains

Romanowsky-type stains are often utilized in practice settings because they work rapidly and are easy to use. They are combinations of basic and acidic dyes dissolved in methyl alcohol. These polychromatic stains impart the basophilic and eosinophilic tinctorial properties observed on blood films. Wright's stain (Wright's Stain Solution, Fisher Scientific) is used widely in most medical and veterinary laboratories because it results in well-stained blood films. Other Romanowsky-type stains used alone or in various combinations include Leishman's, May-Grunwald-Giemsa, and Diff-Quik® (Diff-Quik® Differential Stain Set, American Scientific Products). The latter is a polychromatic stain commonly used in veterinary practice because of its time-saving convenience. For certain specimens such as bone marrow samples, there may be tradeoff in the staining quality. Mast cell granules do not stain reliably with it. If a staining deficiency is suspected during the examination of a discrete cell neoplasm, new methylene blue or Giemsa stain can be used to demonstrate the presence of mast cell granules.

Poorly stained specimens can result from improper staining times, weakened stain from overuse, and improperly managed cytologic preparations. One should become familiar with one kind of Romanowsky-type stain and not switch brands frequently. The composition of dyes in polychromatic stains has been demonstrated to vary considerably among suppliers and from batch to batch from the same supplier. Furthermore, prolonged storage at room temperature (25 °C; 77 °F) can impair staining intensity because of the formation of degradation products in the methanol. It is most convenient to purchase stains in liquid form. Box 1-3 lists the factors that can cause poorly stained specimens with Romanowsky-type stains.

Staining times vary depending on the thickness of the specimen and the freshness of the stain. The frequency with which the solutions are changed or refreshed depends on the number of slides processed. Dull-blue-appearing nuclei that lack sharp chromatin detail is one indication of a weak solution. Solutions should be changed completely whenever infectious agents or cellular elements inappropriately appear on specimens. The staining times for Diff-Quik® stain solutions need to be increased depending on the thickness of the cytologic preparation and the freshness of the stain. A pleural effusion with low cellularity may be stained adequately with three to five dips in each solution. A thick preparation from a lymph node or bone marrow specimen may require 60 to 120 seconds in each solution to obtain optimal staining (Fig. 1-9A&B). Box 1-4 lists staining time guidelines.

At the end of the staining process, the slide is washed with cold running water for 20 seconds to remove stain precipitate and allowed to dry in a nearly vertical position (also see KEY POINT regarding the use of a hair dryer). Any stain film on the back of the slide can be removed with an alcohol-moistened gauze sponge. The stained specimen is examined microscopically using the 10× or 20× objective for staining quality and uniformity. If acceptable, a coverslip is placed on the specimen if a

---

BOX 1-3   Causes of Abnormal Staining

Excessive blue (erythrocytes appear blue green)
  Prolonged contact time with the stain
  Inadequate wash
  Specimen too thick
  Stain or diluent too alkaline—pH >7; check with pH
    paper
  Exposure of specimen to formalin or its fumes
    (e.g., open formalin container)
  Delayed fixation
Excessive pink
  Prolonged washing
  Insufficient contact time with the stain
  Stain or diluent too acidic—pH <7; erythrocytes can
    appear orange or bright red-formic acid can result
    from the oxidation of methyl alcohol with prolonged
    exposure to air; fresh methanol is recommended
  Mounting the coverslip before the specimen is dry
Inadequately stained nucleated cells and erythrocytes
  Insufficient contact time with one or more of the staining
    solutions
  Surface of a second glass slide covers the specimen on
    the first slide (can occur when staining two slides
    back-to-back in Coplin jars)
Precipitate on the stained specimen
  Inadequate washing of the slide at the end of the stain-
    ing period
  Inadequate filtration of the stain
  Unclean slides

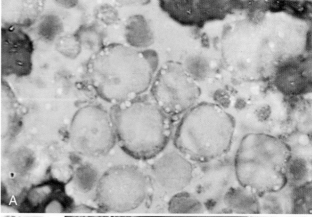
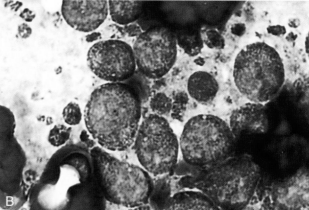

■ **FIGURE 1-9. Staining technique. A,** This aspirate from an enlarged lymph node was stained with approximately five dips in the fixative and each of the staining solutions. Cell outlines can be seen but the detailed cytomorphology cannot be adequately examined. (Diff-Quik®; HP oil.) **B,** The same slide was replaced into the fixative and the staining solutions for approximately 60 seconds in each station while it was slowly moved up and down. A cytologic diagnosis of malignant lymphoma now can be made. A small lymphocyte near center is a helpful size comparator. (Diff-Quik®; HP oil.)

40× objective is to be used. A temporary mount is made by placing a drop of immersion oil on the specimen followed by a coverslip. A permanent mount is made with a commercially available coverslip mounting glue (e.g., Eukitt®, Calibrated Instruments).

KEY POINT A coverslip is always required for sharp focus when the 40× objective is used to examine hematologic and cytologic specimens. A second drop of oil can be placed on the coverslip for use of the oil objective.

KEY POINT Two staining stations are routinely recommended. One is used for "clean" specimens such as blood films, effusions, and lymph nodes aspirates. The other is used for "dirty" specimens such as skin scrapings, fecal and intestinal cytology, and suspected abscesses.

SITE-SPECIFIC CONSIDERATIONS

Cutaneous Nodule and the Lymph Node

The cutaneous nodule and the enlarged lymph node are readily accessible tissues for exfoliative cytology. A minimum of two lymph nodes should be sampled if there is generalized lymphadenopathy. The center of an enlarged lymph node should be avoided to minimize the risk of

---

BOX 1-4   Suggested Procedure for Staining Cytologic Specimens Using Diff-Quik® Solutions*

Fixative: 60 to 120 seconds
Solution 1: 30 to 60 seconds
Solution 2: 5 to 60 seconds†
Rinse under cold tap water: 15 seconds
Examine staining adequacy using low power; eosinophilia
    or basophilia can be enhanced by returning to Solution
    1 or Solution 2, respectively, followed by a rinse.
Air-dry and examine

---

*Suggested times are based on fresh stains; with time and use the stains weaken and longer times will be required. Consistently understained specimens are an indication for replenishing with fresh stain.
†The shortest times are suggested for hypocellular fluids that are low in protein such as transudates, cerebral spinal fluids, and urine sediments.
Modified from Henry MJ, Burton LG, Stanley MW, et al: Application of a modified Diff-Quik® stain to fine needle aspiration smears: rapid staining with improved cytologic detail, *Acta Cytol* 1987; 31:954-955.

obtaining necrotic debris and nondiagnostic cytologic material. The tissue is palpated for consistency and the margins are defined. Softer areas suggestive of fluid or necrotic tissue are identified and separate aspirates of these areas and firmer tissue are planned. The area of interest is clipped and scrubbed before aspiration. The tissue is immobilized firmly between the thumb and forefinger. The needle is inserted into the tissue, an aspiration or nonaspiration technique is used, and the needle is advanced into (but not through) the tissue of interest. The needle is redirected several times (see Fig. 1-1A). The plunger of the syringe is *gently* returned to the start position and the needle is withdrawn. Maintaining vacuum while removing the needle from the tissue causes splattering of the material in the syringe barrel and enhances the potential of blood contamination from a cutaneous vessel. When fluid is encountered, it should be completely removed and handled as a fluid specimen. A separate sampling procedure is executed for the firmer tissue with a new needle and syringe combination.

> **KEY POINT** The exfoliation of cells occurs as a consequence of the needle's passage through the tissue. The repeated movement of the needle through the tissue is the critical component of obtaining diagnostic material from nonfluid tissues.

> **KEY POINT** Not all solid tissues can be adequately sampled with exfoliation cytology. If diagnostic cells are not obtained with FNAB after triaging the stained specimen, consider an excisional biopsy.

Liver, Spleen, Kidney

The use of exfoliative cytology for the investigation of organomegaly of the liver, spleen, and kidney is the most rewarding indication. The cellular or cell-associated causation of the enlarged organ often exfoliates from these tissues. Ultrasonographic examination of these organs has increased the use of FNAB for the examination of focal lesions. The diagnostic efficiency of cytology is reduced in support of this indication. There is a greater possibility that the cell type may not exfoliate or the lesion will be missed and the surrounding tissue examined, resulting in an erroneous impression and misdiagnosis. In addition, greater expertise is required for the examination of FNAB specimens from these organs because nodular hyperplastic lesions of the spleen and canine liver become more prevalent in the geriatric patient (see Chapter 9).

> **KEY POINT** The nonaspiration sampling technique reduces blood contamination from vascular organs such as liver and spleen.

> **KEY POINT** Remember that the liver is a moving target due to its intimate association with the movement of the diaphragm. Consequently, a craniodorsad positioning of the needle reduces the risk of laceration (Fig. 1-10).

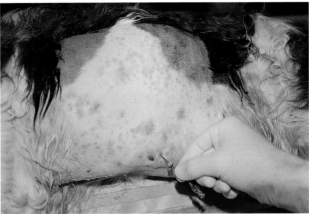

■ **FIGURE 1-10. Liver biopsy.** Fine-needle aspiration biopsy of the liver can be accomplished with the dog in left lateral recumbency. In the picture, the head is to reader's left. The needle is inserted in a craniodorsad direction at the triangle formed by the left lateral edge of the xiphoid process and the union of the last rib with the sternum. Once the needle touches the surface of the liver, the hub of the needle will move in concert with the movement of the diaphragm but in the opposite direction.

> **KEY POINT** Two actions should be taken if a bloody sample is obtained from the liver or spleen. First, place the sample immediately into an EDTA tube. A direct smear (similar to a peripheral blood film) and a buffy-coat preparation should be triaged for diagnostic material such as malignant mesenchymal cells (hemangiosarcoma). Do *not* attempt to "coat" an entire glass slide with the bloody specimen in hopes of a diagnostic specimen. The result will be a dismal diagnostic failure. Second, if no fluid-filled lesion is present upon ultrasound examination, repeat the FNAB with a clean needle and use a nonaspiration technique.

Nose and Lung

Evaluation of the nasal cavity is often compromised by the occult nature of the underlying pathology. Radiography always should precede an attempt to obtain a specimen for cytology or histopathology: it can define the area of the nasal cavity that is predominantly involved and thus suggest the side of the cavity to be sampled. In addition, manipulation within the nasal cavity often results in hemorrhage, which obscures radiographic detail. After radiography, the oropharynx is examined visually and by digital palpation. The dorsal area of the soft palate is examined with a dental mirror and by palpation. If no abnormal tissue is identified for aspiration and/or excisional biopsy, the recesses of the nasal cavity are sampled by a washing or aspiration technique. Examination of the nasal cavity with an otoscope can allow visualization of abnormal tissue and can assist in procuring a tissue specimen.

Superficial lesions, such as eosinophilic or fungal rhinitis, can occasionally be identified by examination of nasal mucus or superficial mucosal scrapings. Most of the time, superficial swab-obtained specimens are nondiagnostic or yield only nonspecific inflammation and bacteria. More aggressive cytologic specimens from the nasal cavity can be obtained by flush or aspiration techniques. A soft, rubber urinary catheter is flexible enough for the retrograde flushing procedure. The saline flush is collected and squash preps made from mucoid globs and bits of tissue. The remaining saline is centrifuged in a conical-tip tube and preps (squash and/or direct smears) made from the pellet. A rigid, large-bore polyurethane urinary catheter or the plastic needle guard from a Sovereign® (Sherwood Medical) intravenous catheter is effective for obtaining a nasal specimen (Fig. 1-11A). The depth of the nasal cavity is approximated, and a corresponding length of catheter is cut at an angle. The catheter is attached to a syringe and firmly advanced into

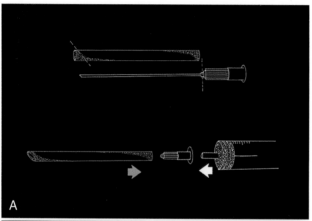

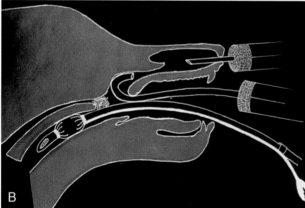

■ **FIGURE 1-11. Nasal biopsy. A,** This schematic representation demonstrates a method of altering an intravenous catheter for use in obtaining nasal cytologic specimens by aspiration. One end of the outer plastic shield is cut at an angle and the needle is cut close to the plastic hub. The outer plastic shield is wedged firmly over the hub. **B,** A sagittal schematic representation of a dog's head, demonstrating two possible techniques for obtaining a cytologic specimen from the nose. The altered intravenous catheter or a relatively rigid large-bore urinary catheter is aggressively inserted via the external nares and aspiration applied when resistance is encountered. Alternatively, a flexible rubber urinary catheter can be inserted above the soft palate and the nasal cavity flushed retrograde. The fluid and solid material are collected in a container. (A and B from Meyer DJ: The management of cytology specimens, *Compend Contin Educ Pract Vet* 9:10-17, 1987.)

the nasal cavity until moderate resistance is encountered. Aspiration is applied while the catheter is manipulated within the nasal cavity (Fig. 1-11B). For this procedure, aspiration and manipulation of the catheter can be more aggressive because of the mucosal and cartilaginous nature of diseased tissue. Another deviation is the maintenance of negative pressure when withdrawing the catheter in an attempt to exteriorize bits of tissues. Fluid and bits of tissue can be used for cytologic preparations. Larger pieces of tissue fragments and clotted blood can be placed in 10% formalin for histopathologic examination to maximize the diagnostic yield.

FNBA of the lung parenchyma is rewarding when the interstitial infiltrative disease is diffuse or large focal lesions are identified radiographically. Unless the cellular infiltrate is radiographically or ultrasonographically notable, the diagnostic yield cannot be expected to be fruitful. Ultrasongraphic guidance of the needle is a more accurate way of ensuring that the desired lesion is sampled. For small or ill-defined lesions guessing the location of needle placement from the radiograph is problematic.

Successful use of the transtracheal wash and brochoalveolar lavage for assessing pulmonary changes depends on the disease process involving the mucosa and/or the alveolar lumen, sampling the diseased region, and adequate collection of the saline lavage. There must be a relatively aggressive attempt to recover the wash or lavage that includes angling the patient's head downward to facilitate a diagnostic yield. Mucosal brushings/scrapings can enhance the cytologic yield of mucosal lesions. (Clercx et al., 1996)

> **KEY POINT** The lung is a dynamic organ prone to laceration by the needle. Momentary apnea can be achieved occasionally by touching or gently blowing on the patient's nose.

Joint

Lameness and swollen joints are the common indications for the examination of the synovial fluid. A review of the skeletal anatomy for the joint of interest is prudent before beginning the sampling procedure. In general, an appropriate interosseous location is determined by digital palpation with the affected joint in a slightly flexed position. The site should be clipped and prepared using sterile technique to avoid contamination of the sample with bacteria. This is especially important if the synovial fluid is also going to be submitted for culture and will ensure its accurate assessment for presence of bacteria. A 22- to 25-gauge needle attached to a 3-cc syringe is used. Normal synovial fluid is viscous and even inflamed synovial fluid may retain this quality. Consequently, gentle aspiration must be linked to patience as the thick fluid slowly rises up the smaller needle. Quantity is less important than quality of the specimen. One drop is adequate for a slide preparation and two or three drops in a sterile tube or applied to a culturette for potential culture will suffice. If nonlocalizing polyarticular disease is suspected, two or more joints, including at least one carpal joint, should be routinely sampled.

Vertebral Body Lesions

Vertebral body pathology may be an incidental finding on radiographs or be suspected based on neurologic abnormalities such as ataxia, inability to rise in either end, or neck pain. Obtaining a cytologic specimen is challenging in such cases due to the difficulty of locating the site by palpation and the proximity to the spinal cord. Experienced radiologists may be successful in obtaining a diagnostic specimen with the use of fluoroscopic guidance of a spinal needle.

SUBMITTING CYTOLOGY SPECIMENS TO A REFERENCE LABORATORY

The busy practitioner often finds it more convenient to submit cytology specimens to a commercial veterinary laboratory for examination. Many of these facilities have personnel specifically trained to make buffy-coat and cytospin preparations of fluid specimens and experienced microscopists to examine cytologic specimens. Their expertise is effective only if the specimen is submitted properly.

Fluid specimens should be placed immediately in EDTA tubes to prevent clot formation. If the fluid will be in transit longer than 24 hours, a direct slide preparation

should be made to accompany the tube. Experience indicates that the red-topped and purple-topped collection tubes are not reliably sterile. Bacterial growth can occur in a "sterile" specimen when transit is prolonged; therefore, an appropriate culture vehicle should be used when the specimen is being submitted for bacterial culture.

As previously indicated, touch imprints can be helpful adjuncts to the histologic examination of formalin-fixed tissues. Formalin vapors can alter the staining characteristics of touch imprints drastically (Fig. 1-12A&B). When touch imprints accompany formalin-fixed tissues, they should be placed in their own air-tight container. Breakage is a common problem when glass slides are mailed in cardboard containers. Rigid plastic or Styrofoam containers offer reliable protection. If there is a lack of familiarity with a particular sample submission procedure, the laboratory always should be contacted for advice before collection.

> **KEY POINT** Formalin fumes are pervasive and rapidly penetrating. They alter the staining and morphology of hematology and cytology specimens. Keep open formalin containers away from these specimens even if opened only momentarily.

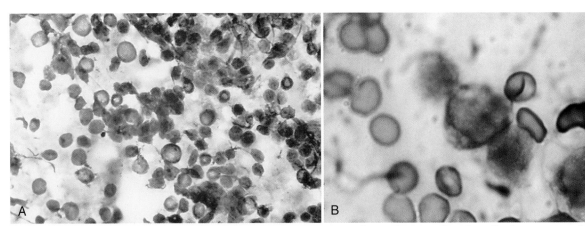

■ **FIGURE 1-12. Formalin effects. A,** This lymph node specimen was inadvertently exposed to formalin fumes. Most of the elements present cannot be recognized as lymphocytes, precluding a cytologic interpretation. Formalin fumes alter the cytomorphology and staining characteristics of nucleated cells; this should be considered as a reason for a nondiagnostic specimen. (Wright; HP oil.) A cytologic diagnosis of lymphoid hyperplasia was made from a second aspirate (not shown). **B,** This sample was also exposed to formalin. Notice how the erythrocyte morphology lacks clarity and has a greenish tint.

REFERENCES

Clercx C, Wallon J, Gilbert S, et al: Imprint and brush cytology in the diagnosis of canine intranasal tumours, *J Sm Anim Pract* 37:423-437, 1996.

Fagelman D, Chess Q: Nonaspiration fine-needle cytology of the liver: a new technique for obtaining diagnostic samples, *Am J Roentgenol* 155:1217-1219, 1990.

Gilson SD, Withrow SJ, Wheeler SL, et al: Pheochromocytoma in 50 dogs, *J Vet Intern Med* 8:228-232, 1994.

Henry MJ, Burton LG, Stanley MW, et al: Application of a modified Diff-Quik stain to fine needle aspiration smears: rapid staining with improved cytologic detail, *Acta Cytol* 31: 954-955, 1987.

Jorundsson E, Lumsden JH, Jacobs RM: Rapid staining techniques in cytopathology: a review and comparison of modified protocols for hematoxylin and eosin, Papanicolaou and Romanowsky stains, *Vet Clin Pathol* 28:100-108, 1999.

Léveillé R, Partington BP, Biller DS, et al: Complications after ultrasound-guided biopsy of abdominal structures in dogs and cats: 246 cases (1984-1991), *J Am Vet Med Assoc* 203(3):413-415, 1993.

Liu YW, Chen CL, Chen YS, et al: Needle tract implantation of hepatocellular carcinoma after fine needle biopsy, *Dig Dis Sci* 52(1):228-231, 2007.

Mair S, Dunbar F, Becker PJ, et al: Fine needle cytology—Is aspiration suction necessary? A study of 100 masses in various sites, *Acta Cytol* 33:809-813, 1989.

Meyer DJ: The management of cytology specimens, *Compend Contin Educ Pract Vet* 9:10-17, 1987.

Meyer DJ, Franks PT: Clinical cytology: Part I: Management of tissue specimens, *Mod Vet Pract* 67:255-259, 1986.

Meyer DJ, Harvey JW: Evaluation of fluids: effusions, synovial fluid, cerebrospinal fluid. In Meyer DJ, Harvey JW (eds): *Veterinary laboratory medicine: interpretation and diagnosis*, Saunders, Philadelphia, 2004, pp 245-259.

Nyland TG, Mattoon JS, Herrgesell EJ, et al: Ultrasound-guided biopsy. In Nyland TG, Mattoon JS (eds): *Small animal diagnostic ultrasound*, ed 2, Philadelphia, 2002a, Saunders, pp 30-48.

Nyland TG, Wallack ST, Wisner ER: Needle-tract implantation following US-guided fine-needle aspiration biopsy of transitional cell carcinoma of the bladder, urethra and prostate, *Vet Radiol Ultrasound* 43(1):50-53, 2002b.

Podell M: Epilepsy and seizure classification: a lesson from Leonardo, *J Vet Intern Med* 13:3-4, 1999.

Yue X, Zheng S: Cytologic diagnosis by transthoracic fine needle sampling without aspiration, *Acta Cytol* 33:806-808, 1989.

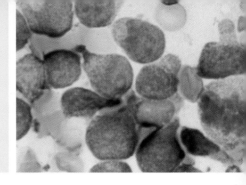

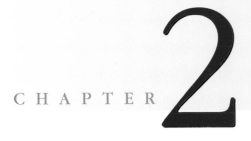

General Categories of Cytologic Interpretation

Rose E. Raskin

One use of cytology is to classify lesions so as to assist with the diagnosis, prognosis, and management of a case. Cytologic interpretations are generally classified into one of five cytodiagnostic groups (Box 2-1). A sixth category can be used for nondiagnostic interpretations. Nondiagnostic samples usually result from insufficient cellular material or excessive blood contamination.

> **KEY POINT** Interpretation of cytologic material may include more than one category, such as inflammation along with a response to tissue injury or neoplasia with inflammation.

NORMAL OR HYPERPLASTIC TISSUE

Normal and hyperplastic tissues are both composed primarily of mature cell types. Normal cells display uniformity in cellular, nuclear, and nucleolar size and shape. Cytoplasmic volume is usually high relative to the nucleus (Figs. 2-1 and 2-2). Hyperplasia is a non-neoplastic enlargement of tissue that can occur in response to hormonal disturbances or tissue injury. Hyperplastic tissue has a tendency to enlarge symmetrically in comparison to neoplasia. Cytologically, hyperplastic

---

BOX 2-1	General Categories of Cytologic Interpretation

Normal or hyperplastic tissue
Cystic mass
Inflammation or cellular infiltrate
Response to tissue injury
Neoplasia
Nondiagnostic sample

---

cells have a higher nuclear-to-cytoplasmic ratio than normal cells. Examples of hyperplastic responses include nodular proliferations within the parenchyma of the prostate (Fig. 2-3), liver, and pancreas (Fig. 2-4).

CYSTIC MASS

Cystic lesions contain liquid or semisolid material. The low-protein liquid usually contains a small number of cells. These benign lesions may result from proliferation of lining cells or tissue injury. Examples include seroma (Fig. 2-5), salivary mucocele, apocrine sweat gland cyst, epidermal/follicular cyst, and cysts associated with noncutaneous glands such as the mammary gland or prostate (Fig. 2-6).

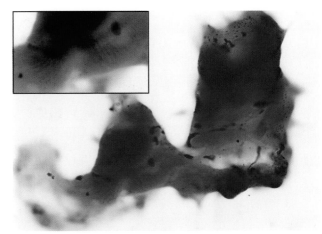

■ **FIGURE 2-1. Normal skeletal muscle. Tissue aspirate. Dog.** Numerous threadlike myofibrils compose each cell whose nucleus is small, condensed, and oval. Cross-striations, characteristic of skeletal muscle, are barely visible against the dark blue cytoplasm but seen in the magnified view (inset). (Wright-Giemsa; IP.)

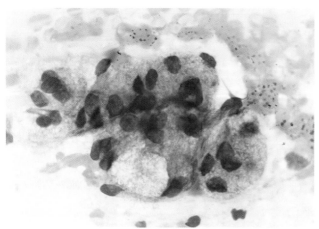

■ **FIGURE 2-2. Normal salivary gland. Tissue aspirate. Dog.** The gland has uniform features of nuclear size, nuclear-to-cytoplasmic ratio, and cytoplasmic content. (Wright-Giemsa; HP oil.)

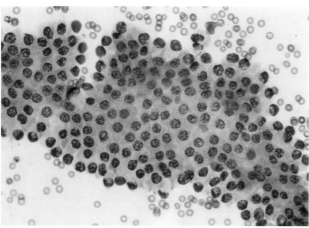

■ **FIGURE 2-3. Canine prostatic hyperplasia. Tissue aspirate. Dog.** The presenting clinical sign in this case involves blood dripping from the prepuce. Cytologically, the nuclear size is uniform; however, the nuclear-to-cytoplasmic ratio is increased as indicated by the close proximity of nuclei to each other. (Wright-Giemsa; HP oil.)

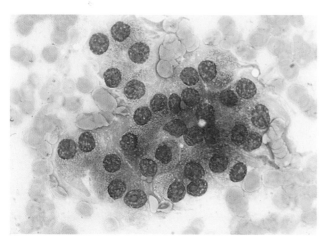

■ **FIGURE 2-4. Nodular hyperplasia of the pancreas. Tissue aspirate. Dog.** Ultrasound examination reveals a hypoechoic mass in the area of the pancreas. Cytologically, hyperplastic parenchymal organs commonly display binucleation. (Wright-Giemsa; HP oil.)

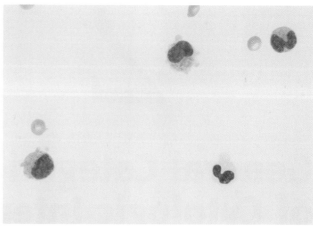

■ **FIGURE 2-5. Seroma. Tissue aspirate. Dog.** Blood-tinged fluid is removed from a swelling on the neck. Cytologically, low cellularity and low protein content is visible in the background. Large mononuclear cells with fine cytoplasmic granularity predominate along with low numbers of erythrocytes. (Wright-Giemsa; HP oil.)

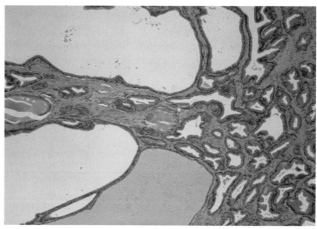

■ **FIGURE 2-6. Prostatic cyst. Histopathology. Dog.** Cuboidal epithelial cells line large cystic spaces that represent dilated ducts. (H&E; LP.)

INFLAMMATION OR CELLULAR INFILTRATE

Inflammatory conditions are classified cytologically by the predominance of the cell type involved. Recognition of the inflammatory cell type often suggests an etiologic condition.

Purulent or suppurative lesions contain greater than 85% neutrophils; they are then classified by the presence or absence of degeneration affecting the neutrophil. Nondegenerate neutrophils are morphologically normal and predominate in relatively nontoxic environments such as immune-mediated conditions, neoplastic lesions (Fig. 2-7), and sterile lesions caused by irritants such as urine and bile. Degenerate neutrophils display nuclear swelling and decreased stain intensity termed *karyolysis* (Fig. 2-8), indicating rapid cell death in a toxic environment (Perman et al., 1979). Increased nuclear staining with coalescence of the nucleus into a single round mass and an intact cellular membrane characterizes *pyknosis*

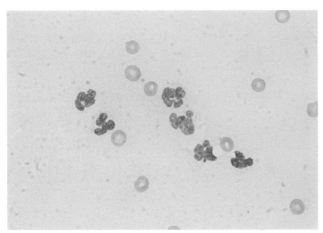

■ **FIGURE 2-7. Nondegenerate neutrophils. Synovial fluid. Dog.** Nonseptic inflammation with well-segmented neutrophils appears secondary to adjacent neoplasia of the bone. (Wright-Giemsa; HP oil.)

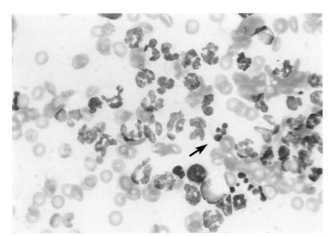

■ **FIGURE 2-8. Karyolysis, karyorrhexis. Tissue aspirate. Dog.** Mild to moderate karyolysis of neutrophils is evident by the decreased nuclear stain intensity and swollen nuclear lobes. Pyknosis of multiple nuclear segments appear as dark, dense, round structures, termed *karyorrhexis (arrow)*, in this case of bacterial dermatitis. (Wright-Giemsa; HP oil.)

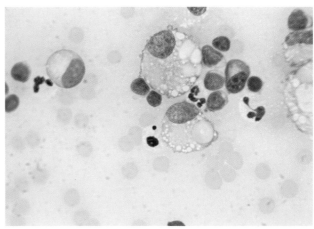

■ **FIGURE 2-9. Pyknosis. Chylous effusion. Dog.** Chronic inflammation of this fluid produces neutrophil nuclei that have condensed into a large, often single, dark, round structure related to the slow progression of cellular change in a nonseptic environment. The pyknotic cell in this case also contains a second, smaller round nuclear fragment. (Wright; HP oil.)

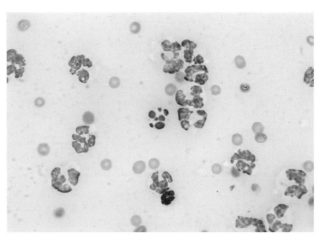

■ **FIGURE 2-10. Karyorrhexis. Tissue aspirate.** Inflammatory response with evidence of multiple pyknotic nuclear segments in the center cell. (Wright-Giemsa; HP oil.)

(Fig. 2-9), a slow, progressive change often within a relatively nontoxic environment. An end stage of cell death, termed *karyorrhexis*, may be seen cytologically as the result of pyknosis of hypersegmented nuclei (Fig. 2-10). Degenerate neutrophils predominate in bacterial infections, particularly gram-negative types. Under septic conditions, bacteria may be found intracellularly (Fig. 2-11).

Histiocytic or *macrophagic* lesions contain a predominance of macrophages, suggesting chronic inflammation (Fig. 2-12). In granulomas, activated macrophages that morphologically resemble epithelial cells are termed *epithelioid macrophages*. These cells may merge to form giant multinucleated forms (Fig. 2-13). The granulomatous lesions are often associated with foreign body reactions and mycobacterial infection.

Pyogranulomatous or *mixed cell* inflammatory lesions contain a mixture of neutrophils and macrophages (Fig. 2-14) that may include increased numbers of

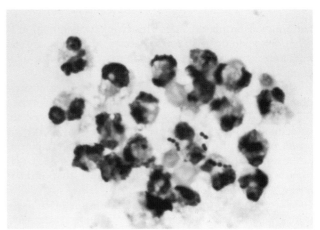

■ **FIGURE 2-11. Bacterial sepsis. Tissue aspirate. Dog.** Markedly karyolytic neutrophils are present with intracellular and extracellular coccoid bacteria. Karyolysis is so severe that the cells are barely recognizable as neutrophils. (Wright; HP oil.)

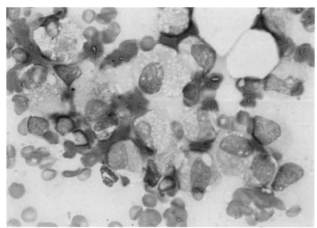

■ **FIGURE 2-12. Macrophagic inflammation. Tissue imprint. Dog.** Nodular lung disease with numerous large mononuclear cells having abundant gray cytoplasm and many cells with multiple cytoplasmic vacuoles. (Wright-Giemsa; HP oil.)

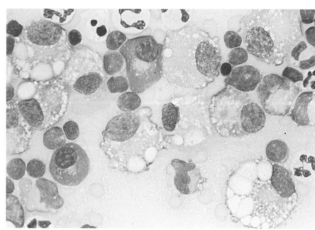

■ **FIGURE 2-14. Pyogranulomatous or mixed cell inflammation. Chylous effusion. Dog.** Chronic chylous effusion contains a variety of cell types, including nondegenerate neutrophils, vacuolated macrophages, small to medium lymphocytes, and two mature plasma cells. (Wright; HP oil.)

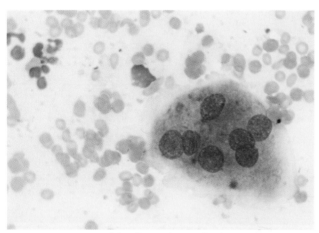

■ **FIGURE 2-13. Multinucleate giant cell. Tissue aspirate. Cat.** Skin lesion with pyogranulomatous inflammation, including many giant cells related to the presence of fungal hyphae. Pictured is a cell with seven distinct nuclei and abundant granular blue-gray cytoplasm. (Wright-Giemsa; HP oil.)

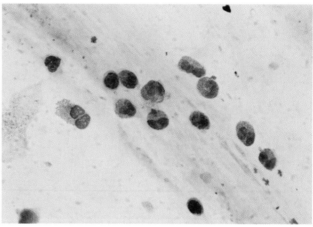

■ **FIGURE 2-15. Eosinophilic inflammation. Transtracheal wash. Cat.** Clinical presentation of a chronic cough in this cat with suspected pulmonary allergy. Fluid contains 95% eosinophils. Pictured are several eosinophils that stain pink to blue-green and adhere to pink mucous material. (Wright-Giemsa; HP oil.)

lymphocytes or plasma cells. This type of inflammation is often associated with foreign body reactions, fungal infections, mycobacterial infections, panniculitis, lick granulomas, and other chronic tissue injuries.

Eosinophilic lesions contain greater than 10% eosinophils in addition to other inflammatory cell types (Fig. 2-15). They are seen with or without mast cell involvement. This inflammatory response is associated with eosinophilic granuloma, hypersensitivity or allergic conditions, parasitic migrations, fungal infections, mast cell tumors, and other neoplastic conditions that induce eosinophilopoiesis.

Lymphocytic or *plasmacytic* infiltration is often associated with allergic or immune reactions, early viral infections, and chronic inflammation. The lymphoid population is heterogeneous, with small or intermediate-sized lymphocytes and plasma cells mixed with other

inflammatory cells (see Fig. 2-14). A monomorphic population of lymphoid cells without other inflammatory cells present suggests lymphoid neoplasia.

RESPONSE TO TISSUE INJURY

Cytologic samples often contain evidence of tissue injury in addition to cyst formation, inflammation, or neoplasia. These changes include hemorrhage, proteinaceous debris, cholesterol crystals, necrosis, and fibrosis.

Hemorrhage that is pathologic can be distinguished from blood contamination encountered during the cytologic collection. Blood contamination is associated with the presence of numerous erythrocytes and platelets. Acute hemorrhage is associated with engulfment of erythrocytes by macrophages termed *erythrophagocytosis* (Fig. 2-16). Chronic hemorrhage is associated with active

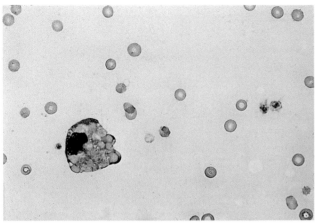

■ **FIGURE 2-16. Erythrophagocytosis. Cerebrospinal fluid. Cat.** Many erythrocytes are in the background along with one large macrophage that engulfed numerous intact red cells. The cat had confirmed infection with feline coronavirus (feline infectious peritonitis). (Wright; HP oil.)

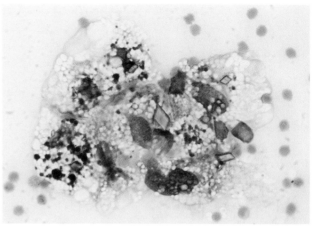

■ **FIGURE 2-18. Hematoidin crystals. Pericardial fluid. Dog.** Activated macrophages with bright yellow rhomboid crystals of variable size appear in this hemorrhagic fluid related to hemoglobin breakdown in an anaerobic environment. Several macrophages also contain black granular material consistent with hemosiderin. (Wright-Giemsa; HP oil.)

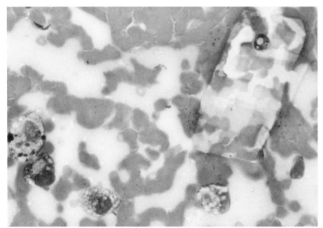

■ **FIGURE 2-17. Chronic hemorrhage. Tissue aspirate. Dog.** Several activated macrophages are present in this follicular cyst lesion. The macrophage directly below the cholesterol crystal contains blue-green granular material in the cytoplasm consistent with hemosiderin, a breakdown product of erythrocytes. On the left edge is a macrophage with large black granules suggestive of hemosiderin. (Wright; HP oil.)

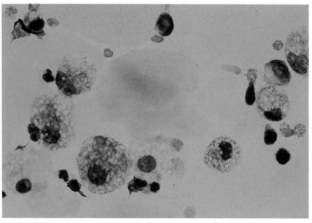

■ **FIGURE 2-19. Mucus. Salivary mucocele. Dog.** The background contains pale pink-blue amorphous material representative of mucus. Numerous activated macrophages or mucinophages compose the predominant population. (Wright; HP oil.)

macrophages containing degraded blood pigment within their cytoplasm—for example, blue-green to black hemosiderin granules (Figs. 2-17 and 2-18) or yellow rhomboid hematoidin crystals (Fig. 2-18). Hemosiderin represents an excess aggregation of ferritin molecules or micelles. This form of iron storage becomes visible by light microscopy and stains blue with the Prussian blue reaction. Hematoidin crystals do not contain iron although they are formed during anaerobic breakdown of hemoglobin such as may occur within tissues or cavities. Hematomas often contain phagocytized erythrocytes if the lesion is acute, or hemosiderin-laden macrophages if the lesion is chronic.

Proteinaceous debris may be seen within the background of the preparation. Mucus stains lightly basophilic and appears amorphous (Fig. 2-19). Lymphoglandular bodies (Fig. 2-20) are cytoplasmic fragments from fragile cells, usually lymphocytes, that are discrete, round, lightly basophilic structures (Flanders et al., 1993). *Nuclear streaming* refers to linear pink to purple strands of nuclear remnants (Fig. 2-21) produced by excessive tissue handling during cytologic preparation or with necrotic material when sampled. Clear to light-pink amorphous strands representing collagen (Fig. 2-22A) may be admixed with spindle cells and endothelium into a fibrovascular stroma. However, when these collagen fibers undergo damage (as in the collagenolysis associated with mast cell tumor), degranulating eosinophils release collagenase that produces dense, hyalinized pink collagen bands (Fig. 2-22B). Amyloid is an uncommon pathologic protein found between cells. It appears amorphous, eosinophilic, and hyaline and may be associated with chronic inflammation.

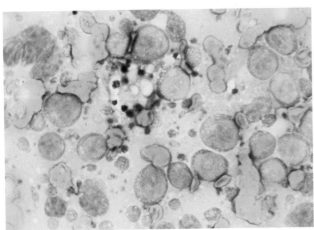

■ FIGURE 2-20. Lymphoglandular bodies. Tissue aspirate. Dog. The background of this lymph node preparation contains numerous small, blue-gray cytoplasmic fragments called *lymphoglandular bodies* that are related to the rupture of the fragile neoplastic lymphocytes. An activated macrophage has phagocytized cellular debris appearing as large blue-black particles. (Wright; HP oil.)

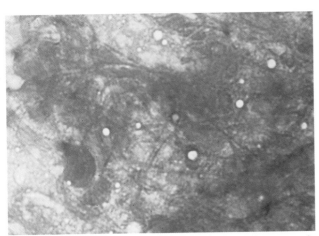

■ FIGURE 2-21. Nuclear streaming. Tissue aspirate. Purple strands of nuclear material are formed from ruptured cells either as an artifact of slide preparation or from fragile cells that are frequently neoplastic. (Wright-Giemsa; HP oil.) (Courtesy of Denny Meyer, University of Florida).

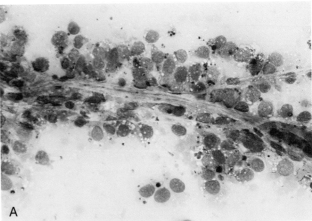

A

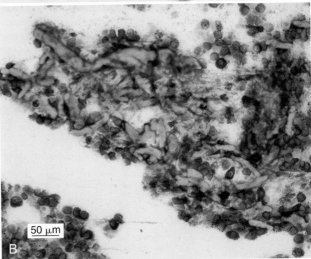

50 μm

B

■ FIGURE 2-22. A, Collagenous fibers. Tissue aspirate. Dog. Clear to light pink strands of intact fibrous connective tissue may resemble fungal hyphae. Collagenous fibers will have poorly defined margins and a variable diameter, unlike hyphae, which have uniform width and distinct borders. (Wright-Giemsa, HP oil.) **B, Collagenolysis. Tissue aspirate. Dog.** Haphazard bands of collagen appear bright pink and hyalinized owing to the breakdown of the fibers through release of collagenase by degranulating eosinophils. This type of connective tissue damage occurs commonly in canine mast cell tumors. Interspersed among tumor cells are eosinophils and their granules. (Wright; IP.)

Cholesterol crystals represent evidence of cell membrane damage that is found in the background of some cytologic preparations. These rectangular, plated crystals are transparent unless background staining is enhanced as, for example, with new methylene blue stain (Fig. 2-23). The crystals are most often associated with epidermal/follicular cysts.

Necrosis and *fibrosis* may occur together or separately in some cytologic preparations. The death of cells is represented by fuzzy, indistinct cell outlines and definition of cell type (Fig. 2-24). A reparative response accompanying tissue injury involves increased fibroblastic activity. It is common to see very reactive fibrocytes (Fig. 2-25) along with severe inflammation. One must be careful not to overinterpret this reactivity as a neoplastic condition.

NEOPLASIA

General Features

Neoplasia is initially diagnosed when a monomorphic cell population is present and significant inflammation is lacking. Further division into benign and malignant types is based on cytomorphologic characteristics. *Benign cells* display uniformity in size, nuclear-to-cytoplasmic ratio, and other nuclear features. *Malignant cells* often display three or more criteria (Box 2-2 and Figs. 2-26 to 2-32) of cellular immaturity or atypia, which should be identified before a diagnosis of malignancy is made. In cases of an equivocal diagnosis or severe inflammation, histopathologic examination is recommended.

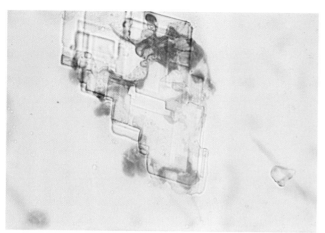

■ **FIGURE 2-23. Cholesterol crystal. Tissue aspirate.** Clear rectangular plates with notched corners are characteristic of cholesterol. This is often associated with degenerate squamous epithelium, as in follicular cysts. Crystals may be highlighted with background cellular debris or stain. (New methylene blue; HP oil.) (Courtesy of Denny Meyer, University of Florida.)

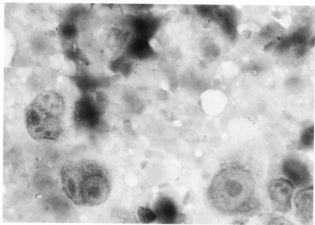

■ **FIGURE 2-24. Necrosis. Tissue aspirate. Dog.** Prominent nucleoli remain visible while other tissue has degenerated into dark blue-gray amorphous debris representative of necrotic material. The sample was taken from a case of prostatic carcinoma in which the necrotic site was focal. (Wright-Giemsa; HP oil.)

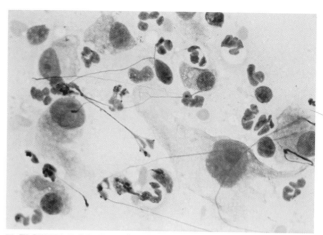

■ **FIGURE 2-25. Reactive fibroplasia. Tissue scraping. Cat.** Oral mass with associated septic inflammation. Pictured are several plump mesenchymal cells with a stellate to spindle appearance and prominent nucleoli along with suppurative inflammation. The severity of the inflammatory response warrants caution in suggesting a malignant mesenchymal mass or sarcoma. Note the nuclear streaming appears as purple strands. (Aqueous-based Wright; HP oil.)

BOX 2-2   Cytologic Criteria Used to Identify Malignant Cells

Pleomorphism of cell size, shape, or maturation state between cells of similar origin (see Fig. 2-26)
High or variable nuclear-to-cytoplasmic ratio (see Fig. 2-27)
Variation in nuclear size, termed *anisokaryosis* (see Fig. 2-27)
Coarse nuclear chromatin clumping (see Fig. 2-28)
Enlarged, multiple, or variably shaped nucleoli (see Fig. 2-29)
Nuclear molding related to the rapid growth of cells (see Fig. 2-30)
Multinucleation (see Fig. 2-31)
Abnormal mitotic figures evident as uneven divisions and isolated or lag chromatin (see Fig. 2-32)

Cytomorphologic Categories

Neoplasms may be divided into four general categories to assist in making the cytologic interpretation by restricting the list of differential diagnoses (Perman et al., 1979, Alleman and Bain, 2000). The categories listed in Table 2-1 are based not on cell origin or function but rather on their general cytomorphologic characteristics. The first two terms are taken from embryology (Noden and de Lahunta, 1985).

Epithelial Neoplasms

This type of neoplasm is associated with a clustered arrangement of cells into ball shapes or monolayer sheets. Cell origin of these neoplasms often involves glandular or parenchymal tissue and lining surfaces. Examples of epithelial neoplasms include lung adenocarcinoma (Fig. 2-33), perianal adenoma (hepatoid tumor), basal cell tumor, sebaceous adenoma, transitional cell carcinoma (Fig. 2-34), and mesothelioma. Specific cytologic features of epithelial neoplasms include the following characteristics:

* Cells exfoliate in tight clumps or sheets
* Cells adhere to each other and may display distinct tight junctions, termed *desmosomes* (Fig. 2-35)
* Cells are large and round to polygonal with distinct, intact cytoplasmic borders
* Nuclei are round to oval

Mesenchymal Neoplasms

Neoplasms with a mesenchymal appearance resemble the embryonic connective tissue, mesenchyme. This tissue is loosely arranged with usually abundant extracellular matrix (Noden and de Lahunta, 1985) and individualized spindle or stellate cells (Bacha 2000). Benign

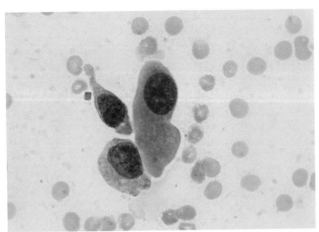

■ **FIGURE 2-26. Pleomorphism. Tissue aspirate. Dog.** Transitional cell carcinoma cells display variability in size and shape supportive of malignancy. (Wright-Giemsa; HP oil.)

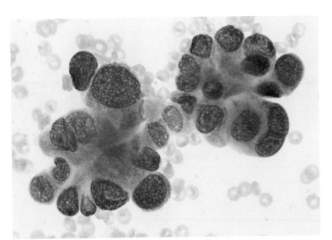

■ **FIGURE 2-27. Anisocytosis, anisokaryosis. Tissue aspirate. Dog.** Lung adenocarcinoma specimen has several features of malignancy. These features include high and variable nuclear-to-cytoplasmic ratio, anisokaryosis, binucleation, and coarse nuclear chromatin. (Wright-Giemsa; HP oil.)

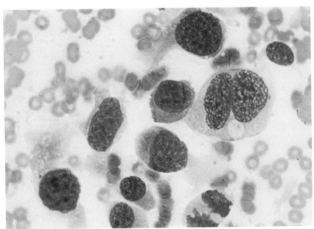

■ **FIGURE 2-28. Coarse chromatin. Tissue aspirate. Dog.** Same case as FIGURE 2-26. The nuclear material is mottled with light and dark spaces clearly evident. This appearance is often associated with neoplastic transitional epithelium but may be seen with other tissues. Binucleation is seen in one cell and a mitotic figure is present on the bottom edge. (Wright-Giemsa; HP oil.)

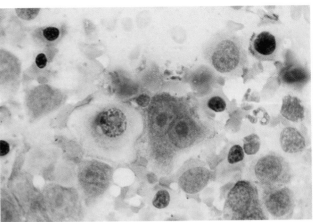

■ **FIGURE 2-29. Prominent nucleoli. Tissue aspirate. Dog.** Same case as FIGURE 2-24. A binucleate cell with very large single nucleoli in each nucleus is present. A prominent nucleolus is noted in the adjacent cell, which also displays coarse chromatin or chromatin clumping. (Wright-Giemsa; HP oil.)

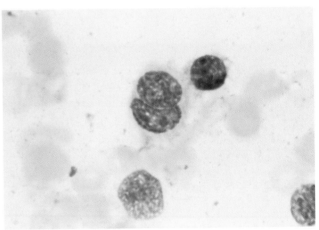

■ **FIGURE 2-30. Nuclear molding. Tissue aspirate. Dog.** Nasal chondrosarcoma pictured with a binucleate cell in which one nucleus is wrapped around the other. This feature is present in malignant tissues and is related to the lack of normal inhibition of cell growth. (Wright-Giemsa; HP oil.)

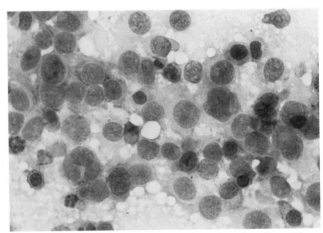

■ **FIGURE 2-31. Multinucleation. Tissue imprint. Dog.** Pheochromocytoma with two multinucleate cells, one in the lower left side with three nuclei and the other to the right of center with an irregularly shaped nuclear region. Multinucleation may be found also in epithelial, mesenchymal, and round cell neoplasms. (Wright-Giemsa; HP oil.)

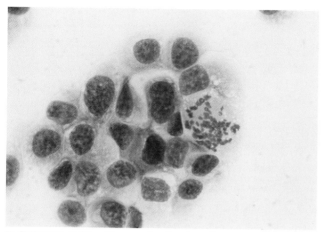

■ **FIGURE 2-32. Abnormal mitosis. Tissue aspirate. Dog.** Same case as Figure 2-26. Chromosomal fragments are dispersed irregularly with some isolated from the rest, termed *lag chromatin*. Increased mitotic activity may be suggestive of malignancy but abnormal division is diagnostic for malignancy. (Wright-Giemsa; HP oil.)

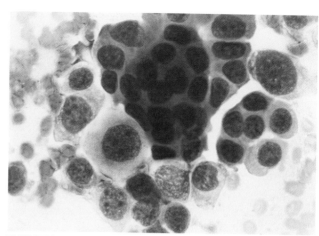

■ **FIGURE 2-34. Epithelial neoplasm. Tissue aspirate. Dog.** Same case as Figure 2-26. Cells are formed into tight balls or as sheets. Nuclei are round to oval and cells are large, round to polygonal with distinct cytoplasmic borders. (Wright-Giemsa; HP oil.)

TABLE 2-1	Cytomorphologic Categories of Neoplasia	
Category	**General Features**	**Examples**
Epithelial	Clustered, tight arrangement of cells	Transitional cell carcinoma, lung tumors
Mesenchymal	Individualized, spindle to oval cells	Hemangiosarcoma, osteosarcoma
Round cell	Individualized, round, discrete cells	Lymphoma, transmissible venereal tumor
Naked nuclei	Loosely adherent cells with free round nuclei	Thyroid tumors, paragangliomas

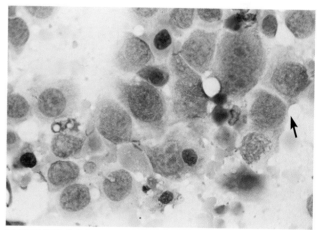

■ **FIGURE 2-35. Desmosomes. Tissue aspirate. Dog.** Same case as Figure 2-24. A sheet of carcinoma cells with prominent desmosomes. These clear lines *(arrow)* between adjacent cells represent tight junctions that are characteristic of epithelial cells. (Wright-Giemsa; HP oil.)

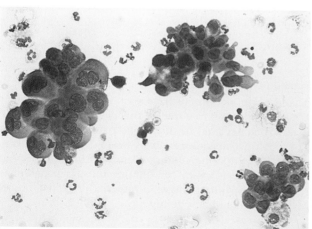

■ **FIGURE 2-33. Epithelial neoplasm. Lung lavage. Dog.** Large clusters of cohesive cells having distinct cell borders from a case of lung adenocarcinoma. (Wright-Giemsa; IP.) (Courtesy of Robert King, Gainesville, FL.)

and malignant mesenchymal neoplasms often originate from connective tissue elements, such as fibroblasts, osteoblasts, adipocytes, myocytes, and vascular lining cells. Examples of mesenchymal neoplasms include hemangiosarcoma (Fig. 2-36), osteosarcoma (Fig. 2-37), hemangiopericytoma, and amelanotic melanoma (Fig. 2-38). Specific cytologic features of mesenchymal neoplasms include the following:

- Cells usually exfoliate individually (however, clumps of cells are seen occasionally)
- Cells are oval, stellate, or fusiform with often indistinct cytoplasmic borders
- Samples are often poorly cellular
- Cells are usually smaller compared with epithelial cells
- Nuclei are round to elliptical

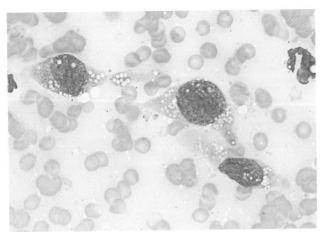

■ **FIGURE 2-36. Mesenchymal neoplasm. Tissue imprint. Dog.** Neoplastic cells exfoliate individually and appear oval, spindle, or fusiform. This bone lesion was confirmed as hemangiosarcoma on histologic examination. Characteristic of hemangiosarcoma cytology is a poorly cellular sample with plump mesenchymal cells that contain numerous small punctate cytoplasmic vacuoles. (Wright-Giemsa; HP oil.)

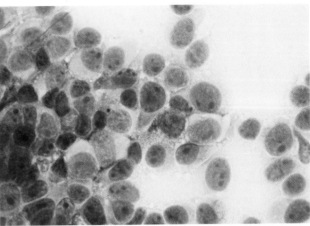

■ **FIGURE 2-38. Mesenchymal neoplasm. Tissue imprint. Dog.** Round to oval nuclei, anisokaryosis, high nuclear-to-cytoplasmic ratio, prominent and variably shaped nucleoli, and individualized cells with poorly distinct cytoplasmic borders suggest a malignant mesenchymal neoplasm. This lesion is from a gum mass with a histologically confirmed diagnosis of amelanotic melanoma. One cell in the center contains small amounts of melanin pigment granules. (Aqueous-based Wright; HP oil.)

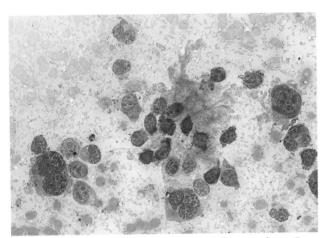

■ **FIGURE 2-37. Mesenchymal neoplasm. Tissue aspirate. Dog.** Individualized pleomorphic cells with abundant extracellular eosinophilic osteoid material is consistent with osteosarcoma. Binucleate and multinucleate forms are common and seen in this sample. (Wright-Giemsa; HP oil.)

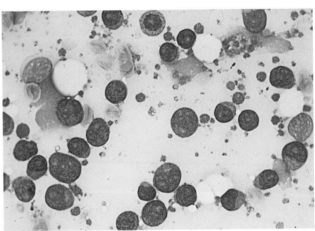

■ **FIGURE 2-39. Round (discrete) cell neoplasm. Tissue aspirate. Dog.** Discrete cells with a round shape, distinct cytoplasmic borders, and a very high nuclear-to-cytoplasmic ratio are characteristic of lymphoid cells. This sample is taken from a lymph node effaced by lymphoma cells. (Wright-Giemsa; HP oil.)

Round Cell Neoplasms

These neoplasms have discrete, round cellular shapes and are often associated with hematopoietic cells. Examples of round cell neoplasms include mast cell tumor, histiocytoma, lymphoma (Fig. 2-39), plasmacytoma, and transmissible venereal tumor (Fig. 2-40). Specific cytologic characteristics of round cell neoplasms include the following:

- Cells exfoliate individually, having distinct cytoplasmic borders
- Cell shape is generally round
- Samples are moderately cellular
- Cells are usually smaller compared with epithelial cells
- Nuclei are round to indented

Naked Nuclei Neoplasms

Naked nuclei neoplasms have a loosely adherent cellular arrangement with free nuclei. This cytologic appearance is an artifact related to the fragile nature of these cells. These neoplasms are usually associated with endocrine and neuroendocrine tumors. Examples include thyroid tumors (Fig. 2-41), islet cell tumors, and paragangliomas (Fig. 2-42). Specific cytologic features of naked nuclei neoplasms include the following:

- Cells exfoliate in loosely attached sheets with many free nuclei present, often having indistinct cytoplasmic borders
- Occasional cell clusters may be present with distinct cell outlines

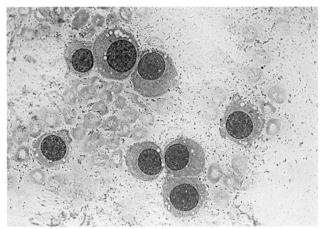

■ **FIGURE 2-40. Round (discrete) cell neoplasm. Tissue aspirate. Dog.** This fleshy vulvar mass is composed of round cells bearing a single prominent nucleolus and moderately abundant cytoplasm with frequent punctate cytoplasmic vacuolation. The cytologic diagnosis is transmissible venereal tumor. (Wright-Giemsa; HP oil.)

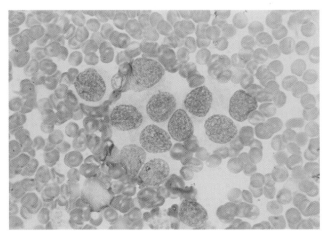

■ **FIGURE 2-41. Naked nuclei neoplasm. Tissue aspirate. Dog.** Cervical mass in the area of the thyroid from an animal with a honking cough. Cytologically the sample presents as a syncytium of round nuclei with relatively uniform features. This is characteristic of an endocrine mass. Typically the distinction between hyperplasia, adenoma, and carcinoma is difficult cytologically and sometimes histologically. (Wright-Giemsa; HP oil.)

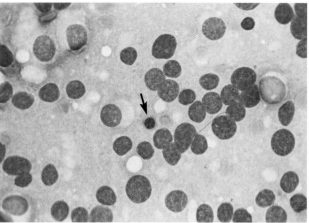

■ **FIGURE 2-42. Naked nuclei neoplasm. Tissue imprint. Dog.** Clinical signs include a head tilt and temporal muscle atrophy. Magnetic resonance imaging suggested a mass involving the osseous bulla. Surgery found a mass at the bifurcation of the common carotid artery. Cytologically, the preparation contains mostly loose or free round nuclei against a finely granular eosinophilic background. Few intact cells remain with pale cytoplasm at the edges and center. Adjacent to the center intact cell is a nucleated red cell *(arrow)* suggestive of extramedullary hematopoiesis. The histologic diagnosis is paraganglioma, specifically a malignant chemodectoma in this case, since it metastasized and was thought to involve the chemoreceptor organ in that site. (Wright-Giemsa; HP oil.)

• Cell shape is generally round to polygonal
• Samples are highly cellular
• Nuclei are round to indented

KEY POINT The use of these four cytomorphologic categories may help to classify neoplastic lesions by their general cellular appearance and suggest specific tumor types. Remember that these categories may not fit well for some neoplasms, especially for poorly differentiated tumors. It is recommended that biopsy specimens for histopathologic examination be taken to determine the specific tumor type and extent of the lesion.

REFERENCES

Alleman AR, Bain PJ: Diagnosing neoplasia: the cytologic criteria for malignancy, *Vet Med* 95:204-223, 2000.

Bacha WJ, Bacha LM: *Color atlas of veterinary histology*, ed 2, Lippincott Williams & Wilkins, Philadelphia, 2000, pp 13-15.

Flanders E, Kornstein MJ, Wakely PE, et al: Lymphoglandular bodies in fine-needle aspiration cytology smears, *Am J Clin Pathol* 99:566-569, 1993.

Noden DM, de Lahunta A: *The embryology of domestic animals*, Williams & Wilkins, Baltimore, 1985, pp 10-11.

Perman V, Alsaker RD, Riis RC: *Cytology of the dog and cat*, American Animal Hospital Association, South Bend, IN, 1979, pp 4-7.

CHAPTER 3

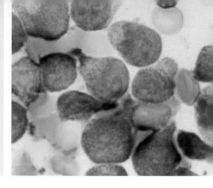

Skin and Subcutaneous Tissues

Rose E. Raskin

NORMAL HISTOLOGY AND CYTOLOGY

There are regional differences in histology of the skin of the dog and cat related to the thickness of the epidermis and dermis (Fig. 3-1A). In general, the epidermis is composed of several layers of squamous epithelium, including a keratinized layer, a granular layer, a spinous layer, and a basal layer. The adnexal structures of the epidermis include hair follicles, sweat glands, and sebaceous glands (Fig. 3-1B). The dermis present below the epidermal layer contains the adnexal structures, smooth muscle bands, blood and lymphatic vessels, nerves, and variably sized collagen and elastic fibers. Beneath the dermis lies the subcutis, composed of loose adipose tissue and collagen bundles. Normal cytology of the dermis and subcutis contains a mixture of epidermal squamous epithelium and well-differentiated glandular elements as well as mature adipose and collagen tissue. Basal epithelial cells are round and deeply basophilic with a high nuclear-to-cytoplasmic ratio. Cells of the other epidermal layers are known as *keratinocytes* because of their composition of keratin. Polygonal cells of the granular layer are evident cytologically by the presence of basophilic to magenta keratohyalin granules within an abundant lightly basophilic cytoplasm having a small, contracted nucleus. The most superficial keratinized layer consists of flattened, sharply demarcated, blue-green hyalinized squames that lack a nucleus. Elongated dark-blue to purple squames are termed *keratin bars,* which represent rolled or coiled cells. Melanocytes from neural crest origin are located within the basal layer of the epidermis or hair matrix. Their brownish-black to greenish-black fine granules may be seen in some keratinocytes. Also present may be a low number of mast cells from perivascular and perifollicular sites.

NORMAL-APPEARING EPITHELIUM

> **KEY POINT** Presence of only mature epithelium in a skin mass most often indicates a non-neoplastic condition.

Non-neoplastic noninflammatory tumor-like lesions account for approximately 10% of skin lesions removed from dogs and cats (Goldschmidt and Shofer, 1992). These include cysts and glandular hyperplasia.

Epidermal Cyst or Follicular Cyst

Also termed *epidermal inclusion cysts* or *epidermoid cysts,* these cysts are found in one third to one half of the non-neoplastic noninflammatory tumor-like lesions removed in dogs and cats, respectively (Goldschmidt and Shofer, 1992). They occur most frequently in middle-aged to older dogs (Yager and Wilcock, 1994). Cysts may be single or multiple, firm to fluctuant, with a smooth, round, well-circumscribed appearance. These are often located on the dorsum and extremities (Goldschmidt and Shofer, 1992). The cyst lining arises from well-differentiated stratified squamous epithelium (Fig. 3-2A). By definition, the lack of adnexal differentiation without a connection to the skin surface seen histologically is termed an *epidermal inclusion cyst.* The more common follicular cyst is characterized by a distended hair follicle infundibulum that opens to the surface via a pore (see Fig. 3-2A). The distinction cannot be made cytologically. Keratin bars, squames, or other keratinocytes predominate on cytology (Fig. 3-2B). Degradation of cells within the cyst may lead to the formation of cholesterol crystals, which appear as negative-stained, irregularly notched, rectangular plates best seen against the amorphous basophilic cellular debris of the background (Fig. 3-2C). They are thought to arise from frictional trauma leading to obstruction of follicular ostia when found on pressure points. Nailbed cysts (Fig. 3-2D) are thought to occur from trauma that allows embedment of germ layer epidermis in underlying tissue creating an epithelial inclusion cyst (Gross et al., 2005). Multiple cysts may have a developmental and/or environmental basis for their formation (Gross et al., 2005). The behavior of these masses is benign, but rupture of the cyst wall can induce a localized pyogranulomatous cellulitis. When this occurs, neutrophils and macrophages

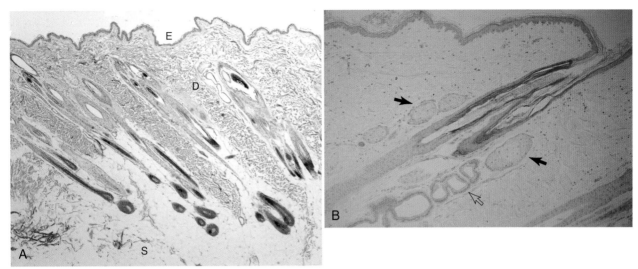

■ **FIGURE 3-1. Normal skin histology. Dog. A,** Section of haired skin from the hip area showing the epidermis *(E)*, dermis *(D)*, and subcutis *(S)*. Note the compound hair follicles common in the dog and cat. (H&E; LP.) **B,** Section of thin skin from the abdomen. The dermis contains the adnexal structures of hair follicles, sebaceous glands *(solid arrows)*, and ducts of the sweat glands *(open arrow)*. In addition, loose and dense collagen bundles are present within the dermis. (H&E; LP.)

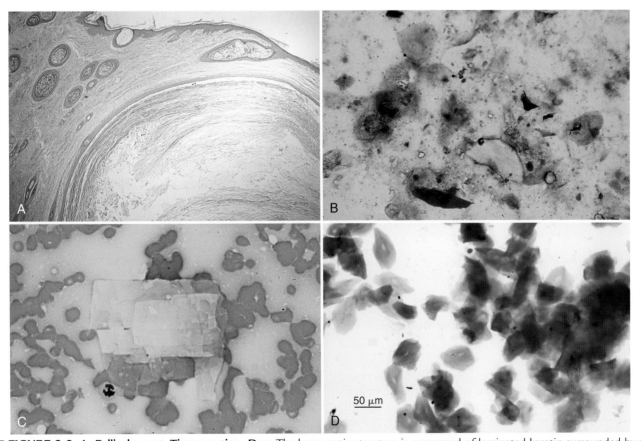

■ **FIGURE 3-2. A, Follicular cyst. Tissue section. Dog.** The large cystic structure is composed of laminated keratin surrounded by a thin rim of stratified squamous epithelium. Note the nearby smaller cysts with pores that open to the surface, suggesting these are of follicular origin. (H&E; LP.) **B-C, Follicular cyst. Tissue aspirate. Dog. B,** Amorphous cellular debris with anuclear squamous epithelium and keratin bars. (Wright; HP oil.) **C,** Cholesterol crystals appear as clear, rectangular plates visible against the proteinaceous background. (Wright; HP oil.) **D, Nailbed cyst. Tissue aspirate. Dog.** A dense collection of keratinized, sometimes pigmented squamous epithelial cells is present as noted by their hyalinized turquoise color and angular shape. (Wright-Giemsa; IP.)

may be frequent. To prevent this inflammatory response, surgery is frequently suggested and the prognosis is excellent.

> *Cytologic differential diagnosis:* infundibular keratinizing acanthoma, dermoid cyst, follicular tumors.

Apocrine Cyst

This is a common lesion in dogs and cats that is formed from occlusion of the apocrine or sweat gland duct. Grossly, it appears as a fluctuant swelling filled with light-brown to colorless fluid that may become brown and gelatinous due to inspissation. On cytology, this fluid is usually acellular, having a clear background. Treatment involves surgical excision and the prognosis is excellent.

> *Cytologic differential diagnosis:* apocrine gland hyperplasia, apocrine gland adenoma.

Nodular Sebaceous Hyperplasia

Grossly, these masses are single to multiple and often resemble a wart. Most are less than 1 cm in diameter. They are firm, elevated, with a hairless, cauliflower or papilliferous surface. Sebaceous hyperplasia is more prevalent than sebaceous adenoma (Yager and Wilcock, 1994). They are very common in old dogs and less common in cats. Distinction cannot be made cytologically and may even be difficult histologically when distinguishing between sebaceous hyperplasia and sebaceous adenoma. Symmetrical proliferation of mature sebaceous lobules grouped around a keratinizing squamous-lined duct is the histopathologic basis used to classify the condition as hyperplasia (Gross et al., 2005). Mature sebaceous epithelial cells are seen cytologically, sometimes in clusters, or as individual pale, foamy cells with a small, dense, centrally placed nucleus, often mistaken for phagocytic macrophages. These are benign proliferations that have an excellent prognosis following surgical excision.

> *Cytologic differential diagnosis:* sebaceous adenoma.

NONINFECTIOUS INFLAMMATION

Acral Lick Dermatitis/Lick Granuloma

This is a chronic inflammatory response to persistent licking or chewing of a limb, producing a thickened, firm, raised plaque lesion that often becomes ulcerated (Fig. 3-3A). Causes include infectious agents, hypersensitivity reactions, trauma, and psychogenesis. Cytologically, there is a mixed population of mononuclear inflammatory cells, including plasma cells, along with intermediate squamous epithelium (Fig. 3-3B) related to acanthosis, i.e., hyperplasia of the epidermal stratum spinosum layer. The healing response to surface erosion may produce fibroblastic cells, which appear in the cytologic specimens

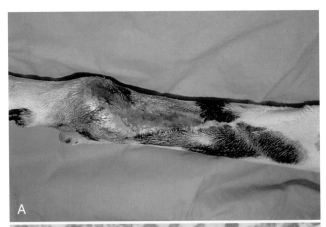

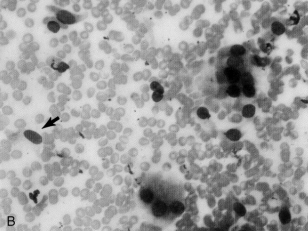

■ **FIGURE 3-3. Lick dermatitis. Dog. A,** Thickened, ulcerated, hairless lesion on the limb. **B, Tissue aspirate.** Sheets of intermediate squamous epithelium predominate related to the thickened epidermis found in these cases. Adjacent to the neutrophil in the lower left is a fibroblastic cell *(arrow)* present in response to stromal reaction. (Wright-Giemsa; HP oil.) (A, Courtesy of Rosanna Marsella, Gainesville, FL.)

as plump, fusiform cells along with numerous erythrocytes related to increased vascularization. Lesions may also involve a secondary bacterial infection with suppuration. Treatment will be determined by the underlying cause, and frequently involves control of the superficial pyoderma.

> *Cytologic differential diagnosis:* foreign body reaction, arthropod bite reaction.

Foreign Body Reaction

These reactions are caused by penetration of plant, animal, or inorganic material into the skin, producing an erythematous wound that progresses to a nodular response that often drains fluid. Cytologically, a mixed inflammatory response is present, composed mostly of macrophages and lymphocytes with smaller numbers of neutrophils and possibly eosinophils (Fig. 3-4A–C). Multinucleated giant cells are frequently present. A

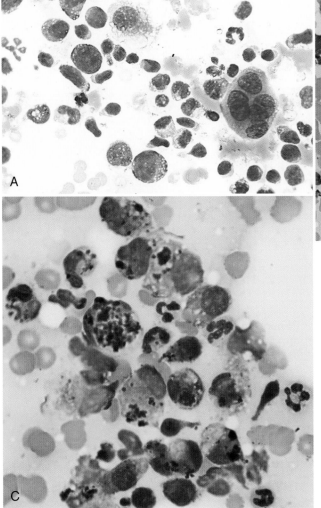

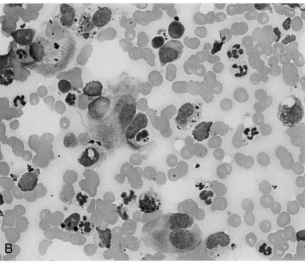

■ **FIGURE 3-4. A, Foreign body reaction. Tissue fluid sediment smear. Dog.** Small lymphocytes and macrophages predominate, with occasional neutrophils found. Note the giant cell, suggesting granulomatous inflammation. The inflammatory reaction was secondary to calcinosis circumscripta that was diagnosed on histopathology. (Aqueous-based Wright; HP oil.) **Same case B-C. Vaccine reaction. Tissue aspirate smear. Dog. B,** Firm subcutaneous swelling between the shoulder blades. A mixed inflammatory cell population composed of nondegenerate neutrophils, macrophages, fibroblasts, eosinophils *(not shown)*, and occasional small and medium lymphocytes against a hemodiluted background. In some cases, a mixed population of lymphocytes may predominate *(not shown)*. (Modified-Wright; HP oil.) **C,** Many macrophages contain variably sized bright magenta globular material. Material that is occasionally present extracellular *(not shown)* is consistent with the vaccine mucopolysaccharide adjuvant. (Modified-based Wright; HP oil.)

fibroblastic response is common. A secondary bacterial infection may occur. Treatment includes surgical exploration or excision with histologic biopsy and culture if warranted.

Cytologic differential diagnosis: fungal, bacterial, noninfectious, or arthropod bite inflammatory lesions.

Arthropod Bite Reaction

Bites from insects, ticks, and spiders, for example, may induce a mild to severe reaction characterized usually by erythema and swelling with acute necrosis that appears as eosinophilic furunculosis or later as a granuloma on histopathology (Gross et al., 2005). Cytology reveals a mixed inflammatory infiltrate composed of neutrophils, macrophages, and usually increased numbers of eosinophils related to a hypersensitivity reaction (Fig. 3-5A–B). These lesions often regress spontaneously, but some may require additional wound care.

Cytologic differential diagnosis: bacterial, fungal, noninfectious, or foreign body reactions.

Nodular Panniculitis/Steatitis

Causes of noninfectious panniculitis include trauma, foreign bodies, vaccination reactions, immune-mediated conditions, drug reactions, pancreatic conditions, nutritional deficiencies, and idiopathy. The condition appears in the cat and dog as solitary or multiple, firm to fluctuant, raised, well-demarcated lesions. These may ooze an oily yellow-brown fluid (Fig. 3-6A). Sites of prevalence include the dorsal trunk, neck, and proximal limbs. Cytologically, nondegenerate neutrophils and macrophages predominate against a vacuolated background composed of adipose tissue (Fig. 3-6B&C). Small lymphocytes and plasma cells may be numerous, especially in lesions induced by vaccination reactions. Frequently macrophages present with abundant foamy cytoplasm or as giant multinucleated forms. When chronic, evidence of fibrosis is indicated by the presence of plump fusiform cells with

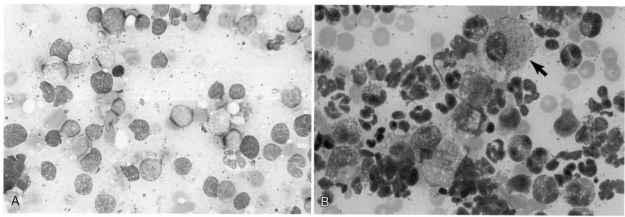

■ **FIGURE 3-5. Arthropod bite reaction. Tissue aspirate. Dog. A,** Small and intermediate-sized lymphocytes infiltrated this mass on the ventral neck in addition to low numbers of eosinophils and neutrophils. (Wright-Giemsa; HP oil.) **B,** A small dermal mass on the muzzle displays a mixed inflammatory cell population with numerous eosinophils and one degranulated mast cell *(arrow)* in addition to many neutrophils, both degenerate and nondegenerate. (Modified-Wright; HP oil.)

nuclear immaturity. The fibrosis may be so extensive as to suggest a mesenchymal neoplasm. Prognosis is usually best for solitary lesions, which respond to surgical excision. Histologically, sterile panniculitis may demonstrate inflammatory cells within the subcutis (Fig. 3-6D) that extend into the dermis. Multiple lesions are often associated with systemic disease in young dogs, and treatment involves glucocorticoid administration. Dachshunds and poodles may be predisposed to this form of the disease. Culture and histopathologic examination are recommended to rule out infectious causes. Fungal stains should be applied to cytologic specimens.

Cytologic differential diagnosis: infectious panniculitis.

Eosinophilic Plaque/Granuloma

Feline eosinophilic plaque presents initially as alopecic focal areas of intense pruritus that progress to ulceration with exudation. It has been associated with flea-bite allergy, food allergy, and atopy. Sites affected include the face, neck, abdomen, and medial thighs. Lesions may become secondarily infected with bacteria. Cytologically, eosinophils and mast cells predominate, with few lymphocytes. When lesions become secondarily infected, neutrophils are prominent. Treatment includes glucocorticoid administration and antibiotics, if necessary.

Eosinophilic granuloma occurs in dogs and young cats in response to a hypersensitivity reaction, similar to plaque formation. Grossly, lesions may appear as raised linear bands of yellow to erythematous tissue along the posterior legs or as papules and nodules on the nose, ears, and feet. Lesions have been seen in the oral cavity. Cytologically, a mixed inflammatory response is seen, with macrophages, lymphocytes, plasma cells, neutrophils, and increased numbers of eosinophils and mast cells (Fig. 3-7A). Rarely multinucleated giant cells may be present. Collagen necrosis may occur as a result of

eosinophil granule release giving rise to the occasional appearance of amorphous basophilic material in the background (Fig. 3-7B). Eosinophil numbers are usually less than are seen in eosinophilic plaque. Surgical excision is recommended for solitary nodular lesions.

Cytologic differential diagnosis: arthropod bite reaction, foreign body reaction.

Pemphigus Foliaceus

This is the most common autoimmune skin disease in dogs and cats. Drugs, chronic disease, and spontaneous causes have been associated with their occurrence. Grossly, lesions appear as erythematous macules that progress to white or yellow pustules and finally to crusts (Fig. 3-8A). The head and feet are preferred sites although the ears, trunk, and neck are also commonly affected in the cat. Direct imprint of the underside of a crust or aspiration of a pustule reveals nondegenerate neutrophils and acantholytic cells appearing as intensely stained individualized oval keratinocytes (Fig. 3-8B). Eosinophils may be present as well, but bacterial infection is usually lacking. Treatment includes antibiotics and immunotherapy. Excisional biopsy of early lesions is recommended. Histologic examination along with direct immunofluorescent antibody tests or direct immunoperoxidase staining tests is necessary to distinguish the different pemphigus subtypes. Antinuclear antibody tests also may be helpful.

Cytologic differential diagnosis: pyoderma.

Cutaneous Xanthoma

Xanthomatosis is an uncommon granulomatous inflammation in cats, birds, and amphibians related to primary or secondary diabetes mellitus, high-fat diets, and hereditary hyperchylomicronemia (Gross et al., 2005). The

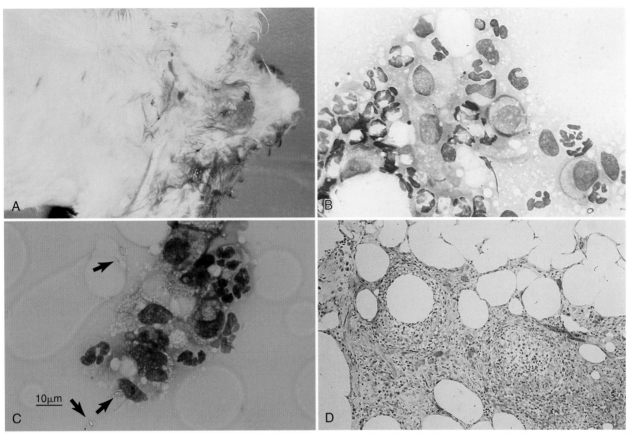

■ **FIGURE 3-6. A-B, Sterile nodular panniculitis. Dog. A,** Wet, draining nodule from the leg. **B, Tissue discharge.** Tracts drained in the lumbar region of this poodle for one year. Infectious agents were not found. Present are numerous degenerate neutrophils, several epithelioid macrophages, and occasional lymphocytes. (Wright-Giemsa; HP oil.) **C, Traumatic panniculitis. Tissue aspirate. Cat.** Subcutaneous mass on the ventral thorax (sternal) displays a background of free lipid and occasional yellow-green crystals, presumed to be mineral *(arrows)*. Shown are several macrophages with fine vacuolation and nondegenerate neutrophils. (Wright-Giemsa; HP oil.) **D, Sterile nodular panniculitis. Tissue section. Dog.** Focal collections of neutrophils and macrophages appear within the subcutis of this animal, which was presented with multiple subcutaneous nodules. No evidence was found for an infectious agent. (H&E; LP.) (A, Courtesy of Leslie Fox, Gainesville, FL.)

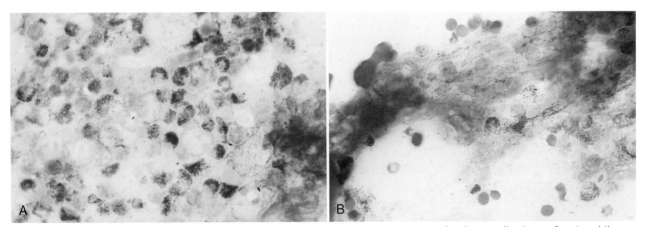

■ **FIGURE 3-7. Eosinophilic granuloma. Tissue aspirate. Cat. Same case A-B. A,** Note the dense collections of eosinophils, many of which have degranulated. (Wright-Giemsa; HP oil.) **B,** Collagenolysis appears as amorphous basophilic material associated with degranulated eosinophils. (Wright-Giemsa; HP oil.)

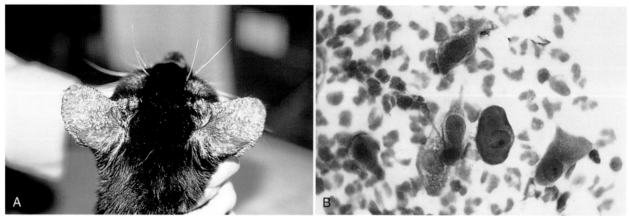

■ **FIGURE 3-8. A, Pemphigus foliaceous. Cat.** Crusty and erythematous lesions on the ear pinnae. **B, Acantholytic cells. Pustule aspirate. Cat.** Densely stained individualized keratinocytes from a skin pustule on an animal with pemphigus foliaceous. These cells are often associated with immune-mediated skin diseases. Numerous neutrophils, mostly nondegenerate, are present in large numbers. (Wright-Giemsa; HP oil.) (A, Courtesy of Janet Wojciechowski, Gainesville, FL.)

deposition of cholesterol and triglycerides in tissues results in lipid-laden macrophages. Grossly, the lesions are single or multiple, white to yellow plaques or nodules that may ulcerate or drain caseous material. Sites preferred are the face, trunk, and foot pads. Cytologically, aspirates contain numerous foamy macrophages (Fig. 3-9A) that stain positive with lipid stains (Fig. 3-9B). Lymphocytes and occasional eosinophils or neutrophils are present as well. Histologically, cholesterol clefts and giant cells may be prominent (Fig. 3-9C). Treatment is aimed at identifying and controlling the underlying cause.

> *Cytologic differential diagnosis:* sterile granuloma, e.g., foreign body reaction.

INFECTIOUS INFLAMMATION

Acute Bacterial Abscess and Pyoderma

The abscess is a common subcutaneous lesion in cats and dogs, often related to bites or other penetrating wounds. This may be localized to the skin or associated with systemic signs. The area is firm to fluctuant, swollen,

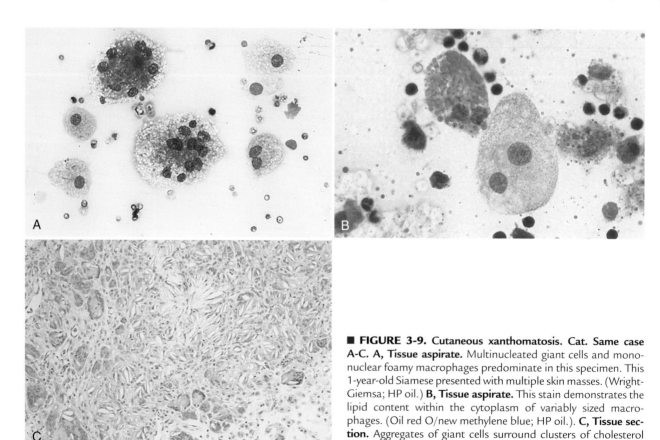

■ **FIGURE 3-9. Cutaneous xanthomatosis. Cat. Same case A-C. A, Tissue aspirate.** Multinucleated giant cells and mononuclear foamy macrophages predominate in this specimen. This 1-year-old Siamese presented with multiple skin masses. (Wright-Giemsa; HP oil.) **B, Tissue aspirate.** This stain demonstrates the lipid content within the cytoplasm of variably sized macrophages. (Oil red O/new methylene blue; HP oil.). **C, Tissue section.** Aggregates of giant cells surround clusters of cholesterol clefts within the dermis. (H&E; IP.)

erythematous, warm, and painful. A creamy white exudate may be aspirated that is characterized cytologically by numerous degenerate neutrophils displaying karyolysis, karyorrhexis, and pyknosis (see Chapter 2). Bacteria may be found in association with the swollen, round nuclei. Case management includes culture and sensitivity tests, with treatment aimed at surgical incision and antibiotics.

Deep pyoderma is manifest as a bacterial inflammation that extends into the dermis and hair follicles with subsequent damage to the follicle (furunculosis). The ruptured follicular wall releases fragments of the hair shaft as well as follicular keratins into the surrounding tissue that creates a foreign body reaction and pyogranulomatous inflammation with formation of a dermal nodule (Gross et al., 2005; Raskin, 2006a). *Staphylococcus intermedius* is typically the primary pathogen but other bacteria and underlying conditions may be occurring to initiate the inflammation. Ulceration is common. Mixed inflammatory cells including neutrophils and macrophages are present (Fig. 3-10A&B).

Clostridial Cellulitis

The infection is usually associated with penetrating wounds. The swollen skin may be crepitant with a serosanguineous wound exudate. Cytologically, tissue aspirates may reveal large rods measuring 1×4 µm, some with a clear, oval, subterminal endospore, occurring singly or in short chains (Fig. 3-11A). This anaerobic organism is gram positive (Fig. 3-11B), but may stain variably as a result of a chronic infection or antibiotic therapy. The specimen background often contains cellular debris and lipid with few, if any, inflammatory cells. Neutrophils, when present, are often degenerate. Anaerobic culture is necessary for diagnosis. Treatment includes surgical management and appropriate antibiotic administration.

Rhodococcus equi Cellulitis

The presence of numerous neutrophils and macrophages with the latter containing small rod to coccoid bacteria should suggest infection from *Rhodococcus* sp. Case reports describe ulcerative swellings that often occur on extremities and involve adjacent lymph nodes (Patel, 2002). These are opportunistic bacteria for which immunosuppressed animals are at higher risk.

Actinomycosis/Nocardiosis

The infection presents as subcutaneous swellings that progress to ulceration with exudation of red-brown fluid. The cause is often related to penetrating wounds. The infections may be associated with systemic signs that often include pyothorax. Cytologically, degenerate neutrophils predominate, with macrophages and small lymphocytes also present. Bacteria may be intracellular or extracellular, the latter often found as dense clusters of organisms (Fig. 3-12A–C). These bacteria are slender, filamentous, branching, lightly basophilic rods with red spotted or beaded areas. They may be highlighted with a silver stain (Fig. 3-12D). Histologically, inflammatory

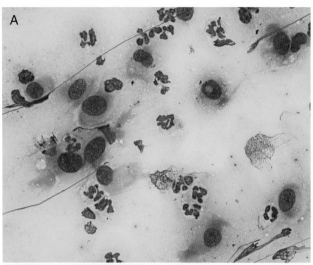

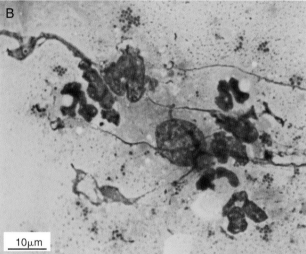

■ **FIGURE 3-10. Pyoderma. Tissue aspirate. Dog. Same case A-B. A,** A persistent dermal mass on the tail consists of a mixed cell population of mostly degenerate neutrophils and plump stromal cells. (Modified Wright; HP oil.) **B,** Note the clusters of large cocci typical of *Staphylococcus* scattered in the background. (Modified Wright; HP oil.)

cells group around dense mats of organisms (Fig. 3-12E). *Actinomyces* sp. are gram positive and acid-fast negative, whereas *Nocardia* sp. are gram positive but variably positive for acid-fast stain. Culture is necessary for diagnosis of the specific type and samples should be obtained anaerobically. Treatment includes surgical drainage and appropriate antibiotics.

> **KEY POINT** Look at the dense areas of the specimen for basophilic mats of bacteria.

Dermatophilosis

This is a rare infection that has been reported in cats and dogs, usually as the result of penetrating wounds contaminated with infected soil or water. The lesion presents as a firm, alopecic, subcutaneous draining mass. The thick gray exudate below the crusted surface is purulent, with

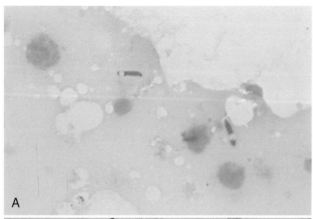

■ **FIGURE 3-11. Clostridial cellulitis. Tissue aspirate. Dog. Same case A-B. A,** Bacilli with terminal spore formation in the subcutis in an animal with subcutaneous emphysema and adjacent bone lysis. (Wright-Giemsa; HP oil.) **B,** Gram-positive rods on aerobic culture were confirmed as *Clostridium* sp. (Gram; HP oil.)

numerous degenerate neutrophils but few eosinophils and macrophages. The organism appears as gram-positive branching filaments that segment horizontally and longitudinally into coccoid forms (Fig. 3-13). Diagnosis is made by morphologic identification of the organism on biopsy or through culture. Treatment involves appropriate antibiotics and appropriate wound management (Carakostas et al., 1984; Kaya et al., 2000).

Mycobacteriosis

Three clinical forms of mycobacteriosis in dogs and cats are recognized, which include internal tuberculous, localized cutaneous nodules (lepromatous), and spreading subcutaneous forms (Greene and Gunn-Moore, 2006). Diagnosis is best performed by tissue culture and histopathology. Definitive identification may be made by polymerase chain reaction (PCR) of tissue specimens. Treatment may include surgical excision and appropriate antibiotics. The tuberculous form is related to *Mycobacterium tuberculosis, Mycobacterium bovis,* or the opportunistic *Mycobacterium avium-intracellulare* complex. Contact with infected people, cattle, birds, or

soil may be documented. The disease may be also associated with immunosuppressed animals. This form is characterized by a systemic disease with weight loss, fever, and lymphadenopathy. While internal organs are most affected, skin nodules can appear on the head, neck, and legs of dogs and cats (Miller et al., 1995). These are slow-growing organisms normally requiring 4 to 6 weeks to culture. Detection may be hastened to 2 weeks and may require PCR and other molecular techniques for identification. Cytologically, macrophages contain few to many beaded bacilli, and some organisms may be extracellular (Fig. 3-14A). Acid-fast staining is helpful in the recognition of the organisms (Fig. 3-14B). Lymphocytes and neutrophils are more abundant than in lepromatous forms.

The lepromatous form in cats is caused by *Mycobacterium lepraemurium* and is common in wet, cooler climates with exposure to infected rodents. A novel, unnamed *Mycobacterium* species has been documented for dogs in Australia, New Zealand, and recently in the United States (Foley et al., 2002). Nonpainful raised nodules are found on the head and distal limbs without systemic signs in cats. These nodules are soft to firm, fleshy, and often localized, with occasional ulceration and little exudation. Spontaneous remission has been reported in a cat (Roccabianca et al., 1996). Nodules in dogs are smooth to ulcerated, occurring frequently on the head, particularly the ears and muzzle. Cultivation of the organism is difficult. Cytologically, macrophages containing numerous intracellular organisms predominate (Twomey et al., 2005) (Fig. 3-14C). Other cells seen include lymphocytes, plasma cells, neutrophils, and occasional multinucleated giant cells.

The more common presentation of cutaneous mycobacteriosis in dogs and cats involves those fast-growing species having an atypical growth pattern or culture characteristic, such as *Mycobacterium fortuitum, Mycobacterium chelonei,* and *Mycobacterium smegmatis.* These are the result of inoculation with contaminated soil or standing water. Lesions are characterized by a spreading subcutaneous pyogranulomatous inflammation having frequent draining tracts. This form also lacks systemic signs. Bacterial culture of deep tissue sites is required and growth may occur within 3 to 5 days. Cytologically, a mixed population of neutrophils and macrophages predominates, with occasional lymphocytes, plasma cells, multinucleated giant cells, or reactive fibroblasts (Fig. 3-14D). Organisms are occasionally found on cytology with the aid of acid-fast staining (Fig. 3-14E&F). On histopathology, lesions appear diffuse and organisms may be found within lipocysts surrounded by inflammatory cells. Prognosis for this form is guarded, as response to antibiotics is often unrewarding.

KEY POINT Mycobacterial organisms are gram positive and acid-fast positive. They appear on cytology as nonstaining, long, thin rods due to the high lipid content of their cell wall.

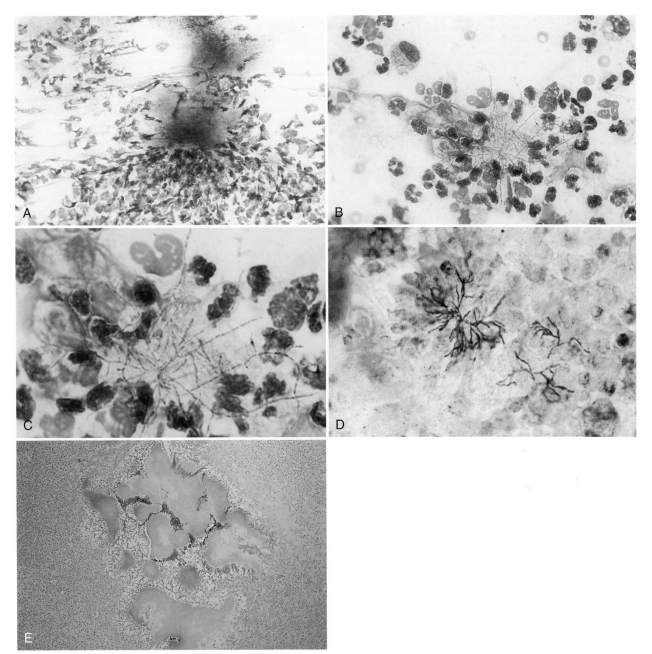

■ **FIGURE 3-12. A, Actinomycosis. Tissue aspirate. Dog.** Note the basophilic clusters of filamentous organisms that resemble amorphous debris. (Wright-Giemsa; HP oil.) **Same case B-C. Nocardiosis. Tissue aspirate. Dog. B,** Cluster of organisms surrounded by many degenerate neutrophils and few macrophages. Culture confirmed presence of *Nocardia* sp. (Wright-Giemsa; HP oil.) **C,** Branching, beaded, slender bacterial filaments are demonstrated in this fluid pocket from a dog with a swollen hind leg. (Wright-Giemsa; HP oil.) **D-E, Actinomycosis. Dog. D, Tissue aspirate.** Branching, beaded, slender bacterial filaments stain with a silver stain. (GMS; HP oil.) **E, Tissue section.** Pyogranulomatous cellulitis surrounding irregular islands of filamentous organisms that are gram positive and acid-fast negative. The periphery of these foci contain densely eosinophilic hyalinized material thought to represent antigen-antibody complexes. This reaction has been termed the *Splendore-Hoeppli phenomenon.* (H&E; LP.)

Localized Opportunistic Fungal Infections

Cutaneous or subcutaneous lesions occur as the result of penetrating wounds contaminated with infected soil or water, commonly in tropical or subtropical climates. One common type is phaeohyphomycosis, caused by a group of dematiaceous (pigmented) fungi such as *Alternaria,* *Curvularia,* or *Bipolaris* spp. (Fig. 3-15A–C). A rare type is hyalohypomycosis, produced by nonpigmented fungi such as *Paecilomyces* spp. (Fig. 3-15D) (Elliott et al., 1984). Nodules develop slowly, usually on extremities, later becoming ulcerated with draining tracts. Cytologically, these produce a pyogranulomatous inflammation

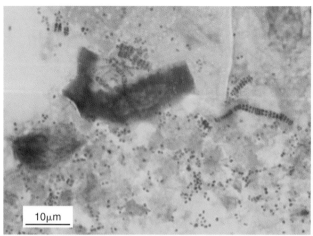

■ **FIGURE 3-13. Dermatophilosis. Tissue scraping. Horse.** *Dermatophilus congolensis* is seen as filamentous strands of paired coccoid bacteria. (Modified Wright; HP oil.)

with degenerate neutrophils, macrophages, multinucleated giant cells, lymphocytes, plasma cells, and mature fibroblasts. Hyphal structures are septate and periodic constrictions may be seen producing globose dilations. Yeast forms rarely occur. Diagnosis involves histopathologic biopsy and tissue culture. Treatment involves surgical excision but prognosis is often poor to guarded.

Cutaneous Lesions from Systemic Fungal Infections

Lesions usually present as single or multiple nodules that ulcerate and drain a serosanguineous exudate. Regional lymphadenopathy is common along with affected organ systems. Examination of the exudate is diagnostic but surgical excision with histopathologic biopsy is recommended. Serum titers and tissue culture are helpful in difficult cases. In general, treatment is aimed at systemic antifungal therapy. Prognosis is guarded.

Blastomycosis

Blastomycosis is a pyogranulomatous or granulomatous inflammation of dogs and, rarely, cats that is related to yeast and rare hyphal forms of *Blastomyces dermatitidis.* The disease is endemic in areas around the Mississippi and Ohio River basins and into Canada. Lesions appear often on the extremities and nose. Cytologically, degenerate neutrophils, macrophages, multinucleated giant cells, and lymphocytes are present. Yeast forms measure 7 to 15 μm in diameter and have a refractile, deeply basophilic, thick cell wall (Fig. 3-16A&B). Organisms may be phagocytized by macrophages or found extracellularly. Cell division occurs by budding that is broad based compared with the narrow-based budding of *Cryptococcus* sp. Structures stain positive with periodic acid-Schiff (PAS) (Fig. 3-16C) and methenamine silver. Definitive diagnosis involves immunostaining of tissue sections and tissue culture. Serum tests involve agar gel immunodiffusion and enzyme-linked immunosorbent assay (ELISA) methods but they have low sensitivity. Confirmation of

organisms found on biopsy may be performed by PCR assays.

Coccidioidomycosis

This disease, caused by *Coccidioides immitis,* produces a pyogranulomatous response similar to that of blastomycosis in dogs and occasionally cats. It is endemic in the southwestern United States. Cytologically, the organism appears as thick-walled spherules measuring 20 to 200 μm diameter (Fig. 3-17A). Within the basophilic spherule (Fig. 3-17B) are uninucleate round endospores measuring 2 to 5 μm in diameter. The free endospores (Fig. 3-17C) may be confused with yeast forms of *Histoplasma.* Empty small spherules resemble *Blastomyces.* Both cell wall and endospores stain positive with methenamine silver, while PAS stains the cell wall purple and the endospores red. Intact spherules are poorly chemotactic for neutrophils compared with free endospores, which attract many neutrophils (see Fig. 3-17A). Serologic tests used include tube precipitin (IgM), complement fixation (IgG), latex agglutination, agar gel immunodiffusion, and ELISA. Fluorescent antibody methods may be used for tissue biopsy. Tissue culture is not recommended because of the public health risk. When results are equivocal, commercial testing using a DNA probe with a chemiluminescent label may be used (Beaudin et al., 2005).

Cryptococcosis

Cryptococcosis is found in several geographic areas, but frequently in tropical or subtropical climates or with soil infected by pigeon droppings. Lesions in dogs and cats may present as crusts or erosions on the nose in addition to nodules. The cellular response is often granulomatous with macrophages predominating (Fig. 3-18A&B). Other cells present include lymphocytes and multinucleated giant cells. There is minimal inflammation in immunocompromised patients and when organisms retain their thick outer capsule. The causative agent, *Cryptococcus neoformans,* is found in cytologic specimens as a round to oval yeast form measuring 4 to 10 μm in diameter. Cell sizes may be variable, ranging from 2 to 20 μm. When present, the thick lipid capsule remains unstained with Romanowsky-type stains (see Figure 5-11B). As a result, the biopsy background appears vacuolated, often with many dense, round cell bodies. Stains such as new methylene blue and India ink are used to enhance visibility of the capsule on unstained specimens (see Figure 5-11C). The internal cell body stains positive with methenamine silver and PAS, while the cell wall requires mucicarmine stain. Cell division involves narrow-based budding compared with the broad-based budding of *Blastomyces.* Definitive diagnosis involves immunostaining in tissue biopsies, latex agglutination test, ELISA, or fungal culture. Confirmation in difficult cases may involve PCR and detection of the CAP59 gene.

Histoplasmosis

This disease produces a pyogranulomatous response by the agent *Histoplasma capsulatum,* and is similar in geographic distribution to blastomycosis. Bird and bat droppings provide an ideal growth medium for the organisms.

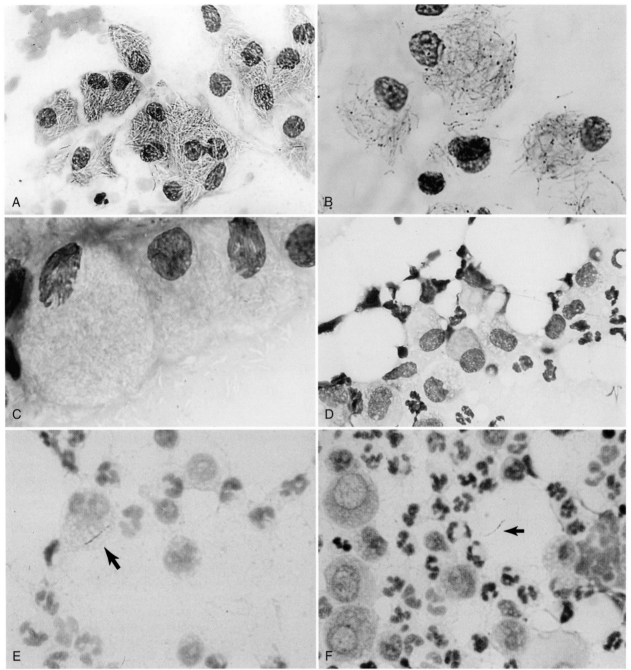

■ **FIGURE 3-14. Same case A-B. Mycobacteriosis. Tissue aspirate. Cat. A,** A swollen area over the nose was confirmed positive for *M. avium-intracellulare* complex. Note the abundance of negative-staining rods with the cytoplasm of macrophages. (Wright-Giemsa; HP oil.) **B,** Acid-fast stain is positive for the beaded linear bacteria. (Ziehl-Neelsen; HP oil.) **C, Feline leprosy. Tissue imprint. Cat.** Negative-stained linear bacteria fill the cytoplasm and appear extracellular, visible against the proteinaceous background. (Giemsa; HP oil.) **Same case D-F. Atypical mycobacteriosis. Tissue aspirate. Dog. D,** Frequent neutrophils and macrophages appear without obvious evidence of sepsis. Neutrophils are mildly degenerate in this 2-cm mass located on the back. (Wright-Giemsa; HP oil.) **E,** Single positive filamentous bacterium found within macrophage *(arrow)*. (Fite's acid-fast; HP oil.) **F,** Tissue aspirate. Single positive filamentous bacterium found within a lipocyst *(arrow)*. (Fite's acid-fast; HP oil.) (C, Glass slide material courtesy of John Kramer, Washington State University; presented at the 1988 ASVCP case review session.)

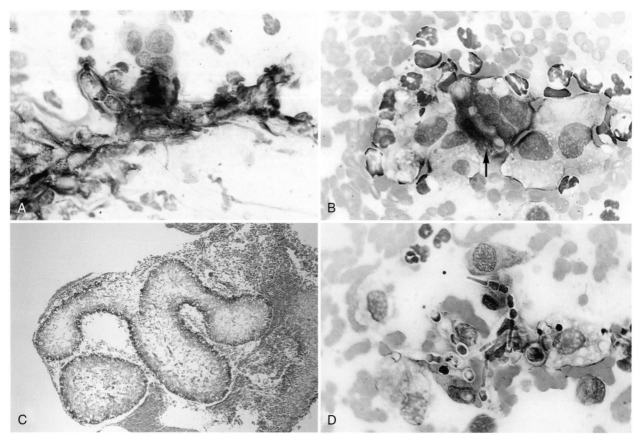

■ **FIGURE 3-15.** **A-B, Phaeohyphomycosis (pigmented fungi). Tissue aspirate. Dog. A,** Small mass on plantar surface of the foot was positive for *Curvularia* sp. on culture. Degenerate neutrophils and macrophages surround the fungal hyphae with yeastlike swellings. (Aqueous-based Wright; HP oil.) **Same case B-C. B,** Mixed inflammation with macrophages, degenerate neutrophils, and lymphocytes surround a hyphal structure (*arrow*) with yeastlike swellings. (Wright-Giemsa; HP oil.) **C, Phaeohyphomycosis. Tissue section. Dog.** Large colonies of brown fungi confirm the diagnosis of dematiaceous or pigmented fungi. (H&E; LP.) **D, Hyalohyphomycosis. Tissue aspirate. Cat.** This swollen digit contained hyphal structures with yeastlike swellings suspected to be caused by *Paecilomyces* sp. Numerous macrophages are noted along with few neutrophils. (Wright-Giemsa; HP oil.)

Cutaneous lesions (Fig. 3-19) are uncommon compared with those in gastrointestinal and hematopoietic organs. Cytologically, macrophages predominate, but lymphocytes, plasma cells, and occasional multinucleated giant cells may be present. Numerous intracellular and extracellular oval yeast forms measuring 2 to 4 μm are frequently found in specimens. They stain positive with PAS and methenamine silver. The yeast structures resemble the protozoan *Leishmania* except *Histoplasma* has a clear halo due to cell shrinkage and the cell body lacks a kinetoplast. Definitive diagnosis of histoplasmosis requires identification by cytology, immunostaining in tissue biopsy, or fungal culture. There are no reliable serologic tests. Molecular tests have been used on a limited basis.

Other systemic infections may involve *Aspergillus* sp., *Candida* sp., or *Paecilomyces* sp. These often occur in immunosuppressed patients.

Dermatophytosis

This is a common infectious and often contagious disease to humans that frequently involves the superficial layers of the skin, hairs, and nails. *Microsporum* and *Trichophyton* sp. are the most common genera of dermatophytes associated with dogs and cats. The lesions typically present with focal alopecia, broken hair shafts, crusts, scales, and erythema on the head, feet, and tail of dogs and cats (Caruso et al., 2002). Less commonly seen are raised or dermal nodules called kerions (Logan et al., 2006). A kerion forms when the infected hair follicle ruptures and both the fungus and keratin spill into the dermis, eliciting an intense inflammatory response. Cytologic specimens reveal a pyogranulomatous inflammation with degenerate neutrophils and large epithelioid macrophages. Arthrospores that measure 2 to 4 μm possess a thin, clear capsule (Fig. 3-20A). The arthrospores and nonstaining hyphae are associated with hair shafts, which are best visualized using clearing agents with plucked hairs (Fig. 3-20B&C) or methenamine silver staining (Fig. 3-20D) or PAS (Fig. 3-20E). Fungal culture is necessary for identification.

An uncommon presentation is a dermatophytic pseudomycetoma, usually seen in Persian cats, that is most often caused by *Microsporum canis* (Zimmerman et al., 2003). It presents as a nodular granuloma with fistulous tracts deep into subcutaneous tissues. Cytologically, this

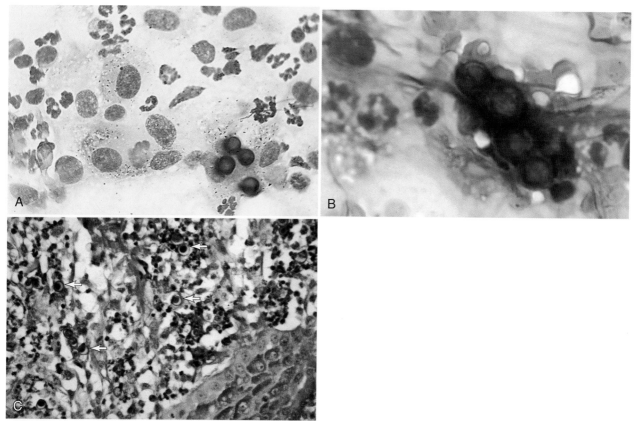

■ **FIGURE 3-16. A-C, Blastomycosis. Dog. A, Tissue imprint.** A mass on the digit revealed several deeply basophilic thick-walled budding yeast forms along with a mixture of macrophages and degenerate neutrophils. (Aqueous-based Wright; HP oil.) **B, Tissue imprint.** Four yeast forms are present that measure approximately the same size as the neutrophils in the field. The thick wall is visible on the deeply basophilic structures. (Modified-Wright; HP oil.) **C, Tissue section.** Dense accumulation of inflammatory cells surround densely stained yeast forms *(arrows)* that collapse on fixation away from the thick cell wall. (PAS; IP.)

involves macrophages with abundant foamy cytoplasm and numerous multinucleated giant cells (Fig. 3-20F). Arthrospores may be present along with fungal hyphae that have an irregular shape and size and may stain variably with Romanowsky-type stains (Fig. 3-20G). Positive staining occurs with PAS and methenamine silver (Fig. 3-20H). Treatment of the nodules involves surgical excision and antifungal drugs.

Malassezia

The causative agent, *Malassezia pachydermatis,* is an opportunistic invader of the skin and ear canal. It is associated with widespread seborrheic dermatitis as well as otitis externa in dogs. Organisms are found in surface scabs or crusts of exudative lesions. Sites of predilection include the face, ventral neck, dorsum of paws, ventral abdomen, and caudal thighs. Cytologically, the skin infection involves primarily a mononuclear inflammation, with lymphocytes and macrophages, but secondary pyoderma may occur with the presence of focal neutrophils (Fig. 3-21A). Typically, the ear infection is minimally inflamed with organisms adhered to squamous epithelium (Fig. 3-21B). Romanowsky stains reveal purple, broad-based budding organisms characterized by a bottle or shoe shape (Fig. 3-21C). Treatment includes surface cleaning and appropriate antifungal agents.

Oomycosis

Two agents, *Pythium insidiosum* and *Lagenidium* sp., are water molds of the oomycete class in the Stromenopila kingdom (Grooters et al., 2003). They differ from true fungi in producing motile, flagellate zoospores, having cell walls without chitin, and having differences in nuclear division and cytoplasmic organelles. This disease is common in dogs and occasional in cats from tropical or subtropical climates, such as the southeastern United States. Animals are infected by standing in or drinking contaminated water. Systemic signs result from gastrointestinal involvement, and are more common than the cutaneous presentation. Dermal ulcerative nodules develop into draining tracts and serosanguineous exudation from sites that include the extremities, tail head, and perineum (Fig. 3-22A). Cytologically, specimens consist of a pyogranulomatous inflammation with increased eosinophils and the presence of broad, poorly septate, and branching hyphal elements. While *Pythium* hyphae are uniform, *Lagenidium* hyphae tend to have larger diameters and more bulbous shapes than *Pythium.*

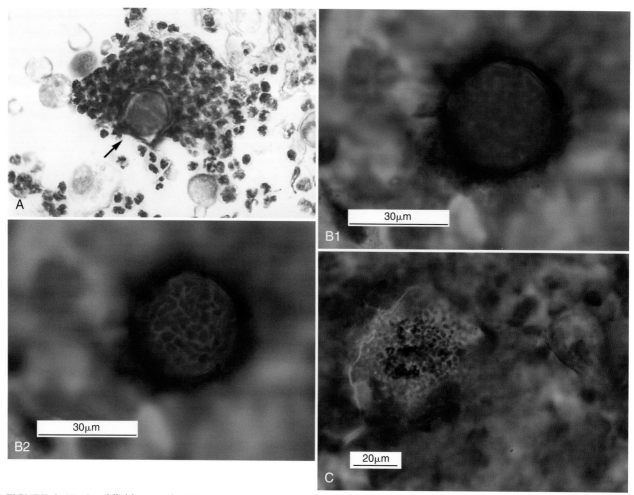

■ FIGURE 3-17. Coccidioidomycosis. Tissue aspirate. Dog. A, Presented with several semifirm skin masses and no systemic signs. Purple, thick-walled spherule (*arrow*) measuring approximately 60 μm in diameter is surrounded by numerous degenerate neutrophils. (Modified Wright; HP oil.) **Same case B-C. B,** Within the scapular mass is a basophilic spherule. 1) Focus is placed on the thick capsule wall with granular contents. 2) Refocusing demonstrates the developing endospores. (Modified Wright; HP oil.) **C,** Present is a small spherule (right) and a larger spherule (left); the latter appears ready to release numerous small (2 microns), round endospores within the poorly defined mixed inflammatory response in the background. (Modified Wright; HP oil.)

Methenamine silver stain is preferred over PAS stain to demonstrate the organisms (Fig. 3-22B). Serum testing for antibodies to oomycete antigens is helpful as a screening test. Culture of infected tissues followed by both morphologic and molecular identification of the pathogen is highly recommended. Immunohistochemistry uses a polyclonal antibody specific for *Pythium insidiosum*, not *Lagenidium*. However, distinction between the two oomycetes is best performed by rRNA gene sequencing or specific PCR amplification. Possible treatment involves wide surgical excision or amputation of affected limbs. Prognosis is guarded to poor.

KEY POINT Organisms stain poorly with Romanowsky stains and are best seen within dense clumps of inflammatory cells at low magnification. The presence of clear, uniformly sized, linear strands suggest hyphal elements (Fig. 3-22C), but these must be distinguished from collagen debris, which may also appear as unstained tissues.

Prototothecosis

This is a rare disease in dogs and cats related to achloric algae, *Prototheca wickerhamii*, that is found in sewage-contaminated food and water. It is frequently associated with immunosuppression or concurrent disease. Cats usually develop a cutaneous disease, while dogs may develop both cutaneous and systemic forms. Systemic involvement primarily includes the gastrointestinal tract, eye, and nervous system. Cutaneous lesions in dogs are chronic, nodular, exudative, and ulcerative, occurring on the trunk and extremities. Large, firm nodules on limbs, feet, head, and tail base have been reported in cats. Cytologically, the inflammation is granulomatous or pyogranulomatous. Epithelioid macrophages predominate, but lymphocytes, plasma cells, and occasional multinucleated giant cells may also be found. Organisms, present outside or within macrophages, measure 5 to 20 μm in diameter (Fig. 3-23A). They are round to oval with internal septation producing 2 to 20 endospores within the

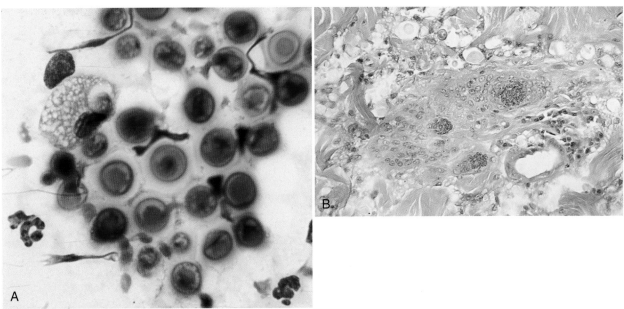

■ **FIGURE 3-18. Cryptococcosis. Cat. A, Tissue aspirate.** Subcutaneous mass in submandibular region contains clusters of yeast with mostly neutrophilic inflammation. Note the variable amount of clear lipid capsule surrounding the structures and the ingested yeast by the foamy macrophage. The scant capsule permits more antigenic stimulation and resulting inflammation to occur. A budding form is shown between the macrophage and a neutrophil. (Aqueous-based Wright; HP oil.) **B, Tissue section.** Perifollicular inflammation related to the presence of numerous clear-walled yeast forms. (H&E; IP.)

cell wall. The endospores are basophilic and granular with a single nucleus, and have a clear halo around them. Both PAS and methenamine silver stains demonstrate the cell wall (Fig. 3-23B). Definitive diagnosis requires culture or tissue biopsy using immunofluorescence or immunoperoxidase techniques. Treatment involves surgical excision for cutaneous lesions. Antimicrobial drugs have been used with limited success in systemic forms. Prognosis is guarded to poor.

Sporotrichosis

This disease is associated with immunosuppression, such as occurs with glucocorticoid administration or concurrent disease. It presents in several clinical forms—cutaneous, systemic, and the most frequent, cutaneolymphatic—usually as the result of penetrating wounds (Welsh, 2003). Grossly, a dermal to subcutaneous nodule progresses into an ulcerated lesion that drains a serosanguineous exudate. In dogs, the skin of the trunk and extremities is preferred, while in cats the large firm nodules appear on the limbs, feet, head, and tail base. The etiologic agent, *Sporothrix schenckii,* is a saprophytic fungus that appears classically as cigar-shaped yeast forms measuring 3 to 5 μm in diameter with a thin, clear halo around the pale-blue cytoplasm (Fig. 3-24A). The shape of the yeast is pleomorphic, with round to oval shapes also observed (Fig. 3-24B). Cytologically, the yeast is located intracellularly or extracellularly, being abundant in cats and infrequent in dogs (Bernstein et al., 2007). In dogs, pyogranulomatous inflammation with degenerative neutrophils is common, while macrophages and lymphocytes predominate in the

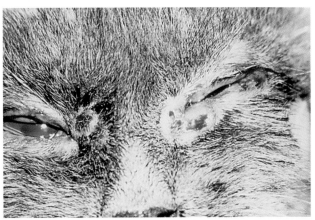

■ **FIGURE 3-19. Histoplasmosis. Cat.** Skin lesions as well as ocular lesions were present around the eyes in this cat. (Courtesy of Heidi Ward, Gainesville, FL.)

cat. The diagnosis may be made from the characteristic cytologic appearance. The organism stains positive with both methenamine silver and PAS. Definitive diagnosis requires fungal culture of the exudate or tissue biopsy using immunofluorescence or immunoperoxidase techniques. Serologic testing is not definitive for current infection. A molecular test has been developed and used in a feline case (Kano et al., 2005). Surgical excision may be performed on single cutaneous lesions. Treatment of the systemic form involves a variety of antimicrobial drugs, which have been used with variable success. Prognosis is poor to guarded. Good response has been obtained with itraconazole (Bernstein et al., 2007).

Text continued on p. 44

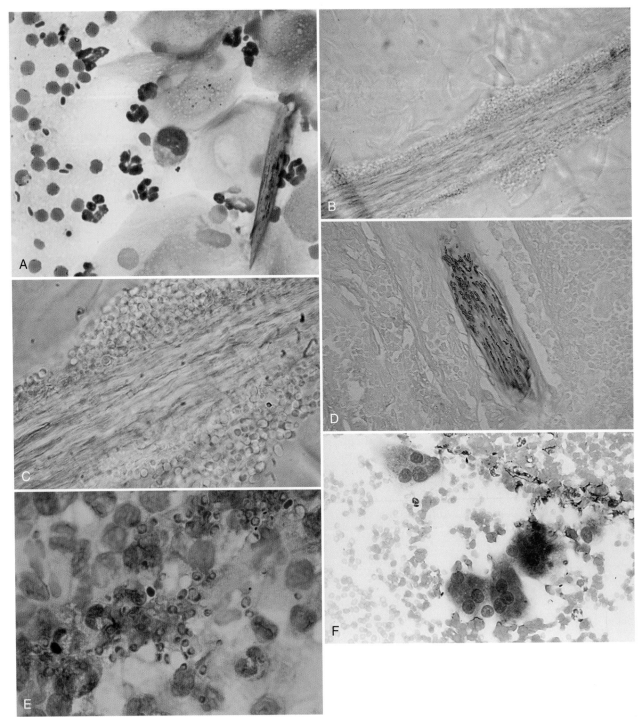

■ **FIGURE 3-20. A-E, Dermatophytosis. A, Tissue imprint. Dog.** Squamous epithelium, remnant hair shaft, and mostly neutrophilic inflammation are present along with moderate numbers of arthrospores. These basophilic, oval to elongate structures with a thin, clear capsule measure 2-3 μm in width and 2-5 μm in length. (Modified Wright; HP oil.) **B, Hair pluck.** Low-magnification view of keratin-cleared hair shaft with attached arthrospores. (Unstained; HP oil.) **C, Hair pluck.** High-magnification view of keratin-cleared hair shaft demonstrating arthrospores outside and fungal hyphae within the hair. (Unstained; HP oil.) **D, Tissue section. Dog.** Note the black stained hyphae within the hair shaft from this tissue section of skin. Diagnosis confirmed as *M. canis* by culture. (Gomori's methenamine silver; HP oil.) **E, Tissue aspirate. Dog.** Dermal nodule (kerion) with multiple pink oval arthroconidia within neutrophils and extracellular. Culture results indicated *Microsporum canis* infection. (Periodic acid-Schiff; HP oil.) **Same case F-H, Dermatophytic pseudomycetoma. Tissue aspirate. Cat. F,** Several multinucleated giant cells are present in this 3-cm superficial mass on the lateral abdomen of a Persian cat. (Wright-Giemsa; HP oil.)

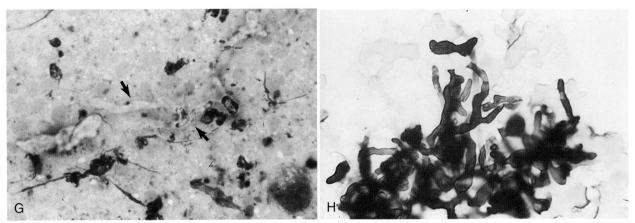

■ **FIGURE 3-20, cont'd. G,** Fungal hyphae are variably visible with Romanowsky staining (*arrows*). Culture confirmed infection by *M. canis.* (Wright-Giemsa; HP oil.) **H,** Hyphal elements are clearly visible with silver staining. (Gomori's methenamine silver; HP oil.) (B-C, Courtesy of the University of Florida Dermatology Section. E, Courtesy of Michael Logan, Purdue University.)

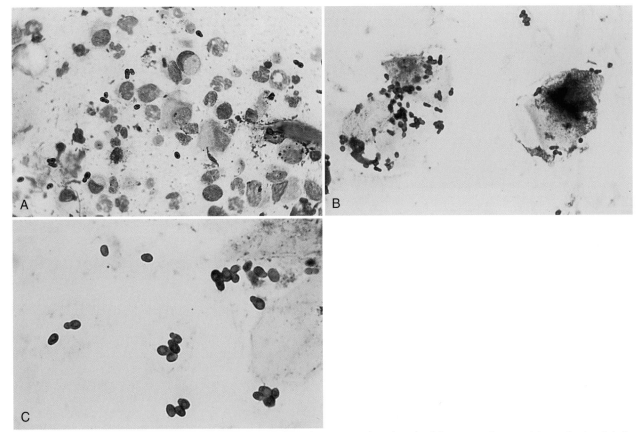

■ **FIGURE 3-21. A,** *Malassezia* **dermatitis. Pustule imprint. Dog.** Abundant budding yeast forms with a mixed-cell inflammatory response were noted in an animal with pustular dermatitis. Mildly degenerate neutrophils are present along with lymphocytes and macrophages. (Wright-Giemsa; HP oil.) **Same case B-C.** *Malassezia* **otitis. Ear swab. Dog. B,** *Malassezia* sp. organisms adhere to keratinized squamous epithelium without evidence of inflammation. (Aqueous-based Wright; HP oil.) **C,** Characteristic shoe print morphology of the broad-based budding yeast form associated with chronic otitis externa. (Aqueous-based Wright; HP oil.)

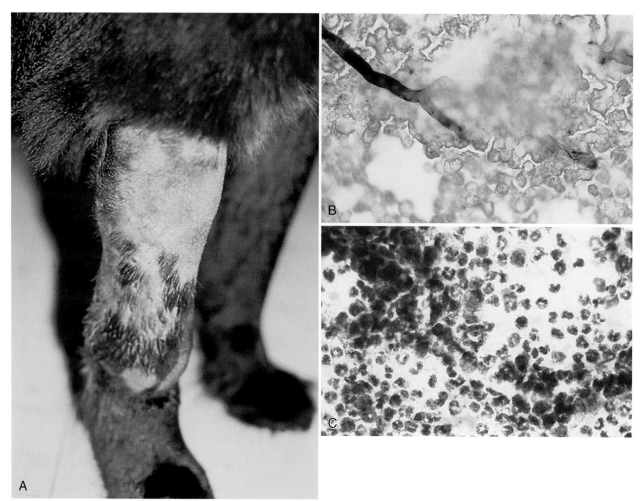

■ **FIGURE 3-22. Oomycetosis. Dog. A,** This draining lesion present on the leg of a longhaired dog was confirmed as pythiosis. **Same case B-C. Tissue discharge. B,** Hyphal elements appear as broad, poorly septate branched structures surrounded by inflammatory cells. (Gomori's methenamine silver; HP oil.) **C,** Clear-staining linear pattern with degenerate neutrophils closely adherent are noted in this draining lesion on the limb and perianal area. Eosinophils are present in significant numbers but are difficult to see in this field. (Aqueous-based Wright; HP oil.) (A, Courtesy of Diane Lewis, Gainesville, FL.)

KEY POINT Organisms resemble those of histoplasmosis, which may be round or oval, but only sporotrichosis has cigar-shaped or slender yeast forms.

KEY POINT The disease may spread to people, usually transmitted by cats.

Cytologic differential diagnosis: histoplasmosis, toxoplasmosis, cryptococcosis.

Leishmaniasis

This is an uncommon multisystemic disease with cutaneous presentation and regional lymphadenopathy. It is caused by the protozoan *Leishmania* spp., which is transmitted by sand flies. The disease is often associated with Mediterranean travel although endemic areas such as Oklahoma and Ohio are found in the United States. It is more likely to occur in dogs than in cats. The condition may begin in the skin and then spread internally. Periorbital alopecia and scaling or ulcerative and erosive lesions of the nose are common signs that may progress to poorly defined cutaneous and mucocutaneous nodules. *Leishmania mexicana* has been associated with a nonsystemic, cutaneous form of the disease in cats from Texas and Mexico (Barnes et al., 1993). On cytology, macrophages predominate but other cells present include lymphocytes, plasma cells, and occasional multinucleated giant cells. The intracellular organisms, termed *amastigotes,* measure 1.5 to 2.0 × 2.5 to 5 μm and possess a red nucleus and characteristic bar-shaped kinetoplasts (Fig. 3-25). In addition to the skin, the bone marrow and lymphoid organs are common sites of involvement. Other laboratory abnormalities include polyclonal or monoclonal gammopathy and nonregenerative anemia. The characteristic cytology or culture is used to obtain a definitive diagnosis. Also immunoperoxidase staining may be performed on tissue biopsies. An indirect fluorescent antibody test is available for *Leishmania donovani*

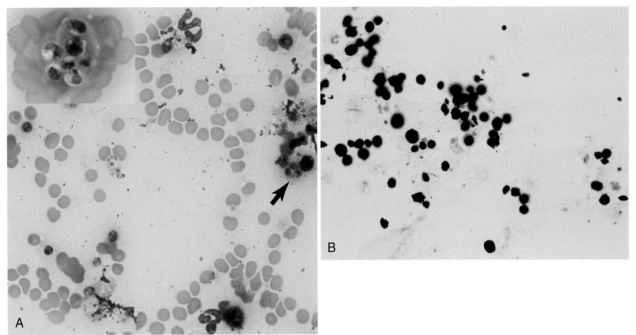

■ **FIGURE 3-23. Protothecosis. Cat. Same case and magnification A-B. A, Tissue aspirate.** This aspirate from a nasal skin nodule contains multiple basophilic round structures (endospores) occurring singly and in clusters *(arrow)* that measure approximately 3-12 µm in diameter. The cutaneous form of protothecosis is unique in the cat. This animal had organisms that extended into the nasal cavity and to a draining mandibular lymph node. This cytology was initially considered to be of a nonencapsulated form of cryptococcosis; however, culture confirmed infection with *Prototheca wickerhamii*. **Inset:** Close-up view of sporulating organism with three endospores. (Wright-Giemsa; HP oil.). **B, Tissue swab.** Numerous silver positive round endospores of variable size are revealed in the nasal cavity swab of a cat with a cutaneous nodule. (Gomori's methenamine silver; HP oil.)

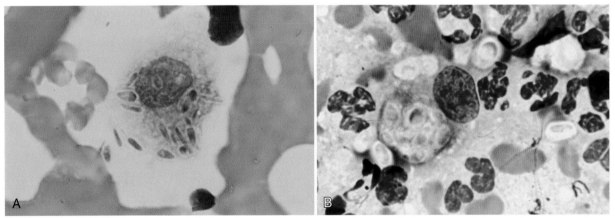

■ **FIGURE 3-24. Sporotrichosis. Tissue imprint. Cat. A,** This 2-cm granulomatous lesion on one digit contains a macrophage with numerous oval to cigar-shaped yeast forms having a thin clear halo around the basophilic center. These structures measure 2 × 5 µm, approximately the width of an erythrocyte. (Wright; HP oil.) **B,** Pyogranulomatous inflammation with engulfed yeast within a macrophage. These forms have a round to oval shape and are difficult to distinguish from *Histoplasma* sp. on the basis of morphology. Culture-confirmed *Sporothrix* sp. (Romanowsky; HP oil.) (B, Courtesy of Peter Fernandes.)

but this only indicates previous exposure. Treatment involves pentavalent antimony compounds, itraconazole, or allopurinol (Lester and Kenyon, 1996) for systemic disease and surgical excision for focal skin lesions. Prognosis is good to guarded; however, this is a zoonotic disease and euthanasia may need to be considered.

Toxoplasmosis

Cutaneous toxoplasmosis is uncommon but has been recently reported in a cat (Park et al., 2007). This single nodule displayed a necrotizing granulomatous panniculitis and vasculitis. Organisms were present within macrophages and other cells. They tested positive for

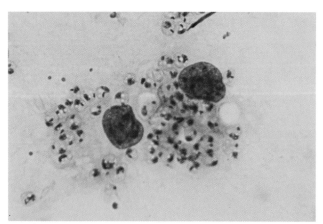

■ **FIGURE 3-25. Leishmaniasis. Tissue aspirate. Cat.** Ear nodule consists of macrophages with intracellular and extracellular organisms having a characteristic appearance of *Leishmania* sp. (Aqueous-based Wright; HP oil.) (Glass slide material courtesy of Ruanna Gossett et al, Texas A & M University; presented at the 1991 ASVCP case review session.)

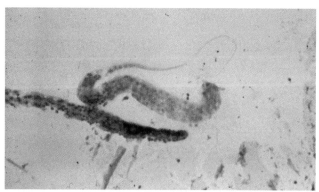

■ **FIGURE 3-26. Dracunculosis. Tissue aspirate. Dog.** A worm-like subcutaneous mass on the thorax contained these large larvae with long, tapered tails. (Romanowsky; IP.) (Courtesy of Judy Radin et al, The Ohio State University; presented at the 1990 ASVCP case review session.)

Toxoplasma gondii and *Neospora caninum* antigens and ultrastructural studies supported *T. gondii*. Furthermore, PCR and DNA sequence analysis was consistent with *T. gondii* infection.

PARASITIC INFESTATION

Dracunculiasis is an uncommon parasitic condition in dogs and potentially in cats that causes pruritic, painful erythematous subcutaneous swellings (Giovengo, 1993) that can be diagnosed by cytologic evaluation of aspirated tissue fluid (Panciera and Stockham, 1988) or imprints from a lesion discharge. First-stage larvae from *Dracunculus insignis* measuring approximately 25 μm wide × 500 μm long appear pale blue when stained (Baker and Lumsden, 2000) or granulated (Fig. 3-26) and have a long, tapered tail. The life cycle involves ingestion of infected water fleas or frogs containing larvae that leave the digestive tract and migrate, usually to the limbs. Surgical excision is used to remove the adult nematode, which often measures 20 cm long (Beyer et al., 1999) but may reach lengths up to 120 cm. Antihelmintics appear ineffective in killing adults.

Another uncommon skin disease caused by parasites includes demodicosis (Neel et al., 2007). In this case, two different populations of demodectic mites were present in skin scrapings.

NEOPLASIA

EPITHELIAL

Squamous Papilloma

These warts are usually solitary lesions, most often affecting older dogs. They are rare in cats. They usually present as a raised growth with keratin-covered, finger-like projections appearing on the head or limbs. On cytology, squamous epithelium in all stages of development is present, but mature forms with benign-appearing nuclei

predominate (Sprague and Thrall, 2001). In younger dogs, papillomas occurring at mucocutaneous sites may be induced by another papovavirus, and these can regress spontaneously. If necessary, surgical excision results in a good to excellent prognosis.

> ***Cytologic differential diagnosis:*** squamous cell carcinoma, infundibular keratinizing acanthoma.

Squamous Cell Carcinoma

This is a common tumor in the dog and cat occurring as solitary or multiple proliferative or ulcerative masses (Fig. 3-27A). It accounts for 15% of skin tumors in cats but only 2% in dogs (Yager and Wilcock, 1994). It is most common on the limbs of dogs and thinly haired areas of the pinnae or face of cats. Tumors are usually locally invasive and may metastasize to regional lymph nodes. Those on the digit are considered to be highly malignant with a greater chance for metastasis. Cytologically, purulent inflammation often accompanies immature or dysplastic squamous epithelium (Fig. 3-27B). Bacterial sepsis may occur if the surface has eroded. A tadpole shape with a tail-like projection and keratinized blue-green hyalinized cytoplasm may be a helpful criterion in determining the cell of origin (Garma-Avina, 1994). The neoplastic epithelium may appear as individual cells or as sheets of adherent cells. Squames and highly keratinized nucleated angular squamous epithelium with nuclear atypia predominate in well-differentiated tumors (Fig. 3-27C). When these cells are concentrically arranged, they correspond to the keratin pearls seen histologically (Fig. 3-27D). The presence of one cell type within the cytoplasm of another, termed *emperipolesis,* may be noted in well-differentiated squamous cell carcinomas (Fig. 3-27E). Moderately differentiated tumors have few angular cells and greater than 50% round or oval dysplastic cells (Fig. 3-27F). Round, individualized cells having a high nuclear-to-cytoplasmic ratio predominate in the poorly differentiated tumors. Cellular and nuclear pleomorphism is marked in the poorly differentiated squamous cell carcinomas. Perinuclear vacuolation is thought to

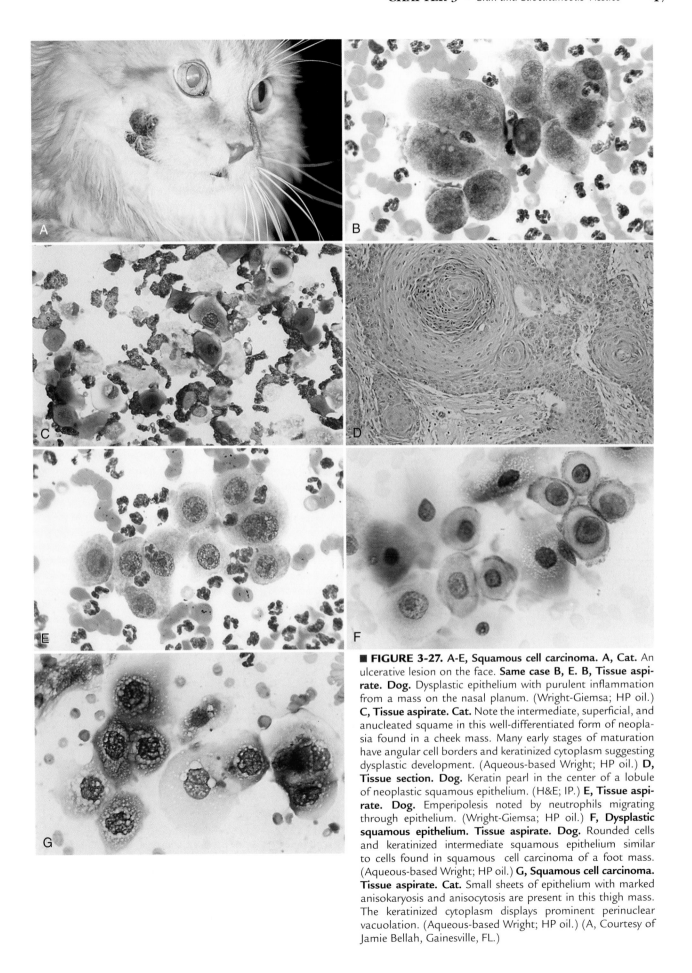

■ **FIGURE 3-27. A-E, Squamous cell carcinoma. A, Cat.** An ulcerative lesion on the face. **Same case B, E. B, Tissue aspirate. Dog.** Dysplastic epithelium with purulent inflammation from a mass on the nasal planum. (Wright-Giemsa; HP oil.) **C, Tissue aspirate. Cat.** Note the intermediate, superficial, and anucleated squame in this well-differentiated form of neoplasia found in a cheek mass. Many early stages of maturation have angular cell borders and keratinized cytoplasm suggesting dysplastic development. (Aqueous-based Wright; HP oil.) **D, Tissue section. Dog.** Keratin pearl in the center of a lobule of neoplastic squamous epithelium. (H&E; IP.) **E, Tissue aspirate. Dog.** Emperipolesis noted by neutrophils migrating through epithelium. (Wright-Giemsa; HP oil.) **F, Dysplastic squamous epithelium. Tissue aspirate. Dog.** Rounded cells and keratinized intermediate squamous epithelium similar to cells found in squamous cell carcinoma of a foot mass. (Aqueous-based Wright; HP oil.) **G, Squamous cell carcinoma. Tissue aspirate. Cat.** Small sheets of epithelium with marked anisokaryosis and anisocytosis are present in this thigh mass. The keratinized cytoplasm displays prominent perinuclear vacuolation. (Aqueous-based Wright; HP oil.) (A, Courtesy of Jamie Bellah, Gainesville, FL.)

represent colorless keratohyalin granules and may be present most frequently in well and moderately differentiated tumor types (Fig. 3-27G). Treatment considerations include surgical excision, cryosurgery, radiotherapy, intralesional chemotherapy, and photodynamic therapy. Prognosis is guarded as recurrence is common, especially in white-faced cats.

> **KEY POINT** It is often difficult to determine if dysplastic changes are the result of the reaction to chronic inflammation or an indication of malignancy.

> *Cytologic differential diagnosis:* infundibular keratinizing acanthoma, squamous papilloma, basosquamous carcinoma.

Cutaneous Basilar Epithelial Neoplasms

Neoplasms that formerly were termed *basal cell tumor* are now classified histologically by evidence supporting differentiation into epidermis, trichofollicular epithelium, or the adnexal structures of sweat and sebaceous glands. Most of previously diagnosed canine or feline basal cell tumors were likely of hair germ origin and therefore best termed *trichoblastoma*. Those diagnosed as basal cell tumor in the cat likely involved apocrine ductular sweat gland neoplasms (Gross et al., 2005). Trichoblastomas are found commonly in dogs and cats and typically present as a benign single, firm, elevated, well-demarcated round intradermal mass that may be ulcerated or pigmented due to abundant melanin (Fig. 3-28A). They are located mostly about the head with frequent occurrence on the neck. Cytologically, basal epithelial cells are small cells characterized by high nuclear-to-cytoplasmic ratios, monomorphic nuclei, and deeply basophilic cytoplasm that may be pigmented (Fig. 3-28B–D). They may be arranged as clusters or in row formation (Fig. 3-28E). Basal cells may predominate in a tumor but foci of scattered keratinocytes (Fig. 3-28F) should suggest the presence of basal tumors with follicular differentiation (Fig. 3-28G). Classification of these basilar neoplasms is difficult on cytology and histopathology is recommended to differentiate the different types (Bohn et al., 2006).

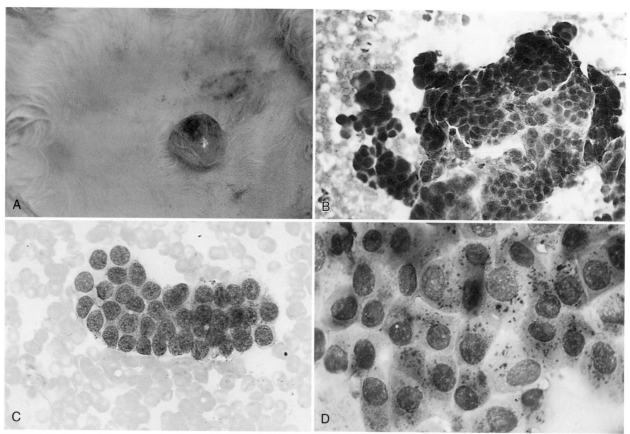

■ **FIGURE 3-28. A-C, Cutaneous basilar epithelial neoplasm. A, Cat.** Note the single, firm, raised, alopecic, well-demarcated round intradermal mass. **B, Tissue imprint. Dog.** Large clusters of tightly adherent uniform-appearing epithelial cells with intensely basophilic cytoplasm are present in this lip mass. Masses with this appearance are most likely termed *trichoblastoma* on histology. (Aqueous-based Wright; HP oil.) **C, Tissue aspirate. Dog.** Tight cluster of uniform cells having a high nuclear-to-cytoplasmic ratio. The cytoplasm is scant and basophilic. This cytologic appearance of this mass is most consistent with a trichoblastoma seen on histology. (Wright-Giemsa; HP oil.) **D-E, Trichoblastoma. Dog. D, Neck mass aspirate.** Sheet of basal epithelium with prominent cytoplasmic granulation and pigmentation, consistent with keratohyalin and melanin. (Wright-Giemsa; HP oil.)

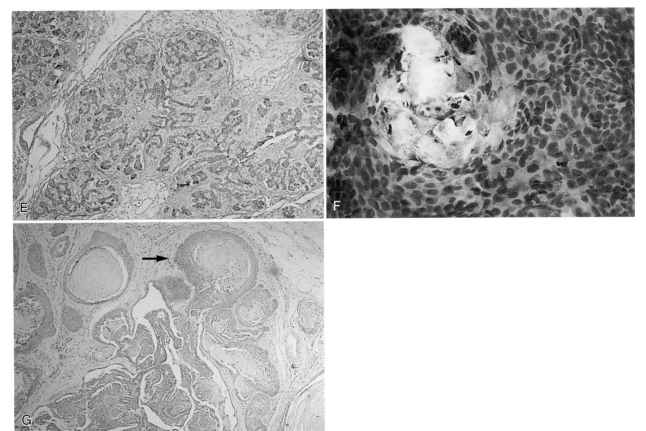

■ **FIGURE 3-28, cont'd. E, Tissue section.** Note the medusoid pattern with cords or ribbons of basal epithelium radiating out from the center. (H&E; LP.) **Same case F-G. F, Basal cell epithelial neoplasm with follicular differentiation. Tissue aspirate. Dog.** Dense clusters of basal epithelium with foci of keratinocytes as evidence of follicular differentiation from a shoulder mass. (Aqueous-based Wright; HP oil.) **G, Trichoblastoma. Tissue section. Dog.** Same case as in F. Note the gradual process of keratinization within the thickened basal epithelium *(arrow)*. This tumor shows areas of follicular differentiation within this trichoblastoma, similar in appearance to a trichoepithelioma. (H&E; LP.) (A, Courtesy of the University of Florida Dermatology Section.)

KEY POINT Because of their common origin, there is considerable overlap cytologically between basal cell tumors and adnexal or follicular tumors.

Cytologic differential diagnosis: follicular tumors, sweat or sebaceous gland tumors.

Hair Follicle Tumors

These benign tumors are usually solitary but may be multiple. They are most often found in older dogs. These are firm, raised, hairless, well-circumscribed masses that may ulcerate. Most often considered are trichoepithelioma (Fig. 3-29) and less commonly pilomatricoma (Masserdotti and Ubbiali, 2002). Cytologically, keratinaceous debris, keratinocytes, and low numbers of germinal epithelium resembling basal cells are present. Histologically, the abrupt keratinization from the basal epithelium forming horn cysts helps to distinguish this tumor from basilar epithelial tumors with follicular differentiation. Treatment consists of surgical excision or cryosurgery. Prognosis is excellent.

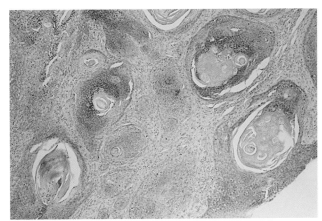

■ **FIGURE 3-29. Trichoepithelioma. Tissue section.** Note the abrupt keratinization in the center surrounded by thickened basal epithelium, suggesting rudimentary hair formation. (H&E; LP.)

Infundibular Keratinizing Acanthoma

This tumor represents a proliferation of the epithelium containing adnexal and follicular structures with a pore to the outside often with numerous horn cysts present (Fig. 3-30). It may be predisposed in some breeds (Norwegian elkhound, keeshond). Pore contents are similar to those of epidermal cyst or follicular cyst. Cytologically, keratinous debris, keratinocytes, and cholesterol crystals characterize this tumor. Low numbers of basal cell epithelia may be found. Treatment consists of surgical excision, cryosurgery, and retinoids, particularly for multiple tumor presentation. Prognosis is good.

Cytologic differential diagnosis: epidermal cyst or follicular cyst, hair follicle tumors.

Sebaceous Adenoma

This appears as a single, smooth, raised, hairless cauliflower lesion or as an intradermal multilobulated mass that usually measures less than 1 cm in diameter (Fig. 3-31A). The overlying skin is alopecic and sometimes ulcerated. These are common in dogs, accounting for approximately 6% of all canine skin and subcutaneous tumors in one survey (Gross et al., 2005). Fifty percent of these tumors in older dogs occur on the head (Goldschmidt and Shofer, 1992). Multiple tumors occur infrequently. Although uncommon in the cat, these tumors are most often found on the head and back. Cystic degeneration and lipogranulomatous inflammation may occur in the center of lobules. Cytologically, mature sebocytes arranged in lobules or clusters predominate and are characterized by pale, foamy

cytoplasm having a small, dense, centrally placed nucleus (Fig. 3-31B&C). A variable number of germinal epithelial cells having basophilic cytoplasm and a higher nuclear-to-cytoplasmic ratio may accompany the secretory cells. Necrotic centers containing amorphous basophilic with cells, remnants of foamy cells, may be found related to cystic degeneration (Fig. 3-31D). Treatment consists of surgical excision or cryosurgery. Prognosis is excellent.

KEY POINT Histologic examination is necessary to distinguish between hyperplastic and adenomatous sebaceous tumors.

Cytologic differential diagnosis: sebaceous hyperplasia.

Sebaceous Epithelioma

This is similar in gross appearance to sebaceous adenoma. When present on the eyelid, it is termed *meibomian adenoma*. Pathologists may classify sebaceous epithelioma in the same category as sebaceous adenoma or basal cell tumor. Histologically, germinal epithelium predominates and small lobules of mature sebaceous epithelium are intermixed (Fig. 3-32A). Cytologically, the tumor resembles a basal cell tumor with small basophilic epithelial clusters along with scattered groups of mature sebocytes (Fig. 3-32B) and low numbers of individualized, well-differentiated squamous epithelial cells. Clinical behavior is benign but the tumors may rarely recur locally. Prognosis is usually excellent following surgical excision.

Cytologic differential diagnosis: sebaceous adenoma, cutaneous basilar epithelial neoplasm.

Sebaceous Carcinoma

This is an uncommon tumor found most frequently on the head of dogs. Cocker spaniels appear predisposed. It presents as a rapidly growing, large, ulcerated, poorly circumscribed mass. Cytologically, pleomorphic glandular epithelium displays malignant nuclear features such as anisokaryosis, prominent nucleoli, and frequent atypical mitotic figures. The finely vacuolated cytoplasm suggests sebaceous differentiation (Fig. 3-33). This malignant tumor is usually locally invasive, but may occasionally metastasize to regional lymph nodes. Treatment consists of wide surgical excision. Prognosis is good.

Cytologic differential diagnosis: squamous cell carcinoma.

Perianal Gland Adenoma

This is a common tumor mostly associated with intact male dogs, suggesting androgen dependency. Goldschmidt and Shofer (1992) reported this tumor involving 9% of skin tumors. Perianal gland tumors are rarely found in the cat. The tumor may be single or multiple, occurring generally near the anus (Fig. 3-34A), but it may also

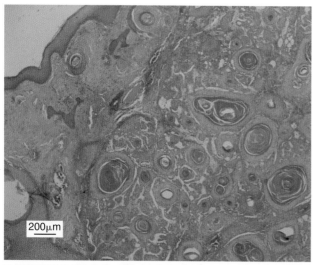

■ **FIGURE 3-30. Infundibular keratinizing acanthoma. Tissue section. Dog.** The proliferation of epithelium with follicular structures is shown. Not visible in this section is the pore to the outside demonstrating the epidermal inversion. (H&E; LP.)

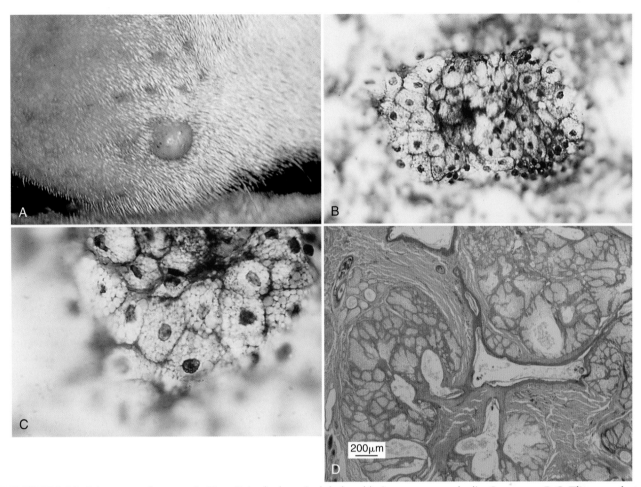

■ **FIGURE 3-31. Sebaceous adenoma. A, Dog.** Raised, alopecic, lobulated lesion present on the lip. **Same case B-C. Tissue aspirate. Dog. B,** The monomorphic population of vacuolated epithelial cells having a small, centrally placed nucleus is consistent with mature sebocytes. (Aqueous-based Wright; HP oil.) **C,** Note the low nuclear-to-cytoplasmic ratio and the foamy cytoplasm with delicate streaks. (Aqueous-based Wright; HP oil.) **D, Tissue section.** Polypoid mass grossly consists of sebaceous lobules, dilated ducts, and areas of cystic degeneration of sebaceous cells. Lack of orientation of lobules around ducts supports the diagnosis of adenomatous growth rather than hyperplasia. (H&E; LP.) (A, Courtesy of the Dermatology Section, University of Florida.)

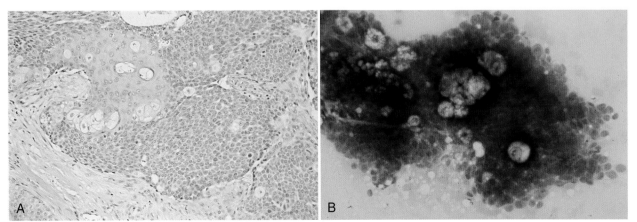

■ **FIGURE 3-32. Sebaceous epithelioma. Dog. A, Tissue section.** Dermal ear mass composed of lobules and islands of neoplastic basal epithelium with occasional foci of sebocytes and keratinocytes. (H&E; IP.) **B, Tissue aspirate.** Clusters of basal epithelium with scattered sebocytes are shown in this shoulder mass. Six months later, this mass was diagnosed as basal cell carcinoma related to progressive infiltration into subcutaneous tissues. (Wright-Giemsa; IP.)

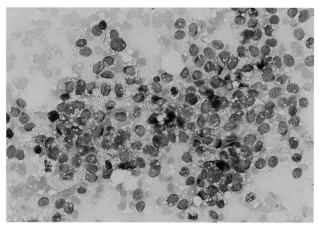

■ **FIGURE 3-33. Sebaceous carcinoma. Tissue aspirate. Dog.** A monomorphic population of cohesive cells in sheets and clumps noted in the shoulder mass. Malignant features include a high nuclear-to-cytoplasmic ratio, anisokaryosis, multinucleation, clumped chromatin, and prominent, variable nucleoli. The cytoplasm is basophilic, with frequent clear, punctate vacuoles suggestive of sebaceous differentiation. Histopathology confirmed the diagnosis. (Wright-Giemsa; HP oil.)

be found on the tail, perineum, prepuce, and thigh, and along the dorsal or ventral midline. Initially they grossly appear as smooth, raised round lesions that lobulate and ulcerate as they enlarge. The tumor arises from modified sebaceous gland epithelium within the dermis that is lined by small basophilic reserve cells (Fig. 3-34B&C). Cytologically, sheets of mature, round hepatoid cells predominate characterized by abundant, finely granular, pinkish-blue cytoplasm (Fig. 3-34D). Nuclei resemble those of normal hepatocytes, appearing round with an often single or multiple, prominent, nucleolus. A low number of smaller basophilic reserve cells having a high nuclear-to-cytoplasmic ratio may also be present, but these lack features of cellular pleomorphism (Fig. 3-34E). Perianal gland adenomas are benign tumors that respond to surgical excision or cryosurgery, coupled with castration. Prognosis is good to excellent. The malignant counterpart of this tumor is infrequently encountered. Nuclear pleomorphism is generally marked in those cases.

Cytologic differential diagnosis: perianal gland hyperplasia, well-differentiated perianal gland carcinoma.

Apocrine Gland Adenocarcinoma of Anal Sac (Anal Sac Adenocarcinoma)

There is an increased incidence of the disease in older, spayed female dogs but a sex predilection has not been confirmed (Goldschmidt and Shofer, 1992). The majority of cases involve dogs, but occasional cases have been reported in the cat. Grossly, this is a subcutaneous mass, firmly fixed around the anal sac, that arises from the glands in the wall of these sacs. A paraneoplastic syndrome of hypercalcemia is associated with 50% to 90% of cases, which may result in renal disease (Ross et al., 1991). Cytologically, dense cell clusters with a papillary shape have poorly defined cell borders in the solid and

anaplastic forms of carcinoma (Fig. 3-35A). Malignant characteristics are easily detected in glandular epithelium, which displays cellular and nuclear pleomorphism, a high nuclear-to-cytoplasmic ratio, and in some cases multiple small cytoplasmic vacuoles (Fig. 3-35B). An acinar arrangement may be detected to aid in the diagnosis and distinguish it from perianal (hepatoid) carcinoma (Fig. 3-35C). Treatment consists of wide surgical excision with postoperative radiation therapy. These malignant tumors commonly metastasize initially to regional lymph nodes. Prognosis is poor to fair.

Cytologic differential diagnosis: perianal gland carcinoma.

Ceruminous Gland Adenoma/Adenocarcinoma

These tumors arise from specialized apocrine sweat glands in the external ear. They are more frequently encountered in cats than dogs, especially in aged cats, and involve approximately 1% of all feline tumors submitted to a diagnostic laboratory (Moisan and Watson, 1996) and 6% of all feline skin tumors (Goldschmidt and Shofer, 1992). The adenoma grossly resembles ceruminous cystic hyperplasia, a non-neoplastic growth also common in the cat that is associated with chronic otitis externa. Both adenoma and hyperplasia present as smooth nodular or pedunculated masses that rarely ulcerate. Brown to black oily fluid collects within the enlarged gland ducts. Cytologically, amorphous debris along with low numbers of inflammatory cells and ductal epithelium may be found. Treatment consists of conservative surgical excision. Prognosis is good. Ceruminous gland adenocarcinoma is found in two thirds of the ceruminous gland tumors in cats (Fig. 3-36A&B). It is invasive locally and frequently metastasizes to regional lymph nodes. Nuclear pleomorphism is expected on cytology and cells in some cases contain fine to coarse black granular material that mimics melanin pigment (Fig. 3-36C). Radical surgical excision is recommended and some suggest postoperative radiotherapy to limit recurrence.

Cytologic differential diagnosis: ceruminous gland hyperplasia (for adenoma).

Sweat Gland Tumors

Of the benign sweat gland tumors found in dogs and cats, most commonly encountered are the apocrine cyst and apocrine ductular adenoma compared with the infrequent apocrine cystadenoma and apocrine secretory adenoma. Cyst cavities lined by cuboidal to columnar cells that contain granular secretory product may be seen with apocrine cystadenoma (Fig. 3-36D&E). Many apocrine ductular adenomas, especially those in the cat, were previously classified as cystic basal cell tumors (Gross et al., 2005). These are noted by the solid basilar epithelium and cystic histologic appearances (Fig. 3-36F). Necrotic cyst material may undergo dystrophic mineralization.

One malignant sweat gland tumor is an uncommon apocrine secretory adenocarcinoma, accounting for up

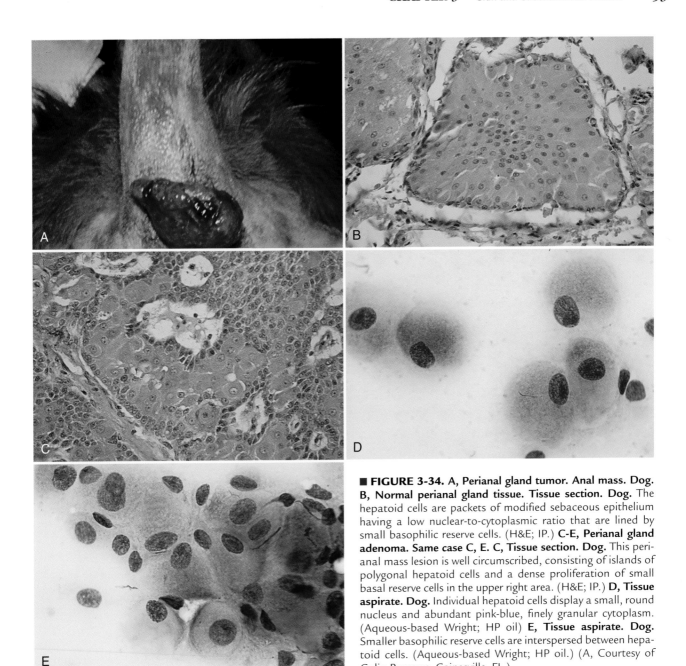

■ **FIGURE 3-34. A, Perianal gland tumor. Anal mass. Dog. B, Normal perianal gland tissue. Tissue section. Dog.** The hepatoid cells are packets of modified sebaceous epithelium having a low nuclear-to-cytoplasmic ratio that are lined by small basophilic reserve cells. (H&E; IP.) **C-E, Perianal gland adenoma. Same case C, E. C, Tissue section. Dog.** This perianal mass lesion is well circumscribed, consisting of islands of polygonal hepatoid cells and a dense proliferation of small basal reserve cells in the upper right area. (H&E; IP.) **D, Tissue aspirate. Dog.** Individual hepatoid cells display a small, round nucleus and abundant pink-blue, finely granular cytoplasm. (Aqueous-based Wright; HP oil) **E, Tissue aspirate. Dog.** Smaller basophilic reserve cells are interspersed between hepatoid cells. (Aqueous-based Wright; HP oil.) (A, Courtesy of Colin Burrows, Gainesville, FL.)

to 2% to 3% of skin tumors of dogs and cats, respectively (Miller et al., 1991; Gross et al., 2005). It is often located on the back, flanks, and feet of dogs and present as solitary, raised, well-circumscribed, and solid mass that often ulcerates. In older cats, most occur on the head and limbs, appearing as a solid, nodular mass. An alternate form observed in the dog and cat is an ulcerative, hemorrhagic, and frequently inflamed lesion that resembles acute dermatitis. Cytologically, ductular epithelium is present as clusters of basophilic cells that display numerous criteria of malignancy. In some cases, significant fibroplasia occurs so aspirates may yield fibroblasts along with epithelium. Treatment consists of wide surgical excision. Prognosis is fair to guarded as local recurrence and metastasis has been reported.

Cytologic differential diagnosis: mammary gland adenocarcinoma, anal sac adenocarcinoma, other adenocarcinomas, cutaneous basilar epithelial neoplasms.

Cutaneous Metastatic Carcinomas

Primary carcinomas that may metastasize to the skin include a duodenal adenocarcinoma (Juopperi et al., 2003), bronchogenic adenocarcinoma (Petterino et al., 2005), and urothelial carcinoma from the bladder and prostate (personal observations). There is a well-recognized association between pulmonary adenocarcinoma and some subtypes to phalangeal metastasis in cats only (Gross et al., 2005). Cytologic features resemble those of the primary site but may appear more anaplastic.

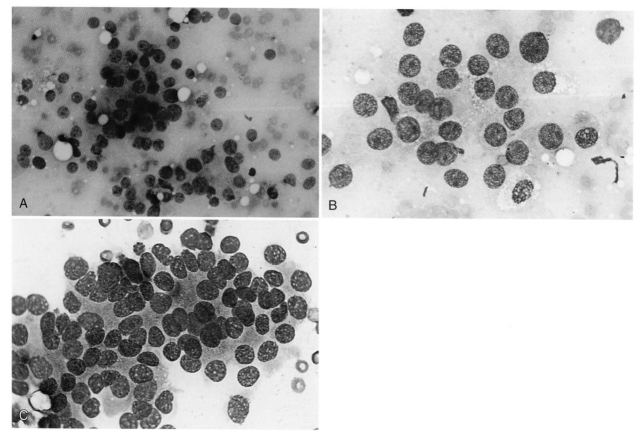

■ **FIGURE 3-35. Anal sac apocrine gland adenocarcinoma. Tissue aspirate. Dog. Same case A-B. A,** Loosely cohesive cell clusters with indistinct cell borders resembling a naked nuclei appearance. (Wright-Giemsa; HP oil.) **B,** Malignant features include high and variable nuclear-to-cytoplasmic ratios, anisokaryosis, coarse chromatin, and prominent nucleoli. (Wright-Giemsa; HP oil.) **C,** An acinar arrangement with nuclei peripheralized within a cluster of cells helps to diagnose this anal mass neoplasm of glandular origin. (Wright-Giemsa; HP oil.)

MESENCHYMAL

Fibroma

This is an uncommon tumor of adult dogs and cats, accounting for approximately 1% of cutaneous neoplasms in dogs (Yager and Wilcock, 1994). It presents as a solitary lesion on the extremities, head, flanks, and groin. Grossly, it is firm to soft, well circumscribed, hairless, and dome shaped or pedunculated. Cytologically, variable numbers of spindle or fusiform cells with small, uniform, dense oval nuclei occur individually or occasionally in small bundles. Generally, few cells exfoliate into cytologic preparations. Cytoplasm is lightly basophilic and cell borders are poorly defined as they form cytoplasmic tails on opposite sides of the nucleus (Fig. 3-37A). Amorphous eosinophilic material representing intercellular collagen protein may be associated with the neoplastic cells. Histologically, spindle cells may be arranged loosely (Fig. 3-37B) or as dense collagen bundles that are found rarely on cytology (Fig. 3-37C). These tumors are benign and treatment consists of surgical excision. Prognosis is generally good except for occasional local recurrence following removal of large tumors.

Cytologic differential diagnosis: myxoma, well-differentiated fibrosarcoma, neural sheath tumors.

Fibrosarcoma

This common tumor of dogs and cats accounts for 15% to 17% of skin neoplasms in the cat and is the fourth most common skin tumor in that species (Miller et al., 1991; Goldschmidt and Shofer, 1992). Those in young cats may be caused by the feline sarcoma virus and may be multiple. In older dogs and cats, tumors are solitary with a predilection for the limbs, trunk, and head. They are poorly circumscribed and sometimes ulcerated (Fig. 3-38A). These malignant tumors are invasive and approximately 25% will metastasize via hematogenous routes. Vaccine-induced fibrosarcomas, possibly related to subcutaneous-administered killed vaccines in cats, are locally invasive and aggressive (Gross et al., 2005). Cytologically, fibrosarcomas consist of abundant numbers of large, plump cells (Fig. 3-38B) occurring individually or in aggregates often associated with pink, collagenous material. Multinucleated giant cells may be present

Text continued on p. 57

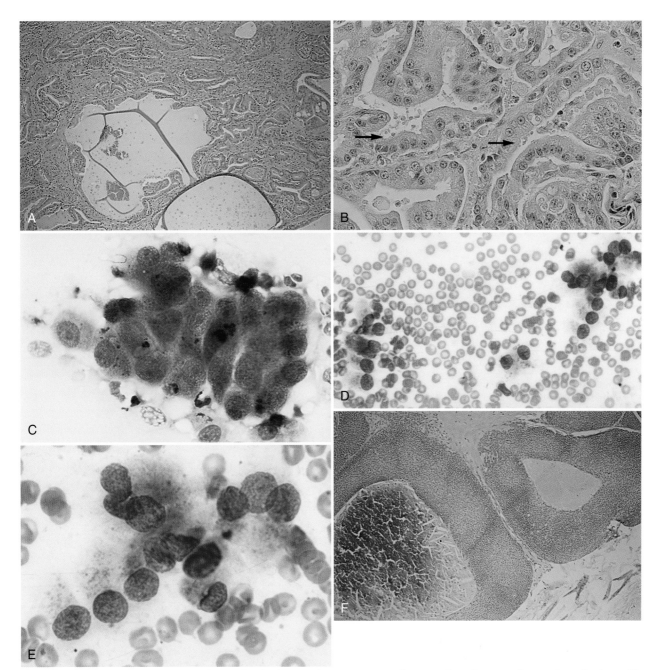

■ **FIGURE 3-36. Same case A-C. Ceruminous gland adenocarcinoma. Cat. A, Tissue section of ear canal mass.** Neoplastic proliferation of ductular epithelium with large cysts formed that contain brown sebum. (H&E; LP.) **B, Tissue section.** Malignant changes noted
by anisokaryosis, vesicular nuclei, prominent nucleoli, and marked anisocytosis of ductular epithelium. Note the apocrine function of
these cells is demonstrated by eosinophilic droplets at the apical surface *(arrows)*. (H&E; HP oil.) **C, Tissue imprint.** Tight clusters
of epithelium demonstrate increased nuclear-to-cytoplasmic ratio, prominent single nucleoli, coarse chromatin, anisokaryosis, and anisocytosis. Note the intracytoplasmic presence of black globular secretory material in some cells, which when finely dispersed in other
cells resembles melanin pigment. (Aqueous-based Wright; HP oil.) **Same case D-E. Apocrine cystadenoma. Tissue aspirate. Dog. D,**
A uniform population of cuboidal to low-columnar epithelium is present. Note the basilar location of the round nucleus. (Wright-
Giemsa; HP oil.) **E,** Higher magnification of A. The epithelial cells contain a dark, granular secretory material. (Wright-Giemsa; HP oil.)
F, Apocrine duct adenoma. Tissue section. Cat. Head mass with basal epithelium proliferation surrounding centers containing choles-
terol, calcium deposits, or liquefactive material. Masses of this nature were previously termed *cystic basal cell tumor,* which is no longer
recognized as appropriate. (H&E; LP.)

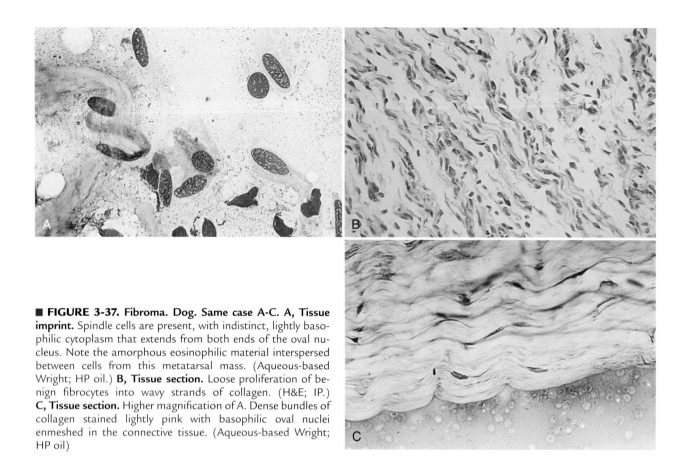

■ **FIGURE 3-37. Fibroma. Dog. Same case A-C. A, Tissue imprint.** Spindle cells are present, with indistinct, lightly basophilic cytoplasm that extends from both ends of the oval nucleus. Note the amorphous eosinophilic material interspersed between cells from this metatarsal mass. (Aqueous-based Wright; HP oil.) **B, Tissue section.** Loose proliferation of benign fibrocytes into wavy strands of collagen. (H&E; IP.) **C, Tissue section.** Higher magnification of A. Dense bundles of collagen stained lightly pink with basophilic oval nuclei enmeshed in the connective tissue. (Aqueous-based Wright; HP oil)

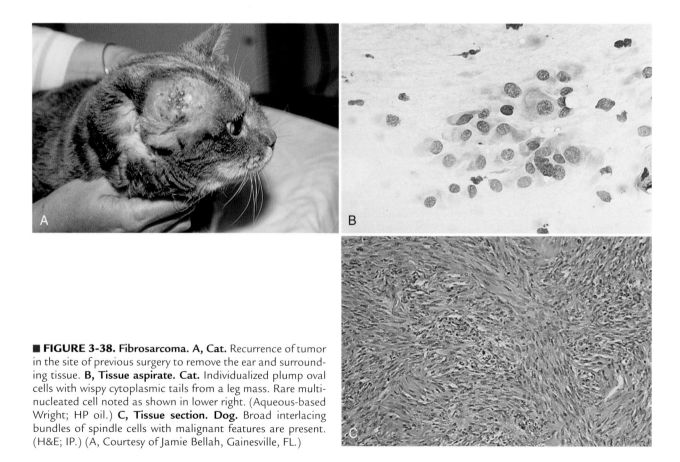

■ **FIGURE 3-38. Fibrosarcoma. A, Cat.** Recurrence of tumor in the site of previous surgery to remove the ear and surrounding tissue. **B, Tissue aspirate. Cat.** Individualized plump oval cells with wispy cytoplasmic tails from a leg mass. Rare multinucleated cell noted as shown in lower right. (Aqueous-based Wright; HP oil.) **C, Tissue section. Dog.** Broad interlacing bundles of spindle cells with malignant features are present. (H&E; IP.) (A, Courtesy of Jamie Bellah, Gainesville, FL.)

occasionally. Nuclear pleomorphism may be marked compared with the benign counterpart. Cells are less uniform and generally have high nuclear-to-cytoplasmic ratios. Treatment consists of wide surgical excision and/ or amputation. Recurrence occurs in 30% of canine cases. Alternately, radiotherapy with or without hyperthermia may be helpful postsurgery. Immunostimulants in combination with surgery and radiotherapy have also shown promising results. Chemotherapy alone has not proven effective in treatment of fibrosarcoma but may be helpful used with other modalities. Prognosis is good to poor depending on the site and degree of anaplasia.

KEY POINT Histologic examination is necessary to distinguish between fibrosarcoma and other spindle cell mesenchymal malignancies or granulation tissue (Fig. 3-38C). Immunohistochemistry may be similarly useful in distinguishing tissue origin.

Cytologic differential diagnosis: granulation tissue, malignant neural sheath tumors, anaplastic sarcoma with giant cells, perivascular wall tumors, myxosarcoma.

Myxoma/Myxosarcoma

Myxomas are rare tumors in dogs and cats, accounting for less than 1% of skin tumors (Goldschmidt and Shofer, 1992). Myxomas are infiltrative growths with a soft, fluctuant feel that present as slightly raised masses. Common sites in the dog and cat include the limbs, thorax, and abdomen. Cytologically, an intercellular matrix is often present in the background as granular eosinophilic amorphous material (Fig. 3-39A&B). Well-differentiated fusiform and stellate cells are found in low numbers in the benign lesion, which increase based on the degree of cellular and nuclear pleomorphism with the malignant form (Fig. 3-39C). Multinucleated cells are occasionally present in myxosarcomas. Alcian blue staining of the ground substance for mucin is diagnostic (Fig. 3-39D). Treatment consists of surgical excision. Prognosis is good to fair since recurrence is common, but it rarely metastasizes.

Cytologic differential diagnosis: fibroma, fibrosarcoma, neural sheath tumors, perivascular wall tumors.

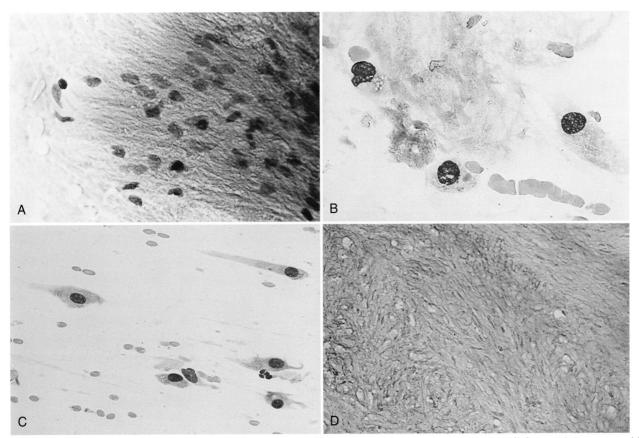

■ **FIGURE 3-39. Same case A, D. A, Myxoma. Tissue aspirate. Dog.** Dense, granular eosinophilic intercellular matrix is present with small, dense nuclei, suggesting a benign proliferation for this carpal mass. (Aqueous-based Wright; HP oil.) **Same case B-C. Myxosarcoma. Tissue aspirate. Dog. B,** An intracellular and extracellular granular eosinophilic matrix is shown with plump individualized mesenchymal cells from a metacarpal mass. (Aqueous-based Wright; HP oil.) **C,** Pleomorphic spindle cells with vesicular oval nuclei characterize the malignant form of myxomatous tumor. (Aqueous-based Wright; HP oil) **D, Myxoma. Tissue section. Dog.** The ground substance stains blue or positive for mucin shown between nuclei staining red. (Alcian blue; IP.)

Perivascular Wall Tumors (Canine Hemangiopericytoma and Myopericytoma)

Tumors originating from this location are common in the dog. They may be present in 7% of skin neoplasms (Goldschmidt and Shofer, 1992). The neoplastic cells are derived from the pericytes (hemangiopericytoma) and myopericytes (myopericytoma), both cells which are located in the wall of blood vessels, adjacent to endothelium. The tumors are often solitary with a predilection for the joints of the limbs, but are found commonly on the thorax and abdomen. They are firm to soft, multilobulated and often well circumscribed. Histologically, it belongs to a broad group of spindle cell tumors with the classic appearance of fingerprint whorls of plump spindle cells and a low mitotic index (Avallone et al., 2007) (Fig. 3-40A). While staghorn vascular patterns are most associated with hemangiopericytoma, whirling and placentoid are best associated with myopericytoma. Cytologically, preparations are moderately to highly cellular (Fig. 3-40B). Plump spindle cells may be individualized or arranged in bundles, sometimes found adherent to the surface of capillaries (Fig. 3-40C). Nuclei are ovoid, with one or more prominent central nucleoli. Multinucleated cells are occasionally seen. Associated with cells may be a pink amorphous collagenous stroma. The cytoplasm is basophilic often with numerous small, discrete vacuoles and occasional eosinophilic globules (Fig. 3-40D). Lymphoid cells have been found in approximately 10% of cases. Treatment should vary by the specific diagnosis with wide surgical excision or amputation, and radiotherapy with or without hyperthermia for the aggressive and recurrent disease termed *hemangiopericytoma*. Prognosis is fair as 20% to 60% will recur locally, especially with conservative excision. Metastasis is rare. Myopericytomas is best distinguished by immunomarkers such as desmin, pan-actin, or calponin (Avallone et al., 2007). Prognosis is good as myopericytomas respond to surgical excision.

> *Cytologic differential diagnosis:* neural sheath tumors, well-differentiated fibrosarcoma, myxomatous tumors, anaplastic sarcoma with giant cells.

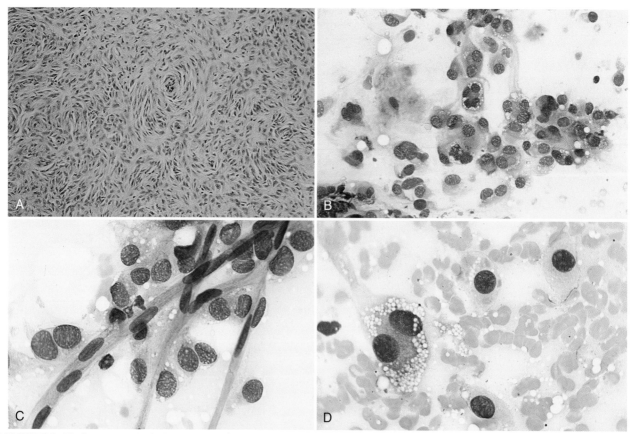

■ **FIGURE 3-40. Same case A, C, D. A, Myopericytoma. Tissue section. Dog.** Classic fingerprint whorls of plump spindle cells around blood vessels from a thigh mass. This histologic pattern of perivascular wall tumor suggests myopericytoma related to the whorling. (H&E; IP.) **B, Perivascular wall tumor. Tissue aspirate. Dog.** Slide preparation from a sternal subcutaneous mass is highly cellular, with aggregates of plump mononuclear or multinucleated mesenchymal cells. (Wright-Giemsa; HP oil.) **C-D, Myopericytoma. Tissue aspirate. Dog. C,** Plump spindle cells are shown adherent to the surface of capillaries. (Aqueous-based Wright; HP oil.) **D,** The cytoplasm is basophilic with numerous small discrete vacuoles, and one cell contains eosinophilic globules. (Aqueous-based Wright; HP oil.)

Anaplastic Sarcoma with Giant Cells (Malignant Fibrous Histiocytoma)

This is an uncommon tumor in dogs, comprising 0.34% of all canine tumors (Waters et al., 1994), and involves up to 3% of skin tumors in cats (Miller et al., 1991). It is a pleomorphic spindle cell tumor (Fig. 3-41A), the origin of which likely involves a primitive dermal pluripotent precursor cell since immunocytochemistry does not support a histiocytic origin (Pace et al., 1994). A subtype of it is known as giant cell tumor of soft parts, in which multinucleated cells are frequent. These tumors may be solitary or multiple, occurring mostly on the limbs of older dogs and cats, but may occur in abdominal organs, lungs, and lymph nodes. The subcutis and skeletal muscle of the shoulder and regional lymph node were diagnosed with malignant fibrous histiocytoma in a report of a dog (Desnoyers and St-Germain, 1994). Tumors are firm and poorly circumscribed. Cytologically, preparations contain a mixed population of multinucleated cells and plump spindle cells (Fig. 3-41B&C). Treatment involves radical excisional surgery with or without radiotherapy, and chemotherapy. Prognosis is guarded as these tumors are locally invasive with frequent recurrence and rarely may metastasize, especially in cases containing higher percentages of giant cells.

Cytologic differential diagnosis: fibrosarcoma, sarcoma of other origins, granulation tissue, histiocytic sarcoma.

Lipoma

This is a very common mesenchymal tumor in dogs, accounting for 8% of skin tumors (Goldschmidt and Shofer, 1992). It is a benign growth affecting generally older, obese female dogs. It is present in 6% of cats (Goldschmidt and Shofer, 1992). The tumor may be single or multiple, occurring mostly on the trunk and proximal limbs. These are dome shaped, well circumscribed, soft, often freely moveable masses within the subcutis that can grow slowly, becoming quite large. Some may infiltrate between muscles. Cytologically, unstained slides appear wet with glistening droplets that do not dry completely. Lipid may be best demonstrated with a water-soluble stain such as new methylene blue (Fig. 3-42A) or the fat stain oil red O. When alcohol fixatives are used with Romanowsky stains, lipid is dissolved, leaving slides often void of cells. When present, intact lipocytes have abundant clear cytoplasm with a small, compressed nucleus to one side of the cell (Fig. 3-42B&C). Treatment involves surgical excision. Prognosis is excellent; however, some infiltrative lipomas may be difficult to completely excise.

Cytologic differential diagnosis: normal subcutaneous fat.

Liposarcoma

Rare tumors of dogs and cats composing less than 0.5% of skin tumors (Goldschmidt and Shofer, 1992), liposarcomas are usually solitary masses occurring anywhere but

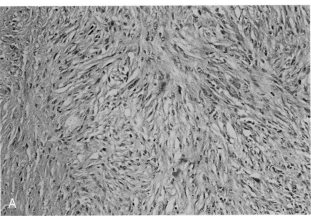
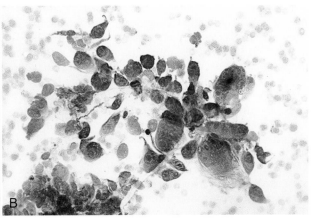
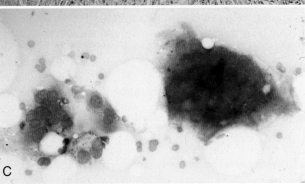

■ **FIGURE 3-41.** Anaplastic sarcoma with giant cells. Same case A, C. **A, Tissue section. Cat.** Pleomorphic spindle cells form tightly swirling or interlacing (storiform) bundles. Note frequent multinucleated cells scattered throughout this thoracic skin mass. This tumor recurred 3 months after previous surgical excision. (H&E; IP.) **B, Tissue aspirate. Dog.** A mixed population of plump spindle cells is present in a flank mass, with multiple criteria for malignancy, including increased and variable nuclear-to-cytoplasmic ratios, prominent nucleoli, anisokaryosis, and multinucleation. (Wright-Giemsa; IP.) **C, Tissue aspirate. Cat.** Several variably sized giant cells are present. The cytoplasm contains fine eosinophilic granulation. (Wright-Giemsa; HP oil.)

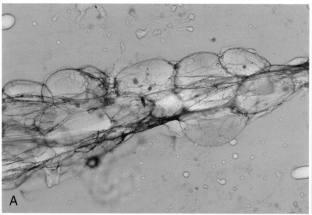

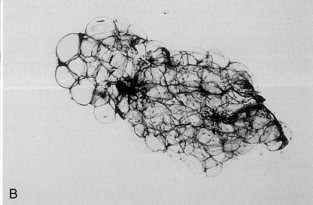

■ **FIGURE 3-42. Lipoma. Tissue mass aspirate. A, Dog.** Adipocytes are not dissolved in the water-soluble stain and are more visible. Note the pyknotic basophilic nucleus in relation to the massive cytoplasmic volume. (New methylene blue; IP.) **B, Dog.** Large aggregate of adipocytes. (Romanowsky; LP.) **C, Cat.** Adipocytes with small, dense nucleus. The pale-blue background material is an artifact likely resulting from incomplete washing of the slide of stain. (Wright-Giemsa; HP oil.)

most often on the ventral abdomen. An association with a foreign body was documented in one report (McCarthy et al., 1996). They are firm, poorly circumscribed, and adherent to underlying tissues (Fig. 3-43A). Ulceration of the epidermis may occur. Cytologically, dense aggregates of mesenchymal cells contain variable amounts of lipid vacuoles (Fig. 3-43B). Cells appear plump, have a spindle shape with large vesicular nuclei and prominent nucleoli, and may contain variably sized intracytoplasmic fat vacuoles (Fig. 3-43C). Multinucleated cells may be present. A myxoid variant may be associated with abundant Alcian blue staining but cytoplasmic vacuoles should still be found within some cells to be considered lipoblasts (Boyd et al., 2005). These are malignant tumors that have moderate metastatic potential. Treatment involves wide surgical excision, but may be coupled with radiation and hyperthermia to control recurrence. Prognosis is guarded as they are likely to recur and may metastasize.

Cytologic differential diagnosis: fibrosarcoma, undifferentiated sarcoma, anaplastic carcinoma.

Hemangioma

These benign tumors are common in dogs but less common in cats, representing about 5% and 2% of skin masses, respectively (Goldschmidt and Shofer, 1992; Miller et al., 1991). They may be solitary or multiple. Hemangiomas are discrete nodules present on the head, trunk, or limbs that appear dark red to purple and

may feel spongy (Fig. 3-44). Cytologically, aspirates appear bloody, resembling blood contamination. Small basophilic endothelial cells are infrequent. Evidence for acute or chronic hemorrhage is often noted, resulting in erythrophagocytosis or hemosiderin-laden macrophages. Platelets are not commonly seen. Treatment involves surgical excision or cryosurgery. Prognosis is excellent.

Cytologic differential diagnosis: hematoma, blood contamination.

Hemangiosarcoma

This is a malignant infiltrative mass of the dermis or subcutis. It is an infrequent tumor of older dogs and cats, occurring in about 1% and 3% of skin tumors, respectively (Goldschmidt and Shofer, 1992). Studies show an association between dermal vascular tumors and solar radiation (Hargis et al., 1992). Tumors are found more frequently in thin-haired areas such as the ventral abdomen of dogs and the ear pinnae of cats (Hargis et al., 1992; Miller et al., 1992). Lesions are raised, poorly circumscribed, ulcerated, and hemorrhagic. Cytologically, slide preparations often have low cellularity with numerous blood cells within the background. Solid, anaplastic cases of hemangiosarcoma may contain large dense aggregates of markedly pleomorphic mesenchymal cells (Fig. 3-45A). Evidence of acute erythrophagia or chronic hemorrhage with hemosiderin-laden macrophages is expected (Fig. 3-45B). Neoplastic cells are pleomorphic, ranging from large

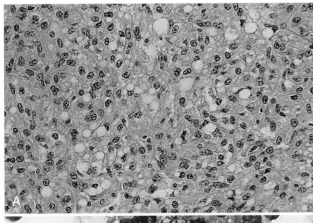

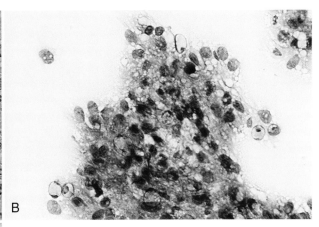

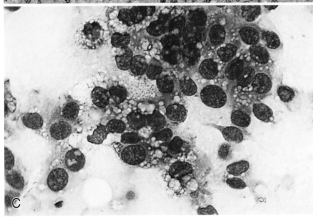

■ **FIGURE 3-43. Liposarcoma. Dog. A, Tissue section.** Lipid vacuoles are scattered between dense sheets of mesenchymal cells with vesicular nuclei. (H&E; IP.) **B, Tissue aspirate.** Large aggregates of mesenchymal cells with scattered lipid vacuoles that appear shrunken and well defined in this leg mass sample. (Aqueous-based Wright; HP oil.). **C, Tissue aspirate.** Cells appear plump and spindle shaped, with large vesicular nuclei and prominent nucleoli with variably sized intracytoplasmic fat vacuoles. (Aqueous-based Wright; HP oil.) (C, Case material courtesy of Peter Fernandes.)

for cytokeratins. Treatment consists of radical surgical excision and, in the case of possible metastatic lesions, combination chemotherapy. Prognosis is guarded because of regional invasion and local recurrence. Metastasis is uncommon but those occurring within the subcutis are more likely to spread.

> *Cytologic differential diagnosis:* fibrosarcoma, undifferentiated sarcoma, perivascular wall tumors, lymphangiosarcoma.

Melanoma

Benign and malignant forms are common, accounting for 5% of canine skin tumors and 3% of feline skin tumors (Yager and Wilcock, 1994). Older animals are usually affected, as are those with dark skin pigmentation. Gross features differ for benign and malignant forms. About 70% of the melanocytic tumors are benign, appearing as mostly dark-brown to black, circumscribed, raised, dome-shaped masses covered by smooth, hairless skin (Fig. 3-46A&B). Malignant tumors are variably pigmented, infiltrative, frequently ulcerated, and inflamed. Cytologically, cells from benign and malignant forms are pleomorphic, ranging from epithelioid (Fig. 3-46C) to fusiform (Fig. 3-46D), or occasionally are discrete and round, resembling those found in cutaneous plasmacytoma (Fig. 3-46E). In well-differentiated tumors, numerous fine, black-green cytoplasmic granules may mask nuclei (Fig. 3-46D, F). Nuclei in benign forms are small and

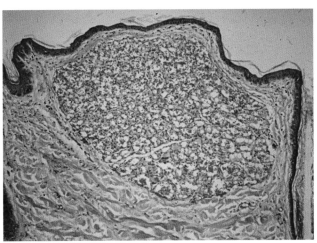

■ **FIGURE 3-44. Hemangioma. Tissue section. Dog.** Well-defined dermal nodule with endothelial proliferation and cavernous spaces filled with blood cells. (H&E; LP.)

spindle to stellate to epithelioid (Wilkerson et al., 2002). Cytoplasm is basophilic, having indistinct cell borders and frequent punctate vacuolation. Cells have high nuclear-to-cytoplasmic ratios, oval nuclei with coarse chromatin, and prominent multiple nucleoli (Fig. 3-45C). Diagnosis may be assisted through immunohistochemistry using von Willebrand's factor (factor VIII–related antigen), CD31, and vimentin (Miller et al., 1992; Bertazollo et al., 2005). The epithelioid angiosarcomas were negative

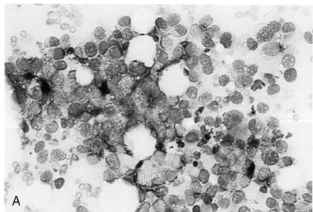
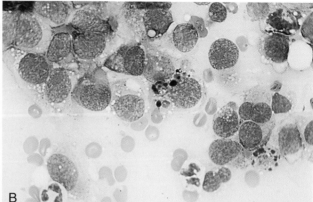

■ **FIGURE 3-45. Hemangiosarcoma. Tissue aspirate. Dog. Same case A-C. A,** Large, dense aggregates of markedly pleomorphic mesenchymal cells from a skin mass. (Wright-Giemsa; HP oil.) **B,** Note the blue-black granules related to chronic hemorrhage. A mitotic figure is shown in the upper right corner. (Wright-Giemsa; HP oil.) **C,** Cells have high nuclear-to-cytoplasmic ratios, oval nuclei with coarse chromatin, and prominent multiple nucleoli. Note the punctate vacuoles in the cytoplasm seen commonly in this tumor. (Wright-Giemsa; HP oil.)

uniform compared with characteristics of anisocytosis, anisokaryosis, coarse chromatin, and prominent nucleoli seen in the malignant melanomas (Fig. 3-46G). Poorly differentiated tumors may contain few or no cytoplasmic granules (see Fig. 3-46C). A gray, dustlike appearance in a few cells may help determine that the tumor is melanocytic (Fig. 3-46H). A balloon cell variant of melanoma is found infrequently that may be difficult to differentiate from sebaceous carcinoma, liposarcoma, or other clear cell tumors without melanocytic markers or ultrastructural evidence of melanosomes (Wilkerson et al., 2003). Treatment usually involves wide surgical excision. Prognosis depends on tumor site of origin and histologic characteristics. Benign skin tumors have a low mitotic rate and frequently have a good prognosis. Malignant forms arise more often from the nail bed, lip, and other oral mucocutaneous junctions in dogs. The latter forms carry a guarded or poor prognosis related to frequent recurrence and metastasis.

KEY POINT The number of melanin granules will vary within a tumor, with deeper regions composed of fusiform cells having fewer granules compared with superficial areas composed of epithelioid cells. Special stains such as the Fontana stain may be used on cytology preparations to detect poorly visible melanin granules, especially useful for amelanotic melanomas. Prussian blue stain will help identify hemosiderin

granules, which appear dark green and may resemble melanocytes. Additionally, the immunohistochemical stains Melan-A and S-100 may help distinguish amelanotic melanoma from plasmacytoma as well as negative expression of CD18 and CD45 (Ramos-Vara et al., 2002) (Fig. 3-46I).

Cytologic differential diagnosis for benign melanoma: normal skin melanocytes, normal pigmented basal cells, melanophages, hemosiderin-laden macrophages.

Cytologic differential diagnosis for malignant melanoma: plasmacytoma, fibrosarcoma, undifferentiated sarcoma, other cutaneous spindle cell tumors.

ROUND OR DISCRETE CELL

Canine Histiocytoma

This is a very common benign, rapidly growing tumor of mostly young dogs, composing about 12% to 14% of skin masses (Goldschmidt and Shofer, 1992; Yager and Wilcock, 1994). Its origin is the Langerhans cell of the epidermis. The tumor appears as a small, solitary, well-circumscribed, dome-shaped, red ulcerated, hairless mass, the so-called button tumor. It occurs commonly on the head, especially the ear pinnae, as well as on the hind

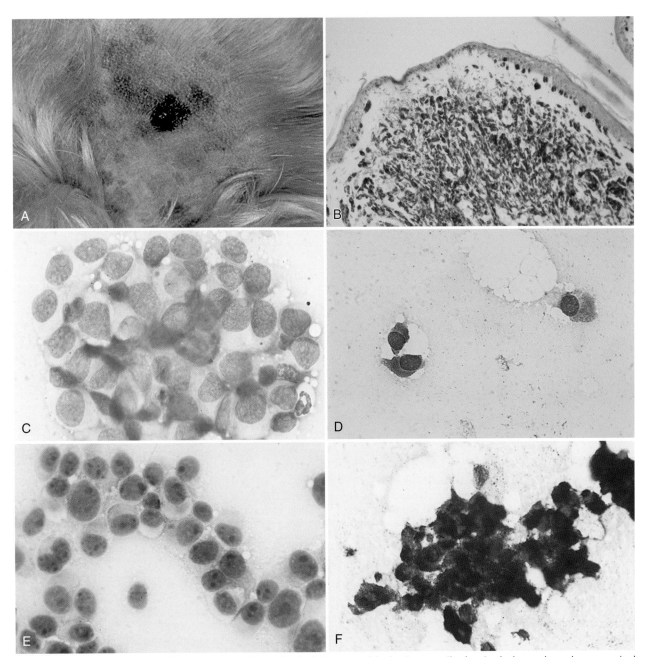

■ **FIGURE 3-46. A, Melanoma. Skin mass. Dog.** Note the dark-brown to black, circumscribed, raised, dome-shaped mass typical of most well-differentiated melanocytic tumors. **Same case B, D, F. B, Benign melanoma. Tissue section. Dog.** Melanocytes are present in the basal layer of the epidermis and within the superficial dermis arranged in clusters and diffusely. Cells are heavily pigmented in this mass on the back. (H&E; IP.) **Same case C, E. C, Amelanotic melanoma. Tissue imprint. Dog.** Cells lacking pigment are clustered, giving a cohesive epithelial appearance. Abundant clear cytoplasm is present in the poorly differentiated type of melanoma. This oral gum mass is associated with a poor prognosis. (Wright-Giemsa; HP oil.) **D, Benign melanoma. Tissue imprint. Dog.** Individual fusiform cells with abundant melanin pigment. (Aqueous-based Wright; HP oil.) **E, Amelanotic melanoma. Tissue imprint. Dog.** In other parts of the slide, individualized cells with a plasmacytoid appearance are evident. Note the prominent and multiple nucleoli, anisokaryosis, coarse chromatin, and oval to round nuclei in the poorly differentiated melanoma. (Aqueous-based Wright; HP oil.) **F, Benign melanoma. Tissue imprint. Dog.** Large aggregates of darkly pigmented cells are found that mask nuclear details. (Aqueous-based Wright; HP oil.)

Continued

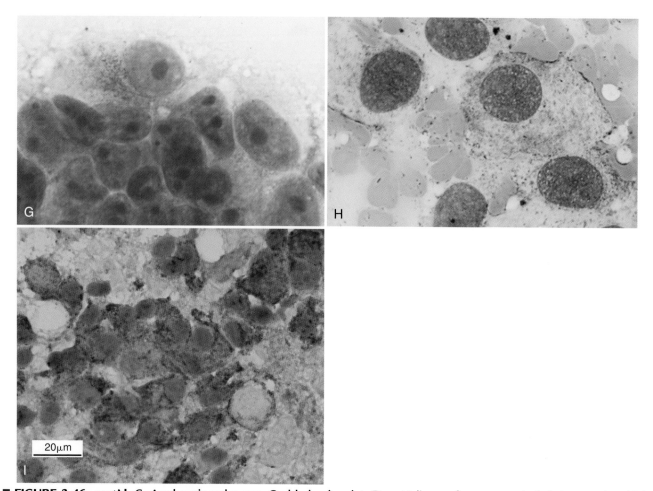

■ **FIGURE 3-46, cont'd. G, Amelanotic melanoma. Oral lesion imprint. Dog.** Malignant features seen include large and multiple nucleoli, anisokaryosis, coarse chromatin, and variable nuclear-to-cytoplasmic ratios. Note the cell with few dustlike, dark granules. (Aqueous-based Wright; HP oil.) **H, Melanoma. Tissue aspirate. Dog.** The uniform fine, gray-black melanin granules help determine the diagnosis in poorly differentiated melanocytic tumors. (Wright-Giemsa; HP oil.) **I, Melanoma. Skin mass aspirate. Dog.** Prominent immunocytochemical staining in the cytoplasm of cells from an multicentric amelanotic melanoma. (Melan-A/AEC; HP oil.) (A, Courtesy of Leslie Fox, Gainesville, FL. I, Courtesy of Michael Logan, Purdue University.)

limbs, feet, and trunk. Histologically, a nonencapsulated dense dermal infiltrate of round cells is closely associated with hyperplastic epithelium (Fig. 3-47A). Mitotic figures are frequently found (Fig. 3-47B). Cytologically, cells have variably distinct cytoplasmic borders (Fig. 3-47C). Nuclei are round, oval, or indented with fine chromatin and indistinct nucleoli (Fig. 3-47D). Cells exhibit minimal anisocytosis and anisokaryosis. The cytoplasm is abundant and clear to lightly basophilic (Fig. 3-47E). A variable number of small, well-differentiated lymphocytes, likely cytotoxic T-cells, are common in regressing lesions and can sometimes appear to be the predominant cell type (Fig. 3-47F). Cytochemical staining and immunostaining of these tumor cells may be positive for histiocytic markers (Fig. 3-47G), including nonspecific esterases, lysozyme, E-cadherin, CD1, CD11c, CD18, CD45, and MHC II (Moore et al., 1996). Treatment involves surgical excision if necessary. Prognosis is excellent to good as the tumor frequently regresses spontaneously within 3 months and recurrence is rare.

> ***Cytologic differential diagnosis:*** lymphoma, plasmacytoma, benign cutaneous histiocytosis, systemic histiocytosis, Langerhans cell histiocytosis, nodular granulomatous dermatitis.

Feline Progressive Dendritic Cell Histiocytosis

A few cases have been identified in cats, presenting as single skin nodules usually around the head, neck, or lower extremities (Affolter and Moore, 2006). These may change into multiple intradermal masses that later become ulcerated. Single or multinucleated histiocytic cells, which can resemble plasma cells, predominate. Cells express CD18, CD1, and MHC II. Since most evaluated lack E-cadherin, it is likely these involve dermal dendritic cells and not Langerhans cells. Chemotherapy or immunosuppressive and immunomodulatory drugs have not been successful. The etiology is not known. The disease is slowly progressive at first, but becomes aggressive in the terminal stage.

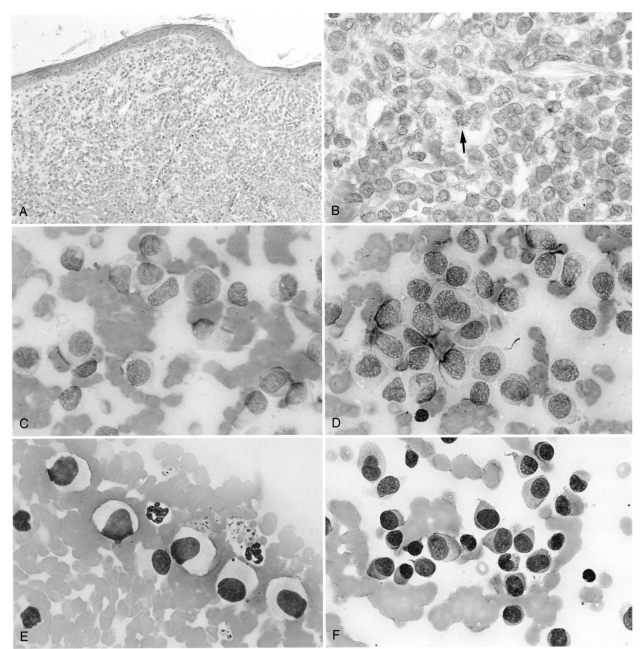

■ **FIGURE 3-47. A-G, Histiocytoma. Dog. Same case A-B. Tissue section. A,** The dermis contains a diffuse nodular and dense infiltrate of round cells that is closely associated with hyperplastic epithelium. (H&E; IP.) **B,** Mitotic figures are frequently found among the pleomorphic histiocytic cells. One mitotic figure is shown in the center *(arrow)*. (H&E; HP oil.) **Same case C-D. C, Tissue aspirate.** Cells have variably distinct cytoplasmic borders in this mass from the dorsum. (Wright-Giemsa; HP oil.) **D, Tissue aspirate.** Nuclei are round, oval, or indented with fine chromatin and indistinct nucleoli. Anisocytosis and anisokaryosis are mild. One small lymphocyte is present at the bottom, left of center. (Wright-Giemsa; HP oil.) **E, Tissue aspirate.** The cytoplasm is abundant and clear to lightly basophilic and cells appear discrete in this lip mass. (Wright-Giemsa; HP oil.) **Same case F-G. F, Tissue aspirate.** Several lymphocytes are present, suggesting regression of the lesion in this elbow mass. (Aqueous-based Wright; HP oil.)

Continued

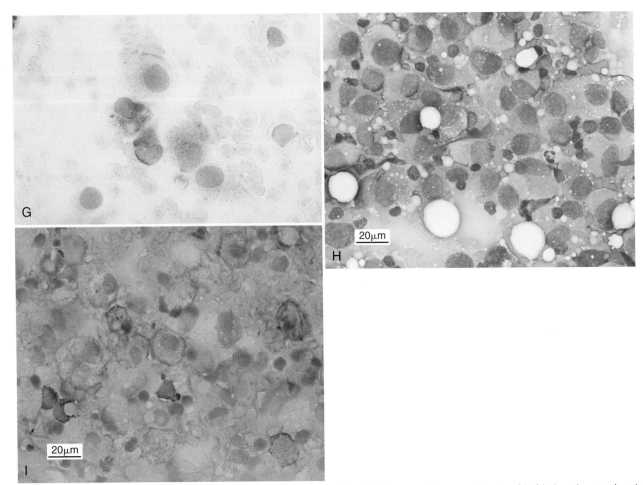

■ **FIGURE 3-47, cont'd. G, Tissue aspirate.** Red cytoplasmic staining indicates positive reaction to this histiocytic cytochemical marker. (Alpha naphthyl butyrate esterase; HP oil.) **Same case H-I. Histiocytic sarcoma. Tissue aspirate. Dog. H,** Skin mass on the flank that one month later progressed to a similar proliferation of cells found around head of the femur. Sample is highly cellular with large (20-30 µm) round cells as the predominant population. These cells have round to indented nuclei that are finely granulated with multiple small nucleoli. The grey cytoplasm is generally abundant with occasional small punctate vacuoles. The background contains free lipid and a mixture of lymphocytes and plasma cells. Anisocytosis, anisokaryosis, and variable nuclear-to-cytoplasmic ratios characterize the population. (Modified Wright; HP oil.) **I,** There is variable red granular membrane staining with immunocytochemistry to the anti-CD1c antigen indicating the cell population is mostly composed of dendritic cells. Another consideration for the histiocytic appearance would be macrophagic origin but CD1 is not expected to be positive.

Cytologic differential diagnosis: lymphoma, plasmacytoma.

Histiocytic Sarcoma

This tumor of neoplastic dendritic cells occurs as a localized or disseminated condition (Affolter and Moore, 2002). Localized histiocytic sarcomas are common in dogs and uncommon in cats. These are firm, often subcutaneous, masses located on the extremities and in periarticular sites. In contrast to histiocytomas and Langerhans cell histiocytosis, both of which originate in the dermis and are E-cadherin positive, histiocytic sarcomas originate within the subcutis from dermal dendritic cells that can extend into the dermis. Cytologically these can have

both a round cell and mesenchymal or spindle cell appearance. Multinucleate giant cells may also occur that resemble the anaplastic sarcoma with giant cell tumor. Individualized round cells contain abundant basophilic cytoplasm that may display vacuolation. Nuclei are vesiculated, round to indented, with one or more nucleoli. Marked anisokaryosis and anisocytosis are often observed (Fig 3-47H). Immunochemical expression is positive for CD45, CD18, CD1, CD11c, and MHC II in the dog and cat (Fig 3-47I). Preliminary studies by the author support expression by BLA.36, a marker often used for B-cells. Tumor cells from dermal dendritic origin lack E-cadherin expression, indicating these are not Langerhans cells. Histiocytic sarcomas are locally invasive with metastasis to draining lymph nodes. Prognosis is favorable with early wide surgical excision or amputation of the limb.

Mast Cell Tumor

This tumor in dogs accounts for about 10% of skin tumors, with higher prevalence in certain breeds such as the boxer, pug, and Boston terrier (Yager and Wilcock, 1994). Tumors in dogs are generally solitary, nonencapsulated, and highly infiltrative into dermis and subcutis (Fig. 3-48A–C). They may occasionally occur in puppies. Tumors are most common on the trunk and limbs in the dog. Cytologically, canine tumor cells vary in the degree of granularity and nuclear atypia. Canine mast cells having numerous distinct metachromatic stained granules with uniform small nuclei are considered grade I (well differentiated). Grade II (intermediate) mast cells have fewer granules and nuclei may vary in size and shape (Fig. 3-48D). Grade III (poorly differentiated) mast cells have few to no cytoplasmic granules, and nuclei display marked atypia with mitotic figures (Fig. 3-48E). This involves anisokaryosis, coarse chromatin, and multiple and prominent nucleoli. Cytoplasmic borders in grade III mast cells are often indistinct. Giant, binucleated cells are more commonly found in grade III forms. Eosinophils are more numerous in canine tumors than feline tumors. The background is usually filled with granules from ruptured cells. Degranulation may be associated with hemorrhage, vascular necrosis, edema, and collagenolysis (Figs. 2-22B and 3-48F). Identification by cytochemistry or immunochemistry involves chloroacetate esterase, antibodies for tryptase and KIT, in addition to Giemsa staining for metachromatic granules (Fernandez et al., 2005). Treatment involves wide surgical excision, cryosurgery, radiotherapy, and chemotherapy. Prognosis for dogs varies with stage and histologic grade. Grade III tumors have a high chance of local recurrence and metastasis to lymph nodes. Less than 10% survive more than 1 year with grade III tumors (Yager and Wilcock, 1994). Tumors occurring on the perineum, scrotum, prepuce, and digits in dogs appear to be more aggressive (Gross et al., 2005). Another prognostic tool in dogs involves the frequency of argyrophilic nucleolar organizer regions and Ki67 as indicators for

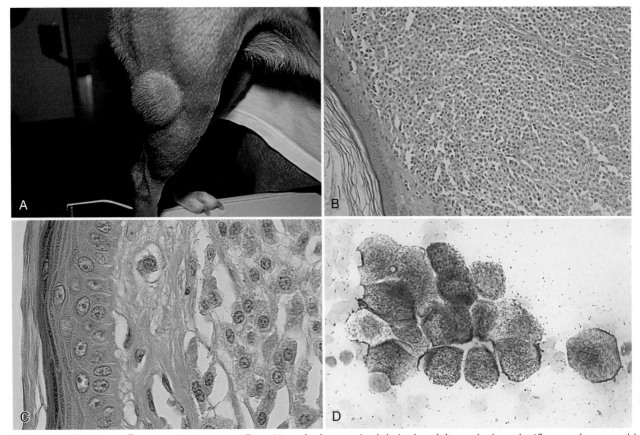

■ **FIGURE 3-48. Mast cell tumor. A, Leg mass. Dog.** Note the large, raised, haired nodule on the lateral stifle area that resembles grossly a lipoma. **Same case B-C. Tissue section. Cat. B,** Diffuse dense dermal infiltration of round cells. (H&E; IP.) **C,** Some granulation is present within the round cells. Nuclear size is uniform in this well-differentiated tumor. (H&E; HP oil.) **Same case D, H. D, Tissue aspirate. Dog.** Variable staining of granules and anisokaryosis suggest a moderately differentiated tumor for this mammary area mass. (Wright-Giemsa; HP oil.)

Continued

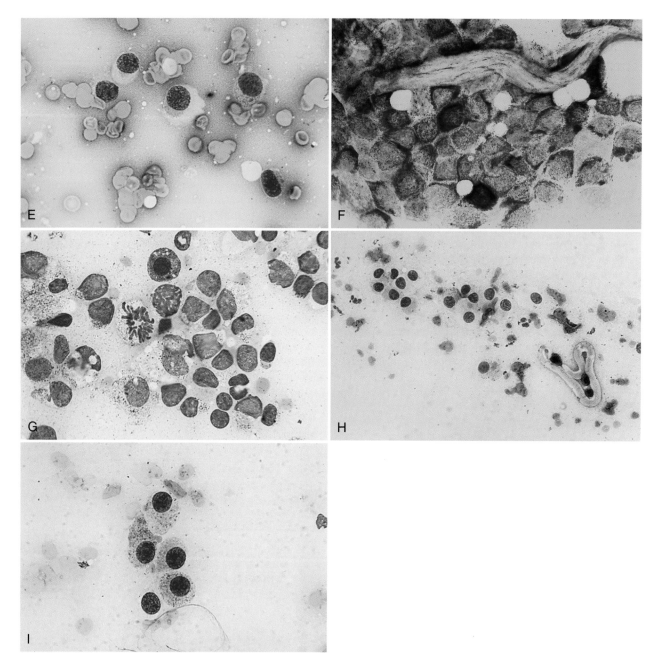

■ **FIGURE 3-48, cont'd. E, Tissue imprint. Dog.** Few scattered fine metachromatic granules are present in cells of this poorly differentiated tumor in the submandibular area of the skin. Malignant nuclear changes include coarse chromatin, anisokaryosis, high and variable nuclear-to-cytoplasmic ratios, and prominent nucleoli. (Wright-Giemsa; HP oil.) **F, Tissue aspirate. Dog.** This moderately differentiated tumor from a thoracic skin mass contains pale-pink collagen strands as a result of collagenolysis. (Wright-Giemsa; HP oil.) **G, Digit mass imprint. Cat.** Note the granular background from released cytoplasmic granules. Cells are pleomorphic with a "histiocytic" appearance and contain a variable number of cytoplasmic granules. This 8-year-old cat had multiple digits on two feet affected by the same tumor. (Wright-Giemsa; HP oil.) **H, Tissue aspirate. Dog.** The water-soluble stain washes out the granular contents so that cytologically the mass appears to be poorly differentiated. Note the *Dirofilaria immitis* microfilaria in the lower right area among the poorly granulated mast cells. (Aqueous-based Wright; HP oil.). **I, Tissue aspirate. Dog.** Higher magnification of D. Note the light dusting of granulation in these cells related to the use of a water-soluble stain. Compare these cells with those in D that retain the granular contents with an alcohol-based Giemsa stain in (Aqueous-based Wright; HP oil.) (A, Courtesy of Leslie Fox, Gainesville, FL.)

cellular proliferation, both of which when increased were associated with decreased survival, as is also the case with KIT protein localization (Webster et al., 2007; Kiupel et al., 2004).

Mast cell tumors in cats represent the second most common skin tumor type, accounting for 12% to 20% of skin tumors (Goldschmidt and Shofer, 1992; Miller et al., 1991). These are usually solitary, well-circumscribed, dermal masses that occur on the head, neck, and limbs. Multiple masses are common in young Siamese cats (Gross et al., 2005). Small, well-differentiated lymphocytes may be associated with the feline tumors. Tumor cells that resemble poorly granulated histiocytes are associated with the multiple form of mast cell tumor (Fig. 3-48G). For cats, the solitary form of the disease is generally considered benign with some exceptions of recurrence and invasion (Johnson et al., 2002). Tumor histopathologic grade involving nuclear pleomorphism, mitotic rate, and deep dermal invasion has no prognostic significance in cats with solitary mast cell tumors (Molander-McCrary et al., 1998). A significant number of young cats with multiple masses respond with spontaneous regression within months.

KEY POINT Giemsa or toluidine blue staining should be used to reveal cytoplasmic granules in poorly differentiated forms. It should be noted that aqueous-based Wright stains, such as Diff-Quik®, often show a lack of granulation, especially in less differentiated forms of mast cell tumor. This is related to the water-soluble nature of the granule contents (Fig. 3-48H&I).

Cytologic differential diagnosis: normal mast cells, chronic allergic dermatitis, lymphoma, balloon cell melanoma, histiocytoma, plasmacytoma.

Plasmacytoma

This tumor is present in about 2% of canine skin tumors and is rare in cats (Yager and Wilcock, 1994). They present as mostly solitary, well-circumscribed masses often on the digits, ears, and mouth. Cytologically, aspirates are moderately to markedly cellular. Individual cells have variable amounts of basophilic cytoplasm in which borders are discrete (Fig. 3-49A&B). Anisocytosis and anisokaryosis are prominent features. Nuclei are round to oval with fine to moderately coarse chromatin and indistinct nucleoli. The nuclei are often eccentrically placed and frequently binucleated. Multinucleated cells may be present (Fig. 3-49C&D). Amorphous eosinophilic material, representative of amyloid, is seen in less than 10% of plasmacytomas (Fig. 3-49E&F). Treatment involves wide surgical excision. Prognosis is generally good, but local recurrences may be common. One study found cases with a polymorphous-blastic type of morphology associated with recurrence and metastasis (Platz et al., 1999). Transition from extramedullary plasmacytoma to myeloma has been documented rarely in the dog and cat, the latter case after five months (Radhakrishnan et al., 2004).

Identification of plasmacytomas can involve cytochemistry (RNA stains magenta with methyl green pyronin) or immunochemistry (CD45, CD79a, lambda chain, MUM1) (Majzoub et al., 2003; Ramos-Vara et al., 2007). The cytologic appearance of a peripheral neural sheath tumor in a cat displayed a morphologic resemblance to plasma cells, which suggests histopathology is best for these cases (Tremblay et al., 2005).

Cytologic differential diagnosis: lymphoma, histiocytoma, amelanotic melanoma, neuroendocrine (Merkel cell) tumor, peripheral nerve sheath tumor.

Cutaneous Lymphoma

The disease may occur as a primary disease of the skin or rarely as a manifestation of generalized lymphoma. It is more common in older dogs and cats, although its presence in juvenile dogs has been reported (Choi et al., 2004). Histologically, this group is divided into nonepitheliotropic and epitheliotropic types. Prevalence of epitheliotropic lymphoma is 1% of skin tumors in dogs and both epitheliotropic and nonepitheliotropic types represent 2.8%. of all feline skin tumors. The epitheliotropic lymphoma is less common in the cat than in the dog (Gross et al., 2005). Lesions are solitary to multiple in the form of nodules, plaques, ulcers, erythroderma, or exfoliative dermatitis in the form of excessive scaling (Fig. 3-50A&B). Pruritus may be common. T-lymphocytes are presumed involved in the infiltration of the dermis and subcutis with nonepitheliotropic lymphomas similar to epitheliotropic lymphoma. B cell lymphoma of the skin is extremely rare (Gross et al., 2005). Epitheliotropic lymphoma, when characterized by neoplastic lymphocyte infiltrates of the epidermis and adnexa, is termed *mycosis fungoides* (Fig. 3-50C). Sometimes focal collections of the neoplastic cells, termed *Pautrier microabscesses,* are formed within the epidermis. The cell of origin is usually a T-lymphocyte with 80% expressing CD8 while the remaining 20% are double negative for CD4 and CD8 (Moore et al., 1994; Gross et al., 2005). When these neoplastic T-lymphocytes are present in the epidermis and peripheral blood, it is then referred to as *Sézary syndrome* (Foster et al., 1997) based on a similar presentation in people. Canine pagetoid reticulosis is a form of CD3+ T-cell lymphoma in which TCRγδ (T-cell receptor gamma delta) positive cells proliferate within the epidermis. Cytologically, lymphocytes are variable ranging in size from small to large with round, indented, or convoluted nuclei (Fig. 3-50D&E). Nucleoli are usually indistinct but may be prominent. Cytoplasm is scant to moderate and lightly basophilic. Uniformity of the lymphoid population without significant inflammation or plasma cell infiltration is suggestive of cutaneous lymphoma. In general, treatment involving chemotherapy, radiotherapy, and immunotherapy has been unsuccessful in achieving long-term remission. Surgical excision may be helpful for solitary lesions (Choi et al., 2004). Prognosis is poor as the disease rapidly progresses, necessitating euthanasia. Nodal involvement, when present, usually occurs late in both types. Laboratory abnormalities such as monoclonal

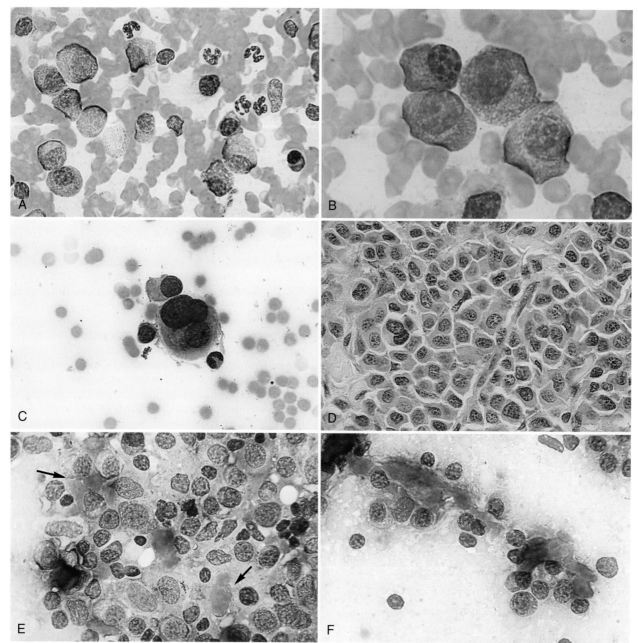

■ **FIGURE 3-49. Plasmacytoma. Smae case A-B. A, Tissue aspirate. Cat.** Cellular specimen with cells that have variable amounts of basophilic cytoplasm in which borders are discrete. Sample taken from a nasal planum mass. (Wright-Giemsa; HP oil.) **B, Tissue aspirate. Cat.** Higher magnification of A. Note the plasmacytoid appearance with eccentrically placed nuclei and variably coarse chromatin. This case had a monoclonal production of gamma globulins. (Wright-Giemsa; HP oil.) **Same case C-D. C, Tissue imprint. Dog.** A digit mass displays multinucleated cells, a frequent finding in this tumor. (Wright-Giemsa; HP oil.) **D, Tissue section. Dog.** There is dense dermal infiltration with pleomorphic round cells. Note the multinucleated cells to the left of center. (H&E; HP oil.) **Same case E-F. Plasmacytoma with amyloid. Tissue imprint. Cat. E,** The specimen from a hock mass is densely cellular with marked anisocytosis and anisokaryosis. Several cells have a plasmacytoid appearance while others appear histiocytic with abundant pale cytoplasm. Small amount of amyloid is present between cells *(arrows)*. (Wright; HP oil.) **F,** Note the abundant pink amorphous material associated with plasmacytoid cells. (Wright; HP oil.) (E-F, Slide material courtesy of Gail Walter et al, Michigan State University; presented at the 1992 ASVCP case review session.)

gammopathy, serum hyperviscosity, and hypercalcemia have been associated with cutaneous lymphoma.

> ***Cytologic differential diagnosis:*** chronic inflammatory dermatitis, histiocytoma.

Canine Transmissible Venereal Tumor

This is a tumor of dogs, most often in free-roaming sexually active animals living in temperate climates, related to transplantation of intact cells. Immunochemistry supports vimentin and CD45 and CD45RA immunoreactivity

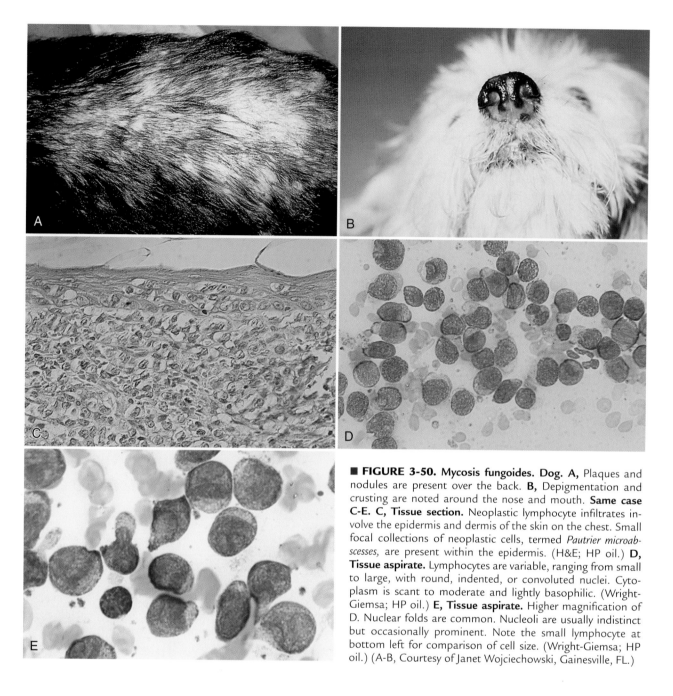

■ **FIGURE 3-50. Mycosis fungoides. Dog. A,** Plaques and nodules are present over the back. **B,** Depigmentation and crusting are noted around the nose and mouth. **Same case C-E. C, Tissue section.** Neoplastic lymphocyte infiltrates involve the epidermis and dermis of the skin on the chest. Small focal collections of neoplastic cells, termed *Pautrier microabscesses,* are present within the epidermis. (H&E; HP oil.) **D, Tissue aspirate.** Lymphocytes are variable, ranging from small to large, with round, indented, or convoluted nuclei. Cytoplasm is scant to moderate and lightly basophilic. (Wright-Giemsa; HP oil.) **E, Tissue aspirate.** Higher magnification of D. Nuclear folds are common. Nucleoli are usually indistinct but occasionally prominent. Note the small lymphocyte at bottom left for comparison of cell size. (Wright-Giemsa; HP oil.) (A-B, Courtesy of Janet Wojciechowski, Gainesville, FL.)

indicating leukocyte origin with positive lysozyme and alpha-1-antitrypsin expression supportive of histiocytic origin (Gross et al., 2005; Park et al., 2006) However, the cells do not appear to be of canine origin, having an abnormal karyotype with 59 chromosomes compared with a normal karyotype of 78 in dogs. PCR and molecular techniques to analyze the sequence of the long interspersed nuclear element (LINE) may be used to identify tumor cells (Park et al., 2006). It appears on the skin of the external genitalia as well as the mucous membranes associated with sexual contact. However, a case of a prepuberal female dog with skin lesions and no mucosal involvement has been reported (Marcos et al., 2006a). Grossly, the tumor is pink to red, poorly circumscribed, multinodular, raised to pedunculated, soft, friable, ulcerated, and hemorrhagic, with frequent necrosis and superficial bacterial infection. The mass exfoliates easily by tissue impression, giving rise to a monomorphic population of large round cells with a round nucleus, coarse chromatin, and one to two prominent nucleoli (see Figs. 12-42 and 12-43). The cytoplasm is abundant and lightly basophilic, and frequently contains multiple punctate vacuoles. Mitotic figures may be seen. Associated with the tumor are small lymphoid cells and inflammatory cells, often with evidence of bacterial sepsis. Treatment involves chemotherapy, particularly with vincristine, radiotherapy, and surgical excision. Prognosis is good with chemotherapy. The tumors may regress spontaneously, presumably related to lymphocyte infiltration. Metastasis may occur (Park et al., 2006) and recurrence is high with surgical intervention.

Cytologic differential diagnosis: other round cell tumors, amelanotic melanoma.

NAKED NUCLEI

Thyroid

Subcutaneous masses located adjacent to the trachea may be confirmed as thyroid glands by fine-needle aspiration. Classically, they consist of small sheets of closely or loosely attached cells, some of which contain black, granular intracytoplasmic material (Fig. 3-51). The cytoplasmic border may or may not be apparent with the appearance of free nuclei. Occasionally the cervical masses may present with no clinical signs other than a subcutaneous paratracheal mass on the neck as demonstrated by a recent report of a C-cell or medullary thyroid carcinoma (Bertazollo et al., 2003). See Chapter 16 for further information about thyroid tumors.

RESPONSE TO TISSUE INJURY

Calcinosis Cutis and Calcinosis Circumscripta

Calcinosis cutis is an uncommon condition of mineral deposition in the dermis, epidermis, or subcutis. It is associated with glucocorticoid use or hyperadrenocorticism (Fig. 3-52A) and iatrogenic administration of calcium products for hypoparathyroid treatment in dogs (Gross et al., 2005). It involves dystrophic mineralization of collagen or elastin of the skin. Sites of predilection include the dorsal neck, inguinal area, and axillary region. Grossly, erythematous papules or firm gritty plaques develop and often ulcerate. Cytologically, the white, gritty material (Bettini et al., 2005) appears densely granular in the background and a mixed inflammatory response occurs, including macrophages, giant multinucleated cells, neutrophils, lymphocytes, and plasma cells. Prognosis

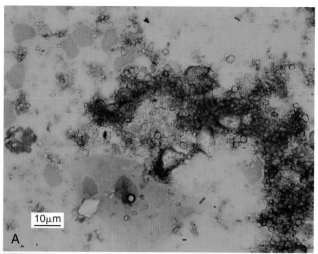

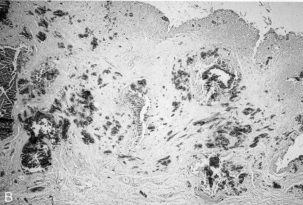

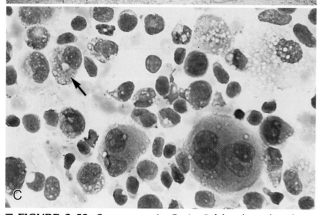

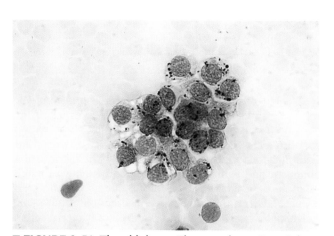

■ **FIGURE 3-51. Thyroid tissue. Tissue aspirate. Dog.** Subcutaneous masses located adjacent to the trachea may be confirmed as thyroid glands by fine-needle aspiration. Note the cohesive sheet of cells, many of which contain black, granular intracytoplasmic material thought to be tyrosine. (Wright-Giemsa; HP oil.)

■ **FIGURE 3-52. Same case A, C. A, Calcinosis cutis. Tissue aspirate. Dog.** This lip mass is taken from a patient with hyperadrenocorticism. A squamous epithelium and a degenerate neutrophil are against a background of variably sized round to irregularly shaped refractile crystals, consistent with dystrophic mineralization. Occasional oral bacterial flora are noted. (Modified Wright; HP oil.) **B-C, Calcinosis circumscripta. Dog. B, Tissue section.** This multinodular dermal and subcutaneous mass is composed of central areas of mineralization that stain intensely red. These areas are surrounded by macrophages, giant cells, and dense, fibrous connective tissue. (H&E; LP.) **C, Tuber coxae mass aspirate.** Fluid from elbows and hip areas contained similar fluid, which was aspirated, sedimented, and smeared onto a slide. Highly cellular sample contained macrophages, giant cells, and lymphocytes. Within the background and phagocytic cells *(arrow)* are numerous clear refractile structures consistent with calcium crystals. (Aqueous-based Wright; HP oil.)

is good as these benign lesions resolve untreated over several months.

A clinical subgroup of calcinosis cutis is calcinosis circumscripta, which is uncommon in dogs and rare in cats. This is a well-circumscribed solitary lesion within the deep dermis and subcutis formed by dystrophic mineralization, the etiology of which is unknown. It is mostly associated with young German shepherd dogs. The lesions often occur over joint areas or pressure points, at sites of previous trauma, or under the tongue (Marcos et al., 2006b; Gross et al., 2005). Mass texture is firm and gritty. Histologically, the lesion is distinguished by large lakes of mineralized deposits surrounded by dense fibrous connective tissue and foreign body giant cells (Fig. 3-52B). Cytologically, it is similar to calcinosis cutis except fibroblasts may be more frequently observed. Mineral deposits often present as refractile yellow-green granules of irregular size and shape that are best observed with a lowered microscope condenser (Fig. 3-52C). Purple fine granular material present in the background likely represents necrotic tissue, which may be prominent. Demonstration of calcium may be enhanced by use of cytochemical stains such as von Kossa and Alizarin red S (Raskin, 2006b; Marcos et al., 2006b). These are benign lesions that may be treated by surgical excision.

Granulation Tissue

Firm subcutaneous swellings may arise from an exuberant fibroblastic response to tissue injury. Histologically, this mass is composed of horizontally arranged proliferating fibroblasts transected by vertically proliferating endothelium from small blood vessels (Fig. 3-53). Mitoses and macrophages are commonly found. The plump, reactive fibroblasts seen on cytology have an ovoid vesicular nucleus and may resemble the fusiform cells seen in fibrosarcoma. Histopathology is recommended to distinguish the two conditions.

Hematoma

Grossly, these blood-filled masses can resemble neoplastic conditions such as hemangioma or hemangiosarcoma. Initially, when formed, the hematoma contains fluid identical in cell content to blood except that it lacks platelets (Hall and MacWilliams, 1988). A short time later, macrophages engulfing erythrocytes (erythrophagocytosis) are common. Over time, the hemoglobin material breaks down, appearing as blue-green to black hemosiderin granules within the macrophage cytoplasm. On occasion, hematoidin crystals, which appear as rhomboid golden crystals, may form from iron-poor hemoglobin pigment. As the healing continues, plump fibroblasts may be seen that can mimic a neoplastic mesenchymal cell population.

Hygroma

This is a swelling within the subcutaneous tissues that forms over bony prominences, commonly the elbow of large-breed dogs, secondary to repeated trauma or pressure. A cystlike structure forms from dense connective tissue that contains a serous to mucinous, clear, yellow, or red fluid, depending on the degree of hemorrhage. Cytologically, the fluid appears clear to lightly basophilic and cells other than those involving blood contamination include macrophages (Fig. 3-54) and reactive fibrocytes. Pathophysiology is similar to that seroma formation.

Mucocele or Sialocele

Duct rupture related to trauma or infection leads to an accumulation of saliva within the subcutaneous tissues. The presence of a fluctuant mass containing clear to bloody fluid with stringlike features grossly suggests a salivary gland duct rupture. The cytologic specimen often stains uniformly purple from the high protein content. The background may contain scattered, pale basophilic, amorphous material, consistent with saliva.

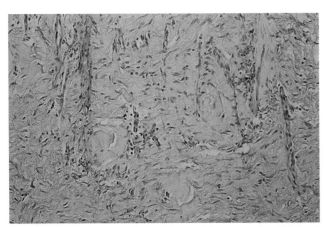

■ **FIGURE 3-53. Granulation tissue. Tissue section. Dog.** A mass on the dorsum contains dense, fibrous connective tissue layered horizontally with capillaries coursing through the tissue vertically. The reaction was secondary to noninfectious panniculitis. (H&E; IP.)

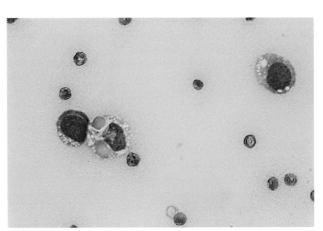

■ **FIGURE 3-54. Hygroma. Aspirate of swelling over elbow. Dog.** The fluid obtained was orange/hazy with WBC < 400/μl and protein 3.3 g/dl. The background is lightly granular related to increased protein content. Cells were mononuclear phagocytes and exhibited erythrophagia as shown. (Wright-Giemsa; HP oil.)

The fluid is often bloody with evidence of both acute and chronic hemorrhage. Erythrophagocytosis is common and occasional yellow rhomboid crystals may be seen. These are termed *hematoidin crystals* and are associated with chronic hemorrhage (Fig. 3-55A). The nucleated cells are predominately highly vacuolated macrophages that display active phagocytosis (Fig. 3-55B). Distinction between these cells and secretory glandular tissue may be difficult, especially when cells are individualized and nonphagocytic. Nondegenerate neutrophils are common, becoming degenerate when bacterial infection occurs.

Seroma

Injury may lead to a seroma, which is composed of clear to slightly blood-tinged fluid. The leaked plasma originates from immature capillaries created during granulation tissue formation. Cytologically, the fluid is poorly cellular and may require sedimentation prior to examination. Phagocytic macrophages will predominate among a mixture of inflammatory cells (Fig. 3-56).

Otic Cytology

Cytology of the ear is a frequently used tool in clinical practice to manage ear conditions and determine an underlying etiology. Specimens should be evaluated for the presence, numbers, and characteristics of cells (leukocytes and nonhematopoietic) and microbiologic or parasitic agents (bacteria, yeast, arthropods) (Angus, 2004). Historically, sample collection of ear swabs have used heat fixation to ensure good-quality smears. This debate has been addressed recently in two separate reports that show that samples taken as swabs for ear cytology do not need heat fixation (Toma et al., 2006; Griffin et al., 2007). For ear masses, it is recommended taking aspirate biopsies, which in cats showed good association with the histopathology (De Lorenzi et al., 2005).

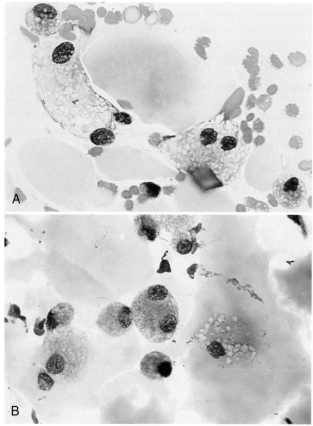

■ **FIGURE 3-55. Sialocele. Cervical mass aspirate. Dog. A,** Chronic hemorrhage is noted by the presence of a large yellow rhomboid crystal, termed *hematoidin*. The background contains pale-pink material and vacuolated mononuclear cells are abundant. (Wright; HP oil.) **B,** The nucleated cells are predominately highly vacuolated mononuclear cells that are not easily identified as salivary gland epithelium or macrophages. Amorphous material in the background is consistent with mucus. (Aqueous-based Wright; HP oil.)

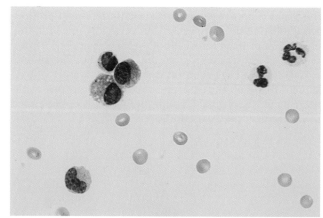

■ **FIGURE 3-56. Seroma. Tissue aspirate. Dog.** Fluid obtained from a swelling on the neck was bloody with WBC 3800/µl and protein 2.5 g/dl. Blood elements composed the majority of cell types found. Mononuclear phagocytes as shown accounted for 24% of the cell population. (Wright-Giemsa; HP oil.)

REFERENCES

Affolter VK, Moore PF: Localized and disseminated histiocytic sarcoma of dendritic cell origin in the dog, *Vet Pathol* 39:74-83, 2002.

Affolter VK, Moore PF: Feline progressive histiocytosis, *Vet Pathol* 43:646-655, 2006.

Angus JC: Otic cytology in health and disease, *Vet Clin North Am Small Anim Pract* 34:411-424, 2004.

Avallone G, Helmbold P, Caniatti M, et al: The spectrum of canine cutaneous perivascular wall tumors: morphologic, phenotypic and clinical characterization, *Vet Pathol* 44:607-620, 2007.

Baker R, Lumsden JH: The skin. In Baker R, Lumsden JH (eds): *Color atlas of cytology of the dog and cat*, St. Louis, 2000, Mosby, pp 39-70.

Barnes JC, Stanley O, Craig TM: Diffuse cutaneous leishmaniasis in a cat, *J Am Vet Med Assoc* 202:416-418, 1993.

Beaudin S, Rich LJ, Meinkoth JH, et al: Draining skin lesion from a desert Poodle, *Vet Clin Pathol* 34:65-68, 2005.

Bernstein JA, Cook HE, Gill AF, et al: Cytologic diagnosis of generalized cutaneous sporotrichosis in a hunting hound, *Vet Clin Pathol* 36:94-96, 2007.

Bertazollo W, Giudice C, Dell'Orco M, et al: Paratracheal cervical mass in a dog, *Vet Clin Pathol* 32:209-212, 2003.

Bertazollo W, Dell'Orco M, Bonfanti U, et al: Canine angiosarcoma: cytologic, histologic, and immunohistochemical correlations, *Vet Clin Pathol* 34:28-34, 2005.

Bettini G, Morini M, Campagna F, et al: True grit: the tale of a subcutaneous mass in a dog, *Vet Clin Pathol* 34:73-75, 2005.

Beyer TA, Pinckney RD, Cooley AC: Massive *Dracunculus insignis* infection in a dog, *J Am Vet Med Assoc* 214:366-368, 1999.

Bohn AA, Wills T, Caplazi P: Basal cell tumor or cutaneous basilar epithelial neoplasm? Rethinking the cytologic diagnosis of basal cell tumors, *Vet Clin Pathol* 35:449-453, 2006.

Boyd SP, Taugner FM, Serrano S, et al: Matrix "blues": clue to a cranial thoracic mass in a dog, *Vet Clin Pathol* 34:271-274, 2005.

Carakostas MC, Miller RI, Woodward MG: Subcutaneous dermatophilosis in a cat, *J Am Vet Med Assoc* 185:675-676, 1984.

Caruso KJ, Cowell RL, Cowell AK, et al: Skin scraping from a cat, *Vet Clin Pathol* 31:13-15, 2002.

Choi US, Jeong SM, Kang M-S, et al: Cutaneous lymphoma in a juvenile dog, *Vet Clin Pathol* 33:47-49, 2004.

De Lorenzi D, Bonfanti U, Masserdotti C, et al: Fine-needle biopsy of external ear canal masses in the cat: cytologic results and histologic correlations in 27 cases, *Vet Clin Pathol* 34:100-105, 2005.

Desnoyers M, St-Germain L: What is your diagnosis? *Vet Clin Pathol* 23:89-97, 1994.

Elliott GS, Whitney MS, Reed WM, et al: Antemortem diagnosis of paecilomycosis in a cat, *J Am Vet Med Assoc* 184:93-94, 1984.

Fernandez NJ, West KH, Jackson ML, et al: Immunohistochemical and histochemical stains for differentiating canine cutaneous round cell tumors, *Vet Pathol* 42:437-445, 2005.

Foley JE, Borjesson D, Gross TL: Clinical, microscopic, and molecular aspects of canine leproid granuloma in the United States, *Vet Pathol* 39:234-239, 2002.

Foster AP, Evans E, Kerlin RL, et al: Cutaneous T-cell lymphoma with Sézary syndrome in a dog, *Vet Clin Pathol* 26:188-192, 1997.

Garma-Avina A: The cytology of squamous cell carcinomas in domestic animals, *J Vet Diagn Invest* 6:238-246, 1994.

Giovengo SL: Canine dracunculiasis, *Comp Contin Educ Pract Vet* 15: 726-729, 1993.

Goldschmidt MH, Shofer FS: *Skin tumors of the dog and cat*, Oxford, UK, 1992, Pergamon Press, pp 1-3, 50-65, 103-108, 271-283.

Greene CE, Gunn-Moore DA: Mycobacterial infections. In Greene CE (ed): *Infectious diseases of the dog and cat*, ed 3, Philadelphia, 2006, Saunders/Elsevier, pp 462-488.

Griffin JS, Scott DW, Erb HN: *Malassezia* otitis externa in the dog: the effect of heat-fixing otic exudate for cytological analysis, *J Vet Med A* 54:424-427, 2007.

Grooters AM, Hodgin EC, Bauer RW, et al: Clinicopathologic findings associated with *Lagenidium* sp. infection in 6 dogs: Initial description of an emerging oomycosis, *J Vet Intern Med* 17:637-646, 2003.

Gross TL, Ihrke PJ, Walder EJ, et al: *Skin diseases of the dog and cat. Clinical and histopathologic diagnosis*, ed 2, Ames, IA, 2005, Blackwell Science.

Hall RL, MacWilliams PS: The cytologic examination of cutaneous and subcutaneous masses, *Semin Vet Med Surg (Sm Anim)* 94-108, 1988.

Hargis AM, Ihrke PJ, Spangler WL, et al: A retrospective clinicopathologic study of 212 dogs with cutaneous hemangiomas and hemangiosarcomas, *Vet Pathol* 29:316-328, 1992.

Johnson TO, Schulman FY, Lipscomb TP, et al: Histopathology and biologic behavior of pleomorphic cutaneous mast cell tumors in fifteen cats, *Vet Pathol* 39:452-457, 2002.

Juopperi TA, Cesta M, Tomlinson L, et al: Extensive cutaneous metastases in a dog with duodenal adenocarcinoma, *Vet Clin Pathol* 32:88-91, 2003.

Kano R, Watanabe K, Murakami M, et al: Molecular diagnosis of feline sporotrichosis, *Vet Rec* 156:484-485, 2005.

Kaya O, Kirkan S, Unal B: Isolation of *Dermatophilus congolensis* from a cat, *J Vet Med B Infect Dis Vet Public Health* 47:155-157, 2000.

Kiupel M, Webster JD, Kaneene JB, et al: The use of kit and tryptase expression patterns as prognostic tools for canine cutaneous mast cell tumors, *Vet Pathol* 41:371-377, 2004.

Lester SJ, Kenyon JE: Use of allopurinol to treat visceral leishmaniasis in a dog, *J Am Vet Med Assoc* 209:615-617, 1996.

Logan MR, Raskin RE, Thompson S: "Carry-on" dermal baggage: a nodule from a dog, *Vet Clin Pathol* 35:329-331, 2006.

Majzoub M, Breuer W, Platz SJ, et al: Histopathologic and immunophenotypic characterization of extramedullary plasmacytomas in nine cats, *Vet Pathol* 40:249-253, 2003.

Marcos R, Santos M, Marrinhas C, et al: Cutaneous transmissible venereal tumor without genital, *Vet Clin Pathol* 35:106-109, 2006a.

Marcos R, Santos M, Oliveira J, et al: Cytochemical detection of calcium in a case of calcinosis circumscripta in a dog, *Vet Clin Pathol* 35:239-242, 2006b.

Masserdotti C, Ubbiali FA: Fine needle aspiration cytology of pilomatricoma in three dogs, *Vet Clin Pathol* 31:22-25, 2002.

McCarthy PE, Hedlund CS, Veazy RS, et al: Liposarcoma associated with a glass foreign body in a dog, *J Am Vet Med Assoc* 209:612-614, 1996.

Miller MA, Greene CE, Brix AE: Disseminated *Mycobacterium avium-intracellulare* complex infection in a miniature schnauzer, *J Am Anim Hosp Assoc* 31:213-216, 1995.

Miller MA, Nelson SL, Turk JR, et al: Cutaneous neoplasia in 340 cats, *Vet Pathol* 28:389-395, 1991.

Miller MA, Ramos JA, Kreeger JM: Cutaneous vascular neoplasia in 15 cats: clinical, morphologic, and immunohistochemical studies, *Vet Pathol* 29:329-336, 1992.

Moisan PG, Watson GL: Ceruminous gland tumors in dogs and cats: a review of 124 cases, *J Am Anim Hosp Assoc* 32: 449-453, 1996.

Molander-McCrary H, Henry CJ, Potter K, et al: Cutaneous mast cell tumors in cats: 32 cases (1991-1994), *J Am Anim Hosp Assoc* 34: 281-284, 1998.

Moore PF, Olivry T, Naydan D: Canine cutaneous epitheliotropic lymphoma (mycosis fungoides) is a proliferative disorder of CD8+ T cells, *Am J Pathol* 144:421-429, 1994.

Moore PF, Schrenzel MD, Affolter VK, et al: Canine cutaneous histiocytoma is an epidermotropic Langerhans cell histiocytosis that expresses CD1 and specific beta-2-integrin molecules, *Am J Pathol* 148:1699-1708, 1996.

Neel JA, Tarigo J, Tater KC, et al: Deep and superficial skin scrapings from a feline immunodeficiency virus-positive cat, *Vet Clin Pathol* 36:101-104, 2007.

Pace LW, Kreeger JM, Miller MA, et al: Immunohistochemical staining of feline malignant fibrous histiocytomas, *Vet Pathol* 31:168-172, 1994.

Panciera DL, Stockham SL: *Dracunculosis insignis* infection in a dog, *J Am Vet Med Assoc* 192:76-78, 1988.

Park C-H, Ikadai H, Yoshida E, et al: Cutaneous toxoplasmosis in a female Japanese cat, *Vet Pathol* 44:683-687, 2007.

Park M-S, Kim Y, Kan M-S, et al: Disseminated transmissible venereal tumor in a dog, *J Vet Diagn Invest* 18:130-133, 2006.

Patel A: Pyogranulomatous skin disease and cellulitis in a cat caused by *Rhodococcus equi*, *J Sm Anim Pract* 43: 129-132, 2002.

Petterino C, Guazzi P, Ferro S, et al: Bronchogenic adenocarcinoma in a cat: an unusual case of metastasis to the skin, *Vet Clin Pathol* 34:401-404, 2005.

Platz SJ, Breuer W, Pfleghaar S, et al: Prognostic value of histopathological grading in canine extramedullary plasmacytomas, *Vet Pathol* 36:23-27, 1999.

Radhakrishnan A, Risbon RE, Patel RT, et al: Progression of a solitary, malignant cutaneous plasma-cell tumour to multiple myeloma in a cat, *Vet Comp Oncol* 2:36-42, 2004.

Ramos-Vara JA, Miller MA, Johnson GC, et al: Melan A and S100 protein immunohistochemistry in feline melanomas: 48 cases, *Vet Pathol* 39:127-132, 2002.

Ramos-Vara JA, Miller MA, Valli VEO: Immunohistochemical detection of multiple myeloma 1/interferon regulatory factor 4 (MUM1/IRF-4) in canine plasmacytoma: comparison with CD79a and CD20, *Vet Pathol* 44:875-884, 2007.

Raskin RE: Applied cytology: canine elbow mass, *NAVC Clinician's Brief* 4:65-67, Feb 2006a.

Raskin RE: Applied cytology: tail mass in a dog, *NAVC Clinician's Brief* 4:13-15, Nov 2006b.

Roccabianca P, Caniatti M, Scanziani E, et al: Feline leprosy: spontaneous remission in a cat, *J Am Anim Hosp Assoc* 32:189-193, 1996.

Ross JT, Scavelli TD, Matthiesen DT, et al: Adenocarcinoma of the apocrine glands of the anal sac in dogs: a review of 32 cases, *J Am Anim Hosp Assoc* 27:349-355, 1991.

Sprague W, Thrall MA: Recurrent skin mass from the digit of a dog, *Vet Clin Pathol* 30:189-192, 2001.

Toma S, Cornegliani L, Persico P, et al: Comparison of 4 fixation and staining methods for the cytologic evaluation of ear canals with clinical evidence of ceruminous otitis externa, *Vet Clin Pathol* 35:194-198, 2006.

Tremblay N, Lanevschi A, Doré M, et al: Of all the nerve! A subcutaneous forelimb mass on a cat, *Vet Clin Pathol* 34:417-420, 2005.

Twomey LN, Wuerz JA, Alleman AR: A "down under" lesion on the muzzle of a dog, *Vet Clin Pathol* 34:161-133, 2005.

Waters CB, Morrison WB, DeNicola DB, et al: Giant cell variant of malignant fibrous histiocytoma in dogs: 10 cases (1986-1993), *J Am Vet Med Assoc* 205:1420-1424, 1994.

Webster JD, Yuzbasiyan-Gurkan V, Miller RA, et al: Cellular proliferation in canine cutaneous mast cell tumors: associations with *c-KIT* and its role in prognostication, *Vet Pathol* 44: 298-308, 2007.

Welsh RD: Sporotrichosis, *J Am Vet Med Assoc* 223:1123-1126, 2003.

Wilkerson MJ, Chard-Bergstrom C, Andrews G, et al: Subcutaneous mass aspirate from a dog [epithelioid hemangiosarcoma], *Vet Clin Pathol* 31:65-68, 2002.

Wilkerson MJ, Dolce K, DeBey BM, et al: Metastatic balloon cell melanoma in a dog, *Vet Clin Pathol* 32:31-36, 2003.

Yager JA, Wilcock BP: *Color atlas and text of surgical pathology of the dog and cat. dermatopathology and skin tumors*, London, 1994, CV Mosby, pp 243-244, 245-248, 257-271, 273-286.

Zimmerman K, Feldman B, Robertson J, et al: Dermal mass aspirate from a Persian cat, *Vet Clin Pathol* 32:213-217, 2003.

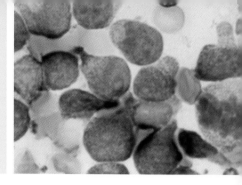

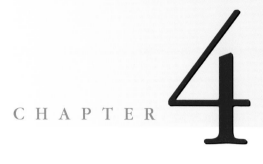

CHAPTER 4

Lymphoid System

Rose E. Raskin

The lymphoid organs commonly examined by cytology include the peripheral and internal lymph nodes, spleen, and occasionally the thymus. As a result of their similar cell populations, the following cytodiagnostic categories are used. It should be noted that more than one presentation might occur in a specimen at a time.

GENERAL CYTODIAGNOSTIC GROUPS FOR LYMPHOID ORGAN CYTOLOGY

- Normal tissue
- Reactive/hyperplastic tissue
- Inflammation
- Metastatic disease
- Primary neoplasia
- Extramedullary hematopoiesis

LYMPH NODES

Indications for Lymph Node Biopsy

- *Lymphadenomegaly,* or enlargement of one or multiple lymph nodes, may be detected by palpation or by radiography and ultrasonography.
- *Evaluation of metastatic disease* involves evaluation of the lymph node(s) draining the primary lesion (Table 4-1).
- *Classification of lymphoma* may be enhanced by the cytologic features stained with Romanowsky stains, or by cytochemical and immunocytochemical stains (see Chapter 17) to distinguish B- and T-cell subtypes; the latter stains may be performed at specialized laboratories.

Aspirate and Impression Biopsy Considerations

Submandibular lymph nodes are frequently enlarged and reactive because of their constant exposure to antigens, making them a poor choice for biopsy in generalized lymphadenopathy.

> **KEY POINT** Popliteal and prescapular lymph nodes are the preferred biopsy sites for generalized lymphadenopathy.

The size of the lymph node should also be considered. Very large nodes may yield misleading information as they frequently contain necrotic or hemorrhagic tissue. A slightly enlarged lymph node is preferred, and a sample from more than one location is desirable. If a large lymph node must be aspirated, the needle should be aimed tangentially to avoid the direct center.

> **KEY POINT** The center of a very large lymph node should be avoided during aspiration.

In performing aspirate smears, a 22-gauge needle is used alone or together with a 6- or 12-ml syringe. The needle is inserted into the node in several directions. With the syringe attached to the needle or butterfly catheter, quick and multiple withdrawal motions of the plunger are made to create negative pressure. The pressure on the plunger is released *before* removing the needle to avoid splattering the material within the syringe. An air-filled syringe is reattached and the needle contents expelled onto the approximate center of a glass slide. The aspirate appears creamy white, watery to viscous, indicating many leukocytes are present. The material is *gently* squashed with a second slide, sliding them apart horizontally. Smears are dried rapidly with a hair dryer to avoid crenation effects.

> **KEY POINT** An alternative method of aspiration biopsy uses no suction but relies on capillary action to draw cells into the needle. This technique (Fig. 4-1) is preferred for lymphoid organs to prevent excess blood contamination.

> **KEY POINT** Aspirates smears must be spread gently since immature lymphoid cells are often quite fragile.

TABLE 4-1   Selected Peripheral Lymph Nodes in the Dog

Lymph Node	Location	Drainage Features
Submandibular	Group of two to four nodes located ventral to the angle of the jaw	Includes most of the head, including the rostral oral cavity
Prescapular	Group of two or three nodes located in front of the supraspinatus muscle	Includes the caudal part of the head (pharynx, pinna), most of the thoracic limb, and part of the thoracic wall
Axillary	One or two nodes located caudal and medial to the shoulder joint	Includes most of the thoracic wall, deep structures of the thoracic limb and neck, and the thoracic and cranial abdominal mammary glands
Superficial inguinal	Two nodes located in the furrow between the abdominal wall and the medial thigh	Includes the caudal abdominal and inguinal mammary glands, ventral half of the abdominal wall, penis, prepuce, scrotal skin, tail, ventral pelvis, and medial part of the thigh and stifle
Popliteal	One node located behind the stifle	Includes areas distal to the stifle

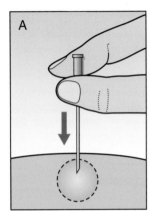 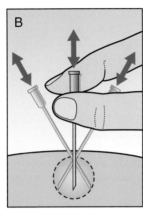 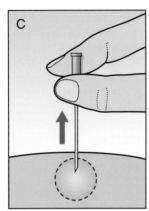 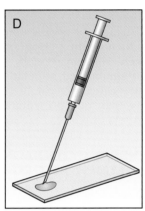

■ **FIGURE 4-1. Fine need biopsy without suction.** Diagrammatic stepwise illustration of biopsy procedure: **A,** Needle inserted into target tissue; **B,** Needle moved back and forth inside target varying the angle; **C,** Needle withdrawn; **D,** Needle attached to syringe and sample blown onto microscopy slide. (From Orell SR, Sterrett GF, Whitaker D: *Fine needle aspiration cytology,* ed 4, Edinburgh, 2005, Churchill Livingstone.)

When preparing impression smears from an excisional biopsy, it is important to blot excessive tissue fluids before touch preparations are made to increase the cellular yield. The cut surface of the excised lymph node is blotted on a paper towel, and then touched gently to a glass slide. To avoid the formalin artifact cytologic and histopathologic samples must be mailed separately when submitted to a referral laboratory.

> **KEY POINT** Keep cytologic preparations away from formalin fumes to avoid premature fixation resulting in poor staining and cytologic detail.

Normal Histology and Cytology

The canine or feline lymph node consists of a thin connective tissue capsule that surrounds cortical and medullary lymphoid tissue and extends inward as trabeculae. The outer cortex contains variably sized lymphatic nodules (Fig. 4-2A) composed primarily of B-lymphocytes surrounded by a thin rim of small T-lymphocytes. The diffuse lymphoid tissue between the nodules composed primarily of T-lymphocytes extends deep into the paracortex, where macrophages and dendritic reticular cells act as antigen-presenting cells. The diffuse lymphoid tissue extends inward to form medullary cords (Fig. 4-2B), which contain B-lymphocytes, plasma cells, macrophages, and other leukocytes. Between the cords are endothelial-lined sinuses in contact with dendritic reticular cells and reticular fibers. Lymph enters the afferent vessels that penetrate the capsule, through the subcapsular and cortical sinuses of the cortex, into the medullary sinuses and exits through efferent vessels at the hilus. Blood flow enters the hilus through arterioles that branch into the cortex to perfuse the lymphatic nodules. In this region, vessels enlarge to form postcapillary or high endothelial venules of the paracortex (Fig. 4-2C). These venules are important sites for the travel of lymphocytes from blood into the lymph node parenchyma that is related to the selective binding of the lymphocyte with receptors on the endothelial cells. The venules drain into larger veins that exit via the hilus region.

Cytologically, small, well-differentiated lymphocytes that measure 1 to 1.5 times the diameter of an erythrocyte

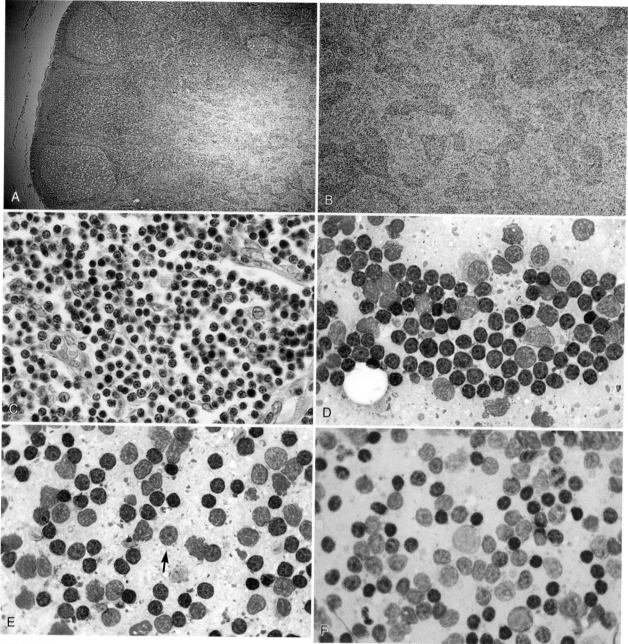

■ **FIGURE 4-2. Same case A-C. Lymph node. Tissue section. Dog. A,** Cortex contains variably sized lymphoid nodules and the medullary area contains cords of cells along endothelial-lined sinuses. (H&E; LP.) **B,** Medullary cords appearing as dark bands are composed of lymphocytes, plasma cells, and macrophages and lie adjacent to pale-stained sinus spaces. (H&E; LP.) **C,** The deep cortex contains high endothelial venules shown in cross section (lower left) and longitudinal section (upper right). Lymphocytes selectively adhere to receptors on endothelium to leave the circulation and enter the lymph node. (H&E; HP oil.) **D, Lymph node. Tissue aspirate. Dog.** This prescapular lymph node contains a majority of small lymphocytes. Low numbers of medium-sized lymphocytes are present as well as several lysed cells that appear light-pink and lack cytoplasmic borders. (Wright-Giemsa; HP oil.) **Same case E-F. Normal lymph node. Tissue aspirate. Dog. E,** This popliteal lymph node contains a majority of small lymphocytes. Note the medium-sized lymphocyte *(arrow)*. (Wright-Giemsa; HP oil.) **F,** A mixed cell population is shown. Note the large lymphocyte in the center and occasional granulocytes. (Wright-Giemsa; HP oil.)

in the dog and cat compose approximately 90% of the population (Fig. 4-2D). The chromatin of these cells is densely clumped with no visible nucleoli. Cytoplasm is scant. These cells are the darkest staining of all the lymphocytes. The medium and large lymphocytes whose nuclei measure two to three times erythrocyte diameter may

be present in low numbers (<5% to 10%) (Fig. 4-2E&F). Their nuclei have a fine, diffuse, and light chromatin pattern. Nucleoli may be prominent. The cytoplasm is more abundant and often basophilic. Mature plasma cells represent a small portion of the cells found. Their chromatin is densely clumped and often the nucleus is eccentrically placed within the abundant, deeply basophilic cytoplasm. A pale area or halo is seen adjacent to the nucleus, which indicates the Golgi zone. Occasional macrophages (histiocytes) appear as large mononuclear cells with abundant light cytoplasm, often containing cellular debris. Nuclear chromatin is finely stippled and nucleoli may be found in activated macrophages. Mast cells and neutrophils also may be present in low numbers (Bookbinder et al., 1992).

Reactive or Hyperplastic Lymph Node

Enlargement of a lymph node under this condition is due to any local or generalized antigenic response, which may include infection, inflammation, immune-mediated disease, or neoplasia from an area that drains into the lymph node. Histologically, lymphoid nodules within the cortex form prominent germinal centers that develop following antigen stimulation (Fig. 4-3A). A light and dark zone compose the germinal center. In addition to small lymphocytes, the center light zone contains reticular dendritic follicular cells, macrophages, and larger lymphoid cells (Fig. 4-3B). In benign hyperplasia, the dark zone or mantle cell cuff expands from proliferation of small B-lymphocytes that surround the pale portion of the germinal center with the thickest portion of the cuff at the apical end (see Fig. 4-3B). The hyperplastic germinal centers often demonstrate polarity (Fig. 4-3C) directed towards the antigen source, so that a dark mantle

Text continued on p. 83

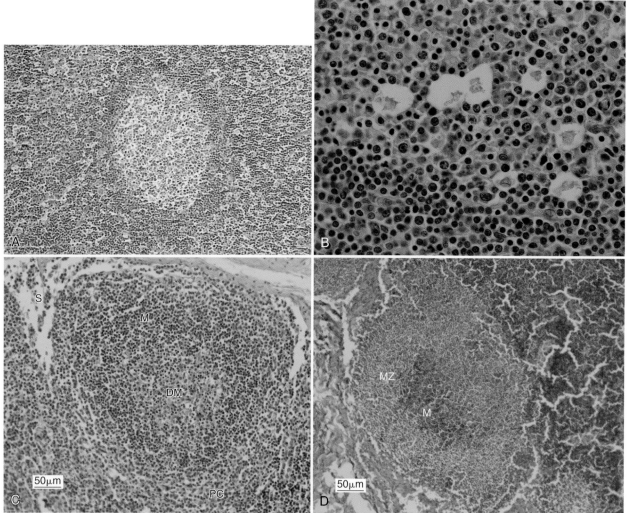

■ **FIGURE 4-3. A-B, Hyperplastic lymph node. Tissue section. Dog. A,** Prominent germinal center composed of two zones, a dark zone with a thin rim of small, dense lymphocytes (mantle cells) and a light middle zone composed of larger lymphocytes, dendritic cells, and macrophages. (H&E; IP.) **B,** Light zone of a germinal center is shown above the dark mantle cell layer. The light zone is composed of large lymphocytes, dendritic cells, and macrophages, the latter cell appearing as large, clear spaces with a shrunken cellular material. The mantle cells are small, round cells with scant cytoplasm and a dense chromatin pattern. (H&E; HP oil.) **C, Reactive lymph node, cortex. Tissue section. Dog.** Germinal center demonstrating polarity with subcapsular sinus *(S)* as the source of antigenic stimulation, cuff of small mantle B-lymphocytes *(M)*, middle area of dendritic cells and lymphophagocytic macrophages or tangible bodies *(DM)*, and an area containing plasma cells *(PC)* below the germinal center. (H&E; IP.) **Same case D-E. Hyperplastic lymph node. Tissue section. Dog. D,** Prominent light-colored marginal zone cuff *(MZ)* surrounds the fading germinal center with residual mantle cells *(M)* recognized by their dark, small cell appearance. (H&E; LP.)

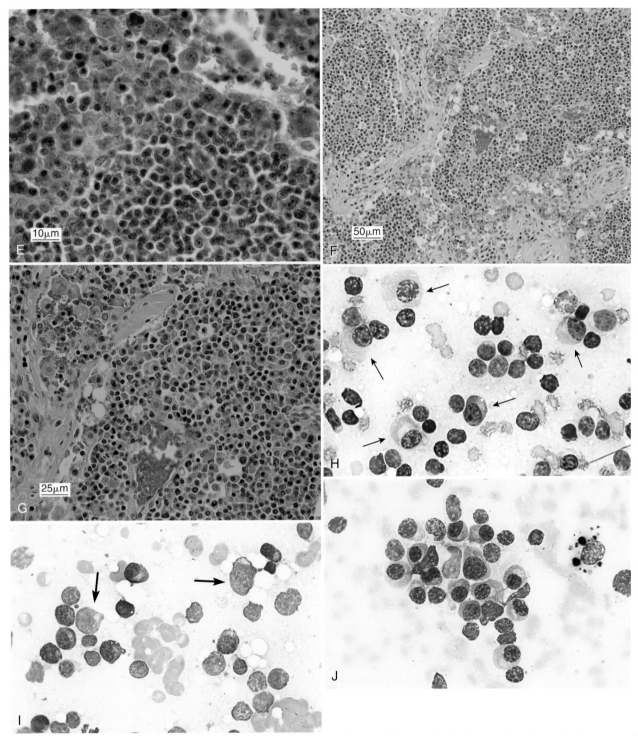

■ **FIGURE 4-3, cont'd. E,** Expanded marginal zone cells at the bottom frequently have vesicular chromatin and a single large, centrally located nucleolus. Note the lack of mitotic activity in this region. At the top is the medullary region filled with abundant macrophages, many of which contain a dark yellow pigment, presumed to be hemosiderin. (H&E; HP oil.) **F-G, Reactive lymph node. Tissue section. Dog. F,** Medullary cords filled with plasma cells and hemosiderin-laden macrophages are expanded and compressing the blood-filled sinuses between the cords. (H&E; IP.) **G,** Higher magnification of F. Medullary cords are filled with plasma cells readily identified by their eccentrically placed nucleus. (H&E; IP.) **H-I, Reactive lymph node. Tissue aspirate. Dog. H,** Many small lymphocytes are present along with several well-differentiated plasma cells *(arrows)*. Higher numbers of medium-sized lymphocytes than expected in normal lymph nodes are noted in the center. (Wright; HP oil.) **I,** Plasma cells are moderately increased in number and two appear shifted toward immaturity *(arrows)*. (Wright-Giemsa; HP oil.) **Same case J-K. J, Reactive lymph node. Tissue imprint. Dog.** Note the marked increase in plasma cell numbers composed of various degrees of differentiation. A hemosiderin-laden macrophage is present to the right of the field. (Aqueous-based Wright; HP oil.).

Continued

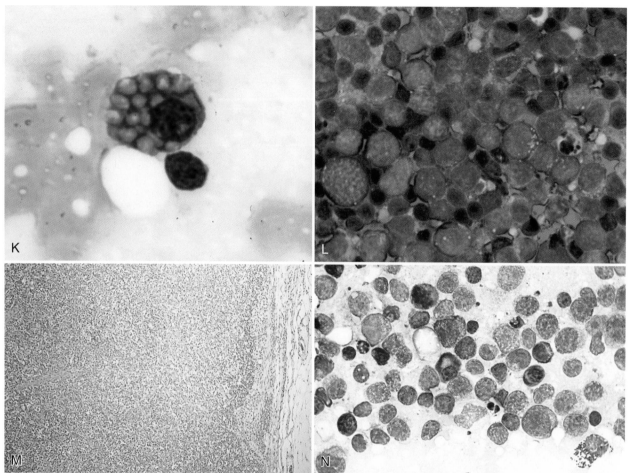

■ **FIGURE 4-3, cont'd. K, Mott cell. Tissue imprint. Dog.** This plasma cell from a reactive lymph node is highly activated with an abundant basophilic cytoplasm that contains multiple large, pale vacuoles. The vacuoles known as Russell bodies represent packets of immunoglobulin secretions. (Aqueous-based Wright; HP oil.) **L, Atypical lymphoid hyperplasia, lymph node. Tissue aspirate. Cat.** Aspirates from both submandibular lymph nodes were similar. This 10-year-old cat was recently treated for hyperthyroidism and presented with ulcerative stomatitis. The cat was otherwise clinically normal and tested negative for FeLV and FIV. The specimen contained a predominant population of medium and large lymphocytes with occasional plasma cells (not shown). It is presumed that this is a paracortical hyperplastic response related to the oral lesion. (Wright; HP oil.) **Same case M-N. M, Hyperplastic lymph node. Tissue section. Cat.** Peripheral node lymphadenopathy in this case is characterized by a paracortical expansion displacing normal lymphoid nodules and creating a homogenous appearance resembling lymphoma. At the right, a thin band of small, dark lymphocytes remains from the normal nodule. (H&E; LP.) **N, Reactive and hyperplastic lymph node. Tissue imprint. Cat.** This sample of prescapular lymph node contains a mixed population of small, medium, and large lymphocytes, plasma cells, and a mast cell (lower right). The majority of the lymphocytes are medium sized with moderately coarse chromatin and indistinct nucleoli. (Aqueous-based Wright; HP oil.)

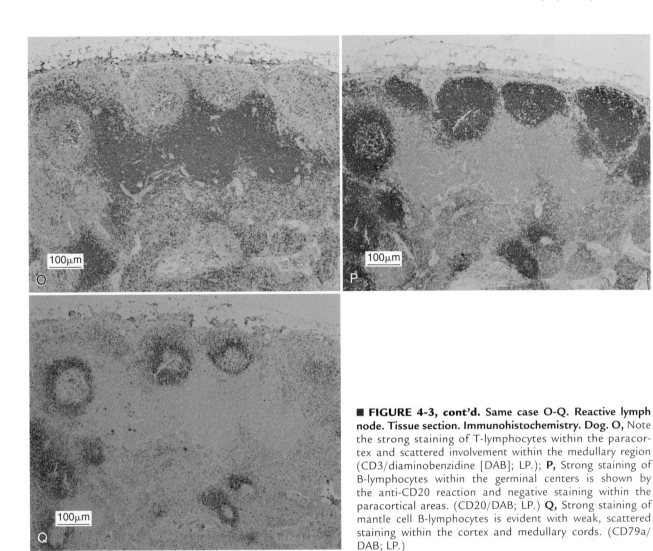

■ **FIGURE 4-3, cont'd. Same case O-Q. Reactive lymph node. Tissue section. Immunohistochemistry. Dog. O,** Note the strong staining of T-lymphocytes within the paracortex and scattered involvement within the medullary region (CD3/diaminobenzidine [DAB]; LP.); **P,** Strong staining of B-lymphocytes within the germinal centers is shown by the anti-CD20 reaction and negative staining within the paracortical areas. (CD20/DAB; LP.) **Q,** Strong staining of mantle cell B-lymphocytes is evident with weak, scattered staining within the cortex and medullary cords. (CD79a/DAB; LP.)

cell cuff is at one end (cortical) and a more pale group of large lymphocytes appears at the other end (medullary). The presence of follicular polarity helps distinguish follicular hyperplasia from follicular lymphoma (Valli, 2007). In contrast to the heterogeneity of the germinal centers, the nodules in follicular lymphoma contain a monomorphic population of neoplastic lymphocytes. The expanded follicles may press against the capsule, producing a thin mantle zone, but there is no destruction of the subcapsular sinus as occurs with lymphoma. With expanded hyperplasia, marginal zone cells that surround the mantle cell cuff may increase in number producing a heterogeneous population that expands into the paracortical region and mixes with resident T-lymphocytes (Fig. 4-3D). Sampling these areas cytologically displays cell size variability without a marked increase in plasma cells. The marginal zone cells are unique in their appearance with a medium cell size (nucleus about 1.5 times the erythrocyte diameter) and abundant cytoplasm contributing to the lighter color on histopathology. Marginal zone cells may be transformed to have marginated chromatin and contain a single large, centrally located nucleolus, but mitotic activity is low despite the immaturity of these cells (Fig. 4-3E). Specialized paracortical blood

vessels termed *high endothelial venules* in view of their cuboidal or rounded nucleus increase in prominence and number. The T-lymphocytes from circulating blood enter the paracortex transmurally through these venules. Retention of these venules between follicles helps distinguish histologically paracortical hyperplasia from lymphoma in which they may be incorporated within the nodular or follicle-like neoplasia. In response to antigenic stimulation, plasma cells move from the paracortex and accumulate within the medullary cords (Fig. 4-3F&G), where they produce antibodies.

Cytologically, small lymphocytes predominate in reactive or hyperplastic lymph nodes, but there is an increase (>15%) in medium and/or large cell types of the total cell population (Fig. 4-3H). Plasma cells are mildly to markedly increased in number and may be shifted toward immaturity (Fig. 4-3I&J). Some highly activated plasma cells, termed *Mott cells,* are characterized by abundant cytoplasm filled with multiple large, spherical, pale vacuoles that represent immunoglobulin secretions known as *Russell bodies* (Fig. 4-3K). Macrophages, neutrophils, eosinophils, and mast cells also may mildly increase in response to antigen stimulation; however, these cells occur in lower numbers than expected for lymphadenitis.

During early antigenic stimulation before germinal centers have developed, the paracortex responds with expansion and crowding of the cortex (Fig. 4-3L). Paracortical hyperplasia may precede plasma cell proliferation, and two weeks may pass before the appearance of prominent germinal centers. During this time, aspirate smears may contain a variably sized lymphoid population without significant numbers of plasma cells.

A benign condition in young cats has been reported (Moore et al., 1986; Mooney et al., 1987) in which peripheral lymph nodes show marked enlargement that histologically resembles lymphoma (Fig. 4-3M). Cells may be primarily medium and large lymphocytes with low numbers of small lymphocytes and plasma cells (Fig. 4-3N). High endothelial venules are prominent in the paracortex in this condition (Valli, 2007). These cases generally regress spontaneously in 1 to 17 weeks (Mooney et al., 1987). In one study, the majority of cats were feline leukemia virus (FeLV) positive and 1 of 14 cats progressed to lymphoma (Moore et al., 1986). Generalized lymphadenopathy is known to occur in cats infected with feline immunodeficiency virus (FIV) and *Bartonella* sp. (Kordick et al., 1999).

Immunostaining of reactive lymph nodes demonstrates the paracortical expansion of T-lymphocytes (Fig. 4-3O) and the development of the germinal centers (Fig. 4-3P&Q).

Lymphadenitis

The predominant inflammatory cell population categorizes the type of inflammation in a lymph node.

Neutrophilic Lymphadenitis

Purulent or suppurative (Fig. 4-4A) lymphadenitis involves greater than 5% neutrophils and may be associated with bacterial (Fig. 4-4B&C), neoplastic, or immune-mediated conditions.

Eosinophilic Lymphadenitis

Greater than 3% eosinophils of the nucleated cell population are often related to flea bite hypersensitivity, feline eosinophilic skin disease (Fig. 4-5A), hypereosinophilic syndrome, and paraneoplastic syndrome for mast cell tumor (Fig. 4-5B), as well as certain lymphomas (Thorn and Aubert, 1999) and carcinomas (Fig. 4-5C).

Histiocytic or Pyogranulomatous Lymphadenitis

Inflammation of the lymph nodes may involve increased numbers of macrophages, which is termed *histiocytic lymphadenitis* (Fig. 4-6A), or involve a mixture of neutrophils and macrophages, referred to *pyogranulomatous lymphadenitis* (Fig. 4-6B), even though a granuloma is best appreciated on histologic sections. Conditions associated with these inflammatory responses include systemic fungal infections, other fungal infections (Walton et al., 1994) (Fig. 4-6C), mycobacteriosis (Grooters et al., 1995), leishmaniasis, salmon

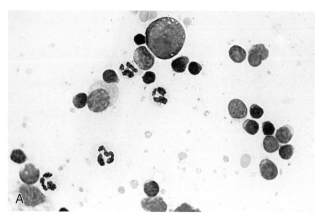
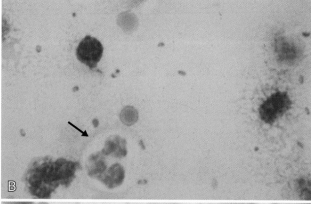
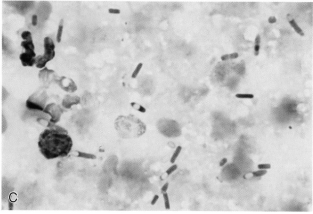

■ **FIGURE 4-4. A, Neutrophilic lymphadenitis. Tissue aspirate. Cat.** Four nondegenerate neutrophils are present along with small and medium lymphocytes. One large lymphocyte is also noted. (Wright; HP oil.) **B, Septic suppurative lymphadenitis. Tissue aspirate. Cat.** Bipolar coccobacillus bacteria confirmed as *Yersinia pestis* are present extracellularly adjacent to a degenerate neutrophil *(arrow)*. (Wright-Giemsa; HP oil.) **C, Septic suppurative lymphadenitis. Tissue imprint. Dog.** The history included a dog fight 2 months prior to the present lymphadenomegaly. Most of the lymphoid cells are necrotic and appear as amorphous basophilic material. Note two intact degenerate neutrophils and one small lymphocyte. Large bacilli with subterminal and terminal swellings are numerous in the background, which culture confirmed as *Clostridium* sp. (Wright-Giemsa; HP oil.) (B, Photo courtesy of Kyra Royals et al, Colorado State University; presented at the 1996 ASVCP case review session.)

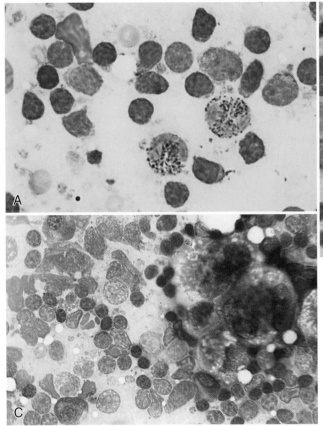

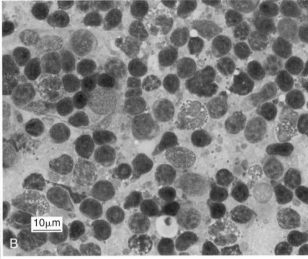

■ **FIGURE 4-5. A-C, Eosinophilic lymphadenitis. A, Tissue aspirate. Cat.** Two eosinophils are shown within a population of small lymphocytes from an animal with a rodent ulcer of the mouth. (Wright-Giemsa; HP oil.) **B, Tissue aspirate. Dog.** Submandibular lymph node is examined for evidence of spread from a mast cell tumor on the nose. The lymphoid population is predominately small with low numbers of intermediate lymphocytes. Frequent eosinophils are present but no evidence of metastatic tumor is found. (Wright; HP oil.) **C, Tissue imprint. Dog.** Small lymphocytes predominate along with increased numbers of medium lymphocytes and eosinophils. On the right is a cluster of pleomorphic epithelium from an animal with metastatic transitional cell carcinoma found within the sublumbar lymph node. (Wright-Giemsa; HP oil.)

fluke poisoning disease (Fig. 4-6D&E), prototheosis (Fig. 4-6F&G), pythiosis, vasculitis (Fig. 4-6H–J), and hemosiderosis (Fig. 4-6K&L) (see Fig. 4-3G). The systemic fungal diseases include blastomycosis (Fig. 4-6M), cryptococcosis (Lichtensteiger and Hilf, 1994) (Fig. 4-6N), histoplasmosis (Fig. 4-6O), and coccidioidomycosis.

Metastasis to the Lymph Node

Metastasis is suggested by the presence of a cell population not normally expected in a lymph node, which for epithelial cells is relatively easier to detect because of their large cell size and clustered appearance (Fig. 4-7A&B). These foreign cells often appear larger than surrounding lymphocytes and abnormal, displaying several cytologic features of malignancy (Fig. 4-7C). Histologically, metastasis to the lymph node may occur at the peripheral sinus or medullary sinuses related to lymphatic spread (Fig. 4-7D).

Mesenchymal-appearing neoplasms are most difficult to recognize because of their individualized cell presentation. The presence of anaplastic round to spindle-shaped cells in a lymph node aspirate can support a diagnosis of malignancy (Desnoyers and St-Germain, 1994). Tumors such as melanoma may be easily confused with hemosiderin-laden macrophages (Grindem, 1994) (see Fig. 4-6K) related to the dark blue-black granules. Hemosiderin granules tend to be variable in size, large, and coarse compared

with melanin granules that are small and finely granular (Fig. 4-7E). Cytochemical staining may be necessary to distinguish the two, such as Fontana stain for melanin and Prussian blue for iron (Fig. 4-7F). Furthermore, immunochemistry may be helpful in amelanotic cases that lack visible granules (Fig. 4-7G) using markers such as S-100, Melan-A (Fig. 4-7H), and others (see Chapter 17).

Metastatic hematopoietic neoplasms such as granulocytic leukemia cause mild to moderate lymphadenomegaly. The cell population appears mixed (Fig. 4-7I) and dysplastic cells or granulated precursors may be present (Fig. 4-7J). In some cases myeloblasts may be indistinguishable from lymphoid precursors (Fig. 4-7K) and cytochemical staining for granulocytic origin may be indicated (Fig. 4-7L). Well-granulated mast cells may appear in low numbers, up to 6 per slide in clinically healthy dogs (Bookbinder et al., 1992), but increased cell numbers and the appearance of poorly granulated mast cells suggest metastasis (Fig. 4-7M&N). The presence of eosinophils, especially in the dog, suggests degranulation and release of histamine. Lymphoid malignancies originating from the bone marrow or solid tissue sites such as the spleen or gastrointestinal tract (Fig. 4-7O) may be easily recognized in lymph nodes when cells are granulated (Goldman and Grindem, 1997). The immunophenotypic features of feline large granular lymphocytes (LGL)

Text continued on p. 88

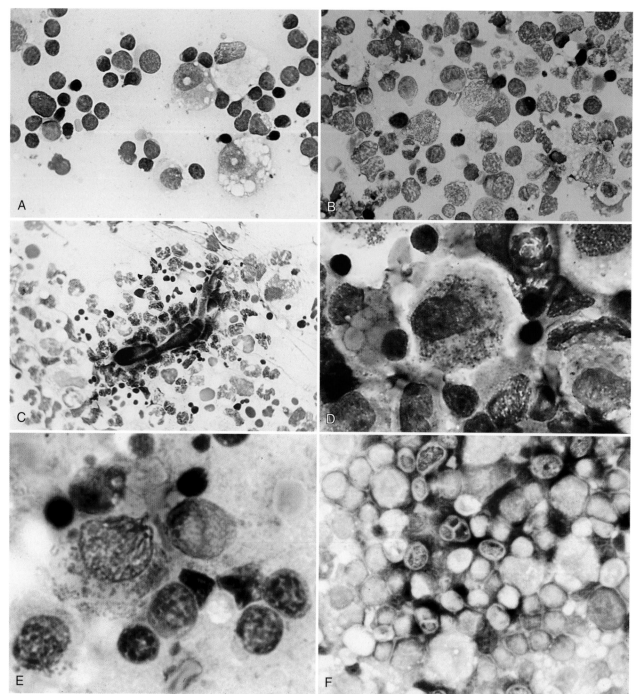

■ **FIGURE 4-6. A, Histiocytic lymphadenitis. Tissue aspirate. Cat.** Several macrophages are present along with small and medium-sized lymphocytes. (Wright; HP oil.) **B-C, Pyogranulomatous lymphadenitis. Tissue aspirate. Dog. B,** Numerous macrophages and neutrophils appear among a mixed population of lymphocytes. (Wright-Giemsa; HP oil.) **C,** A mixed inflammatory cell infiltrate of degenerate neutrophils and macrophages is shown from an inguinal lymph node draining a mass on the digit. Note the septate fungal hyphae with bulbous appearance that was confirmed by culture as *Fusarium* sp. (Wright-Giemsa; HP oil.) **Same case D-E. Salmon fluke poisoning disease. Dog. D, Peripheral lymph node aspirate.** Numerous small basophilic granules are shown within a macrophage infected with *Neorickettsia helminthoeca*. (Romanowsky; HP oil.) **E, Lymph node aspirate.** Lymph nodes display increased numbers of medium lymphocytes and plasma cells in addition to the inflammatory response. Note the rickettsial organism within the macrophage. (Romanowsky; HP oil.) (Case material courtesy of Jocelyn Johnsrude) **F-G, Protothecosis. Dog. F, Colonic lymph node imprint.** Several round to oval structures are present that measure approximately 6 to 10 μm in length. These endospores have a basophilic granular cytoplasm and thin, clear cell wall. Note the sporulated forms with multiple endospores. (Aqueous-based Wright; HP oil.)

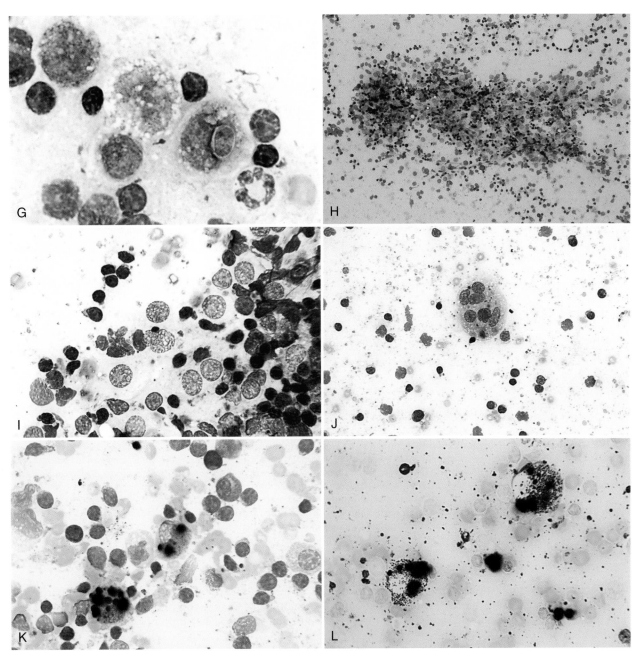

■ **FIGURE 4-6, cont'd. G, Lymph node imprint.** Note the single endospore engulfed by a macrophage. (Aqueous-based Wright; HP oil.) **Same case H-J. H, Histiocytic lymphadenitis with prominent vascular elements. Submandibular lymph node aspirate. Dog.** Several aggregates of fibrohistiocytic elements surrounding blood vessels are noted in this lymph node draining an inflamed skin mass. Histopathology supported the clinical diagnosis of an immune-mediated disease by finding lymphoplasmacytic and suppurative vasculitis in several subcutaneous tissues. (Wright-Giemsa; IP.) **I-J, Histiocytic lymphadenitis. Tissue aspirate. Dog. I,** Higher magnification displays a cohesive mass of large mononuclear cells having abundant clear cytoplasm. Small lymphocytes are present in the background. (Wright-Giemsa; HP oil.) **J,** Multinucleated giant cells were present in low numbers in this generalized histiocytic proliferation within the lymph node. Mixed lymphoid cell population is noted in the background. (Wright-Giemsa; HP oil.) **Same case K-L. K, Histiocytic lymphadenitis with hemosiderosis. Lymph node aspirate. Dog.** Numerous hemosiderin-laden macrophages are shown, characterized by large, coarse, black granules. The background contains several small dark granules consistent with hemosiderin. The lymphoid cell population is mixed, which is consistent with immune stimulation. A malignant neoplasm was previously diagnosed in this area drained by this submandibular lymph node. (Aqueous-based Wright; HP oil.) **L, Hemosiderosis. Lymph node aspirate. Cytochemistry. Dog.** Iron stain demonstrates a large amount of coarse, blue-black, granular material both intra- and extracellularly. Note the small, positively stained granules in the background. (Prussian blue; HP oil.)

Continued

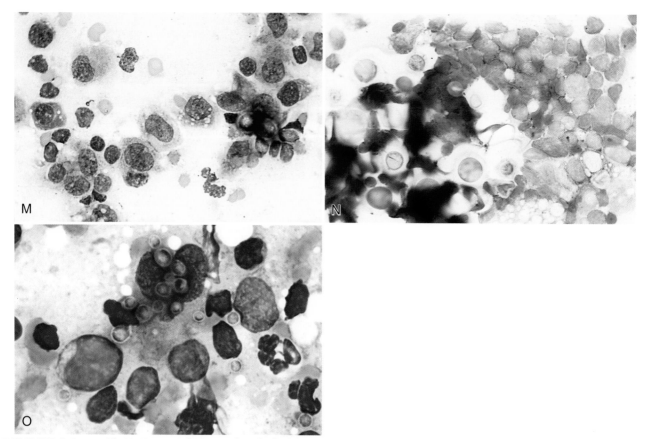

■ **FIGURE 4-6, cont'd. M, Pyogranulomatous lymphadenitis with blastomycosis. Tissue aspirate. Dog.** Two round basophilic yeast structures are surrounded by a mixed inflammatory response, including macrophages, degenerate neutrophils, small and medium lymphocytes, and plasma cells. (Wright; HP oil.) **N, Histiocytic lymphadenitis with cryptococcosis. Lymph node aspirate. Cat.** A subcutaneous mass behind the ear is present in this animal. A periauricular lymph node demonstrates numerous encapsulated yeast forms, consistent with *Cryptococcus* sp. Note the lymphocytes in the background with few inflammatory cells present. (Wright-Giemsa; HP oil.) **O, Pyogranulomatous lymphadenitis in histoplasmosis. Lymph node aspirate. Cat.** Several intracellular small, oval yeast forms are present within a macrophage. Extracellular yeast structures are also found, including a mixed population of lymphoid cells and degenerate neutrophils. (Aqueous-based Wright; HP oil.) (D, Case material courtesy of Jocelyn Johnsrude; F, Case material courtesy of Karyn Bird et al, Texas A&M University; presented at the 1988 ASVCP case review session; G, Photo courtesy of Peter Fernandes.)

are similar to the small intestinal intraepithelial lymphocytes and hence may be the site of origin of this lymphoma in cats. In dogs, by contrast, the spleen is the site of origin (Roccabianca et al., 2006). The prognosis is poor for cats with LGL lymphoma, with median survival in treated animals of 57 days (Krick et al., 2008). Metastases from sarcomas are often difficult to discern among the normal fibrohistiocytic elements. However, angiosarcomas have distinctive, large, individualized cells that may be prominent against the small lymphocytes (Fig. 4-7P).

Inflammation may accompany metastasis to lymphoid tissue, with eosinophils most commonly present as a paraneoplastic syndrome in canine mast cell tumors (Fig. 4-7Q) or some carcinomas (see Fig. 4-5C). Neutrophils commonly occur with squamous cell carcinoma and may involve bacterial sepsis. The remaining lymphoid population often appears immune stimulated, with cell types present as described under Reactive or Hyperplastic Lymph Node. Early in the disease process, metastatic lesions will usually involve a small proportion of the entire cell population, usually less than 50%. In some cases, often late in the disease, the metastatic

neoplasm may replace the lymph node parenchyma completely so as to interfere with the cytologic recognition of the tissue as lymph node (Fig. 4-7R–U).

Primary Neoplasia

These tumors originate from the lymph node and usually involve the lymphocyte population; rarely vascular tumors arising from the lymph node have been reported. HogenEsch and Hahn (1998) described eight hemangiomas and one lymphangioma, mostly in the popliteal lymph node of aged dogs from a research colony, which were found as incidental lesions at postmortem.

Lymphoma

Lymphoma is a very common spontaneous neoplasm in dogs and cats. One study found an incidence of 103 cases within a pet population of 130,684 insured dogs in the United Kingdom (Edwards et al., 2003). Within this population boxers had significantly higher relative risks compared with other breeds. The other breeds with increased relative risk included basset hound, St. Bernard,

Text continued on p. 93

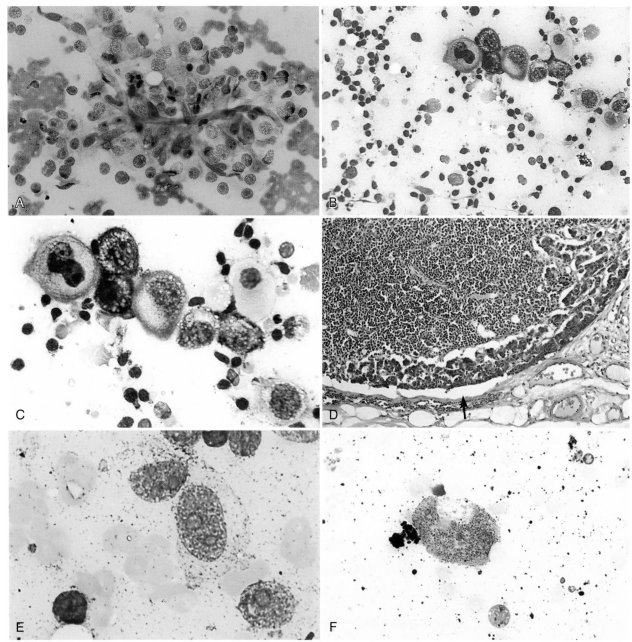

■ **FIGURE 4-7. A, Metastatic renal carcinoma. Lymph node aspirate. Dog.** An aggregate of capillaries are entwined around the malignant epithelial population. (Wright-Giemsa; HP oil.) **Same case B-C. Metastatic squamous cell carcinoma. Lymph node aspirate. Dog. B,** A sheet of neoplastic squamous epithelium is surrounded by numerous small lymphocytes. (Wright-Giemsa; HP oil.) **C,** Higher magnification demonstrates the marked pleomorphism of the nuclei, coarse chromatin staining, and multiple, prominent, variably sized nucleoli. (Wright-Giemsa; HP oil.) **D, Metastatic carcinoma. Lymph node. Tissue section. Dog.** Neoplastic population has infiltrated the cortex beginning at the subcapsular sinus region *(arrow)*. (H&E; IP) **E-F, Metastatic melanoma. Lymph node aspirate. Dog. E,** Fine black granules define the cell of origin. Prominent multiple nucleoli are also noted. Small lymphocytes are present in the background. (Aqueous-based Wright; HP oil.) **F, Cytochemistry.** An iron stain helps to distinguish positive-staining background hemosiderin from a nonstaining cell containing melanin granules. Hemorrhage is often present in metastatic lesions. (Prussian blue; HP oil.)

Continued

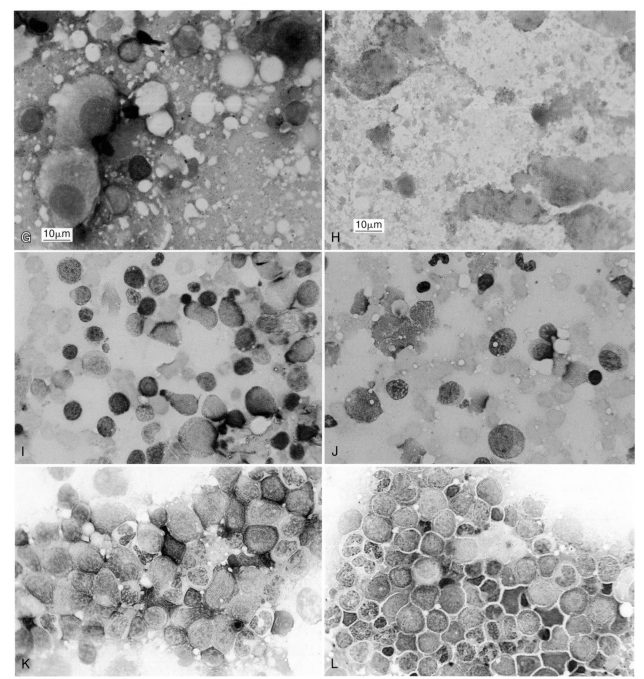

■ **FIGURE 4-7, cont'd. Same case G-H. Metastatic amelanotic melanoma. Lymph node aspirate. Cat. G,** Multiple masses on the leg and back with metastasis to regional lymph nodes. Shown are three large, poorly differentiated melanoma cells with prominent nucleoli against a background of small and medium lymphocytes. (Wright; HP oil.) **H, Immunocytochemistry.** The cytoplasm of several large neoplastic cells with prominent nucleoli is positive for Melan-A, a sensitive marker for melanin. A few small lymphocytes are unstained. (Melan-A/AEC; HP oil.) **Same case I-J. Granulocytic leukemia. Lymph node aspirate. Dog. I,** A mixed cell population is present, with many large irregularly shaped cells. (Wright-Giemsa; HP oil.) **J,** Small granules are present in the granulocytic precursor in the cell at bottom of the field. Note the hyposegmented Pelger-Huet-type neutrophils at the top, indicating morphologic abnormalities in that cell line. (Wright-Giemsa; HP oil.) **Same case K-L, Granulocytic leukemia. K,** Prescapular lymph node aspirate. **Dog.** Numerous large granulocytic precursors are present with irregularly shaped nuclei. (Wright-Giemsa; HP oil.) **L, Lymph node aspirate. Cytochemistry. Dog.** Cytochemical staining is positive for this granulocytic marker. (Chloroacetate esterase; HP oil.)

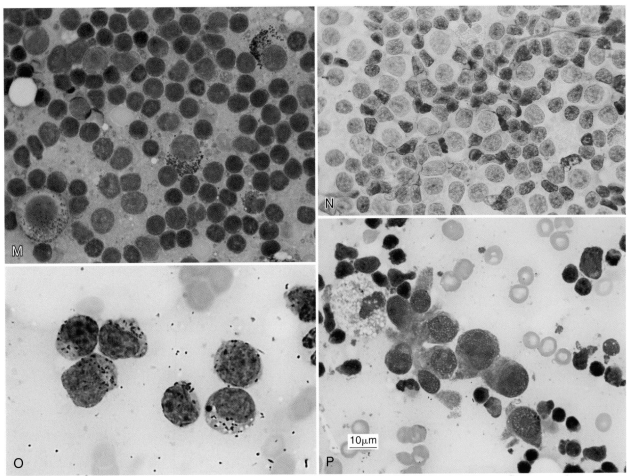

■ **FIGURE 4-7, cont'd. M-N, Metastatic mast cell tumor. Lymph node aspirate. M, Dog.** Three mast cells and one eosinophil are shown in this submandibular lymph node draining an ulcerated mast cell tumor on the muzzle. These mast cells are moderately differentiated having prominent nucleoli and minimal granulation. The surrounding lymphoid cells are predominately small lymphocytes. (Wright; HP oil.) **N, Cat.** Note the poorly granulated, round cells among the small lymphocytes, suggesting a poorly differentiated mast cell tumor. (Aqueous-based Wright; HP oil.) **O, Metastatic large granular lymphoma. Intestinal lymph node aspirate. Cat.** Nearly all cells present in this lymph node are medium sized with moderately basophilic cytoplasm containing prominent purple granules. (Wright-Giemsa; HP oil.) **P, Metastatic angiosarcoma. Popliteal lymph node aspirate. Dog.** Several large, individualized pleomorphic cells are surrounded by the normal lymphoid population of mostly small lymphocytes. The original hock mass was removed 9 months earlier but now the leg is swollen with evidence of metastasis to the draining lymph node. (Wright; HP oil.)

Continued

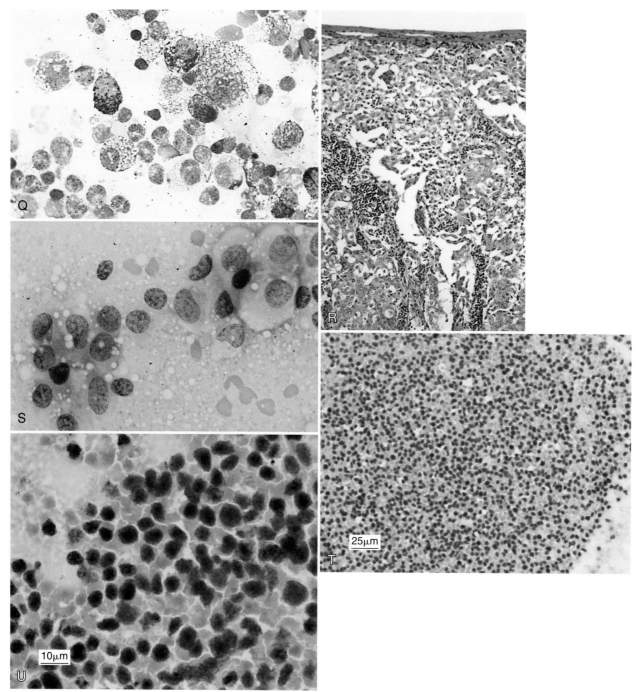

■ **FIGURE 4-7, cont'd. Q, Eosinophilic lymphadenitis. Tissue aspirate. Dog.** Numerous eosinophils are present along with several mast cells displaying variable degrees of degranulation and pleomorphism in an animal with a mast cell tumor. (Aqueous-based Wright; HP oil.) **Same case R-S. R, Metastatic islet cell tumor. Gastric lymph node. Tissue section. Dog.** There is nearly complete effacement of the lymph node by an expansion of neoplastic cells. Note the remaining small, dark-staining lymphocytes at left center. (H&E; IP.) **S, Metastatic islet cell tumor. Gastric lymph node imprint. Dog.** Clusters of intact cells are occasionally found, with most cells present resembling those on the left side, having naked nuclei with indistinct cell borders, typical of endocrine tissue. (Wright-Giemsa; HP oil.) **T-U, Metastatic neuroblastoma. Iliac lymph node aspirate. Dog. T,** Under low magnification, the cytologic preparation appears highly cellular with many individualized cells suggestive of lymphoid cells. (Wright; IP.) **U,** Higher magnification of material from case in T. Cells appear to have more abundant pink cytoplasm than expected for lymphocytes and there is moderate anisokaryosis. The loss of crisp nuclear features is related to necrosis occurring within this lymph node. The lack of cytoplasmic borders supports a naked nuclei appearance to the metastatic neoplasm. The primary neoplasm was found during an abdominal exploratory in which a large mass located beneath the lumbar spine incorporated the vena cava, kidney, and part of the pancreas. The mass was diagnosed as neuroblastoma in this 1.5 year old boxer. (Wright; HP oil.) (R-S, Case material courtesy of Robin Allison et al, Colorado State University; presented at the 1998 ASVCP case review session.)

Scottish terrier, Airedale terrier, bulldog, Labrador retriever, Bouvier des Flandres, and Rottweiler (Edwards et al., 2003). Others with observed increased risk include Golden retrievers and bull mastiffs.

Primary neoplasia most often involves the lymphocytes of the lymph node and is termed *lymphoma* (formerly termed *lymphosarcoma*). It is generally recognized as lymphadenomegaly (Fig. 4-8A). The predominant neoplastic cell in dogs and cats is usually a medium or large immature lymphocyte; however, the cat may display a small cell lymphoma within the alimentary tract (Twomey and Alleman, 2005). Medium-sized or large lymphocytes often compose >50% of the total cells in lymphoma (Fig. 4-8B). An exception is the infrequent presentation of a T-cell–rich B-cell lymphoma in which reactive T lymphocytes represent the majority of the cell population. A report by Steele et al. (1997) demonstrated by using immunohistochemistry that a parotid mass in a cat contained low numbers of large, atypical B-cells among many small reactive T-lymphocytes.

A micrometer such as an erythrocyte is used to determine the size of the lymphocytes present (Fig. 4-8C). The nucleus of a small, medium, and large canine lymphocyte is 1 to 1.5, 2 to 2.5, and > 3 times a red blood cell (RBC) diameter, respectively (Box 4-1).

Within the background of the preparation are lymphoglandular bodies (see Fig. 4-8C) that result from the rupture of lymphocytes and appear as small platelet-sized basophilic cytoplasmic fragments. Although they may be seen in benign lymph node conditions, a higher frequency is expected in lymphoma because of the immaturity and fragility of these cells. Lysed nuclei may appear as lacy, amorphous eosinophilic material (see Fig. 4-8B&C).

The population is often homogenous (Fig. 4-8D&E), although early in the disease there may be incomplete effacement of the lymph node. When cell populations are mixed, including different cell sizes present such as small and large lymphocytes, the diagnosis of lymphoma may require additional procedures. Surgical removal and

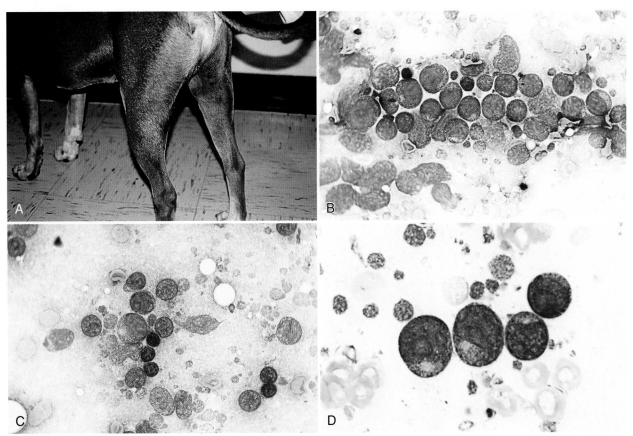

■ **FIGURE 4-8. A-C, Lymphoma. Dog. A,** Popliteal lymph node enlargement. **B, Lymph node aspirate.** B-cell, high grade. Centroblastic, monomorphic subtype. Medium and large lymphocytes compose 60% to 90% of the total cells in this B-cell, high-grade, monomorphic subtype of the centroblastic category in the Kiel classification. (Wright-Giemsa; HP oil.) **C, Lymph node aspirate.** A micrometer such as the erythrocyte at the top of the field is used to determine the size of the lymphocytes present. Note the three dark-staining, small lymphocytes in the center along with two intact medium and one intact large lymphocyte. Basophilic cytoplasmic fragments termed *lymphoglandular bodies* and pink remnants of lysed nuclei surround the intact cells. (Wright-Giemsa; HP oil.) **D, Lymphoglandular bodies. Lymph node aspirate. Dog.** Prominent basophilic round structures of variable size indicate fragmentation of the cytoplasm. This appearance is often associated with lymphoma but may be found in other conditions having fragile cells. (Wright-Giemsa; HP oil.)

Continued

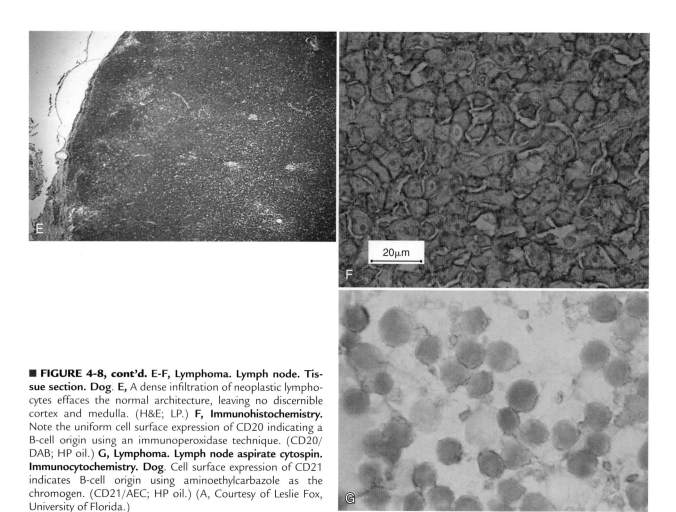

■ **FIGURE 4-8, cont'd. E-F, Lymphoma. Lymph node. Tissue section. Dog. E,** A dense infiltration of neoplastic lymphocytes effaces the normal architecture, leaving no discernible cortex and medulla. (H&E; LP.) **F, Immunohistochemistry.** Note the uniform cell surface expression of CD20 indicating a B-cell origin using an immunoperoxidase technique. (CD20/DAB; HP oil.) **G, Lymphoma. Lymph node aspirate cytospin. Immunocytochemistry. Dog.** Cell surface expression of CD21 indicates B-cell origin using aminoethylcarbazole as the chromogen. (CD21/AEC; HP oil.) (A, Courtesy of Leslie Fox, University of Florida.)

histologic examination of the lymph node is recommended in all equivocal cases to make a definitive diagnosis and classify the cell type of lymphoma for treatment and prognostic purposes. Clinical staging, particularly involving the blood, bone marrow, or miscellaneous sites (stage V), has prognostic importance for time to relapse following a complete remission and survival time (Teske et al., 1994).

Immunophenotyping the lymphoma into B-cell and T-cell types has been shown to assist in prognosis of canine lymphomas (Teske et al., 1994; Ruslander et al., 1997). Antibodies against antigens (e.g., CD20, CD21, CD79a, BLA.36) may be used to determine B-cell origin (Fig. 4-8F&G) (Jubala et al., 2005) while those against CD3, CD4, CD8 are useful for T-cell neoplasms. Chapter 17 expands on the methodology and application of leukocyte immunophenotyping. In one study, B-cell types involved 76%, T-cell types involved 22%, and null cells involved 2% of the canine lymphoma cases (Ruslander et al., 1997). In this same report, dogs with T-cell lymphomas were at significantly higher risk of relapse (52 vs. 160 days) and early death (153 vs. 330 days) compared with B-cell lymphomas following therapy. However, other studies (Chiulli et al., 2003; Ponce et al., 2004) demonstrated that while the T-cell phenotype was associated in general with a poor prognosis, significant prognostic

differences were evident within the B- and the T-cell subtypes of canine lymphoma. Therefore B-cell types are not always "Best" and T-cell types are not always "Terrible." These studies support the use of a clinicomorphologic characterization of the disease in dogs, similar to the current hematopoietic neoplasm classification scheme for humans, which is based on clinical presentation, immunophenotype, anatomic site, morphology, cytogenetics, and clinical aggressiveness (Jaffe et al., 2001). An updated edition for the World Health Organization (WHO) classification of hematopoietic neoplasms is expected soon (Swerdlow et al., 2008). Description of some of the veterinary WHO subtypes shown in Table 4-2 may be found in textbooks and articles (Fry et al, 2003; Cienava et al., 2004; Valli et al., 2006; Valli, 2007).

Immunophenotyping is necessary initially to characterize the type of lymphoma and may be accomplished through a variety of techniques. Canine and feline lymphoid neoplasia may be immunophenotyped by flow cytometry including use of fine-needle aspirates (Dean et al., 1995; Ruslander et al., 1997; Grindem et al., 1998; Culmsee et al., 2001; Gibson et al., 2004), or by immunostaining of tissue sections (Teske et al., 1994; Fournel-Fleury et al., 1997a; Vail et al., 1998; Kiupel et al., 1999, Fournel-Fleury et al., 2002), or by immunostaining of cytologic preparations obtained by fine-needle aspiration

BOX 4-1 Cytologic Protocol and Terms Used to Evaluate Lymphoma Cases

- Determine the cell size based on comparison of the nucleus to the size of an erythrocyte.
    - Small: 1-1.5 3 RBC
    - Medium: 2-2.5 3 RBC
    - Large: .3 3 RBC
- Determine the shape of the nucleus and its placement within the cytoplasm.
    - Round: Circular with no indentations
    - Irregularly round: Few indentations or convolutions
    - Convoluted: Several deep indentations
    - Clefted: Single deep indentation
    - Central vs. eccentric placement
- Determine the number, size, visibility, and location of nucleoli within the neoplastic lymphocytes.
    - Single vs. multiple
    - Large vs. small
    - Indistinct: Not visible or barely perceivable
    - Prominent: Easily visible
    - Central vs. marginal or peripheral placement
- Describe the cytoplasm by amount and color. Be sure to note presence of Golgi zone or granulation.
    - Scant: Small rim around nucleus
    - Moderate size: Amount intermediate between scant and abundant
    - Abundant: Nearly twice the size of the nucleus
    - Pale: Light basophilia or clear
    - Moderate basophilia: Color intermediate between pale and dark blue
    - Deep basophilia: Royal blue or darker
- Estimate the mitotic index by looking at 5 cellular fields under 40× or 50× objectives.
    - Low: 0-1 mitotic figures per 5 fields
    - Moderate: 2-3 mitotic figures per 5 fields
    - High: >3 mitotic figures per 5 fields
- Tumor grade is morphologically based on cell size and mitotic index.
    - Low grade: Low mitotic index and small cell size
    - High grade: Moderate or high mitotic index and medium or large cell size

(Fisher et al., 1995; Caniatti et al., 1996). The study by Fisher et al. (1995) demonstrated an excellent correlation of immunophenotype between immunostained canine cytologic and histologic samples. From the evidence of several studies (Teske and van Heerde, 1996; Fournel-Fleury et al., 1997a; Ponce et al., 2004; Raskin, 2004), B-cell lymphomas accounted for approximately 60% of the cases, while T-cell types involve 40%. Neoplasms of natural killer cell origin are rarely encountered in veterinary medicine and are often considered by exclusion.

At times, conventional immunophenotyping falls short of determining cellular origin, particularly with immature cell populations. As an alternative, use of molecular methods such as PCR for antigen receptor rearrangement (PARR) to determine clonality and cellular origin have gained much favor (Vernau and Moore, 1999; Burnett et al., 2003; Avery, 2004). Readers should see Chapter 17 for further information on methodology and application in dogs and cats.

Morphologic appearance of the neoplastic cells has been used along with immunophenotype to further classify the lymphomas for prognostic value (Ponce et al., 2004). The classification scheme currently used is the modified or updated Kiel Classification (Lennert and Feller, 1992; Callanan et al., 1996; Teske and van Heerde, 1996; Fournel-Fleury et al., 1997a). Teske and van Heerde (1996) found the classification from needle-aspiration biopsies closely correlated to that from histologic samples. Classification into low and high grades of malignancy has been shown to have prognostic importance for canine lymphoma cases (Teske et al., 1994). High grade is morphologically defined as moderate or high mitotic index and a medium or large cell size (see Box 4-1). Use of this scheme indicates that the morphologic types of lymphoma with a high grade of malignancy are most frequently encountered in dogs.

Another prognostic indicator involves use of cell proliferation markers in histologic and cytologic specimens to evaluate active cell turnover. The most commonly

TABLE 4-2 Recognized Subtypes for Canine and Feline Lymphoid Malignancies Using the Current World Health Organization Classification

	B-Cell	T-Cell
Precursor	Lymphoblastic leukemia/lymphoma	Lymphoblastic leukemia/lymphoma
Mature	Lymphocytic lymphoma/CLL Prolymphocytic leukemia Mantle cell lymphoma Marginal zone lymphoma types Follicular lymphoma Lymphoplasmacytic lymphoma/ Waldenstrom macroglobulinemia Plasma cell neoplasms: myeloma, plasmacytoma Diffuse, large B-cell lymphoma Mediastinal (thymic) lymphoma Primary effusion lymphoma	Large granular lymphocytic leukemia/lymphoma Prolymphocytic leukemia Adult T-cell leukemia/lymphoma Hepatosplenic T-cell lymphoma Subcutaneous panniculitis-like lymphoma Mycosis fungoides/Sezary syndrome Peripheral T-cell lymphoma Enteropathy-type T-cell lymphoma Angioimmunoblastic T-cell lymphoma Anaplastic large cell lymphoma

used are mitotic index, percent positive for Ki-67 antigen, percent positive for proliferation cell nuclear antigen (PCNA), and argyrophilic nucleolar organizing regions (AgNOR) quantitation (Vail et al., 1996; Vail et al., 1997; Fournel-Fleury et al., 1997b; Kiupel et al., 1998; Kiupel et al., 1999; Dank et al., 2002; Hipple et al., 2003; Whitten and Raskin, 2004; Vajdovich et al., 2004; Bauer et al., 2007). Ki-67 recognizes an antigen expressed in all cell cycle phases except the resting stage (G0). PCNA increases during G1, becomes maximal at DNA synthesis (S), and decreases during G2, mitosis (M), and G0. Mitotic index reflects only the M phase. The most comprehensive marker appears to be AgNOR, which indicates proteins associated with loops of DNA involved in ribosomal RNA transcription. The quantity of AgNOR not only reflects the percentage of cells cycling but also it increases when the cell cycle is faster. AgNOR counts correlated well with tumor grade (Kiupel et al., 1998). Studies on AgNOR frequency and area parameters demonstrated significant predictive potential for remission and survival time in treated and untreated cases of

canine lymphoma (Vail et al., 1996; Kiupel et al., 1998; Kiupel et al., 1999). A later study found that use of nucleolar AgNOR counts may be more reliable prognostically than mean AgNOR or percent proliferative AgNOR counts for certain forms of canine lymphoid neoplasia (Whitten and Raskin, 2004).

B-Cell Neoplasms. Of dogs displaying a high grade of malignancy, the most common morphologic type, representing approximately half of all lymphoma cases, is the centroblastic form of B-cell lymphoma, as it is called in the updated Kiel classification. Centroblasts are medium to large cells that originate from the follicular areas. A monomorphic subtype is composed of greater than 60% centroblasts (see Fig. 4-8B). These cells have a round nucleus, fine chromatin pattern, and two to four small basophilic and prominent marginally placed nucleoli (Fig. 4-9A). The cytoplasm is scant to moderate and basophilic. Other follicular cell types such as centrocytes and immunoblasts may be present to a lesser extent.

Text continued on p. 100

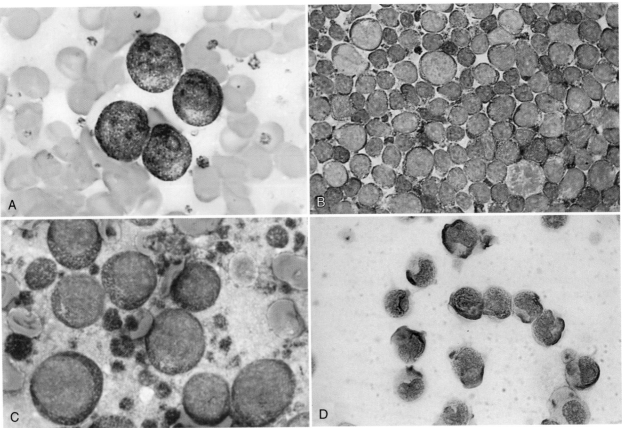

■ **FIGURE 4-9.** B-cell neoplasms. A-J, Diffuse large B-cell lymphoma. Dog. A-C, Lymph node aspirate. High grade, centroblastic. **A, Monomorphic subtype (Kiel).** These medium to large cells have a round nucleus, fine chromatin pattern, two to four small prominent, and generally marginally placed nucleoli. The cytoplasm is scant and deeply basophilic. Immunostaining was positive for CD21, CD79a, and IgG. (Wright-Giemsa; HP oil.) **B-C, Polymorphic subtype (Kiel). B,** This population contains an increased number of immunoblasts. Note the mitotic figure at the bottom of the field. Mitotic activity was high in this case. Immunostaining was positive for CD79a and IgG. (Wright-Giemsa; HP oil.) **Same case C-D. C,** A single prominent nucleolus can be seen in several cells. Numerous lymphoglandular bodies are present in the background. Immunostaining was positive for CD21, CD79a, and IgG. (Wright-Giemsa; HP oil.) **D, Lymph node aspirate cytospin preparation. Immunocytochemistry.** Immunostaining is positive as indicated by dark-brown granular staining within the cytoplasm. (IgG/DAB; HP oil.)

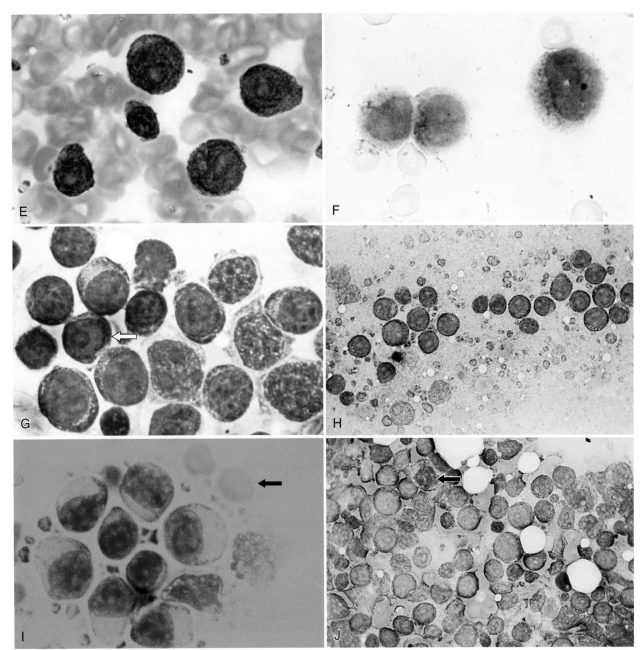

■ **FIGURE 4-9, cont'd. Same case E-F, J. B-cell neoplasms. E, Lymph node aspirate.** Several medium to large lymphoid cells are present, each containing one large centrally placed nucleolus. Immunostaining was positive for CD79a. (Wright-Giemsa; HP oil.) **F, Lymph node aspirate cytospin prep. Immunocytochemistry.** Immunostaining is positive as indicated by diffuse brown granular staining cytoplasmic staining. Note that this marker may show a nonspecific nuclear reaction which should not be considered as positive. (CD79a/DAB; HP oil.) **G, Lymph node aspirate. High grade, centroblastic, centrocytoid subtype (Kiel).** Several medium-sized cells are present that contain one or more nucleoli. A dense, small centrocyte *(arrow)* is seen to the left of a medium-sized centrocytoid cell that has a single large, centrally placed nucleolus. This centrocytoid cell sometimes has been referred to as a *macronucleated medium-sized cell*, which likely represents a cell from the marginal zone of the germinal follicle. Immunostaining was positive for CD21, CD79a, and IgG. (Wright-Giemsa; HP oil.) **H, Lymph node aspirate. High grade, centroblastic, centrocytoid subtype (Kiel).** In this subtype, medium-sized centrocytoid cells exceed 30% of the cell population. Immunostaining was positive for CD21 and CD79. (Wright-Giemsa; HP oil.) **I, Lymph node aspirate. High grade, centroblastic, centrocytoid subtype (Kiel).** The nuclei measure 1.5 to 2 times RBC diameter, indicating these are medium-sized lymphocytes. Compare the size of these cells against a faint-staining erythrocyte in the field *(arrow)*. The abundant cytoplasm in several cells produces a plasmacytoid appearance, which leads to the mistaken identification of these cells as immunoblasts, noting many have a single prominent, centrally placed nucleus present. (Wright-Giemsa; HP oil.) **J, Lymph node aspirate.** The population is predominantly composed of large lymphoid cells that have a single large, centrally placed nucleolus. A mitotic figure *(arrow)* is present at the top of the field. (Wright-Giemsa; HP oil.)

Continued

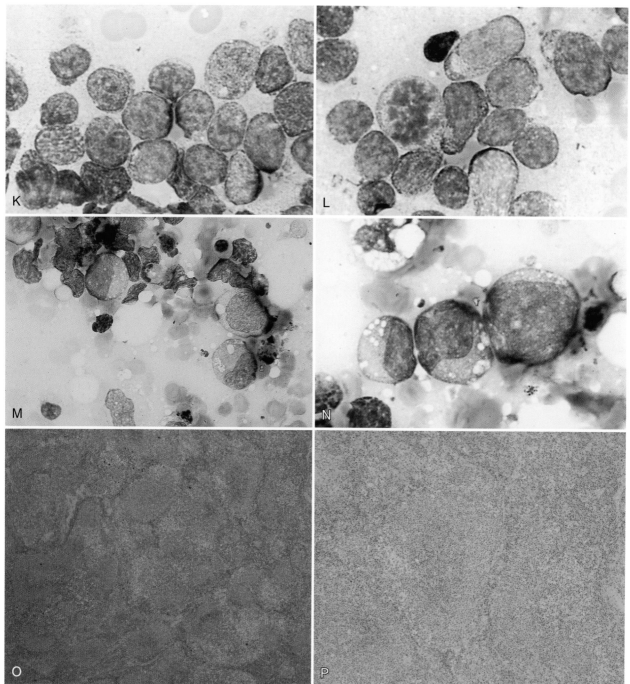

■ **FIGURE 4-9, cont'd. B-cell neoplasms. Same case. K-L. B-cell. Lymphoblastic lymphoma. Lymph node aspirate. Dog. K,** Cells are small to medium-sized with round nuclei measuring 1.5 to 2.5 times RBC diameter. Nucleoli are generally indistinct. The cytoplasm is scant and moderately basophilic. Immunostaining was positive for CD21 and CD79a. These cells were present in the bone marrow and spleen as well in this 7-year old cocker spaniel who survived only 29 days once diagnosed. (Wright-Giemsa; HP oil.) **L,** Mitotic activity is high for the lymphoblastic category. Note the small, dark-staining lymphocyte for size comparison. Most cells are medium sized with indistinct nucleoli and scant cytoplasm. (Wright-Giemsa; HP oil.) **Same case M-N. B-cell. Mediastinal lymphoma. Tissue aspirate. High grade, large cell anaplastic (Kiel). Dog. M,** Among the necrotic debris several large intact cells are found that have histiocytic features. This 3-year old Bassett hound was found to have a mediastinal mass with pleural fluid as well as lung and peripheral node involvement. Immunostaining was positive only for IgG. (Wright-Giemsa; HP oil.) **N,** Note the large, histiocytic-appearing cells with cytoplasmic vacuolation. Mitotic index was high (not shown) (Wright-Giemsa; HP oil.) **O-R, B-cell. Marginal zone lymphoma. Dog. Same case O-P. Mesenteric lymph node histologic section. O,** Multiple follicles are expanded with a loss of normal architecture. (H&E; LP.) **P,** A higher magnification of a single follicle is shown with remnant small, dense-staining mantle cells within the center of a pale proliferation of larger lymphoid cells. Note the poorly demarcated follicular margin with the expansion of malignant cells into the surrounding interfollicular areas compared with well-defined follicle with marginal zone expansion in Figure 4-3D. (H&E; LP.)

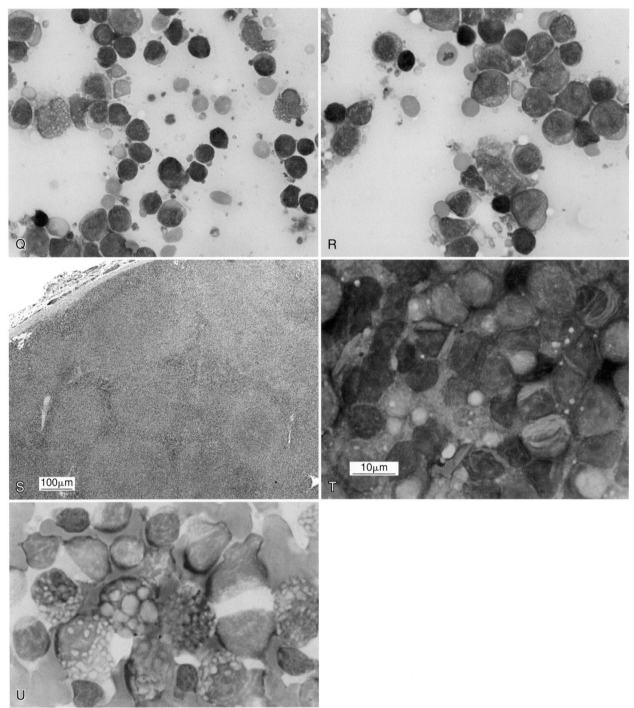

■ **FIGURE 4-9, cont'd. B-cell neoplasms. Same case Q-R. Mesenteric lymph node imprint**. **Q,** There is a mixed opulation of lymphoid cells, most of which are small in this field. The few remaining cells are medium lymphocytes, smudged cells, and cellular remnants in the background along with the low numbers of erythrocytes. (Wright-Giemsa; HP oil.) **R,** Another field in this case demonstrates an increased number of medium-sized lymphocytes, most of which contain a single large, prominent nucleolus and moderate amounts of basophilic cytoplasm consistent with the marginal zone cell. The remaining nucleated cells are small and medium lymphocytes having scant cytoplasm. (Wright-Giemsa; HP oil.) **S-U, B-cell. Lymphoplasmacytic lymphoma. Dog**. Same case S-T. **S, Inguinal lymph node histologic section.** Loss of normal lymph node architecture is indicated by expansive follicular areas having a uniform pale-staining appearance. This animal was clinically staged as IVa and had an indolent course of disease with more than 2 years survival despite the presence of a malignant clonal proliferation that was verified by PARR. (H&E, LP.) **T, Inguinal lymph node imprint.** A mixture of small and intermediate lymphocytes is present. Frequently observed within the cytoplasm are threadlike needle and splinter crystals, consistent with an atypical form of Russell bodies. Immunostaining was positive for CD21, CD45RA, and CD79a. (Wright-Giemsa; HP oil.) **U, Prescapular lymph node aspirate**. A mixture of small and intermediate lymphocytes is present, some of which appear plasmacytoid. Frequently observed within the cytoplasm are variably sized, coarse, pebble-like inclusions, consistent with an atypical form of Russell bodies. The animal was clinically staged as Vb and had an aggressive course of disease with survival of 49 days. These cells were present in other sites such as the kidney and rectum suggesting a widely disseminated lymphoma. (Wright; HP oil.)

A polymorphic subtype of the centroblastic category (Fig. 4-9B–D) contains an increased number of immunoblasts that account for greater than 10% and less than 90% of the cell population. Immunoblasts are large cells with abundant basophilic cytoplasm and a nucleus that measures at least three times the size of an erythrocyte. There is one large, centrally placed nucleolus (Fig. 4-9E) and immunophenotyping supports B-cell origin (Fig. 4-9F). Callanan et al. (1996) evaluated eight natural and experimental cases of FIV-associated lymphomas in cats, finding a high prevalence of B-cell types that, under the updated Kiel classification, relate to the centroblastic, polymorphic subtype in five of the eight cases.

A third subtype of the centroblastic category is termed *centrocytoid* because it is intermediate in size between the small centrocyte and the large centroblast (Fig. 4-9G). Generally the nucleus of this medium-sized cell contains two to five small, basophilic, centrally placed nucleoli. The cytoplasm is scant and moderately basophilic. In this subtype, centrocytoid cells should exceed 30% of the cell population. A unique-appearing cell type found in dogs and not recognized separately in human lymphoma cases resembles the centrocytoid cell except it contains only one large nucleolus instead of multiple nucleoli (Fig. 4-9G–I). This cell has been labeled *macronucleated medium-sized cell* (MMC) by Fournel-Fleury et al. (1997a), who suggest the cell arises from the marginal perifollicular zone. On the basis of low mitotic activity and low expression of the Ki-67 (Fournel-Fleury et al., 1997b), MMC was considered to have a low grade of malignancy. However, cases with a predominant MMC appearance clinically present in stages IV or V at the time of initial diagnosis. Therefore it may be more appropriate to place them in the high grade of malignancy category based on their aggressive clinical behavior and larger cell size compared with other cases having a low grade of malignancy. It is further possible that despite the low Ki-67 expression, the cell may have a short cell cycle length when evaluated using nucleolar-organizing regions.

Immunoblastic is another B-cell high-grade morphologic type that may be associated with the canine and feline follicular or diffuse large B-cell lymphomas (Fig. 4-9J). The morphologic categories of centroblastic and immunoblastic are derived from cells of the follicular germinal centers. These categories are frequently encountered, as shown in a canine study (Raskin and Fox, 2003) in which 30 of 62 lymphomas with these morphologies were diagnosed as *diffuse large B-cell lymphoma* (DLBCL) using the WHO classification. In this same study, prognosis of DLBCL defined as survival following diagnosis differed within this group based on clinical substaging. Those dogs without signs of illness (substage a) had an indolent course with a median of 314 days compared with those displaying signs of illness (substage b) having a highly aggressive course and only 24 days median survival.

Neoplastic B-lymphoid cells arising from precursor cells within the bone marrow may quickly spread to lymph nodes and appear as lymphoblastic lymphoma when evaluated in solid tissues (Fig. 4-9K&L). Cases of *B-lymphoblastic leukemia/lymphoma* had a highly aggressive course with a median of 48 days survival (Raskin and Fox, 2003).

An uncommon form of lymphoma thought to arise from thymic B-cells from the medulla of the thymus is *mediastinal B-cell lymphoma*. These masses are composed of large anaplastic cells (Fig. 4-9M&N) having a histiocytic appearance and high mitotic activity, but they can have long survival with chemotherapy.

A common but poorly recognized B-cell lymphoma arises from the marginal zone layer surrounding the germinal center. These *marginal zone lymphomas* are among the indolent forms of lymphoma (Valli et al., 2006) that are best diagnosed by histopathology (Fig. 4-9O&P). In a study of 9 cases in which follow-up data were available, median survival was 9 months. Cases most often involved lymph nodes only but several cases involved the spleen as well. Cytologically, a mixture of small and intermediate lymphocytes is found with an increased percentage of immature, intermediate-size lymphocytes, some with a single prominent nucleolus and others that appear more monocytoid (Fig. 4-9Q&R).

Another peripheral B-cell neoplasm with an indolent course is *lymphoplasmacytic lymphoma*. Cytologically, cells are similar to those in marginal zone lymphoma with a mixture of small and intermediate lymphocytes that often have plasmacytoid appearance. Needle-like stacks, thick splinters of immunoglobulin (Fig. 4-9S&T), or round (Fig. 4-9U) cytoplasmic inclusions have been recognized in a low percentage of these lymphoma cases.

T-Cell Neoplasms. Diagnostic testing should confirm T-cell origin with minimal immunostaining for the CD3 antigen (Fig. 4-10A). Additionally cytochemical staining for focal acid phosphatase reaction may be used (Fig. 4-10B). See Chapter 17 for more complete information on methodology and application of immunochemistry.

The boxer breed has been shown statistically to have a higher frequency of T-cell lymphomas than rottweilers or golden retrievers (Lurie et al., 2004).

Within the *peripheral T-cell lymphoma* category, the pleomorphic medium- and large-cell category is a common morphology and accounted for nearly 40% of all T-lymphoma cases evaluated in one study (Fournel-Fleury et al., 2002). Twelve of 30 cases with peripheral T-cell lymphoma in the above study presented with hypercalcemia, a common paraneoplastic condition with lymphomas of T-cell origin. This tumor is composed of medium, large, or mixed medium and large cells that display considerable nuclear pleomorphism (Fig. 4-10C–G). Often the nucleus is convex and smooth on one side while the opposite side is concave with many irregular indentations or serrations and may be described as cerebriform. Nucleoli are large and of variable shape and number. The cytoplasm is moderately abundant and moderately basophilic. A few eosinophils may be present within these lesions in people. A hand-mirror or single cytoplasmic extension called a uropod may be observed with T-lymphocytes (see Fig. 4-10D–F). In the human WHO classification most forms of nodal T-cell lymphomas fall into the peripheral T-cell lymphoma, unspecified category,

Text continued on p. 104

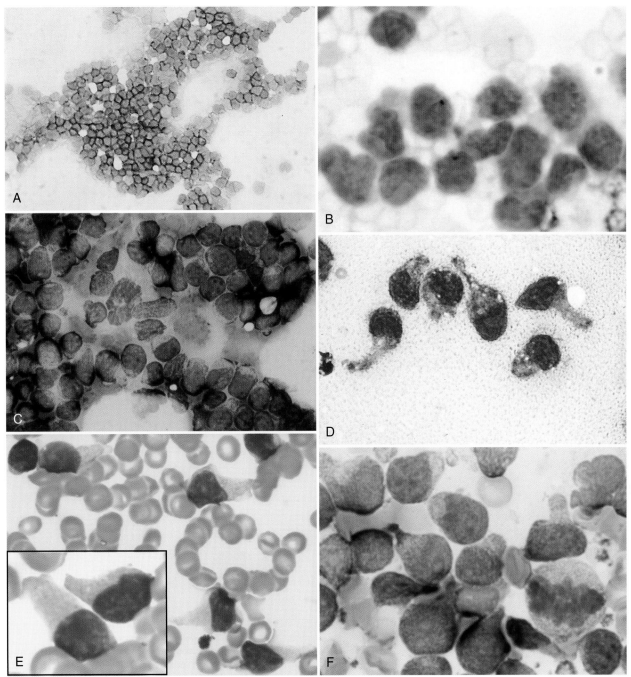

■ **FIGURE 4-10. T-cell neoplasms. A, Peripheral T-cell lymphoma. Lymph node aspirate cytospin. Low grade, T-zone lymphoma (Kiel). Immunocytochemistry. Dog.** A strong positive reaction is indicated by the brown cytoplasmic stain. (CD3/DAB; HP oil.) **B, T-cell lymphoma. Cytologic preparation. Cytochemistry. Dog.** A strong positive reaction is indicated by focal red staining that is associated with T-cells. (Acid phosphatase; HP oil.) **C-F, Peripheral T-cell lymphoma. High grade, pleomorphic medium/large cell subtype (Kiel). Dog. C-E, Lymph node aspirate. C,** Medium-sized lymphocytes predominate displaying nuclear pleomorphism. Note the irregular nuclear shape often having multiple indentations or serrations on one side. Chromatin is finely granular and nucleoli are prominent in the large lymphocytes. The cytoplasm is moderately abundant and lightly basophilic. Immunostaining was positive for CD3. (Wright-Giemsa; HP oil.) **D,** Animal also has cutaneous nodules, which appear similar cytologically, and on histopathology these lymphocytes infiltrate the epidermis. Cells display a hand-mirror shape with cytoplasmic pseudopods that extend in different directions. (Wright-Giemsa; HP oil.) **E,** Uropod formation is frequent in this sample with individual cells extended in different directions. Uropods are thought to help in binding the T-cells to other cells and permit release of cytoplasmic contents. *Inset:* The pale cytoplasm in this case demonstrates the presence of few fine granules. (Romanowsky; HP oil.) **Same case F-G. F, Lymph node cytologic preparation.** Notice the frequent serrated margins of the nuclei. This convoluted appearance of the nucleus is a distinctive morphologic feature of some T-cells. Nucleoli are also prominent in this case. (Wright-Giemsa; HP oil.)

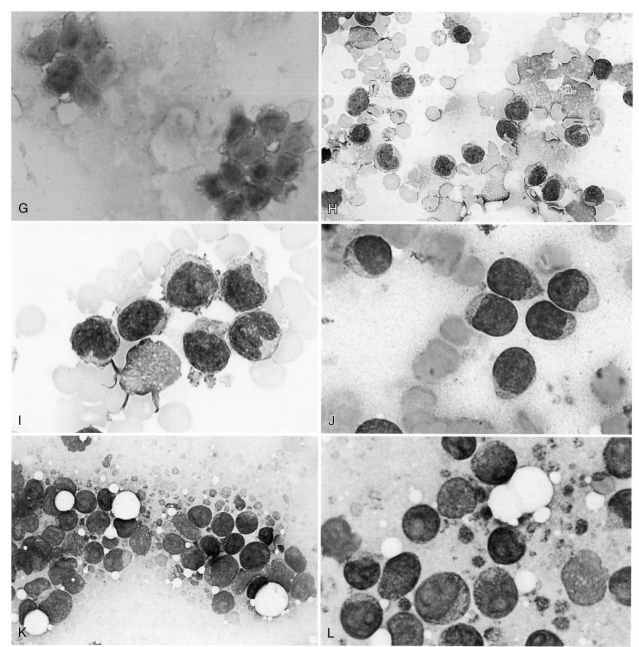

■ **FIGURE 4-10, cont'd.** T-cell neoplasms. **G, Peripheral T-cell lymphoma. Lymph node cytospin preparation. Immunocytochemistry. Dog.** The cell surface CD3 is expressed using aminoethylcarbazole reaction. These cells also expressed CD45RA, an isoform of CD45 which is found on some B-cells and nodal T-cell lymphomas. (CD3/AEC; HP oil.) **H-L, Peripheral T-cell lymphoma. Lymph node aspirate. Dog. Same case H-I. Low grade, Pleomorphic small cell (Kiel). H,** A relatively monomorphic population of small cells with scant gray cytoplasm. Immunostaining was positive for CD3. (Wright-Giemsa; HP oil.) **I,** The nucleus is characterized by a smooth surface on one side and serrations on the opposite side. (Wright-Giemsa; HP oil.) **J, Low grade, T-zone lymphoma (Kiel).** The tumor cells are small and monomorphic with small nucleoli. The nuclear surface is round to irregularly round without indentations. Immunostaining was positive for CD3. (Wright-Giemsa; HP oil.) **Same case K-L. High grade, T-cell immunoblastic (Kiel). K,** There are several large cells present, with a single large, centrally placed nucleolus. Immunostaining was positive for CD3. (Wright-Giemsa; HP oil.) **L,** Higher magnification to demonstrate the irregularly round nuclear shape and prominent nucleolus. The cytoplasm is moderately abundant and basophilic. (Wright-Giemsa; HP oil.)

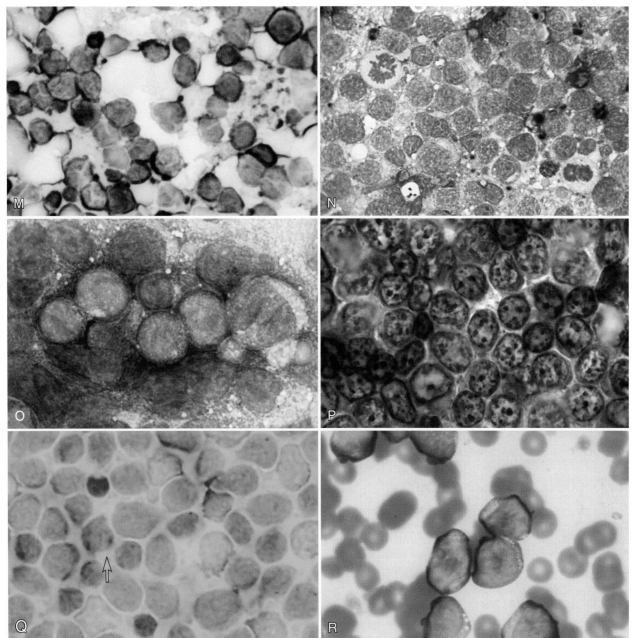

■ **FIGURE 4-10, cont'd. T-cell neoplasms. M, Peripheral T-cell lymphoma. Lymph node cytologic preparation. Immunocytochemistry. Dog.** A strong positive reaction for expression of CD45RA is indicated by the brown cytoplasmic stain. This 8-year old Shetland sheepdog was clinically staged as Vb and had an aggressive course of disease with 56 days of survival. There was disease involvement of the spleen and bone marrow in addition to the lymph nodes. (CD45RA/DAB; HP oil.) **N-Q, T-cell lymphoblastic lymphoma. Lymph node aspirate. Dog. N-P, High grade, Lymphoblastic (Kiel). N,** The number of mitotic figures often exceeds three per five fields at 40× or 50× objectives. Cells have scant cytoplasm and nucleoli that are indistinct. (Wright-Giemsa; HP oil.) **O,** The predominant cell population is medium sized with multiple convolutions of the nucleus. Nucleoli are indistinct. Immunostaining was positive for CD3 and CD8. (Wright-Giemsa; HP oil.) **P,** Use of a wet mount procedure easily demonstrates the round or irregularly round nuclear shape and the presence of small multiple nucleoli. (New methylene blue; HP oil.) **Q, Cytochemistry.** Note the prominent focal staining of some lymphocytes such as the one identified with an arrow. Most of the other lymphocytes have trace focal staining. (Acid phosphatase; HP oil.) **R, T-cell lymphoblastic lymphoma. Peripheral blood smear. Dog.** This 6-month-old English bulldog presented with anemia, thrombocytopenia, and marked leukocytosis (298,000/μl) of which most were immature lymphoid cells with irregularly round nuclei. Note the small, prominent nucleoli and fine chromatin within the nucleus. Besides the blood, involvement included the bone marrow and several peripheral lymph nodes. Clinical staging was Vb and the disease was highly aggressive with survival of 17 days following initial diagnosis. (Wright-Giemsa; HP oil.) (E, Case material courtesy of Harold Tvedten.)

including those with a small cell and low grade appearance, and immunoblastic appearance (Fig. 4-10H–L). Immunocytochemistry for the CD45RA isoform is often positive in nodal lymphomas (Fig. 4-10M), whereas T-cell lymphomas in the skin or mucosal sites are generally negative.

Other T-cell high-grade types that may be encountered include the lymphoblastic (Fig. 4-10N–R). The lymphoblastic type was associated with a mediastinal mass in 8 of 13 cases (Ponce et al., 2003) and a paraneoplastic syndrome of hypercalcemia with 4 of 13 cases (Ponce et al., 2003). The morphologic features of the lymphoblast involve a small to medium cell size with nuclei measuring 1.5 to 2.5 times RBC diameter. The nucleus may be round or convoluted and the nucleoli are small and indistinct, best appreciated with a new methylene blue wet mount (see Fig. 4-10P). The cytoplasm is often scant. Mitotic activity is high (see Box 4-1). Another diagnostic tool is cytochemical staining that is distinctive with a focal or dot appearance with alpha naphthyl acetate esterase, alpha naphthyl butyrate esterase, and acid phosphatase (Raskin and Nipper, 1992). Prognosis for this morphologic type is poor owing to renal failure, which results from the hypercalcemia or from the diffuse and expansive infiltration of the bone marrow (see Fig. 4-10R).

T-cell low-grade types are more frequent than B-cell low-grade types. They include mycosis fungoides or small cerebriform (see Fig. 3-50C–E) as well as pleomorphic small and T-zone lymphoma, using the Kiel classification (see Fig. 4-10H–J). Further immunostaining of cytologic specimens may demonstrate reactivity with antibodies against CD4 and/or CD8 (Fournel-Fleury et al., 2002).

EXTRAMEDULLARY HEMATOPOIESIS

Infrequently evidence for extramedullary hematopoiesis is found in the lymph node (Fig. 4-11). It is more likely to occur in animals having severe bone marrow disease, so hematopoietic activity in other organs such as the spleen, lung, or lymph node should not be unexpected.

CYTOLOGIC ARTIFACTS

In attempting to aspirate the submandibular lymph node, it is quite common to sample salivary gland tissue (Fig. 4-12A&B). The submandibular lymph node is found directly ventral from the prominent part of the zygomatic arch, which is behind and below the eye, midway between the eye and ear. The mandibular salivary gland is located within the bifurcation of the external jugular vein and is more posterior and dorsal to the lymph node (Fig. 4-12C).

SPLEEN

Indications for Splenic Biopsy

- *Splenomegaly* may be detected by palpation or by radiography and ultrasonography.
- *Abnormal imaging features* suggest the presence of hyperplasia or infiltrative processes.
- *Evaluation of hematopoiesis* may be indicated when bone marrow disease is present.

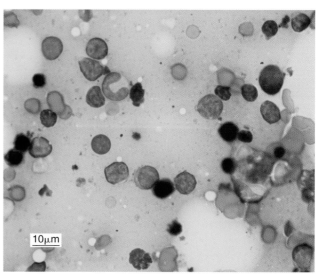

■ **FIGURE 4-11. Extramedullary hematopoiesis. Lymph node aspirate. Cat.** Among the small and medium-sized lymphocytes are variably sized, dense-staining erythroid precursors, some of which are closely associated with a macrophage displaying erythrophagocytosis. The CBC indicated pancytopenia with a hematocrit of 20% with lack of regeneration (i.e., polychromasia) in the blood smear. (Wright; HP oil.)

Aspirate Biopsy Considerations

Aspiration may be performed in cases of thrombocytopenia, but body movements should be minimized, either by manual restraint or sedation. The needle and syringe may be coated with sterile 4% disodium EDTA prior to aspiration to reduce the clotting potential of the specimen. A 1- to 1.5-inch, 21- or 22-gauge needle may be used alone or attached to a hand-held 12-ml syringe or aspiration gun. In some cases, it may be preferable to use a 2.5- to 3.5-inch spinal needle. The animal is placed in right lateral or dorsal recumbency and the area over the site is prepared surgically. The site is carefully determined by palpation or ultrasonography.

> **KEY POINT** The nonaspiration method of biopsy is preferred with vascular sites such as the spleen to reduce blood contamination and increase cellularity (LeBlanc et al., 2008).

Normal Histology and Cytology

The spleen is enclosed by a thick, smooth muscle capsule that extends inward as trabeculae. The splenic parenchyma is divided into white pulp and red pulp. The white pulp consists of dense, periarterial lymphatic sheaths and lymphatic nodules and the red pulp consists of erythrocytes contained within a reticular meshwork, within endothelial lined sinuses, or within blood vessels (Fig. 4-13A). The splenic artery enters the hilus of the spleen and branches into arteries that become the central arteries of the lymphatic sheaths. These vessels branch into pulp capillaries that are surrounded by concentric layers of macrophages within a reticular meshwork. The pericapillary macrophage sheaths, termed *ellipsoids*, are abundant in the marginal zone

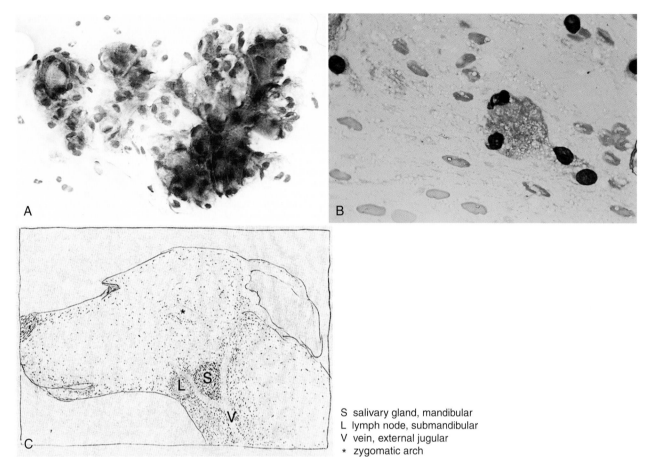

S salivary gland, mandibular
L lymph node, submandibular
V vein, external jugular
* zygomatic arch

■ **FIGURE 4-12. A-B, Salivary gland. Tissue aspirate. Dog. A,** Attempted aspirate of the submandibular lymph node resulted in the collection of epithelial clusters. (Wright-Giemsa; HP oil.) **B,** Individual salivary gland cell with abundant foamy basophilic cytoplasm. Free nuclei in the background are easily mistaken for small lymphocytes. Note the basophilic granular background consistent with mucin and the manner erythrocytes are caught in it resembling a string of cells. (Wright-Giemsa; HP oil.) **C, Diagram showing the location of the mandibular salivary gland and submandibular lymph node. Dog.** The asterisk (*) indicates the bony prominence of the zygomatic arch. The submandibular lymph node (L) is directly ventral or perpendicular to the arch. Note the more posterior and dorsal location of the mandibular salivary gland (S) located within the bifurcation of the external jugular vein (V).

surrounding periarterial lymphatic sheaths adjacent to the red pulp (Fig. 4-13B).

On cytology, aspirate preparations contain large amounts of blood contamination, as evidenced by many intact erythrocytes and platelet clumps. Lymphoid cells present are similar to those of the normal lymph node (see Fig. 4-2E). Small lymphocytes predominate with occasional medium and large lymphocytes present. A few macrophages and plasma cells may be seen along with rare neutrophils and mast cells. Macrophages may contain small amounts of blue-green to black granular debris, compatible with hemosiderin. Occasional groups of macrophages may be admixed with the reticular stroma representing the ellipsoids (Fig. 4-13C). In aged dogs, it is not uncommon to aspirate sidero-calcific plaques or nodules, also called Gamna-Gandy nodules, that lie along the splenic margins within the fibrous capsule. These firm, sometimes calcified, masses mostly contain a form of blood pigment either as hemosiderin (blue-black) or hematoidin (golden yellow) that may be found within the associated macrophages or extracellularly. They can result from previous hemorrhage as well as represent a senile change in dogs. Prussian blue staining will help determine the presence of hemosiderin while hematoidin that lacks iron will be negative.

Reactive or Hyperplastic Spleen

Grossly the reactive or hyperplastic spleen may present with nodular or diffuse enlargement. Lymphoid hyperplasia may result from antigenic reaction to infectious agents or the presence of blood parasites. Small lymphocytes still predominate but there is an increase in medium-sized and large lymphocytes. Macrophages and plasma cells are commonly observed (Fig. 4-14A). Frequent large collections of reticular stroma with increased numbers of mast cells may be observed at low magnification (Fig. 4-14B). Hemosiderosis may be present with large amounts of coarse, dark granules (Fig. 4-14C). Capillaries may be more commonly observed with increased endothelial elements in the spleen (Fig. 4-14D).

Another condition responsible for a nodular presentation and lymphoid hyperplasia in the canine spleen is fibrohistiocytic nodule. Within the firm, raised nodules are focal proliferations of spindle cells, macrophages, lymphocytes, and plasma cells (Fig. 4-14E–H). It is thought that these lesions represent a continuum between splenic

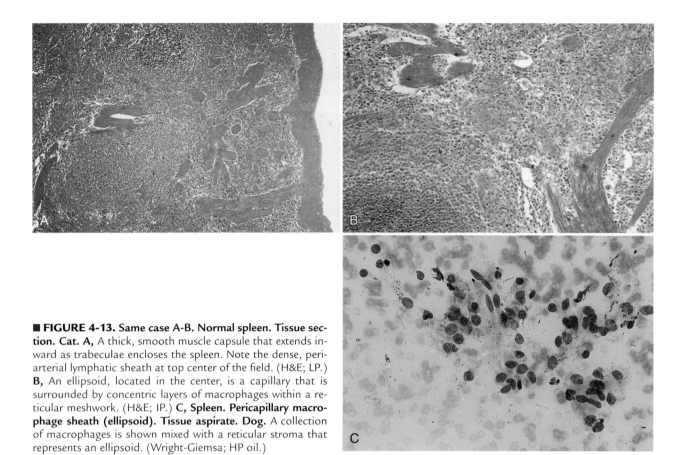

■ **FIGURE 4-13.** **Same case A-B. Normal spleen. Tissue section. Cat. A,** A thick, smooth muscle capsule that extends inward as trabeculae encloses the spleen. Note the dense, periarterial lymphatic sheath at top center of the field. (H&E; LP.) **B,** An ellipsoid, located in the center, is a capillary that is surrounded by concentric layers of macrophages within a reticular meshwork. (H&E; IP.) **C, Spleen. Pericapillary macrophage sheath (ellipsoid). Tissue aspirate. Dog.** A collection of macrophages is shown mixed with a reticular stroma that represents an ellipsoid. (Wright-Giemsa; HP oil.)

lymphoid nodular hyperplasia and malignant splenic stromal neoplasms (Spangler and Kass, 1998).

Splenitis

In addition to the macrophagic response associated with splenic hyperplasia, inflammatory cells will increase in number with other noninfectious or infectious causes of disease. Noninfectious causes such as malignancy or immune reaction can incite neutrophilic or eosinophilic infiltration (Thorn and Aubert, 1999) (Fig. 4-15A). The

diagnosis of splenitis must be made cautiously if circulating neutrophilia or eosinophilia are present. Macrophagic or histiocytic inflammation often occurs with the presence of systemic fungal infections such as histoplasmosis (Fig. 4-15B–D) or protozoal infections such as cytauxzoonosis (Fig. 4-15E) and leishmaniasis (Fig. 4-15F). Mild to moderate histiocytic hyperplasia may be associated with immune-mediated hemolytic anemia and immune-mediated thrombocytopenia as well as with other etiologies for hemolytic anemia (Christopher, 2003).

Text continued on p. 109

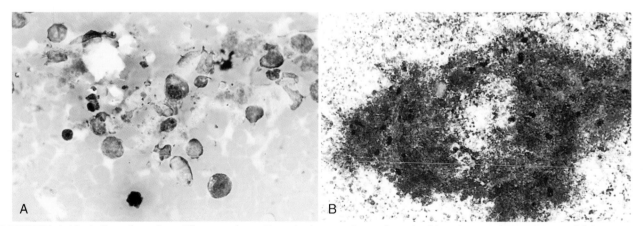

■ **FIGURE 4-14. A, Reactive spleen. Tissue aspirate. Dog.** An increase in medium-sized lymphocytes is present. In addition, several plasma cells are noted along with a macrophage. (Wright-Giemsa; HP oil.) **B-D, Hyperplastic spleen. Tissue aspirate. Dog. B,** This animal was being treated with chemotherapy for lymphoma. A very large aggregate of reticular stroma is shown dotted by an increased number of mast cells that appear as dark-purple cells evenly dispersed throughout. (Wright-Giemsa; IP.)

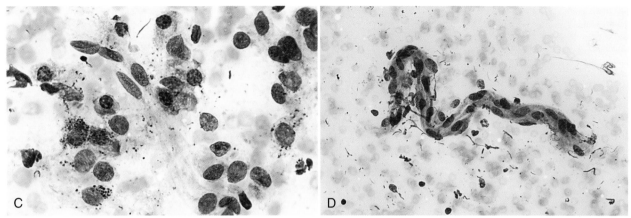

■ **FIGURE 4-14, cont'd. Same case C-D. C,** Hemosiderosis is recognized by the presence of hemosiderin-laden macrophages containing large amounts of coarse dark granules. (Wright-Giemsa; HP oil.) **D,** An endothelial-lined capillary is noted as a result of endothelial hyperplasia. (Wright-Giemsa; HP oil.)

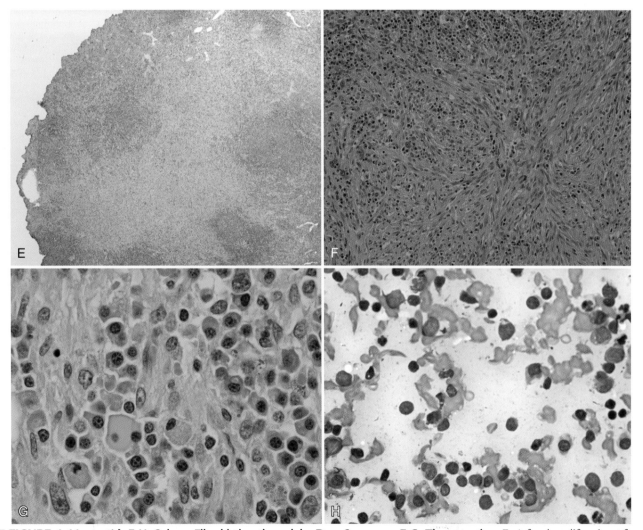

■ **FIGURE 4-14, cont'd. E-H, Spleen. Fibrohistiocytic nodule. Dog. Same case E-G. Tissue section. E,** A focal proliferation of eosinophilic connective tissue is shown placed between the multiple basophilic lymphoid follicles. The normal architecture is distorted by this proliferation of spindle cells. (H&E; LP.) **F,** There are intersecting dense bands of plump spindle cells and connective tissue with scattered basophilic lymphoid cells. (H&E; IP.) **G,** This is a close-up of the basophilic cellular areas that are composed primarily of numerous plasma cells, small lymphocytes, and few hemosiderin-laden macrophages. The background is composed of eosinophilic stroma. (H&E; HP oil.) **H, Tissue imprint.** The sample is cellular, composed of mostly small and medium lymphocytes with increased numbers of plasma cells against a hemodiluted background. Scattered plump, mononuclear cells are present, a few of which have indistinct cytoplasmic borders that resemble the spindle cells in the tissue sections. (Wright; HP oil.)

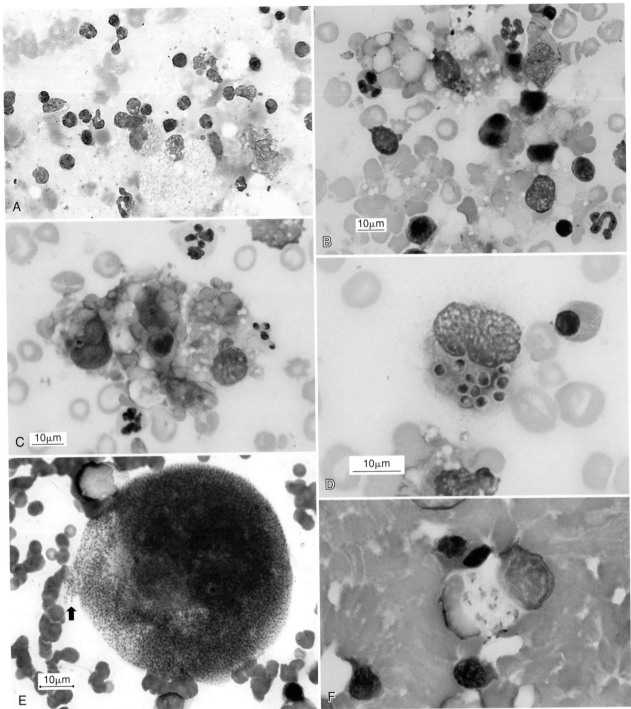

■ **FIGURE 4-15. A, Splenitis. Tissue aspirate. Dog.** Neutrophils, eosinophils, and activated macrophages compose the severe inflammatory response in this animal with a necrotizing splenitis. (Wright-Giemsa; HP oil.) **Same case B-D. Macrophagic splenitis. Histoplasmosis. Tissue aspirate. Dog. B,** A macrophage at the top contains yeast forms while a concurrent extramedullary erythropoiesis is present. Note the many rubricytes and metarubricytes along with polychromatophils. (Wright; HP oil.) **C,** The frequent erythrophagocytosis supports the presence of a hemophagic syndrome in light of the marked red cell destruction. This may occur with infection such as in this case. The hematocrit decreased to 12.5% during this period of infection. (Wright; HP oil.) **D,** Multiple oval yeast forms measuring approximately 3 × 2 μm are present within a macrophage. (Wright; HP oil.) **E, Cytauxzoonosis. Mature schizont. Cytologic preparation. Cat.** This mature schizont from the bone marrow involves a parasitized mononuclear phagocyte similar to those found lining the endothelium of splenic vessels. Imprints of affected tissues may reveal schizonts that have plugged blood vessels and represent the tissue phase of the infection. Along the edge the mature schizont shown are small, about 1 μm, merozoites *(arrow)* that will infect erythrocytes following release from the ruptured schizont. (Wright-Giemsa; HP oil.) **F, Macrophagic splenitis. Leishmaniasis. Tissue imprint. Dog.** Macrophage with engulfed protozoal organisms confirmed as *Leishmania* sp. Note the organism contains a small, round nucleus and a short, rod-shaped kinetoplast. Various stages of erythroid precursors support a diagnosis of extramedullary hematopoiesis. (Wright-Giemsa; HP oil.) (Photo courtesy of Cheryl Swenson and Gary Kociba, The Ohio State University; presented at the 1987 ASVCP case review session.)

Lymphoid Neoplasia

Differentiation between primary and metastatic neoplasia may not always be possible, especially if multiple organs are involved. To help distinguish between hyperplasia and neoplasia, a blast cell count above 40% is often indicative of splenic lymphoma as demonstrated by use of PARR for verification (Williams et al., 2006). Lymphoma will appear morphologically similar to that of the lymph node (Fig. 4-16A).

Marginal zone lymphoma may be recognized in the spleen with the appearance of a mixed cell population including those with a monocytoid appearance (Fig. 4-16B). In rare cases, PAS positive round cytoplasmic inclusions (Fig. 4-16C) may be seen in cases of marginal zone lymphoma as well as other forms of B-cell lymphoma. More often an increase or predominance of medium-sized lymphocytes with a single, large, centrally located nucleolus is found (Fig. 4-16D&E).

Granular lymphocytic leukemia is thought to originate from the spleen (McDonough and Moore, 2000; Workman and Vernau, 2003). The patient often presents with marked granular lymphocytosis in circulation that is present also within the spleen (Fig. 4-16F). The bone marrow is usually not infiltrated by the neoplastic population (Lau et al., 1999). Clinical signs are variable and progression of the neoplastic disease may be slow. Granules may be very small and difficult to see with use of aqueous-based Wright stains (Fig. 4-16G&H). Immunophenotyping of these neoplastic granular lymphocytes usually indicates positivity for CD3, CD8α, and CD11d antigens (Fig. 4-16I&J). Nonneoplastic conditions may produce a reactive granular lymphocytosis, which should first be ruled out.

A less common form of chronic lymphocytic lymphoma/leukemia of B-cell origin may be seen with an indolent course. Cells are uniform, being small with scant cytoplasm. Nuclei are round with moderately dense clumped chromatin (Fig. 4-16K). Monoclonal gammopathy may be associated with this leukemia in a low percentage of patients (Fig. 4-16L). These CD5-positive cells

Text continued on p. 112

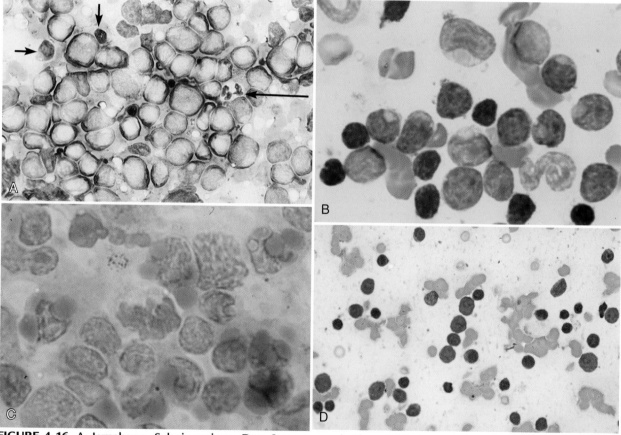

■ **FIGURE 4-16. A, Lymphoma. Splenic aspirate. Dog.** Same case as in Figure 9-26. A population of neoplastic lymphocytes was aspirated from an enlarged spleen. The neutrophil *(long arrow)* and small lymphocyte *(short arrows)* are useful cell micrometers. (Wright; HP oil.) **Same case B-C. Marginal zone lymphoma. Bone marrow aspirate. Dog. B,** This 5-year-old pit bull terrier presented with a late form of this lymphoma with dissemination to the spleen, liver, lymph nodes, blood, and bone marrow. Lymphoid cells are variable in size, some of which display monocytoid features. Several medium-sized lymphocytes have a pale blue-gray inclusion that appears to indent the nucleus. This dog was clinically staged as Vb but had an indolent course of disease with 162 days of survival. (Wright-Giemsa; HP oil.) **C, Cytochemistry.** The cytoplasmic inclusions stain positive indicating the presence of glycogen, consistent with immunoglobulin deposition. (PAS; HP oil.) **Same case D-E. Marginal zone lymphoma. Splenic imprint. Dog. D,** A mixed population of small and medium lymphocytes are present in the spleen. Same case as in Figures 4-9O-R. (Wright; HP oil.)

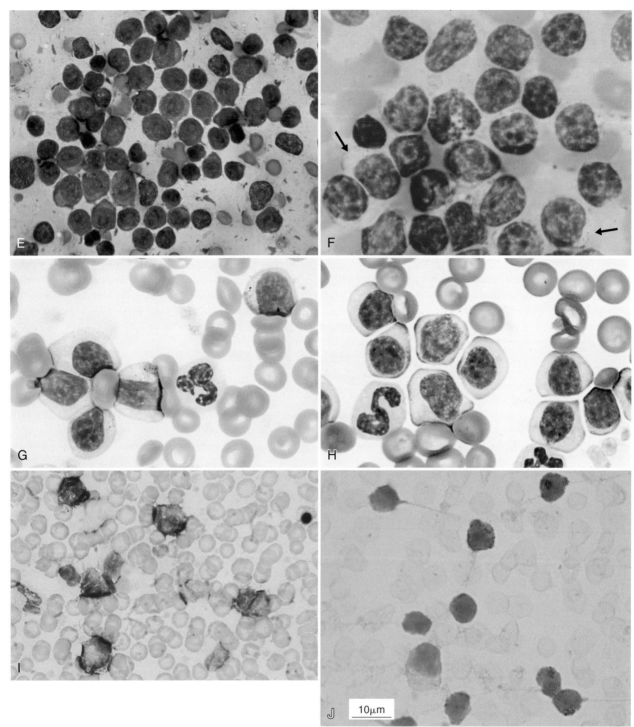

■ **FIGURE 4-16, cont'd. E,** Many of the medium lymphoid cells have a single, prominent, centrally located nucleolus. (Wright; HP oil.) **F, Granular lymphocyte lymphoma. Splenic aspirate. Dog.** One small lymphocyte and an eosinophil surrounded by a mono-morphic population of medium lymphocytes with clumped chromatin and moderately abundant clear cytoplasm. Some of the cells visibly contain several fine azurophilic granules that is best demonstrated by the cells indicated *(arrows)*. The spleen was considered to be the primary organ of involvement and stained with CD3, a T-cell marker. (Wright-Giemsa; HP oil.) **Same case G-J. Granular lym-phocyte leukemia. Blood smear. Dog. G,** The history involved 2 months of persistent lymphocytosis of counts exceeding 20,000/μl. Rickettsial infections were ruled out by titer tests. Note the typical abundant clear cytoplasm with small red granules arranged in a focal paranuclear manner. The bone marrow was not infiltrated by this cell population. (Wright-Giemsa; HP oil.) **H,** Use of this aqueous-base stain did not demonstrate the cytoplasmic granules. Alcohol-based Romanowsky stains are recommended. (Aqueous-based Wright; HP oil.) **I-J, Immunocytochemistry. I,** Same case and specimen as in G. Several lymphoid cells stain diffusely positive for the cell surface antigen. (CD8α/DAB; HP oil.) **J,** Several lymphoid cells stain positive in a focal to diffuse manner for leukocyte integrin CD11d, also called alpha D. These positive cells come from the red pulp region of the spleen. (CD11d/AEC; HP oil.)

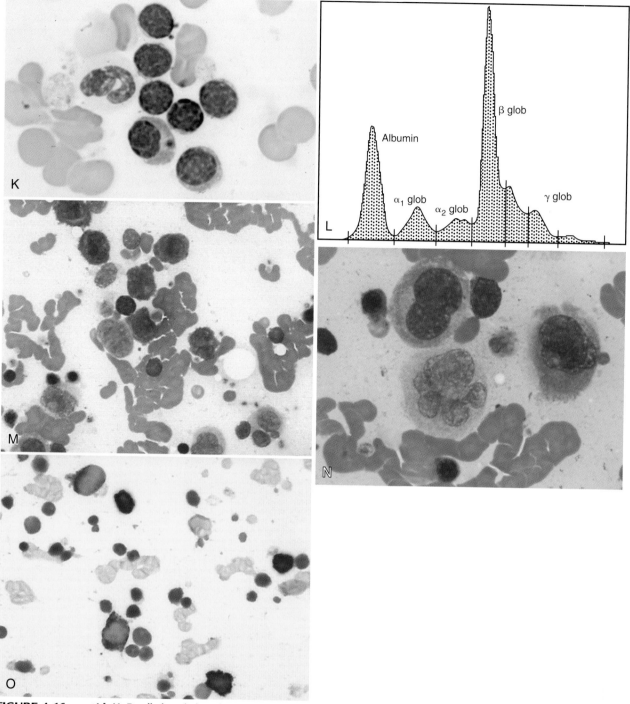

■ **FIGURE 4-16, cont'd. K, B-cell chronic lymphocytic leukemia/lymphoma. Bone marrow aspirate. Dog.** Both the bone marrow and spleen were involved in this case of a 13-year-old mixed breed dog with Va clinical staging. The neoplastic cells were uniformly round with generally scant cytoplasm, and a low mitotic index. Cells expressed CD79a, CD21, and sIg. This disease had an indolent course with 160 days of survival. (Wright-Giemsa; HP oil.) **L, B-cell chronic lymphocytic leukemia/lymphoma with paraproteinemia. Serum electro-phoresis scan. Dog.** Same case as in K. The densitometer scan indicates a monoclonal spike in the beta region indicative of IgA or IgM. Immunoelectrophoresis confirmed IgA production in the M-component. **Same case M-O. Diffuse large B-cell lymphoma, atypical variant. Cytologic preparation. Cat. M,** This animal had atypical and pleomorphic neoplastic cells in the spleen, liver, bone marrow, and abdominal fluid. Shown are several large cells measuring approximately 25 to 20 μm in diameter. Nuclei are highly lobulated and cells resemble histiocytic cells. (Wright-Giemsa; HP oil.) **N,** Notice the uneven lobulation. (Wright-Giemsa; HP oil.) **O, Immunocyto-chemistry.** Many of large, pleomorphic, neoplastic cells stain diffusely red indicating expression of CD79a, a marker for the B-cell receptor on the cell surface. (CD79a/AEC; HP oil.)

in people are thought to arise from follicular mantle cells or circulating naïve cells (Jaffe et al., 2001).

An uncommon presentation of splenic lymphoid neoplasia includes an anaplastic variant of diffuse large B-cell lymphoma. These cells are highly pleomorphic with variable nuclear shapes that may be mistaken for histiocytic neoplasia (Fig. 4-16M&N). The presence of CD79a expression supports the diagnosis of B-cell origin (Fig. 4-16O).

Non-Lymphoid Neoplasia

In the study by Day et al. (1995), hematoma occurred in six cases and nonspecific changes such as extramedullary hematopoiesis, congestion, and hemosiderosis occurred in 16 of 87 canine biopsies. Hemangiosarcoma was the most commonly diagnosed splenic neoplasm (Day et al., 1995), involving 17 of 87 canine splenic biopsies. Hemangiosarcoma cells are similar to those in other sites. Scattered large, mesenchymal-appearing cells may be found scanning on low magnification (Fig. 4-17A&B). Extramedullary hematopoiesis, chronic hemorrhage, and lymphoid reactivity may accompany the tumor. Neoplastic cells are large

with abundant cytoplasm having wispy, indistinct borders and. Frequently. multiple punctate vacuoles (Fig. 4-17C). The nucleus is round with coarse chromatin and multiple prominent nucleoli.

Other mesenchymal-appearing tumors in the canine spleen involve primarily fibrosarcoma, undifferentiated sarcoma (Fig. 4-17D), leiomyosarcoma, osteosarcoma, liposarcoma, myxosarcoma, and malignant fibrous histiocytoma (Spangler et al., 1994; Hendrick et al., 1992).

In cats, the most important cause of splenomegaly is mastocytoma, accounting for 15% of the total pathologic conditions submitted for diagnosis (Spangler and Culbertson, 1992). Diffuse enlargement of the spleen is detected on palpation or diagnostic imaging (Fig. 4-17E). Often a nearly pure population of highly granulated mast cells is present, several of which may display erythrophagocytosis (Fig. 4-17F). Other discrete cell tumors found in the spleen include myeloid leukemia, extramedullary myeloma or plasmacytoma (Fig. 4-17G), and histiocytic sarcoma (Fig. 4-17H&I). Splenic involvement of plasma cell myeloma with paraproteinemia was common in a

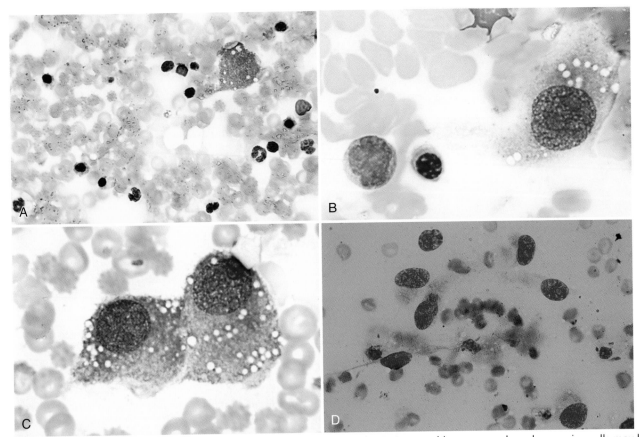

■ **FIGURE 4-17. Same case A-C. Hemangiosarcoma. Splenic aspirate. Dog. A,** Scattered large mesenchymal-appearing cells may be found scanning on low magnification such as the one shown. (Wright-Giemsa; HP oil.) **B,** Medium lymphocyte, rubricyte, and large malignant cell. Note the round nucleus with coarse chromatin, multiple large nucleoli, and vacuolated cytoplasm with indistinct cell borders. Extramedullary hematopoiesis and lymphoid reactivity are commonly found in this condition. (Wright-Giemsa; HP oil.) **C,** Multiple punctate vacuoles are commonly found in the stellate cells of this neoplasm. (Wright-Giemsa; HP oil.) **D, Poorly differentiated sarcoma. Splenic aspirate. Dog.** Mesenchymal-appearing cells with wispy cell borders, round to oval nuclei, coarse chromatin, anisokaryosis, and prominent nucleoli are present. (Wright-Giemsa; HP oil.)

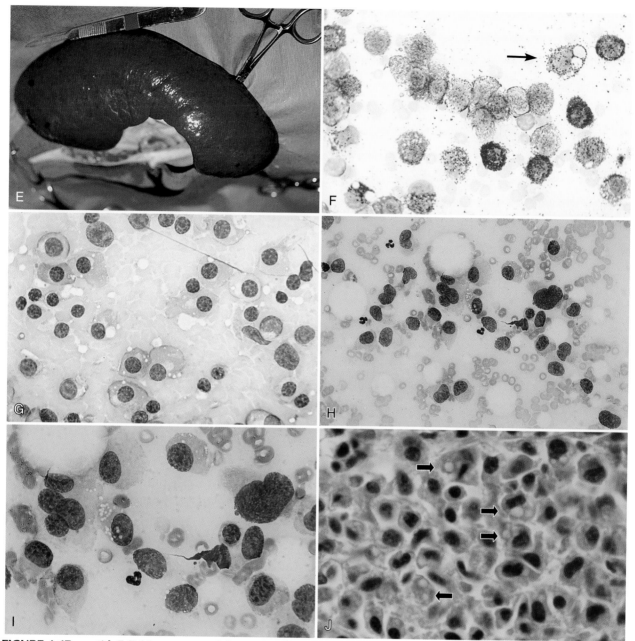

■ **FIGURE 4-17, cont'd. E-F, Mastocytoma. Spleen. Cat. E,** Diffuse enlargement of the spleen is commonly found for this neoplasm. **F, Cytologic preparation.** A monomorphic population of moderately to highly granulated mast cells is present. Note the cell *(arrow)* demonstrating erythrophagocytosis, a feature common for splenic mastocytoma. (Wright-Giemsa; HP oil.) **G, Plasmacytoma. Splenic imprint. Dog.** Plasma cells composed the majority of cells present. Note the abundant eosinophilic cytoplasm typical for a "flame cell." Serum protein electrophoresis indicated a monoclonal gammopathy, which immunoelectrophoresis confirmed as an abnormal amount of IgA. (Romanowsky; HP oil.) (Case material courtesy of Christine Swardson and Joanne Messick, The Ohio State University; presented at the 1989 ASVCP case review session.) **Same case H-I. Histiocytic sarcoma. Splenic aspirate. Dog. H,** A cellular specimen shows a monomorphic population of individually arranged cells. The cells are round to oval with a moderate amount of basophilic cytoplasm, several of which contain few punctate vacuoles. (Wright-Giemsa; HP oil.) **I,** Higher magnification demonstrates a lobulated cell (right) and a multinucleated cell (left). (Wright-Giemsa; HP oil.) **Same case J-L. J-K, Hemophagocytic histiocytic sarcoma. Dog. J, Splenic tissue section.** The spleen was replaced by a neoplastic population of histiocytic cells several of which are shown displaying erythrophagocytosis *(arrows)*. This 10-year old Rottweiler presented with marked anemia and thrombocytopenia along with clinical signs of lethargy and anorexia. (H&E; HP oil.) (Photo courtesy of Tricia Bisby, Purdue University)

Continued

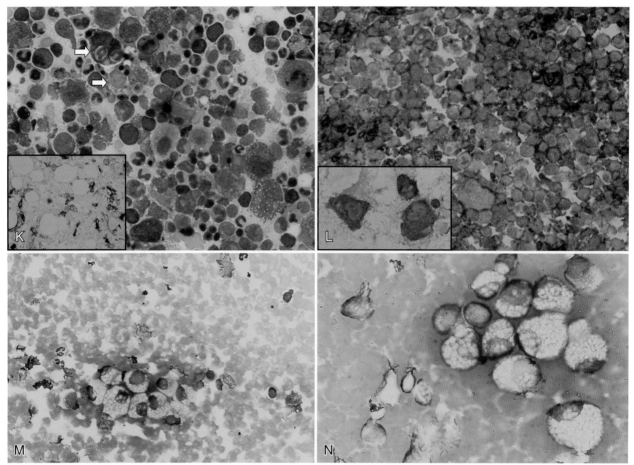

■ **FIGURE 4-17, cont'd. K, Bone marrow.** Cellular bone marrow aspirate with large histiocytic cells, some of which display leukocyto-phagia and erythrophagia *(arrows)*. (Wright; HP oil.). *Inset:* Bone marrow core section demonstrating frequent expression of CD11d, a marker of splenic macrophages. (CD11d/DAB; IP.) **L, Hemophagocytic histiocytic sarcoma. Spleen tissue section. Bone marrow aspirate. Immunochemistry. Dog.** Nearly all cells in the spleen express BLA.36 on their cell surface in this tissue section. (BLA.36/DAB; IP.) *Inset:* Three large bone marrow cells strongly express BLA.36 in this aspirate sample (BLA.36/AEC; HP oil.) **Same case M-N. Metastatic prostatic carcinoma. Splenic aspirate. Dog. M,** Cluster of individualized epithelial cells with marked anisokaryosis. (Wright-Giemsa; HP oil.) **N,** Higher magnification demonstrates the secretory nature of the tumor cells from the presence of abundant vacuolated cyto-plasm. A carcinoma with similar-appearing cells was found in the prostate and thought to be the origin of the splenic mass. (Wright-Giemsa; HP oil.) (K, Photos courtesy of Tricia Bisby, Purdue University. L, Spleen photo courtesy of Tricia Bisby, Purdue University.)

study of 16 cats (Patel et al., 2005). Histiocytic sarcoma may be localized to the spleen or disseminated to other sites (Affolter and Moore, 2002). This tumor arises from dendritic cells that are CD1+, CD4-, CD11c+, CD11d-, MHC II+, ICAM-1+ in comparison to the hemophago-cytic histiocytic sarcoma that arises from macrophages and is associated with a rapid decline in health (Moore et al., 2006). Marked erythrophagocytosis by CD11d+ macrophages usually occurs in the spleen and bone mar-row (Fig. 4-17J&K). Studies suggest BLA.36 (Fig. 4-17L) may be a useful immunochemical marker for neoplastic histiocytic cells when positive in addition to negative expression for CD3 and CD79a surface antigens (Publica-tion pending Bisby et al., 2009).

Occasionally, highly disseminated epithelial malig-nancies will be found in the spleen. An example of secretory epithelium with anaplastic features is shown (Fig. 4-17M&N).

Extramedullary Hematopoiesis

Extramedullary hematopoiesis was the most common cytologic abnormality in one study, accounting for 24% of the patients (O'Keefe and Couto, 1987). While precursors from all three cell lines may be observed, erythroid cells are the most common, with metarubricytes, rubricytes, and prorubricytes present (Fig. 4-18A&B). Care must be taken as erythroid precursors and lymphoid precursors appear very similar and occasional late-stage erythroid precursors may be encountered normally on splenic cytology. The finding of erythroid islands (Fig. 4-18C) with developing rubricytes in contact with a macrophage for exchange of iron is strong evidence for extramedullary erythropoiesis. Mature megakaryocytes are easily observed during scan-ning because of their large size. Conditions associated with extramedullary hematopoiesis include acute and chronic hemolytic anemia, myeloproliferative disorders, and lym-phoproliferative disorders (Fig. 4-18D).

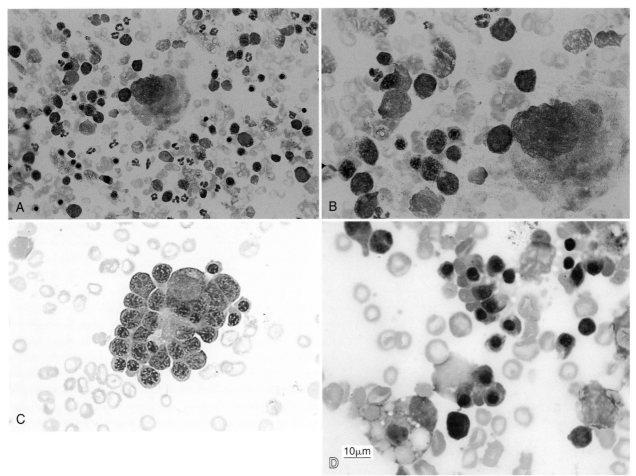

■ **FIGURE 4-18. Same case A-D. Extramedullary hematopoiesis. Splenic aspirate. Dog. A,** A megakaryocyte and numerous erythroid precursors are detected in this sample from an animal that received chemotherapy 2 weeks earlier for lymphoma. (Wright-Giemsa; HP oil.) **B,** Higher magnification demonstrates low numbers of medium-sized lymphocytes with many rubricytes in addition to the mature megakaryocyte. (Wright-Giemsa; HP oil.) **C,** A nurse cell or a macrophage surrounded by various stages of erythroid development may be found in areas of increased erythropoiesis. (Wright-Giemsa; HP oil.) **D, Extramedullary hematopoiesis with hemophagocytosis.** Same case as in Figure 4-15B. Mild hematopoiesis with erythroid predominance is occurring in this case with *Histoplasma* sp. infection. Hemophagocytosis may be a normal activity in the spleen or accelerated as in this case, where the hematocrit was 12.5%. (Wright; HP oil.)

Appearing similar to extramedullary hematopoiesis is myelolipoma, an uncommon tumor in both dogs and cats, occurring in the liver or spleen. The presence of hematopoietic precursors with large amounts of lipid vacuoles in the background is strongly suggestive of this benign neoplasm (Fig. 4-19A–C). It is often found unassociated with hematologic abnormalities. Ultrasound examination may demonstrate a small focal hyperechoic mass in the spleen.

Cytologic Artifacts

Samples collected with the assistance of ultrasound often produce magenta debris in the background. This granular material represents ultrasound gel particles (Fig. 4-20) and can mimic necrotic tissue when mixed with blood. The material also may cause lysis or cellular swelling and therefore may create unsuitable preparations for cytologic examination. See Chapter 1 for more information about imaging concerns.

Care should be taken when an incisional biopsy is taken of the spleen and impression smears are made.

When the capsular surface is mistakenly imprinted instead of the parenchyma, uniform sheets of loosely attached mesothelium are seen (Fig. 4-21A&B).

THYMUS

Indications for Thymic Biopsy

- *Enlargement* may be detected by radiography and ultrasonography, often producing signs of dyspnea, pleural effusions, and dysphagia (swallowing difficulties).
- *Abnormal imaging features* suggest the presence of hyperplasia or infiltrative processes.

Normal Histology and Cytology

Before puberty, the thymus has a prominent parenchyma divided into cortical and medullary regions (Fig. 4-22A). The outermost cortex is composed of small, densely packed lymphocytes without formation of lymphoid

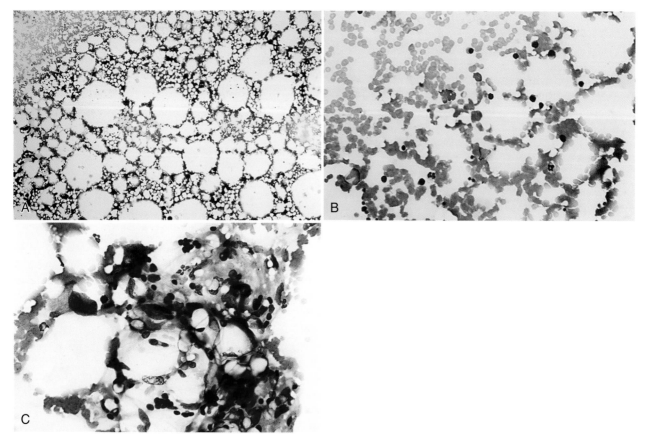

■ **FIGURE 4-19. Myelolipoma. Splenic aspirate. Cat. Same case A-C. A,** Low magnification demonstrates the massive amounts of variably sized clear vacuoles, consistent with lipid. (Wright-Giemsa; LP.) **B,** Dark-staining erythroid precursors are associated with the lipid material. (Wright-Giemsa; HP oil.) **C,** A megakaryocyte and collections of reticuloendothelial stroma are present within the small discrete nodule on the splenic tail. (Wright-Giemsa; HP oil.)

nodules. The central medulla is continuous between lobules that are formed by the inward extension of the thin connective tissue capsule. The medulla contains fewer and larger vesicular lymphocytes. The thymus is supported by a reticular network of stellate epithelium that forms loose cuffs around small vessels, termed

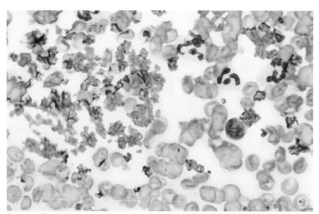

■ **FIGURE 4-20. Ultrasound gel. Transabdominal needle aspirate. Dog.** An attempt to sample the spleen produced a cytologic artifact. Note the pink to magenta, coarse, granular material in the background. (Wright; HP oil.) (Case material courtesy of Kurt Henkel et al, Michigan State University; presented at the 1996 ASVCP case review session.)

Hassall's corpuscles. These concentric whorls of flattened reticular cells may become keratinized or calcified (Fig. 4-22A&B). The reticular epithelium also gives rise to a ductal system within the medulla that may become cystic and lined by ciliated epithelium. After puberty, the thymic parenchyma begins to atrophy, becoming replaced by adipose tissue.

Cytologically, the cell population of the cortex is similar to that of the lymph node with the predominance of small, dense-staining lymphocytes (Fig. 4-22C&D). Occasional mast cells are present. Large stellate cells with round vesicular nuclei representing the thymic epithelium may be found scattered between the lymphocytes or in tight balls (Fig. 4-22E&F), the latter arrangement become Hassall's corpuscles. These dense collections of epithelium resemble epithelioid macrophages having abundant pale-blue cytoplasm with cellular attachment to each other.

Primary Neoplasia

The two different cell populations, lymphocytes and reticular epithelium, become the origin for the two types of neoplasia that develop within the thymus. Neoplasia of the lymphoid cells of the thymus is termed *thymic lymphoma,* having the appearance of lymphoma in other lymphoid organs like the lymph node (see Figs. 4-8 to 4-10). The cell type involved most often

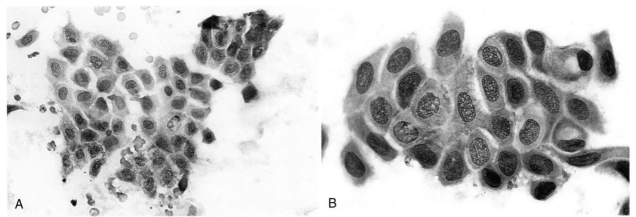

■ **FIGURE 4-21. Mesothelium. Splenic imprint. Dog. Same case A-B. A,** Splenomegaly from suspected hypersplenism necessitated removal of the spleen. The outside surface was inadvertently imprinted on the slide. Note a large sheet of interlocking cells. (Aqueous-based Wright; HP oil.) **B,** Higher magnification demonstrates a uniform population of adherent cells with abundant basophilic cytoplasm. Clear spaces between cells represent cytoplasmic junctions. This benign sheet of cells is typical for mesothelial lining. The capsule on this spleen was prominently thickened grossly and histologically. (Aqueous-based Wright; HP oil.)

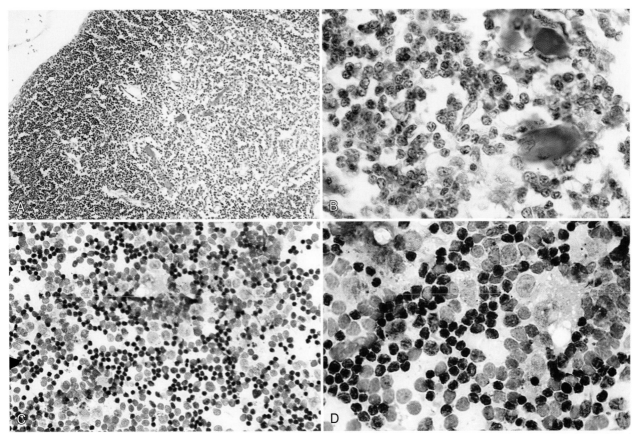

■ **FIGURE 4-22. A-F, Normal thymus. Young dog. Same case A-B. Tissue section. A,** The dense cortical area is composed of packed lymphocytes (left), while the medulla is more pale staining (right). Note the dark-staining structures in the medulla called *Hassall's corpuscles.* (H&E; IP.) **B,** The medulla contains eosinophilic Hassall's corpuscles that represent perivascular cuffs of flattened reticular stroma that becomes keratinized or calcified. The medullary lymphocytes are larger with vesicular nucleus. (H&E; HP oil.) **C-F, Tissue aspirate. Same case C-D. C,** Many small, dark-staining lymphocytes are the predominant population, with fewer medium lymphocytes. Note the two large epithelial cells in the top center of the field. (Wright-Giemsa; HP oil.) **D,** Higher magnification to demonstrate the large stellate reticular epithelium with vesicular nuclei. (Wright-Giemsa; HP oil.)

Continued

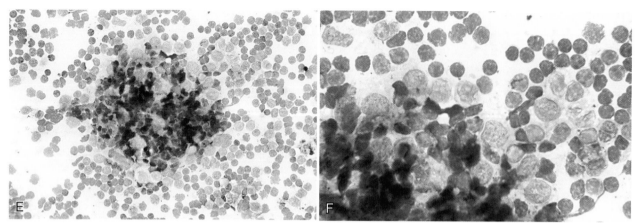

■ **FIGURE 4-22, cont'd. Same case E-F. E,** Thymic epithelium may be found in tight balls, possibly representing perivascular cuffs. (Wright-Giemsa; HP oil.) **F,** Higher magnification to demonstrate the small lymphocytes and thymic epithelium. (Wright-Giemsa; HP oil.)

is the lymphoblastic type and these tumors have been associated with hypercalcemia.

Neoplasia of the thymic epithelial cells is termed *thymoma* and usually takes one of three forms in dogs and cats; epithelial thymoma, mixed lymphoepithelial thymoma, or lymphocyte-predominant thymoma. The relative numbers of these two cell types histologically determine the specific diagnosis. In the epithelial thymoma, the reticular epithelium predominates, with low numbers of mostly small lymphocytes remaining. The epithelial cells appear as large cohesive, pale, mononuclear cells that resemble epithelioid macrophages. In the mixed cell thymoma, variably sized clusters of neoplastic epithelium appear with many small lymphocytes and fewer medium or large lymphocytes (Figs. 4-23 and 4-24). A lymphocyte-predominant thymoma contains many small lymphocytes and only scattered thymic epithelium with a loss of normal architecture (Fig. 4-25A–E).

Large numbers of well-differentiated mast cells are commonly found within thymomas and may give the false impression of a mast cell tumor or metastatic mast cells into a lymph node. Eosinophilic material may be associated with cells in a thymoma (Andreasen et al., 1991), which closely resembles the colloid found in a thyroid tumor and may present a diagnostic dilemma. Immunohistochemistry, when performed, often indicates positive stain reactions for CD3 and cytokeratin markers (see Fig. 4-25E).

Clinically, increased survival has been demonstrated for dogs older than 8 years of age, dogs with the histologic subtype lymphocyte-predominant, and dogs without concurrent megaesophagus (Atwater et al., 1994). Myasthenia gravis and pure red cell aplasia are paraneoplastic syndromes associated with thymoma in addition to hypercalcemia. Elevated serum antibodies against acetylcholine receptor have been demonstrated in a dog

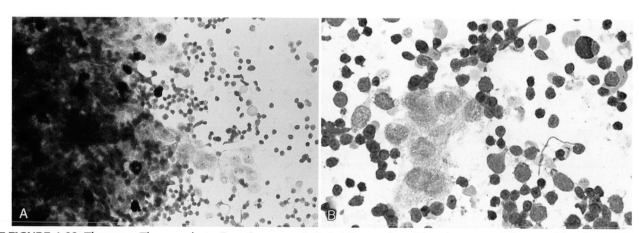

■ **FIGURE 4-23. Thymoma. Tissue aspirate. Dog. Same case A-B. A,** Mixture of small lymphocytes and clusters of thymic epithelium suggests the lymphoepithelial histologic type. Note the scattered mast cells throughout the stroma at the left side seen as dark cells. (Wright-Giemsa; HP oil.) **B,** This animal presented with no clinical signs except radiographic evidence of an anterior mediastinal mass during screening for elective surgery. Note the small cluster of reticular epithelium that resembles spindle cells. A well-differentiated mast cell is shown in the upper right corner. (Wright-Giemsa; HP oil.)

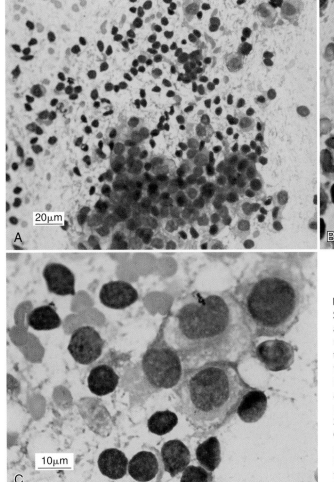

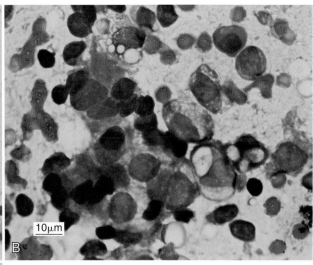

■ **FIGURE 4-24. Malignant thymoma. Tissue imprint. Dog. Same case A, C. A,** A mixed population of small lymphocytes and thymic epithelial cells is present from a cranial mediastinal mass from a 9-year-old German Shorthaired Pointer. Notice the large cluster of the thymic cells at the bottom of the field. These cells expressed cytokeratin (not shown) supporting the epithelial origin of these cells. (Wright; IP.) **B,** This is a higher magnification of the case in A. Notice the pleomorphism and variability in the nuclear-to-cytoplasmic ratio. Small but prominent nucleoli are seen. (Wright; HP oil.) **C,** Features of malignancy include anisokaryosis, prominent multiple nucleoli, variable nuclear-to-cytoplasmic ratio, and binucleation. The presence of increased mitotic activity and tissue necrosis indicates rapid cell turnover and supports an interpretation of malignancy. (Wright; HP oil.)

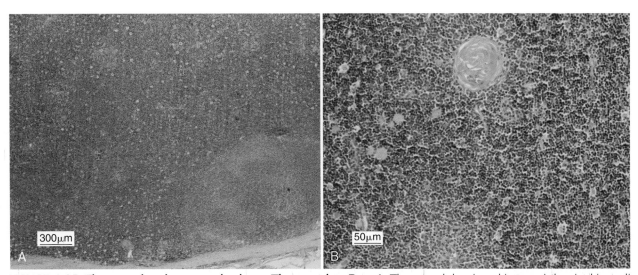

■ **FIGURE 4-25. Thymoma, lymphocyte predominant. Tissue section. Dog. A,** The normal thymic architecture is lost in this mediastinal mass from a 3-year old mixed breed dog. There is disruption of the normal cortex by a focal proliferation of pale pink cells just under the thick, fibrous capsule. The majority of the cell population appears basophilic and diffuse. (H&E; LP.) **Same case B-D. B, Hassall's Corpuscle.** This is a higher magnification of the dense basophilic and cellular area from the case shown in A. Notice the circular pink area, called Hassall's corpuscle, which is composed of keratinized stromal cells that surround a blood vessel. (H&E; IP.)

Continued

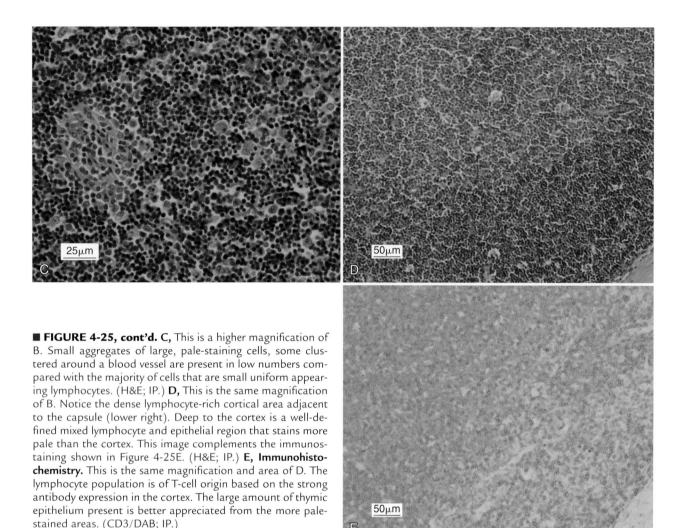

■ FIGURE 4-25, cont'd. C, This is a higher magnification of B. Small aggregates of large, pale-staining cells, some clustered around a blood vessel are present in low numbers compared with the majority of cells that are small uniform appearing lymphocytes. (H&E; IP.) **D,** This is the same magnification of B. Notice the dense lymphocyte-rich cortical area adjacent to the capsule (lower right). Deep to the cortex is a well-defined mixed lymphocyte and epithelial region that stains more pale than the cortex. This image complements the immunostaining shown in Figure 4-25E. (H&E; IP.) **E, Immunohisto-chemistry.** This is the same magnification and area of D. The lymphocyte population is of T-cell origin based on the strong antibody expression in the cortex. The large amount of thymic epithelium present is better appreciated from the more pale-stained areas. (CD3/DAB; IP.)

with megaesophagus (Lainesse et al., 1996). Because of the close association between megaesophagus and myasthenia gravis, it is recommended that all dogs with megaesophagus and thymoma be tested for myasthenia gravis (Scott-Moncrieff et al., 1990). Metastasis to the lung and liver is uncommon but has been reported in three of eight malignant canine cases in one study (Bellah et al., 1983). Cats with thymoma were reported to have exfoliative skin lesions (Scott et al., 1995; Day, 1997). Reports of an uncommon occurrence of cystic thymomas in cats demonstrated metastasis in several of the cases (Patnaik et al., 2003). A recent case in a cat was present in an ectopic location and diagnosis involved histopathology with immunochemistry of the mass and flow cytometry of the lymphocyte population. Lymphocytes were double positive for CD4 and CD8, supporting the diagnosis of thymoma (Lara-Garcia et al., 2008). Thymoma masses are often large (Fig. 4-26), but because of their localized and often encapsulated appearance, surgical excision is recommended. Chylous effusion has also been associated with thymoma related to the infiltration of the tumor into the lymphatics.

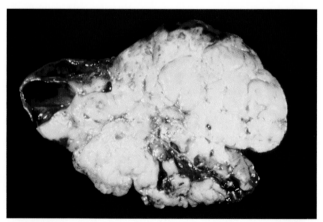

■ FIGURE 4-26. Thymoma. Gross specimen. German shepherd dog. This large cranial mediastinal mass measured 12 × 10 × 8 cm. It was partially encapsulated, slightly firm, and tan with occasional mucus-containing cysts. (Photo courtesy of Lois Roth, Angell Memorial Hospital; presented at the 1997 ASVCP case review session.)

REFERENCES

Affolter VK, Moore PF: Localized and disseminated histiocytic sarcoma of dendritic cell origin in dogs, *Vet Pathol* 39:74-83, 2002.

Andreasen CB, Mahaffey EA, Latimer KS: What is your diagnosis? *Vet Clin Pathol* 20:15-16, 1991.

Atwater SW, Powers BE, Park RD et al: Thymoma in dogs: 23 cases (1980-1991), *J Am Vet Med Assoc* 205:1007-1013, 1994.

Avery PR, Avery AC: Molecular methods to distinguish reactive and neoplastic lymphocyte expansions and their importance in transitional neoplastic states, *Vet Clin Pathol* 33:196-207, 2004.

Bauer NB, Zervos D, Moritz A: Argyrophilic nucleolar organizing regions and Ki67 equally reflect proliferation in fine needle aspirates of normal, hyperplastic, inflamed, and neoplastic canine lymph nodes (n=101), *J Vet Intern Med* 21:928-935, 2007.

Bellah JR, Stiff ME, Russell RG: Thymoma in the dog: Two case reports and review of 20 additional cases, *J Am Vet Med Assoc* 183:306-311, 1983.

Bookbinder PF, Butt MT, Harvey HJ: Determination of the number of mast cells in lymph node, bone marrow, and buffy coat cytologic specimens from dogs, *J Am Vet Med Assoc* 11:1648-1650, 1992.

Burnett RC, Vernau W, Modiano JF et al: Diagnosis of canine lymphoid neoplasia using clonal rearrangements of antigen receptor genes, *Vet Pathol* 40:32-41, 2003.

Callanan JJ, Jones BA, Irvine J et al: Histologic classification and immunophenotype of lymphosarcomas in cats with naturally and experimentally acquired feline immunodeficiency virus infections, *Vet Pathol* 33: 264-272, 1996.

Caniatti M, Roccabianca P, Scanziani E et al: Canine lymphoma: immunocytochemical analysis of fine-needle aspiration biopsy, *Vet Pathol* 33: 204-212, 1996.

Chiulli FM, Raskin RE, Fox LE et al: The clinical and pathological characteristics influencing the prognosis of 50 canine patients with lymphoid malignancies, *Vet Pathol* 40:619, 2003 (abstract).

Christopher MM: Cytology of the spleen, *Vet Clin Small Anim* 33:135-152, 2003.

Cienava EA, Barnhart KF, Brown R et al: Morphologic, immunohistochemical, and molecular characterization of hepatosplenic T-cell lymphoma in a dog, *Vet Clin Pathol* 33:105-110, 2004.

Culmsee K, Simon D, Mischke R: Possibilities of flow cytometric analysis for immunophenotypic characterization of canine lymphoma, *J Vet Med Ass* 47:199-206, 2001.

Dank G, Lucroy MD, Griffey SM et al: bcl-2 and MIB-1 labeling indexes in cats with lymphoma, *J Vet Intern Med* 16:720-725, 2002.

Day MJ: Review of thymic pathology in 30 cats and 36 dogs, *J Sm Anim Pract* 38:393-403, 1997.

Day MJ, Lucke VM, Pearson H: A review of pathological diagnoses made from 87 canine splenic biopsies, *J Sm Anim Pract* 36:426-433, 1995.

Dean GA, Groshek PM, Jain NC et al: Immunophenotypic analysis of feline haemolymphatic neoplasia using flow cytometry, *Comp Haematol Int* 5:84-92, 1995.

Desnoyers M, St-Germain L: What is your diagnosis? *Vet Clin Pathol* 23:89,97, 1994.

Edwards DS, Henley WE, Harding EF et al: Breed incidence of lymphoma in a UK population of insured dogs, *Vet Comp Oncology* 1:200-206, 2003.

Fisher DJ, Naydan D, Werner LL et al: Immunophenotyping lymphomas in dogs: a comparison of results from fine needle aspirate and needle biopsy samples, *Vet Clin Pathol* 24: 118-123, 1995.

Fournel-Fleury C, Magnol JP, Bricaire P et al: Cytohistological and immunological classification of canine malignant lymphomas: comparison with human non-Hodgkin's lymphomas, *J Comp Pathol* 117:35-59, 1997a.

Fournel-Fleury C, Magnol JP, Chabanne L et al: Growth fractions in canine non-Hodgkin's lymphomas as determined *in situ* by the expression of the Ki-67 antigen, *J Comp Pathol* 117:61-72, 1997b.

Fournel-Fleury C, Ponce F, Felman P et al: Canine T-cell lymphomas: a morphological, immunological, and clinical study of 46 new cases, *Vet Pathol* 39:92-109, 2002.

Fry MM, Vernau W, Pesavento PA et al: Hepatosplenic lymphoma in a dog, *Vet Pathol* 40:556-562, 2003.

Gibson D, Aubert I, Woods JP et al: Flow cytometric immunophenotype of canine lymph node aspirates, *J Vet Intern Med* 18:710-717, 2004.

Goldman EE, Grindem CB: What is your diagnosis? Seven-year-old dog with progressive lethargy and inappetence, *Vet Clin Pathol* 26:187, 195-197, 1997.

Grindem CB: What is your diagnosis? *Vet Clin Pathol* 23:72, 77, 1994.

Grindem CB, Page RL, Ammerman BE et al: Immunophenotypic comparison of blood and lymph node from dogs with lymphoma, *Vet Clin Pathol* 27:16-20, 1998.

Grooters AM, Couto CG, Andrews JM et al: Systemic *Mycobacterium smegmatis* infection in a dog, *J Am Vet Med Assoc* 206:200-202, 1995.

Hendrick MJ, Brooks JJ, Bruce EH: Six cases of malignant fibrous histiocytoma of the canine spleen, *Vet Pathol* 29:351-354, 1992.

Hipple AK, Colitz CMH, Mauldin GH et al: Telomerase activity and related properties of normal canine lymph node and canine lymphoma, *Vet Comp Oncol* 1:140-151,2003.

HogenEsch H, Hahn FF: Primary vascular neoplasms of lymph nodes in the dog, *Vet Pathol* 35:74-76, 1998.

Jaffe ES, Harris NL, Stein H et al (eds): *WHO classification of tumours: pathology and genetics of tumours of haematopoietic and lymphoid tissues*, Lyon, France, 2001, IARC Press, pp 109-235.

Jubala CM, Wojcieszyn JW, Valli VEO et al: CD 20 expression in normal canine B cells and in canine non-Hodgkin lymphoma, *Vet Pathol* 42:468-476, 2005.

Kiupel M, Bostock D, Bergmann V: The prognostic significance of AgNOR counts and PCNA-positive cell counts in canine malignant lymphomas, *J Comp Pathol* 119:407-418, 1998.

Kiupel M, Teske E, Bostock D: Prognostic factors for treated canine malignant lymphoma, *Vet Pathol* 36:292-300, 1999.

Kordick DL, Brown TT, Shin K et al: Clinical and pathologic evaluation of chronic *Bartonella henselae* or *Bartonella clarridgeiae* infection in cats, *J Clin Microbiol* 37:1536-1547, 1999.

Krick EL, Little L, Patel R et al: Description of clinical and pathological findings, treatment and outcome of feline large granular lymphocyte lymphoma (1996-2004), *Vet Comp Oncol* 6:102-110, 2008.

Lainesse MFC, Taylor SM, Myers SL et al: Focal myasthenia gravis as a paraneoplastic syndrome of canine thymoma: Improvement following thymectomy, *J Am Anim Hosp Assoc* 32: 111-117, 1996.

Lara-Garcia A, Wellman M, Burkhard MJ et al: Cervical thymoma originating in ectopic thymic tissue in a cat, *Vet Clin Pathol* 37:397-402, 2008.

Lau KWM, Kruth SA, Thorn CE et al: Large granular lymphocytic leukemia in a mixed breed dog, *Can Vet J* 40:725-728, 1999.

LeBlanc CJ, Head L, Fry MM: Comparison of aspiration and non-aspiration techniques for obtaining cytology samples from the canine spleen, *Vet Pathol* 45:735, 2008 (abstract).

Lennert K, Feller AC: *Histopathology of non-Hodgkin's lymphoma (based on the updated Kiel classification)*, ed 2, New York, 1992, Springer-Verlag, pp 13-18, 22-39, 115-126.

Lichtensteiger CA, Hilf LE: Atypical cryptococcal lymphadenitis in a dog, *Vet Pathol* 31:493-496, 1994.

Lurie DM, Lucroy MD, Griffey SM et al: T-cell-derived malignant lymphoma in the boxer breed, *Vet Comp Oncol* 2:171-175, 2004.

McDonough SP, Moore PF: Clinical, hematologic, and immuno-phenotypic characterization of canine large granular lymphocytosis, *Vet Pathol* 37:637-646, 2000.

Mooney SC, Patnaik AK, Hayes AA et al: Generalized lymphadenopathy resembling lymphoma in cats: six cases (1972-1976), *J Am Vet Med Assoc* 190:897-899, 1987.

Moore FM, Emerson WE, Cotter SM et al: Distinctive peripheral lymph node hyperplasia of young cats, *Vet Pathol* 23:386-391, 1986.

Moore PF, Affolter VK, Vernau W: Canine hemophagocytic histiocytic sarcoma: a proliferative disorder of CD11d+ macrophages, *Vet Pathol* 43:632-645, 2006.

O'Keefe DA, Couto CG: Fine-needle aspiration of the spleen as an aid in the diagnosis of splenomegaly, *J Vet Int Med* 1:102-109, 1987.

Patel RT, Caceres A, French AF et al: Multiple myeloma in 16 cats: a retrospective study, *Vet Clin Pathol* 34:341-352, 2005.

Patnaik AK, Lieberman PH, Erlandson RA et al: Feline cystic thymoma: a clinicopathologic, immunohistologic, and electron microscopic study of 14 cases, *J Feline Med Surg* 5:27-35, 2003.

Ponce F, Magnol JP, Blavier A et al: Clinical, morphological and immunological study of 13 cases of canine lymphoblastic lymphoma: comparison with the human entity, *Comp Clin Path* 12:75-83, 2003.

Ponce F, Magnol J-P, Ledieu D et al: Prognostic significance of morphological subtypes in canine malignant lymphomas during chemotherapy, *The Veterinary Journal* 167:158-166, 2004.

Raskin RE, Nipper MN: Cytochemical staining characteristics of lymph nodes from normal and lymphoma-affected dogs, *Vet Clin Pathol* 21:62-67, 1992.

Raskin RE: Canine lymphoid malignancies & the new clinically relevant WHO classification, *Proceedings of the 22nd annual meeting of American College of Veterinary Internal Medicine*, Minneapolis, Minnesota, pp 632-633, June 2004.

Raskin RE, Fox LE: Clinical relevance of the World Health Organization classification of lymphoid neoplasms in dogs, *Vet Clin Pathol* 32:152, 2003 (abstract).

Roccabianca P, Vernau W, Caniatti M et al: Feline large granular lymphocyte (LGL) lymphoma with secondary leukemia: primary intestinal origin with predominance of a CD3/CD8aa phenotype, *Vet Pathol* 43:15-28, 2006.

Ruslander DA, Gebhard DH, Tompkins MB et al: Immunophenotypic characterization of canine lymphoproliferative disorders, *In Vivo* 11:169-172, 1997.

Scott DW, Yager JA, Johnston KM: Exfoliative dermatitis in association with thymoma in three cats, *Feline Pract* 23:8-13, 1995.

Scott-Moncrieff JC, Cook JR, Lantz GC: Acquired myasthenia gravis in a cat with thymoma, *J Am Vet Med Assoc* 196:1291-1293, 1990.

Spangler WL, Culbertson MR: Prevalence and type of splenic diseases in cats: 455 cases (1985-1991), *J Am Vet Med Assoc* 201:773-776, 1992.

Spangler WL, Kass PH: Pathologic and prognostic characteristics of splenomegaly in dogs due to fibrohistiocytic nodule: 98 cases, *Vet Pathol* 35:488-498, 1998.

Spangler WL, Culbertson MR, Kass PH: Primary mesenchymal (nonangiomatous/nonlymphomatous) neoplasms occurring in the canine spleen: anatomic classification, immunohistochemistry, and mitotic activity correlated with patient survival, *Vet Pathol* 31:37-47, 1994.

Steele KE, Saunders GK, Coleman GD: T-cell-rich B-cell lymphoma in a cat, *Vet Pathol* 34:47-49, 1997.

Swerdlow SH, Campo E, Harris NL et al: *WHO classification of tumours of haematopoietic and lymphoid tissues*, ed 4, Geneva, Switzerland, 2008, WHO Press.

Teske E, van Heerde P: Diagnostic value and reproducibility of fine-needle aspiration cytology in canine malignant lymphoma, *Vet Quart* 18:112-115, 1996.

Teske E, van Heerde P, Rutteman GR et al: Prognostic factors for treatment of malignant lymphoma in dogs, *J Am Vet Med Assoc* 205:1722-1728, 1994.

Thorn CE, Aubert I: Abdominal mass aspirate from a cat with eosinophilia and basophilia, *Vet Clin Pathol* 28:139-141, 1999.

Twomey LN, Alleman AR: Cytodiagnosis of feline lymphoma, *Compend Contin Educ Pract Vet* 27:17-31, 2005.

Vail DM, Kisseberth WC, Obradovich JE et al: Assessment of potential doubling time (Tpot), argyrophilic nucleolar organizing regions (AgNOR) and proliferating cell nuclear antigen (PCNA) as predictors of therapy response in canine non-Hodgkin's lymphoma, *Exp Hematol* 24:807-815, 1996.

Vail DM, Kravis LD, Kisseberth WC et al: Application of rapid CD3 immunophenotype analysis and argyrophilic nucleolar organizer region (AgNOR) frequency to fine needle aspirate specimens from dogs with lymphoma, *Vet Clin Pathol* 26:66-69, 1997.

Vail DM, Moore AS, Ogilvie GK et al: Feline lymphoma (145 cases): proliferation indices, cluster of differentiation 3 immunoreactivity, and their association with prognosis in 90 cats, *J Vet Intern Med* 12:349-354, 1998.

Vajdovich P, Psader R, Toth ZA, Perge E: Use of the argyrophilic nucleolar region method for cytologic and histologic examination of the lymph nodes in dogs, *Vet Pathol* 41:338-345, 2004.

Valli VEO: *Veterinary comparative hematopathology*, Ames, IA, 2007, Blackwell Publishing, pp 9-117, 109-235.

Valli VE, Vernau W, DeLorimier LP et al: Canine indolent nodular lymphoma, *Vet Pathol* 43:241-256, 2006.

Vernau W, Moore PF: An immunophenotypic study of canine leukemias and preliminary assessment of clonality by polymerase chain reaction, *Vet Immunol Immunopath* 69:145-164, 1999.

Walton R, Thrall MA, Wheeler S: What is your diagnosis? *Vet Clin Pathol* 23:117, 128, 1994.

Whitten BA, Raskin RE: Evaluation of argyrophilic nucleolar organizer regions (AGNORS) as a prognostic indicator for canine lymphoproliferative diseases, *Vet Pathol* 41:552, 2004 (abstract).

Williams M, Avery A, Olver CS: Diagnosing lymphoid hyperplasia vs lymphoma in canine splenic aspirates, *Vet Pathol* 43:809, 2006.

Workman HC, Vernau W: Chronic lymphocytic leukemia in dogs and cats: the veterinary perspective, *Vet Clin North Am Small Anim Pract* 33:1379-1399, 2003.

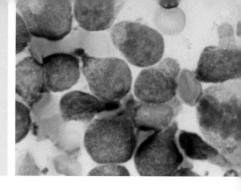

Respiratory Tract

Mary Jo Burkhard and Laurie M. Millward

Cytologic evaluation of the respiratory tract in correlation with history, clinical data, and imaging results provides invaluable diagnostic information that directly impacts patient management. Cytologic features seen in the respiratory tract following injury, disease, and primary or metastatic neoplasia depend largely on the normal underlying structure and function of the cellular elements. Thorough examination of a high-quality sample is critical for obtaining meaningful cytology results. This chapter describes appropriate sampling techniques and cytologic interpretation of samples from the respiratory tract, including the nasal cavity, larynx, airways, and lung parenchyma.

THE NASAL CAVITY

Normal Anatomy and Histologic Features

Beginning at the nares, the nasal cavity is divided by the nasal septum, and terminates caudally as the osseous ethmoid plate. The passages that traverse through bony and cartilaginous sinuses are lined by a mucous membrane. The entrance to the nasal cavity, or vestibule, encompasses the nares and a narrow section of the anterior nasal cavity. The posterior portion, or nasal cavity proper, consists of extensive, delicate, mucous membrane–lined turbinates. The nasolacrimal duct opens through the ventral lateral wall of the vestibule allowing serous secretions from the conjunctival sac to flow into the rostral nasal cavity. Communicating with the nasal cavity are several paired, air-filled, mucosa-lined paranasal sinuses.

The vestibule is contiguous with the external skin and is lined by keratinized squamous epithelium at the nares that briefly transitions into a nonkeratinized squamous epithelium in the front of the nasal cavity. In the dog, this transitional nonciliated nasal epithelium consists of round to cuboidal cells that layer on each other and are thought to play a role in metabolizing inhaled and circulating xenobiotics related to their endowment with cytochrome P450 monoxygenase enzymes. The nasal cavity proper, nasal septum, and paranasal sinuses are lined by a ciliated, pseudostratified, columnar epithelium. Serous, mucous, and mixed tubuloalveolar glands are present in the rostral nasal cavity, while olfactory glands, albeit in low numbers in carnivores, are found in the caudal nasal cavity. Nasal-associated lymphoid tissue (NALT) and lymphoid follicles are found in the submucosa of the caudal nasal cavity and are especially numerous in the nasopharynx.

The vomeronasal organ is bilaterally symmetric and located along the base of the nasal septum in the rostral part of the nasal cavity. The organ is comprised of various components including epithelium, ducts, glands, and connective tissue (Salazar et al., 1996) and, at least in dogs, is also rich in tissue of neuronal origin (Dennis et al., 2003). In addition to neuron cell bodies and axon fascicles, the sensory epithelium also expresses neuronal markers.

Collection Techniques and Sample Preparation

When history and clinical signs suggest disease of the nasal cavity, the first diagnostic step is a thorough inspection of the external and internal nasal cavity, pharynx, hard and soft palates, and oral cavity including examination of the gingiva and upper dental arcade for oronasal fistulation and periodontal disease. Additionally, palpation for enlarged regional lymph nodes and subsequent aspiration and/or biopsy may provide a valuable indirect means of achieving a diagnosis if disseminated or metastatic disease is present. Magnetic resonance imaging (MRI) and computed tomography (CT) provide additional data regarding the extent of the lesion, airway involvement, and three-dimensional localization (e.g., of foreign bodies). However, in most cases radiographs remain a reliable tool to localize mass lesions for diagnostic sampling (Jones and Ober, 2007; Petite and Dennis, 2006) although they are less sensitive for differentiating inflammatory and neoplastic rhinitis (Kuehn, 2006). Adequate visual inspection of the nasal cavity endoscopically and localization of lesions via radiographs or other imaging techniques will enable the appropriate collection techniques to be employed. However, it should be noted that rhinoscopic assessment does not uniformly predict the presence or absence of inflammatory disease; thus obtaining a sample for microscopic evaluation is critical (Johnson et al., 2004; Windsor et al., 2004). Examination by flexible endoscope is preferred as approximately 50% to 80% of the nasal cavity cannot be visualized through examinations by either a rigid endoscope or an otoscope (Elie and Sabo, 2006). If an endoscope is unavailable, an otoscope may be used to examine the rostral nasal cavity, and with aid of a dental mirror and light, a portion of the nasopharynx can also be visualized. Radiography and rhinoscopy should be performed prior to sampling as hemorrhage may hinder radiographic interpretation and obscure visualization during endoscopy.

A complete blood count (CBC) and coagulation profile should be performed prior to sampling as the majority of collection techniques result in hemorrhage owing to the rich venous plexuses underlying the nasal mucosa. Appropriate anesthetic restraint is tantamount for safe and successful procurement of tissue samples. General anesthesia allows appropriate restraint, placement of a properly inflated endotracheal tube, packing of the oropharynx with gauze, and tilting the patient's nose downward to protect against aspiration during sample collection.

Nasal Swabs

The presence of an acute or chronic nasal discharge indicates upper respiratory disease but is nonspecific and may be present with inflammatory, infectious, or neoplastic disorders. Nasal discharge may be unilateral or bilateral and range from serous, suppurative, mucoid, to serosanguineous depending on the underlying cause(s). Superficial and deep nasal swabs are easy to obtain and relatively nontraumatic, but often do not provide much information beyond identifying superficial inflammation, secondary bacterial infection, hemorrhage, necrosis, and mucus, while the underlying disease process remains obscure. As a general rule, invasive techniques allowing collection of tissue deep to the nasal mucosa increase diagnostic potential. For example, successful detection of aspergillosis increases from positive detection of 13% to 20% of samples examined by a direct smear or blinds swab to 93% to 100% positive detection in samples obtained by brush cytology or biopsy (DeLorenzi et al., 2006a). However, occasionally the simplest technique can be rewarding, such as the cytologic examination of a nasal swab for the diagnosis of cryptococcosis infection in cats. Therefore, cytologic examination of nasal exudate should be performed initially in any nasal disease.

Nasal Flush

Nasal flushing methods have been reviewed elsewhere (Smallwood and Zenoble, 1993). In general, invasive and aggressive techniques are more likely to yield diagnostic material. Nontraumatic nasal flushes only produce material for a definitive diagnosis in approximately 50% of the cases. A 6 to 10 French polypropylene or soft red rubber urinary catheter is inserted into the external nares to flush sterile, nonbacteriostatic, physiologic saline or lactated Ringer's solution through the nasal cavity (Fig. 5-1A). A traumatic nasal flush can be accomplished by beveling or nicking the tubing or catheter, creating a rough surface to aid in dislodging tissue. As with any instrument placed into the nasal cavity, penetration through the cribriform plate into the cranial vault can be avoided by measuring the distance from the external nares to the medial canthus of the eye and cutting the tubing or catheter to the appropriate length, or marking the instrument with tape.

Small aliquots (5 to 10 ml) of fluid are introduced into the nasal cavity via a 20- to 35-ml syringe with alternating positive and negative pressure. As the fluid enters the cavity, the tubing or catheter is aggressively moved back and forth against the nasal turbinates in an attempt to free tissue fragments that can be collected on gauze sponges held below the external nares or reaspirated into the collection syringe. An alternative method

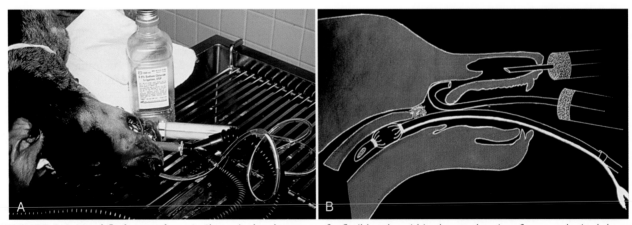

■ **FIGURE 5-1. Nasal flush procedure. A,** Shown is the placement of a flexible tube within the nasal cavity of an anesthetized dog and use of sodium chloride irrigation fluid. **B,** Diagram of an alternate technique demonstrating placement of a flexible tube retroflexed below and around the soft palate with collection of fluid from the external nares. (A, Courtesy of Robert King, University of Florida. B, From Meyer DJ: The management of cytology specimens, *Compend Contin Educ Pract Vet* 9:10-16, 1987.)

involves directing a Foley catheter into the oral cavity and retroflexing around the soft palate into the naso-pharynx, inflating the bulb, and lavaging the saline so that the fluid passes through the nasal cavity and out the external nares for collection (Fig. 5-1B).

The fluid and particulate matter retrieved should be placed into an EDTA-anticoagulated tube. If the fluid is turbid, direct smears can be prepared for cytologic evaluation by placing a drop of the fluid on a clean glass slide and placing a second slide on top. After the fluid has spread between the slides, the two slides are pulled apart in a horizontal fashion, with a slight amount of vertical pressure applied if small tissue fragments are present. If the fluid is relatively clear, the sample can be concentrated by centrifugation, and smears are pre-pared from the sedimented material resuspended in a small volume of remaining supernatant similar to urine sediment preparation. Further concentration of the sample may be achieved via cytocentrifugation, if avail-able. If large tissue chunks are retrieved, touch prepara-tions may be prepared for cytologic evaluation. A small aliquot of fluid can be placed in a tube without any additives for culture and sensitivity, or the fluid may be applied to a culturette.

Fine Needle Aspiration

Fine-needle aspiration (FNA) biopsy is most rewarding when mass lesions are present. If a visible external nasal mass is present, direct aspiration may be performed. To sample masses within the nasal cavity, the location is best identified by imaging techniques prior to aspira-tion. For FNA, a 1- to 1½-inch 22- to 23-gauge needle is attached to a 3- to 12-ml syringe. The needle is intro-duced into the mass while strong negative pressure is applied and released several times. The needle should be redirected and the procedure repeated; negative pressure is released before withdrawing the needle from the mass. Frequently, only minimal material is col-lected into the needle hub. Collected material should be expelled onto slides for cytologic preparation and evaluation.

Imprint and Brush Cytology

Alligator biopsy forceps are used to obtain a pinch biopsy for impression cytology and histopathology, while an en-doscopic brush is used to collect tissue to roll on a glass slide for cytology. Both sampling techniques are typically performed with endoscopic guidance. Imprint cytology can also be performed on core biopsy samples obtained using a Tru-Cut Disposable Biopsy Needle (Cardinal Health Allegiance, Deerfield, IL). Similarly, the polypropylene por-tion of an indwelling catheter with the needle removed, or a polypropylene urinary catheter with the end cut at a 45-degree angle can also be used to obtain tissue speci-mens. The catheter is pushed into the mass and rotated while applying negative pressure. Tissue can then be rolled on a glass slide or used to make touch imprints for cytologic evaluation before placing in 10% neutral buff-ered formalin. Brush cytology often misses the deeper inflammatory cells and may not correlate well with histo-logic results (Michiels et al., 2003). Therefore, deeper,

more invasive samples are preferred wherever possible. In one study of 54 dogs with nasal tumors, brush and imprint cytology correctly identified neoplasia of epithe-lial origin in 88% and 90% of the cases, respectively (Clercx et al., 1996). However, in the same study, the abil-ity to diagnose mesenchymal tumors was significantly less. Histologic diagnosis correlated with 50% of imprint cytology impressions and only 20% of those made by brush cytology.

If the above procedures do not yield diagnostic sam-ples, or cannot be performed because of the nature of the lesion or small patient size, exploratory rhinotomy may be necessary to obtain an excisional biopsy from which impression smears for cytology can be prepared before the remainder of the tissue is preserved for histo-pathologic examination.

Normal Cytology and Common Cytologic Changes

Normal Nasal Cytology

Nasal swabs and flushes of healthy animals contain few cells, small amounts of mucus, and low numbers of a mixed population of extracellular bacteria (normal flora) found colonizing the surface of epithelial cells. Ciliated columnar respiratory epithelial cells from the posterior nasal cavity typically predominate; however, small num-bers of squamous epithelial cells originating from the anterior nasal cavity may also be present. Respiratory epithelial cells can be seen singly or in small clusters, are columnar and contain a round, basally located nucleus. Cilia, if present, are located opposite the nucleus and can be seen as an eosinophilic brush border (Fig. 5-2A). While also columnar with a basally located nucleus, goblet cells lack cilia, are more plump, and contain a moderate amount of cytoplasm with numerous prominent, round, purple-staining cytoplasmic mucin granules (Fig. 5-2B). Occasionally, basal epithelial cells may be seen. When present, these cells are round to cuboidal with scant, deeply basophilic cytoplasm and round, centrally placed nuclei. On cytologic specimens, mucus appears as an eosinophilic amorphous extracellular material that often entraps cells. Nasal-associated lymphoid tissue (NALT) can be found in the nasal cavity of both the dog and the cat and responds similarly to organized lymphoid tissue in other location (Fig. 5-3). The canine and feline nasal cavity contains NALT and lymphoid follicles, particularly in the nasopharynx. These islands of lymphocytes can respond similarly to other organized lymphoid tissue such as lymph nodes. The degree of hemorrhage ob-served is contingent on the collection procedure. Eryth-rocytes with platelet clumps and white blood cells in numbers and proportions consistent with blood (approximately one white cell per 500 to 1000 red cells) indicate iatrogenic contamination of the sample or peracute hemorrhage. The nasal cavity of the dog and cat harbor large numbers of a mixed population of both aerobic and anaerobic bacteria that are considered normal microflora including *Streptococcus* sp., *Staphylo-coccus* sp., *Escherichia coli*, *Pseudomonas* sp., *Proteus* sp., and *Bordetella bronchiseptica*.

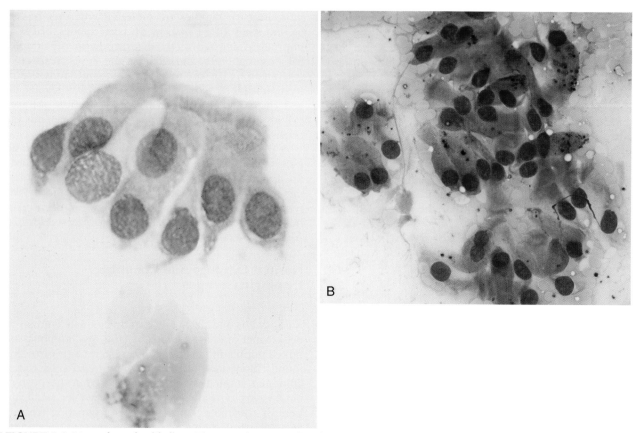

■ **FIGURE 5-2. Normal nasal epithelium. Tissue aspirate. A,** Ciliated columnar epithelium having basally located nuclei is found normally in the upper respiratory tract. (Wright-Giemsa; HP oil.) **B,** Goblet cells containing large, globular, magenta granules admixed in with ciliated columnar epithelial cells. (Wright-Giemsa; HP oil.)

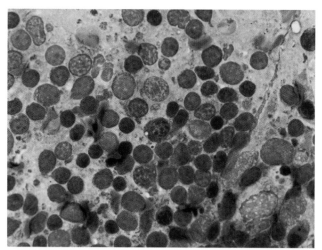

■ **FIGURE 5-3. Nasal associated lymphoid tissue. Tissue aspirate. Dog.** This aspirate contains a heterogeneous mixture of small and medium lymphocytes, lymphoblasts, and increased numbers of plasma cells indicating mild reactive lymphoid hyperplasia. (Wright-Giemsa; HP oil.)

Oropharyngeal Contamination

Oropharyngeal contamination is seen most frequently in samples collected by flushing techniques. The presence of *Simonsiella* sp. is a hallmark of oropharyngeal

contamination. *Simonsiella* sp. are large, rod-shaped bacteria that align in a row after division resulting in a distinctive pattern that resembles stacked coins (Fig. 5-4A&B). Oropharyngeal contamination is also characterized by the presence of a mixed population of bacteria found extracellularly that colonize the surface of keratinized squamous epithelial cells. If oropharyngeal inflammation is present (e.g., periodontal disease), inflammatory cells may be seen associated with the oropharyngeal contamination (Fig. 5-4C).

Hyperplasia/Dysplasia

Chronic inflammation secondary to various infectious and noninfectious etiologies (e.g., trauma, chronic irritation, or neoplasia) is common in the nasal cavity and can have a profound effect on the integrity and function of normal cellular constituents. Several adaptive mechanisms are employed by cells to survive amid the inflammatory stimulus. Increased numbers of cells, or hyperplasia, is one such mechanism and is often accompanied by dysplasia (Fig. 5-5A). Dysplasia is readily identified histologically as a loss of architectural organization but is more difficult to identify in cytologic preparations, which typically lack structural features. Samples from an inflamed nasal cavity with hyperplasia and dysplasia are likely to contain numerous clusters and sheets of epithelial cells with an increased nuclear-to-cytoplasm ratio,

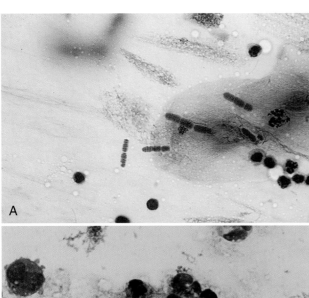

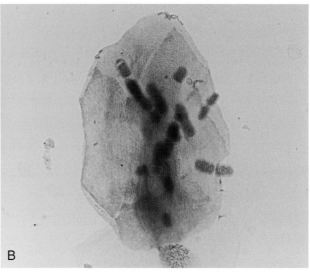

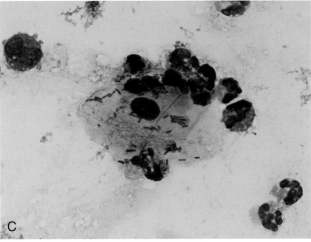

■ **FIGURE 5-4. A, Oropharyngeal contamination. TTW.** Presence of squamous epithelial cells with closely associated *Simonsiella* bacteria suggests contamination by normal microflora or an oronasal fistula. (Wright-Giemsa; HP oil.) **B, Oropharyngeal contamination. TTW.** Degenerating squamous epithelial cell with adherent *Simonsiella* bacteria and chains of cocci. (Wright-Giemsa; HP oil.) **C, Suppurative inflammation with oropharyngeal contamination. BAL.** In this case, the source of the inflammation can be difficult to determine. There is obvious suppurative inflammation, and some neutrophils appear to have phagocytized several rod bacteria. However, the presence of squamous epithelial cells with adherent rod bacteria indicates oropharyngeal contamination, which suggests that the inflammation and infection may be localized to the oral cavity. (Wright-Giemsa; HP oil.)

mild to moderate anisocytosis, and increased cytoplasmic basophilia (Fig. 5-5B). Mitotic figures, while normal in appearance, may be increased as well. Hyperplasia and dysplasia are reversible but may represent early neoplastic changes and can be difficult to differentiate cytologically from well-differentiated carcinoma.

Metaplasia

Another adaptive response to chronic irritation/inflammation is metaplasia. Metaplasia involves a change in cellular differentiation such that a susceptible specialized normal cell type is transformed to one that is better able to endure the environmental stress while losing specialized function. In the respiratory system, metaplasia is often characterized by the transformation of columnar respiratory epithelial cells to a more squamous phenotype resulting in a loss of the ability to produce and secrete protective mucus. Cytologically, squamous metaplasia is detected by the presence of squamous epithelial cells either as the primary cell type or admixed with more normal respiratory epithelial cells (French, 1987). Cells may be present in sheets or individually depending on the degree of keratinization. Basilar cells tend to remain in clusters, while more

keratinized squamous cells often appear individually and have angular borders, abundant hyalinized, basophilic cytoplasm and small, and occasionally pyknotic or karyorrhectic nuclei. As with hyperplasia, neoplastic transformation of the squamous cells may occur.

Nasal melanosis has also been suggested as a metaplastic transformation of the nasal respiratory mucosa and has been reported rarely in dogs with odontopathic rhinitis (DeLorenzi et al., 2006b).

Noninfectious Inflammatory Disease

Foreign Bodies

Nasal foreign bodies occur most commonly in dogs and often originate from plants such as plant awns, foxtails, or twigs. Foreign bodies may be directly inhaled into the nasal cavity, or they may enter the cavity traumatically (e.g., buckshot) through the nares, nasal planum, or via the oral cavity by penetrating the palate. Cytologically, specimens are characterized by marked inflammatory reactions ranging from suppurative to pyogranulomatous often with significant hemorrhage and foreign material such as plant material or fibers. Secondary bacterial infection is common.

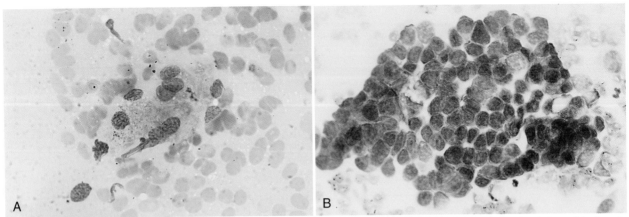

■ **FIGURE 5-5. A, Serous mucous glands of frontal sinus. Tissue imprint. Dog.** Clusters of hyperplastic glandular epithelium have an abundant, pale-blue to gray, foamy cytoplasm. (Wright-Giemsa; HP oil.) **B, Epithelial dysplasia. Tissue aspirate.** This cluster of cells is characterized by increased cytoplasmic basophilia and moderate anisocytosis and anisokaryosis. (Wright-Giemsa; HP oil.) (A, Courtesy of Rose Raskin, University of Florida.)

Allergic Rhinitis

Hypersensitivity may occur in the nasal cavity alone or concurrent with involvement of the lower airways. The inflammatory infiltrate associated with an allergic rhinitis is characterized predominantly by eosinophils, with lesser numbers of neutrophils, occasional mast cells, and occasional plasma cells (Fig. 5-6). Increased numbers of goblet cells and abundant mucus may also be seen along with rafts of hyperplastic respiratory epithelial cells. Differentials for eosinophilic inflammation include parasitic and fungal infection. Mast cell tumors should also be considered; however, the numbers of mast cells often helps to differentiate these two processes. Typically, mast cells comprise only a small proportion of the inflammatory infiltrate in allergic rhinitis, whereas mast cells tend to be the predominant cell present in mast cell tumors.

Lymphoplasmacytic Rhinitis

Until recently, only occasional cases of idiopathic lymphoplasmacytic rhinitis had been described (Burgener et al., 1987; Tasker et al., 1999b). This chronic nasal disease in

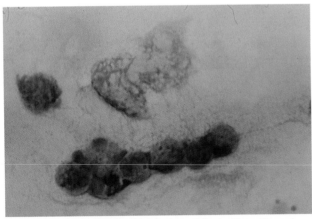

■ **FIGURE 5-6. Allergic rhinitis. Nasal flush. Dog.** Several eosinophils are enveloped in basophilic mucus that affects the stain quality of the cells. (Wright-Giemsa; HP oil.)

dogs was thought to be immune mediated rather than allergic in origin. However, a more recent study has identified that idiopathic lymphoplasmacytic rhinitis may be more common than previously suspected (Windsor et al., 2004) and may be associated with, and even contribute to, chronic nasal disease in dogs, ultimately resulting in turbinate remodeling and even bony destruction. Despite histologic evidence of bilateral disease in most dogs, a unilateral discharge was seen in some of the cases indicating the need to examine both sides of the nasal cavity even in cases that appear localized in origin. Lack of response to glucocorticoid therapy in the latter report (Windsor et al., 2004) suggests mechanisms other than immune-mediated disease, although multifactorial disease including an immune-mediated component cannot be excluded. Other proposed etiologies include immune dysregulation, allergies, or disruption of the normal microbial flora. Because aspergillosis can also induce a lymphoplasmacytic rhinitis (see Fig. 5-3), there has been concern that idiopathic lymphoplasmacytic rhinitis represents occult aspergillosis. However, analysis of cytokine profiles from nasal biopsies from dogs with these two diseases indicates that the immunologic pattern is quite different. Aspergillosis induces a predominantly T-helper type 1 (Th1) response while a partial Th2 response was detected in cases of idiopathic lymphoplasmacytic rhinitis (Peeters et al., 2007). This type 2 response is in contrast to the type 1 cytokine profile reported in cats with chronic inflammation of the nasal cavity (Johnson et al., 2005), which suggests different underlying etiologies and pathogenesis between these species.

Nasal Polyps

Nasal polyps are occasionally reported in dogs but occur most commonly in cats and are characterized by hyperplasia of the mucous membranes or exuberant proliferation of fibrous connective tissue. Polyps originate within the nasopharyngeal region from the Eustachian tube, middle ear, or nasopharynx. The majority of affected cats are young, often less than 1 year of age (Moore and Ogilvie, 2001). Nasal polyps are speculated to develop secondary to chronic irritation. Although occasional reports have suggested an underlying infectious etiology, the cause of nasal polyps remains unclear in most cases. Inflammatory polyps have the same epithelial and/or connective tissue hyperplasia but also contain a prominent inflammatory infiltrate. Polyps appear grossly as small, smooth, well-circumscribed, pedunculated masses arising from the mucosal surface of the nasal cavity. Clinical signs are usually apparent when the polyp enlarges enough to occlude the nasopharynx. Cytologically, mature lymphocytes and plasma cells are often admixed with rafts of epithelial cells (Fig. 5-7A). Small numbers of neutrophils and macrophages may also be present. Squamous metaplasia and/or dysplasia are frequently seen and, when present, can make the distinction from epithelial neoplasia difficult.

Chronic Sinusitis

Recurrent clinical signs of sneezing and nasal congestion may be related to infectious agents, parasites, allergies, foreign bodies, or neoplasia. A cause may not be demonstrated on cytology or histology in some of these cases.

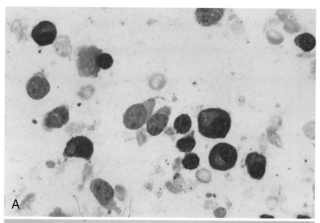

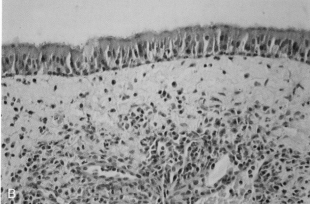

■ **FIGURE 5-7. A, Chronic inflammation. Tissue aspirate.** This mononuclear cell population is composed of small and medium-sized lymphocytes and well-differentiated plasma cells. (Wright-Giemsa; HP oil.) **B, Chronic rhinitis. Nasal mucosa. Cat.** Tissue section demonstrating intact respiratory epithelium with mild to moderate infiltration of mononuclear cells into the lamina propria. (H&E; IP) (B, Courtesy of Rose Raskin, University of Florida.)

Cytologically, respiratory epithelium appears reactive as evidenced by hyperplasia, dysplasia, or metaplasia. Inflammatory infiltrates often consist of mixed mononuclear cells, including small to medium-sized lymphocytes, plasma cells, and macrophages (Fig. 5-7B).

Infectious Causes

Bacteria

With the exception of *Bordetella bronchiseptica* and *Pasturella multocida,* which may cause acute rhinitis in the dog, primary bacterial rhinitis is rare. However, secondary bacterial infection is common and may accompany nasal neoplasia, viral infection, fungal infection, parasitic infection, trauma, foreign bodies, dental disease, or oronasal fistulation (Fig. 5-8). Infection with *Mycoplasma* sp. and *Chlamydia* sp. in cats may cause mild upper respiratory signs concurrently with conjunctivitis.

Primary bacterial infection of the nasal cavity is determined cytologically by finding large numbers of a primarily monomorphic bacteria accompanied by a marked suppurative inflammatory response with numerous phagocytized bacteria (Fig. 5-9A). Mucus may be abundant and can obscure identification of bacteria in some cases (Fig. 5-9B&C). Culture of the nasal exudate reveals heavy growth of one type of organism. However, a uniform population of organisms can also be detected with secondary or opportunistic pathogens. Therefore, because bacterial rhinitis is uncommon, significant effort should be made to identify any possible underlying causes. PCR may also be useful for detection of certain organisms, such as *Mycoplasma* sp. Identification of the bacteria as bacilli or cocci may aid initial institution of antimicrobial therapy as cocci are typically gram-positive and bacilli are typically gram-negative. The presence of filamentous organisms forming mats of colonies suggests *Actinomyces* and *Nocardia* spp. Regardless, culture and sensitivity are necessary for proper identification of microorganisms. In addition, whether bacteria are present

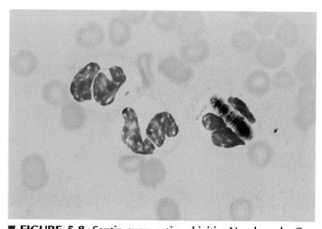

■ **FIGURE 5-8. Septic suppurative rhinitis. Nasal swab. Cat.** Three karyolytic neutrophils are present, one of which has phago-cytized *Simonsiella* sp. bacteria. An active bacterial infection was present in this animal with chronic sneezing and nasal discharge. (Wright-Giemsa; HP oil.) (Courtesy of Rose Raskin, University of Florida.)

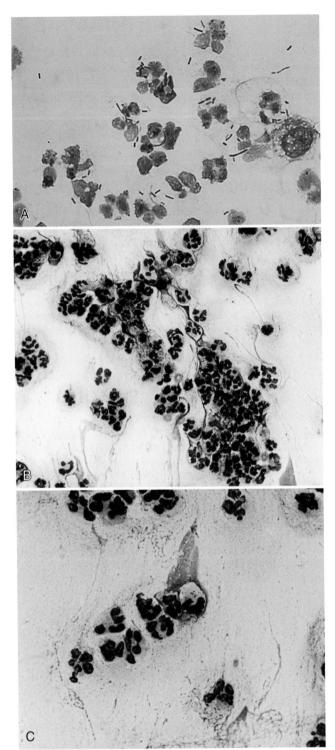

■ **FIGURE 5-9. A, Bacterial rhinitis. Nasal flush.** Large numbers of degenerate neutrophils and a monomorphic population of intracellular and extracellular rod bacteria, consistent with septic suppurative inflammation. (Wright-Giemsa; HP oil.) **B, Mucopurulent inflammation. Nasal flush.** Degenerate and nondegenerate neutrophils admixed with streams of mucous and nuclear debris. (Wright-Giemsa; HP oil.) **C, Septic mucopurulent inflammation. Nasal flush.** Closer view of B reveals the presence of intracellular short rod to cocci bacteria that can be difficult to differentiate from the extracellular mucus and cellular debris. (Wright-Giemsa; HP oil.)

as a primary or secondary pathogen or as an asymptomatic inhabitant of the nasal cavity, antimicrobial resistance may be of concern.

Viral

Viral infection of the upper airways often manifests as an acute and transient inflammatory process unless a secondary bacterial infection develops. However, if the viral infection results in turbinate damage and/or epithelial and glandular hyperplasia, chronic rhinitis may follow. Canine distemper virus, adenovirus types 1 and 2, and parainfluenza are the most common etiologies of canine viral rhinitis. Rarely disease may result from infection with herpes virus and reovirus. In cats, feline rhinotracheitis virus (feline herpesvirus I) and feline calicivirus tend to induce moderate to severe upper respiratory signs while reovirus is more often associated with milder symptoms. Severe and recurrent rhinitis is common in cats infected with feline leukemia virus (FeLV) and feline immunodeficiency virus (FIV). Diagnosis of viral rhinitis is based on patient signalment, history (lack of appropriate vaccination, contact with other animals), clinical signs (mucopurulent nasal discharge, the presence of oral ulcers, conjunctivitis, and fever), direct fluorescent antibody testing of cells obtained from conjunctival scrapings, virus isolation, and/or serology. Cytologic findings associated with viral rhinitis are typically nonspecific with variable numbers and types of inflammatory cells. In addition, the cytology of viral rhinitis is often confounded by the effects of secondary bacterial infection. Viral inclusions are very rarely observed within the epithelial cells.

Fungal

The diagnosis of fungal rhinitis can be complicated because while fungal infection can be a primary disease, fungal organisms may also be found as secondary and opportunistic invaders. In addition, fungi such as *Aspergillus* sp. and *Penicillium* sp. can occasionally be cultured from the nasal cavity of clinically normal dogs. *Aspergillus* sp. and *Penicillium* sp. are the most common fungal agents in mycotic rhinitis in the dog, whereas *Cryptococcus* sp. occurs most frequently in cats. Upper respiratory involvement with *Histoplasma capsulatum* and *Blastomyces dermatitidis* has also been reported but is rare (Table 5-1).

Aspergillosis and penicilliosis can occur as focal or disseminated respiratory infections in dogs and cats. Both fungi are morphologically similar, necessitating culture for differentiation. Because these two fungi are frequent contaminants of the respiratory tract, diagnosis should be supported by a combination of culture, cytologic, or histologic identification of the organism, and the presence of an inflammatory reaction. German shepherd dogs are frequently afflicted with systemic aspergillosis. While aspergillosis often appears as an opportunistic infection, there are reported cases without obvious predisposing factors.

Infection with *Aspergillus* sp. can be associated with purulent, granulomatous, or pyogranulomatous inflammation. Infection and inflammation may be present in

TABLE 5-1 Mycotic and Protozoal Organisms Commonly Seen in the Respiratory Tract of Dogs and Cats

Organism	Common Locations	Forms Seen	Size	Typical Cellular Location	Typical Inflammation	Cytologic Features
Fungal						
Aspergillus sp.	Nasal cavity Lung	Hyphae	5–7 μm	Extracellular	Granulomatous Pyogranulomatous	Septate, branching hyphae
Blastomyces dermatitidis	Airways Lung	Yeast	5–20 μm	Extracellular	Granulomatous Pyogranulomatous	Broad-based budding
Coccidioides immitis	Lung	Spherules Endospores	10–100 μm 2–5 μm	Extracellular	Granulomatous Pyogranulomatous	Spherules often seen
Cryptococcus neoformans	Nasal cavity Lung	Yeast Unencapsulated forms	8–40 μm 4–8 μm	Extracellular Intracellular (rare)	Variable	Narrow-based budding Mucoid capsule
Histoplasma capsulatum	Nasal cavity Airways Lung	Yeast	1–4 μm	Intracellular Extracellular	Granulomatous Pyogranulomatous	Thin, clear capsule
Penicillium sp.	Nasal cavity	Hyphae	5–7 μm	Extracellular	Granulomatous Pyogranulomatous	Cytologically similar to *Aspergillus*
Pneumocystis carinii	Lung	Cysts Trophozoites	5–10 μm 1–2 μm	Intracellular Extracellular	Granulomatous Pyogranulomatous	Free trophozoites difficult to identify
Sporothrix schenkii	Airways Lung	Yeast	2–7 μm	Intracellular Extracellular	Granulomatous Pyogranulomatous	Cigar-shaped organisms
Rhinosporidium seeberi	Nasal cavity	Endospores Sporangia	5–15 μm 30–300 μm	Extracellular	Mixed	Sporangia rare
Protozoa						
Neospora caninum	Lung	Tachyzoites	1–7 μm	Intracellular Extracellular	Mixed	Cytologically similar to *Toxoplasma* Suppurative
Toxoplasma gondii	Airways Lung	Tachyzoites	1–4 μm	Intracellular Extracellular	Mixed	Banana-shaped forms, single or clustered Suppurative

the nasal cavity alone, the frontal sinus alone, or both sites (Johnson et al., 2006). Cytologically, fungal hyphae are branching, septate, 5-7µm in width, with straight, parallel walls and globose terminal ends. Hyphae can stain either intensely basophilic with a thin, clear outer cell wall or appear as negatively staining images against a cellular background (Fig. 5-10). Hyphae may be difficult to identify when found in low numbers or in dense mats admixed with mucus, inflammatory cells, and cellular debris. Occasionally, round to ovoid blue-green fungal spores may also be observed. Periodic acid-Schiff or silver stains (GMS) are useful when fungal organisms are suspected but not readily identified in the sample. While cytologic characteristics may suggest aspergillosis, culture is necessary for a definitive diagnosis. Similar to bacterial rhinitis, the presence of fungal elements does not rule out underlying neoplasia or other disorders.

Cryptococcus sp. is a common cause of chronic upper respiratory disease in cats and is also occasionally reported in dogs. However, both *Cryptococcus neoformans* and *Cryptococcus gattii* have been reported in the nasal passages of dogs and cats in the absence of local or systemic infection (Duncan et al., 2005; Malik et al., 1997), suggesting that subclinical infection or asymptomatic carriage needs to be considered when the organism is detected in an otherwise normal animal. Inhalation is the suspected route of infection. Concurrent ocular, cutaneous, or neurologic disease may also be seen in animals with *Cryptococcus* rhinitis. Immunity is speculated to play a role in the development of infections as well as in dissemination of infection throughout the body. Corticosteroid therapy during infection worsens the symptoms as well as the disease progression (Greene, 1998; Medleau and Barsanti, 1990). However, underlying diseases, in particular those that are immunosuppressive (e.g., FeLV, FIV), have not been proven to be predisposing factors to infection (Flatland et al., 1996; Medleau and

Barsanti, 1990). Organisms are readily identified in swabs of nasal exudates or imprints/aspirates from nasal masses (Fig. 5-11A&B). Positive identification of the organism via cytology is diagnostic; however, serologic testing and fungal culture may also be useful. New methylene blue (Fig. 5-11C) and India ink can be used to demonstrate the negative staining capsule; however, care must be taken not to mistake air bubbles and fat droplets for organisms. *Cryptococcus* sp. are round to oval yeast that range in diameter from 8 to 40 µm (including the capsule). The organism has a granular internal structure that stains eosinophilic to purple and is surrounded by a thick, nonstaining, mucoid capsule. The capsule material can give the sample a mucinous texture. Occasionally, narrow-based budding may be seen. Unencapsulated or rough forms are 4 to 8 µm and are difficult to distinguish from *H. capsulatum*. Fungal culture and serology are useful in this case. The presence and type of inflammation range from the observation of a few to no inflammatory cells amid a field full of organisms to pyogranulomatous inflammation. The degree and type of inflammation may be related to characteristics of the capsule.

Rhinosporidium seeberi occasionally infects the nasal cavity of dogs resulting in single to multiple polyps in which numerous small, miliary sporangia can be observed on the surface. The pathogenesis of infection is unclear, but contact with water and trauma to the nasal mucous membranes are predisposing factors. Cytologically, preparations contain variable numbers of magenta-staining spores that range in diameter from 5 to 15µm. They have slightly refractile capsules and contain numerous, round, eosinophilic structures (spherules). In some cases, the spores stain deeply eosinophilic, preventing visualization of the internal structures. Sporangia are variably sized. They are often very large (range 30 to 300µm) (Fig. 5-12A), well-defined, globoid structures that undergo sporulation to contain numerous small, round

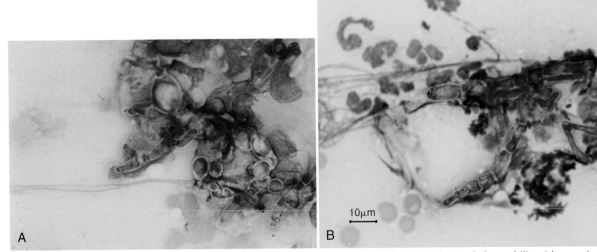

■ **FIGURE 5-10. A, Fungal rhinitis. Tissue aspirate.** Mat of branching fungal hyphae stain intensely basophilic with prominent septations and globose terminal ends. (Wright-Giemsa; HP oil.) **B, Fungal rhinitis. Nasal flush. Dog.** *Aspergillus fumigatus* hyphae shown with degenerate neutrophils is cultured from a secondary infection following treatment for cryptococcosis. (Wright; HP oil.) (B, Courtesy of Rose Raskin, Purdue University.)

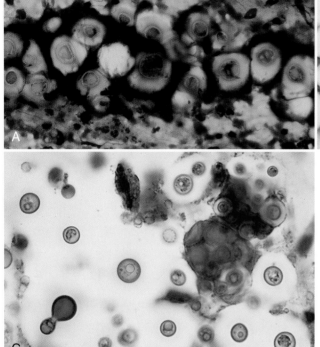

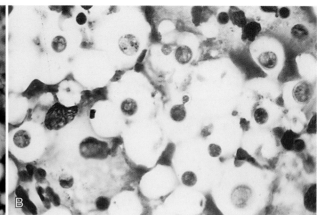

■ **FIGURE 5-11. Cryptococcal rhinitis. A, Nasal swab.** Numerous yeast forms with distinctive nonstaining, variably thick, mucoid capsules surrounding granular internal structures. The presence of inflammatory cells is variable. (Wright-Giemsa; HP oil.) **B, Nasal swab.** Narrow-based budding is a feature of Cryptococcus. (Wright-Giemsa; HP oil.) **C, Nasal discharge. Cat.** Prominent budding and internal structure along with the capsule are highlighted by a water-soluble stain. (New methylene blue; HP oil.) (C, Courtesy of Rose Raskin, University of Florida.)

endospores (Fig. 5-12B&C). Sporangia are not commonly observed in stained smears because the wall of the sporangia are slightly refractile and do not stain. Sporangia can be observed in unstained direct preparations (Caniatti et al., 1998). Endospores within the sporangia are brown when observed microscopically before staining and appear as three different basophilic forms or stages of maturation with Romanowsky stains (Meier et al., 2006). Immature endospores are approximately 2 to 4 μm in diameter with lightly basophilic cytoplasm and a pink-purple nucleus encompassing ⅓ to ½ of the endospore and 1 to 2 smaller round magenta structures. Intermediate endospores are rarely described but appear to be spherical, granular, basophilic structures approximately 5 to 8 μm in diameter with eosinophilic to globular internal structures and a variably sized, clear halo. Mature endospores tend to predominate in cytologic preparations. These structures are 8 to 15 μm in diameter, with a thick, hyalinized cell wall and a pale, magenta to nonstaining halo. Internal structure can be difficult to visualize in thick areas of the prep, but when endospores are spread out, numerous small spherical eosinophilic globular internal structures can be seen. PAS staining enhances the chance of finding the spores in cytologic or histologic specimens (Fig. 5-12D). Rhinosporidiosis incites a mixed inflammatory response consisting of neutrophils, plasma cells, and lymphocytes. Macrophages, mast cells, and eosinophils are less commonly observed.

Rosetting of inflammatory cells, particularly neutrophils, around the spores has been observed and is considered a useful feature in finding the spores during cytologic examination under low magnification (Gori and Scasso, 1994).

Sporotrichosis has been rarely identified in samples from the nasal cavity of dogs (Cafarchia et al., 2007; Whittemore and Webb, 2007). The paucity of organisms and cytologic appearance is similar to that reported for *Sporothrix schenckii* from other canine samples. *Sporothrix schenckii* has also been isolated in the nasal cavity of cats with sporotrichosis and is more commonly detected in those with cutaneous lesions (Leme et al., 2007).

Nasal mycosis due to infection of cats by *Alternaria* species, one of the dematiaceous fungi that induce phaeohyphomycosis, has been recently reported in three cats from the United Kingdom (McKay et al., 2001; Tennant et al., 2004). Cytologic findings include the presence of pyogranulomatous inflammation, lymphocytes, and plasma cells. Fungal organisms are pale staining, oval to round with septate hyphae of approximately 7 to 14 μm having a narrow peripheral clear area and finely stippled eosinophilic internal material.

Parasitic

Parasitic rhinitis is uncommon in dogs and cats and may or may not be associated with clinical signs (King et al., 1990). Infection with *Eucoleus aerophilus* (formerly

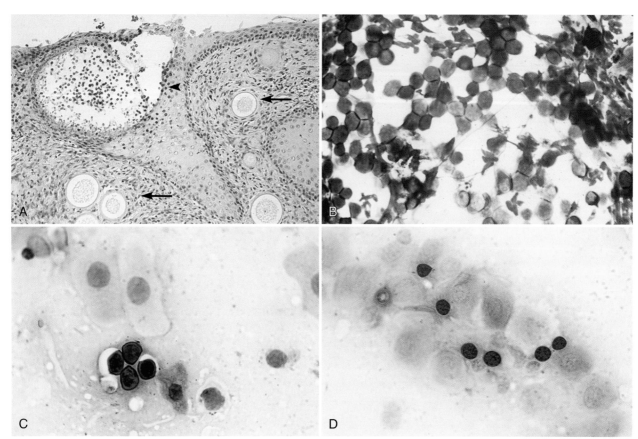

■ **FIGURE 5-12. Same case A, C, D. A, Rhinosporidia sporangia. Nasal mass. Dog.** Large mature sporangium with numerous endospores expels its contents to the surface *(arrowhead)*. Smaller, variably sized sporangia *(arrows)* are present within the lamina propria. (H&E; IP.) **B, Rhinosporidia endospores. Nasal flush. Dog.** Large numbers of round, eosinophilic staining endospores of *Rhinosporidium seeberi*. Sporangia are rarely seen cytologically. (Wright-Giemsa; HP oil.) **C, Rhinosporidia endospores. Tissue imprint.** The capsule outline of four endospores is visible along with associated squamous epithelium. (Wright; HP oil.) **D, Rhinosporidia endospores.** Seven magenta-stained endospores are prominent. (Periodic acid-Schiff; HP oil.) (A, Glass slide material courtesy of John Bentinck-Smith et al, Mississippi State University; presented at the 1984 ASVCP case review session.)

Capillaria aerophila) is diagnosed by finding the adult nematodes or characteristic ova in nasal secretions. The ova are large (60 × 35 µm), ovoid in shape, with two asymmetrical terminal plugs. Mixed inflammation often containing eosinophils is present. The nasal cavity and frontal sinuses of dogs may be inhabited by several forms of the arthropod parasite *Linguatula serrata*. Because the ova are infrequently seen in nasal exudates, this parasite is most readily diagnosed by direct visualization via rhinoscopy. The ova measure 90 × 70µm, larvae up to 500 µm, and nymphs measure 4 to 6 mm. Infection with this parasite most commonly elicits mild signs such as sneezing and nasal discharge, but occasionally severe clinical signs occur. The nasal mite *Pneumonyssoides caninum* is best diagnosed by direct rhinoscopic visualization of the off-white, 1- to 2-mm adult mites inhabiting the nasal cavity and paranasal sinuses of dogs. Infection results in a mild, transient rhinitis.

Protozoal

Leishmania sp. may induce masses in the nasal cavity of dogs. Amastigotes can be identified in aspirates or biopsies from dogs with leishmaniasis (Llanos-Cuentas et al., 1999).

Algal

Prototheca sp. may produce a nasal mass in cats near the nares resulting from a cutaneous infection. Cytologically, aspirate or swab preparations reveal a mixture of inflammatory cells, mostly degenerate neutrophils and macrophages along with numerous sporulated and nonsporulated endospores. The endospores present as variably sized spheres having a thin, clear rim and a granular, dense center (see Fig 3-23A&B).

Neoplasia of the Nasal Cavity and Paranasal Sinuses

While neoplasia of the nasal cavity and paranasal sinuses is uncommon in dogs and cats, a diagnosis of upper respiratory neoplasia usually carries a poor prognosis as the majority of nasal tumors are malignant. Carcinomas predominate in both dogs and cats. Neoplasia is more commonly diagnosed in older animals (lymphoma and transmissible venereal tumor are notable exceptions). Although no sex predilection has been observed in dogs, male cats are more often affected than females.

Tumors can arise from any of the numerous tissue types found in the nasal cavity and paranasal sinuses (Table 5-2). Identification of the site of origin can be difficult, as most malignant tumors are locally invasive, destructive, and have extended into surrounding tissues by the time of diagnosis. The majority of tumors involve the caudal two thirds of the nasal cavity near or adjacent to the cribiform plate. Less commonly, tumors may be located in the paranasal sinuses. Malignant neoplasia often involves the nasal turbinates and septum and can extend through the maxilla into the oral cavity. Extension into the orbit and cranial vault via erosion through the cribiform plate is less common but does occur. Metastasis to regional lymph nodes tends to occur late in the disease and is most often associated with epithelial tumors.

Cytologic and histopathologic diagnosis of malignant neoplasia depends on obtaining high-quality diagnostic samples. Emphasis should be placed on evaluation of samples obtained from deep tissues because secondary necrosis, inflammation, and hemorrhage are often prominent features of tumors involving the upper airways, which can confound the diagnosis.

Epithelial Neoplasia

Malignant epithelial tumors of the nasal cavity occur more frequently than their benign counterparts. The most common epithelial tumors of the nasal cavity include adenocarcinomas, squamous cell carcinomas, transitional carcinomas, and anaplastic or undifferentiated carcinomas. Adenocarcinomas are common in dogs and cats, while SCC are more common in cats (Carswell and Williams, 2007). Cytologic samples from carcinomas tend to be moderately cellular. Neoplastic epithelial cells are present in small aggregates to larger sheets (Fig. 5-13A&B).

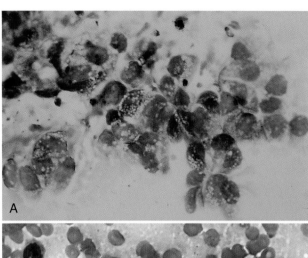

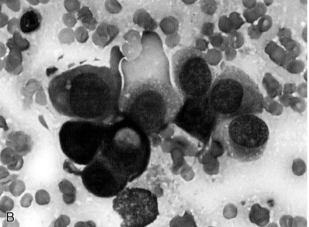

■ **FIGURE 5-13.** Nasal carcinoma. **A, Nasal flush.** Demonstration of cohesive sheets of pleomorphic cells with highly vacuolated cytoplasm. (Wright-Giemsa; HP oil.) **B, Nasal aspirate. Cat.** Poorly cohesive pleomorphic epithelial cells. Notice variation in cell and nuclear size. (Wright-Giemsa; HP oil.)

Adenocarcinomas can be identified by the presence of ring or rosette acinar arrangements that are best visualized at low magnification (e.g., 10×) (Fig. 5-14). Malignant epithelial cells are round to polygonal and typically display numerous criteria of malignancy. Such features include macrocytosis, moderate to marked anisocytosis, anisokaryosis, an increased nuclear-to-cytoplasm ratio, and deeply basophilic cytoplasm that may contain numerous discrete, clear cytoplasmic vacuoles or one large, clear vacuole (signet ring form) suggestive of secretory product. Nucleolar criteria of malignancy should also be assessed, evaluating for the number of nucleoli per nucleus and any size or shape variations. Anaplastic cells may individualize and appear similar to lymphoid cells but large cell size and periodic sheet formation are helpful in distinguishing the two types of neoplasms (Fig. 5-15A&B). Extracellular secretory material such as mucus may also be identified as eosinophilic, amorphous to fibrillar material.

SCC are distinguished by the presence of cells with angular borders containing abundant, homogenous, glassy cytoplasm and centrally placed nuclei. The neoplastic cells display a wide range in maturation, ranging from immature, small, cuboidal, nucleated, epithelial

TABLE 5-2	Neoplasia of the Nasal Cavity	
Tissue of Origin	**Benign Neoplasia**	**Malignant Neoplasia**
Epithelial	Adenoma	Adenocarcinoma[*]
	Papilloma	Squamous cell carcinoma[*]
		Transitional carcinoma
		Undifferentiated carcinoma
Mesenchymal	Fibroma	Fibrosarcoma[*]
	Chondroma	Chondrosarcoma[*]
	Osteoma	Osteosarcoma
	Leiomyoma	Leiomyosarcoma
		Undifferentiated sarcoma[*]
		Fibrous histiocytoma
		Hemongiosarcoma
		Liposarcoma
		Melanoma
Round cell (discrete)		Lymphoma[*]
		Transmissible venereal tumor[*]
		Mast cell tumor[*]
		Plasmacytoma

*Indicates most common tumor types.

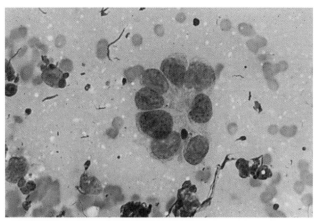

■ **FIGURE 5-14. Adenocarcinoma. Tissue imprint.** Glandular origin may be identified by the presence of acinar arrangements. (Wright-Giemsa; HP oil.)

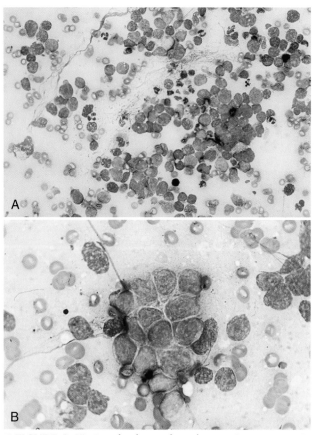

■ **FIGURE 5-15. Anaplastic nasal carcinoma. Same case A-B. A, Mass imprint. Dog.** Many individualized cells with minimal cohesiveness are present in this highly invasive nasal cavity tumor giving it a "round cell" appearance. (Wright-Giemsa; HP oil.) **B,** Areas of the slide demonstrate a cohesive, sheetlike epithelial appearance. (Wright-Giemsa; HP oil.) (A and B, Courtesy of Rose Raskin, University of Florida.)

cells with deeply basophilic cytoplasm to more mature cells, identified as anucleate, fully keratinized cells containing abundant, pale, basophilic cytoplasm and sharply angulated borders. Evidence of asynchronous development may be present such as the identification of fully

keratinized cells with retained large nuclei (Fig. 5-16A). Prominent anisokaryosis and variable chromatin patterns ranging from smooth (immature) to clumped (mature) may be seen. A few neoplastic squamous cells may also show a perinuclear clearing (perinuclear "halo") or even a few, small, clear, punctate, perinuclear vacuoles. Abundant keratinaceous debris represented as amorphous, basophilic extracellular material is often scattered about the slides. A common characteristic of SCC is the presence of a moderate to marked accompanying neutrophilic inflammatory response.

Similar in cytologic appearance to SCC is a neoplasm termed *transitional carcinoma*. This neoplasm arises from nonciliated nasal respiratory epithelium (Carswell and Williams, 2007). It may display a moderately abundant cytoplasm with numerous punctate vacuoles. Malignant features often involve anisokaryosis, multinucleation, coarse chromatin clumping, prominent nucleolus, and variable nuclear-to-cytoplasmic ratios (Fig. 5-16B&C).

Careful documentation of the above characteristics with abundant criteria of malignancy is critical to a diagnosis of neoplasia of the nasal cavity. If criteria of malignancy are not readily apparent, diagnosticians should be cautious as cytologic differentiation of a well-differentiated carcinoma from benign epithelial neoplasia, epithelial hyperplasia, or squamous metaplasia may be impossible, particularly in the presence of inflammation.

Neuroendocrine Carcinoma

Neuroendocrine carcinomas or carcinoids have been rarely described in the nasal cavity of dogs (Patnaik et al., 2002; Sako et al., 2005). Histologically their features appear to be similar to those described elsewhere in the body. Cytologic characteristics have not been reported.

Mesenchymal Neoplasia

Mesenchymal neoplasia of the nasal cavity is uncommon. However, when present, osteosarcoma, fibrosarcoma, and chondrosarcoma are the mesenchymal tumors most often seen (Fig. 5-17). When present, chondrosarcomas are more likely to occur in young dogs with a possible increased risk in medium to large breeds (Lana and Withrow, 2001). Cytologic samples are typically of low cellularity consisting of individualized and occasionally small, loose aggregates of oval, plump, or spindle-shaped cells (Figs. 5-18A&B). Cytoplasmic borders are typically ill defined and neoplastic cells may contain few to moderate numbers of fine eosinophilic to purple cytoplasmic granules. Matrix may be observed as streaming, brightly eosinophilic, fibrillar material often intimately associated with the neoplastic cells. However, this material is easily confused with mucus, and the presence or absence of streaming eosinophilic material on a cytologic preparation should not be used to differentiate the type of neoplasia.

A cytologic diagnosis of mesenchymal neoplasia is complicated by several factors. Mesenchymal neoplasia often exfoliates poorly resulting in a hemodiluted sample that contains only a few pleomorphic spindle-shaped

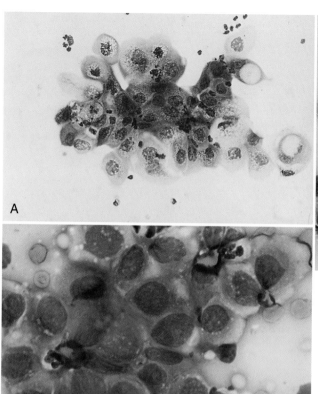

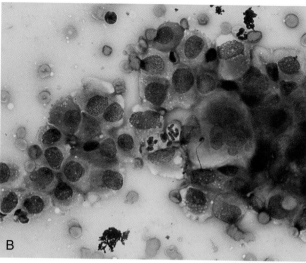

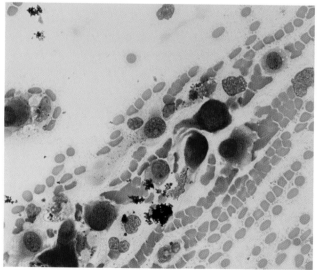

■ **FIGURE 5-16. A, Squamous cell carcinoma. Nasal flush.** Asynchronous keratinization, moderate pleomorphism, and perinuclear vacuolation are typical features of squamous cell carcinoma. The associated suppurative inflammation is commonly seen with this type of tumor. (Wright-Giemsa; HP oil.) **Same case B-C. Transitional carcinoma. Nasal mass imprint. Dog. B,** This appearance is similar to squamous cell carcinoma. Shown is a multinucleate cell with mild neutrophilic inflammation. Notice the pleomorphism of the transitional or nonciliated respiratory epithelium. (Wright-Giemsa; HP oil.) **C,** Notice the moderately abundant cytoplasm with numerous punctate vacuoles. Malignant features involve anisokaryosis, coarse chromatin clumping, prominent nucleoli, and variable nuclear-to-cytoplasmic ratios (Wright-Giemsa; HP oil.) (B and C, Courtesy of Rose Raskin, Purdue University.)

■ **FIGURE 5-17. Frontal sinus sarcoma. Aspirate. Dog.** Several individualized oval-to spindle-shaped pleomorphic cells are present in a background of erythrocytes. Several cells contain a faint dusting of azurophilic granules seen in some mesenchymal neoplasias. (Wright-Giemsa; HP oil.)

cells for evaluation. Also, significant inflammation can induce reactive fibroplasia that can be difficult to distinguish from fibrosarcoma. In this case, cytologic evaluation coupled with physical exam and historical and radiographic information raises the index of suspicion for mesenchymal neoplasia, warranting biopsy with histopathologic examination for definitive diagnosis. Additionally, histopathology is often necessary for classification of mesenchymal neoplasia, as the more commonly seen mesenchymal tumors often lack distinguishing cytologic features. Other types of mesenchymal tumors involving the upper airways (see Table 5-2) are uncommon but have cytologic features resembling soft tissue sarcomas in more common sites.

Discrete Cell Neoplasia

Discrete cell (round cell) tumors such as lymphoma, plasmacytomas, mast cell tumors, and transmissible venereal tumors can occur in the nasal cavity. These tumors yield highly cellular preparations composed of individualized, neoplastic, and discrete, round cells with distinct cytoplasmic borders. The morphology resembles that seen in other sites.

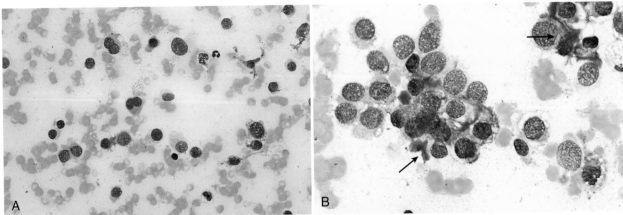

■ **FIGURE 5-18. Nasal chondrosarcoma. Tissue imprint. Dog. Same case A-B. A,** There was a 3-month history of serous nasal discharge and gurgling sounds from nares. Present are pleomorphic individualized cells that display high nuclear-to-cytoplasmic ratios. Several binucleate forms are noted. (Wright-Giemsa; HP oil.) **B,** Matrix is observed as streaming magenta, fibrillar material intimately associated with the aggregated neoplastic population *(arrows)*. (Wright-Giemsa; HP oil.) (A, Courtesy of Rose Raskin, University of Florida.)

Lymphoma is the most common discrete cell tumor reported in the nasal cavity of dogs and cats. In cats, the majority of nasal lymphomas are of B-cell origin, although T-cell lymphoma of the nasal cavity has also been reported (Day et al., 2004; Mukaratirwa et al., 2001). Lymphoma of the nasal cavity tends to be characterized by a monomorphic population of medium-sized or large, immature lymphoblasts with scant, deeply basophilic cytoplasm, large round nuclei, finely granular chromatin, and single to multiple nucleoli (Fig. 5-19). Anaplastic nasal carcinomas (see Fig. 5-15A) can individualize and resemble lymphoma but the presence of very large cells and occasional sheet formation will assist in making the proper diagnosis. Care should be taken to distinguish lymphoma from lymphoid hyperplasia or an inflammatory polyp (see Fig. 5-7A). In lymphoid hyperplasia, a heterogeneous population of lymphocytes and plasma cells are present, with a predominance of small, mature lymphocytes and fewer intermediate-sized lymphocytes and lymphoblasts. In some cases, lymphoma is characterized by a predominance of intermediate-sized lymphocytes with an increased amount of cytoplasm and smooth chromatin lacking nucleoli. Even more problematic are cases where the neoplastic population consists of small, well-differentiated lymphocytes. In such questionable cases, histopathology is imperative for definitive diagnosis of lymphoma.

Canine transmissible venereal tumor (TVT) is a contagious neoplasm involving the external genitalia of both sexes with a low occurrence of metastasis. Spread to the nasal cavity is thought to occur secondary to implantation from a primary genital tumor; however, there are several reports of primary intranasal TVT (Ginel et al., 1995; Papazoglou et al., 2001; Perez et al., 1994). Cytologic preparations reveal large numbers of a monomorphic population of large, round cells with abundant, light to moderately basophilic cytoplasm containing numerous, distinct, small vacuoles. Nuclei are round with coarse to ropy chromatin with 1 or 2 large, prominent nucleoli. Mitoses are frequently observed (Fig. 5-20).

Histiocytic Sarcoma

Canine histiocytic neoplasia can present as either a local or disseminated process. Localized histiocytic sarcomas tend to arise from the subcutis but occasionally originate from other sites including the nasal cavity (Affolter and Moore, 2002). The morphology of cells in this report varied from site to site, as well as within different nodules of the same tumor; however, it was similar in phenotype and variation to those previously described.

Miscellaneous Neoplasia

Oncocytoma of the nasal cavity has been rarely reported in dogs and cats (Doughty et al., 2006) (see section on laryngeal oncocytoma for discussion of cytologic features).

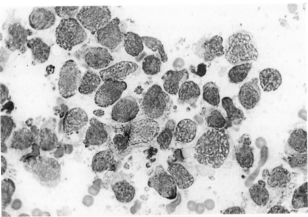

■ **FIGURE 5-19. Nasal lymphoma. Mass imprint. Cat.** Monomorphic population of large round cells with scant cytoplasm, irregularly round nuclei, and single prominent single nucleolus. History included 1-year duration of nasal congestion. (Wright-Giemsa; HP oil.) (Courtesy of Rose Raskin, University of Florida.)

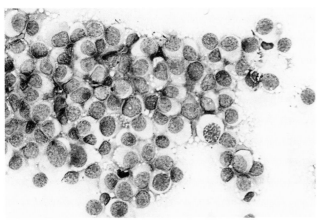

■ **FIGURE 5-20. Transmissible venereal tumor. Nasal mass imprint. Dog.** Highly cellular, moderately pleomorphic population of discrete cells with abundant pale cytoplasm, ropy chromatin, and distinct nucleoli. (Wright-Giemsa; HP oil.)

Intranasal and sinus melanoma appears to be uncommon, but has been reported in both dogs (Hicks and Fidel, 2006) and cats (Mukaratirwa et al., 2001).

LARYNX

Anatomic and Histologic Features

The larynx is a musculocartilaginous portion of the upper respiratory tract that encompasses the vocal folds, arytenoid cartilage, and glottis. The larynx is composed of an elastic cartilage that is lined by a stratified squamous epithelium with collections of lymphoid tissue scattered throughout the lamina propria.

Sample Collection

Respiratory stridor, dyspnea, and changes in or loss of vocal tone suggest laryngeal disease. Cytologic evaluation of the larynx is most useful for the characterization of mass lesions, infiltrative processes, or inflammatory disease and depends on obtaining adequate, representative samples. Laryngeal masses, while uncommon, may be detected and stabilized for sampling by palpation. Radiographs may help detect and localize mass lesions, but may be difficult to interpret due to breed variations and superimposition of soft tissues. Ultrasonographic evaluation affords superior visualization of laryngeal masses and guidance for FNA. Ultrasound-guided aspiration through the ventral laryngeal cartilage has not been associated with significant complications, even in cats (Rudorf and Brown, 1998).

Laryngoscopy allows direct visualization and sampling of laryngeal masses but requires anesthesia. Lidocaine spray may be necessary for complete examination and sampling because of laryngospasm, especially in cats. Masses observed during laryngoscopy can be sampled directly by FNA or brush cytology, or alligator biopsy forceps may be used to obtain pinch biopsies for cytologic touch imprints. Intraluminal sampling

may be associated with significant hemorrhage and edema, particularly in cats, which can result in laryngeal obstruction.

Normal and Inflammatory Cytologic Features

Normal

Samples from the normal larynx typically are sparsely cellular with only scattered squamous epithelial cells observed. Occasional aspirates or brush samples may demonstrate small aggregates of well-differentiated lymphocytes in addition to the epithelial cells.

Inflammation

The most common causes of laryngitis in dogs and cats are infectious (e.g., infectious tracheobronchitis, rhinotracheitis) or to the result of local irritation from inhalation, intubation, or chronic coughing. The laryngeal mucosa and vocal folds are reddened, thickened, and frequently edematous without evidence of mass lesions. Suppurative inflammation is commonly present, although observation of etiologic agents is rare. Hemorrhage is identified by the presence of erythrophagocytic macrophages, while edema is characterized by a basophilic granular proteinaceous fluid background. In chronic inflammation, fibrosis or ossification of the larynx often occurs, resulting in sparsely cellular aspirates containing rare spindle-shaped cells.

Granulomatous laryngitis

Granulomatous laryngitis is a distinct, but uncommon syndrome seen in dogs and cats that may mimic the appearance of neoplasia both grossly and cytologically (Oakes and McCarthy, 1994; Tasker et al., 1999a). Mass lesions can be large and may obstruct the laryngeal lumen. The cytologic appearance is similar to other granulomatous lesions and is characterized by the presence of large numbers of epithelioid macrophages. Lymphocytes may also be present. In chronic lesions, fibroplasia is prominent and aspiration reveals increased numbers of plump, moderately pleomorphic, spindle-shaped cells easily confused with mesenchymal neoplasia. Etiologic agents are not observed and the underlying cause of granulomatous laryngitis is unknown.

Reactive Lymphoid hyperplasia

Reactive lymphoid hyperplasia may occur secondary to infectious, inflammatory, or neoplastic disorders of the larynx. Reactive hyperplasia is differentiated from lymphoma by the heterogeneity of the lymphocyte population, orderly progression from lymphoblasts to small lymphocytes, and the presence of plasma cells and/or other inflammatory cells such as neutrophils, macrophages, and eosinophils.

Laryngeal Neoplasia

Tumors of the larynx are uncommon in small animals; however, primary laryngeal tumors have been identified in both dogs and cats. These tumors can arise from the epithelial or musculocartilagenous components of the larynx, or from the lymphoid nodules. Lymphoma is the most commonly reported laryngeal tumor in the cat, followed by squamous cell carcinoma. In dogs, carcinomas and SCC predominate.

Lymphoma

Lymphoma of the larynx has the same diversity of appearance as lymphoma in other sites. Typically, a uniform population of lymphoblasts is observed (Fig. 5-21). Cytologic diagnosis of intermediate or small cell lymphoma is difficult because of the uniform, well-differentiated appearance of the lymphocytes. In these cases, a biopsy and histologic examination is necessary for diagnosis.

Squamous Cell Carcinoma

Because the larynx is lined by squamous epithelial cells, it is necessary to ensure that a deep sample is obtained as swabs, scrapings, or shallow aspiration will result in exfoliation of the surface squamous lining. Aspirates from SCC tend to be of moderate cellularity. Individual cell morphology ranges from basal to fully keratinized squamous epithelial cells (Fig. 5-22A&B). Basal cells are immature, cuboidal to round, epithelial cells with deeply basophilic cytoplasm, large central nuclei, coarse chromatin, and prominent nucleoli. Mature squamous cells are large with angular borders and contain abundant homogenous cytoplasm and pyknotic or karyorrhectic nuclei. The presence of mature squamous cells alone in a laryngeal sample should not be interpreted as SCC. Multiple stages of epithelial cell development, cellular pleomorphism, and the presence of asynchronous cytoplasmic and nuclear maturation are necessary for a cytologic diagnosis of SCC. Suppurative inflammation is commonly associated with SCC and can confound the diagnosis as inflammation can induce squamous dysplasia.

Carcinoma

Carcinoma of the larynx is more prevalent in dogs than in cats. Aspirates are moderately cellular and contain small clusters or sheets of cohesive epithelial cells with round, centrally located nuclei, coarsely clumped

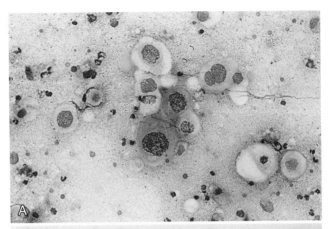

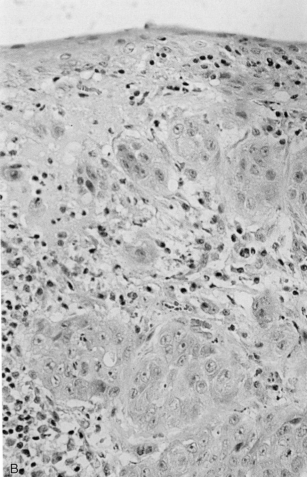

■ **FIGURE 5-22. Squamous cell carcinoma. A, Tissue aspirate.** Pleomorphic squamous epithelium in several stages are evident in association with suppurative inflammation. (Wright-Giemsa; ×50.) **B, Laryngeal mass. Cat.** Clinical signs included brief duration of dyspnea. Tissue section demonstrates islands of neoplastic squamous cells that extend into the deeper tissues. Lymphocytes, plasma cells, and neutrophils are also present indicating chronic active inflammation. (H&E; IP.) (B, Courtesy of Rose Raskin, University of Florida.)

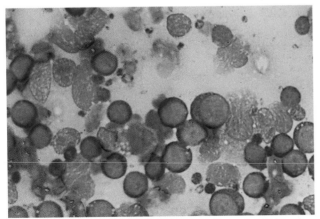

■ **FIGURE 5-21. Lymphoma. Tissue aspirate.** Large lymphoblasts with scant, deeply basophilic cytoplasm, smooth chromatin, and prominent nucleoli. (Wright-Giemsa; HP oil.)

chromatin, and basophilic cytoplasm. Well-differentiated carcinomas are characterized by a relatively uniform population of epithelial cells with only mild to moderate anisocytosis and anisokaryosis and single or indistinct nucleoli. Poorly differentiated carcinomas show moderate to marked pleomorphism between clumps of cells as well as within cells of the same cluster. Laryngeal adenocarcinomas are extremely rare; thus acinar formation or ductular structures are not expected cytologic features of laryngeal carcinomas.

In addition to tumors arising from the larynx, perilaryngeal thyroid carcinomas (see Chapter 16) can invade the larynx and should be considered as a differential.

Laryngeal oncocytoma

Oncocytoma is a relatively common tumor of the larynx in small animals, especially younger dogs. A laryngeal oncocytoma typically presents as a well-circumscribed mass projecting from the laryngeal ventricle. Early reports of laryngeal oncocytomas in dogs (Bright et al., 1994; Pass et al., 1980) were later reviewed (Meuten et al., 1985) and found to be of muscle origin. Oncocytomas are benign tumors arising from oncocytes (oxyphil cells) that appear to be neuroendocrine in origin although the exact genesis of these cells remains unclear. Others believe that these cells originate from transformation of ductular or seromucous gland epithelial cells (Doughty et al., 2006). Cytologically, the tumor is comprised of moderately pleomorphic, large, pale-staining, epithelial cells with abundant foamy to vacuolated cytoplasm. Nuclei are large, round to oval, and centrally located with finely clumped chromatin and typically contain a single, indistinct nucleolus. Anisocytosis and anisokaryosis are common. The tumor frequently contains large areas of hemorrhage that may result in hemodiluted specimens with few neoplastic cells. Rhabdomyomas and granular cell tumors can also originate from the larynx and may require examination by electron microscopy for definitive diagnosis (Tang et al., 1994). Oncocytomas possess abundant numbers of mitochondria in the cytoplasm and express cytokeratin (Doughty et al., 2006) while granular cell tumors stain positive for vimentin, S-100, and NSE (Patnaik, 1993). See Table 5-3 for a list of distinguishing features between several similar laryngeal neoplasms.

Mesenchymal Neoplasia

Tumors arising from the musculocartilagenous component are rare but include leiomyoma, leiomyosarcoma, fibrosarcoma (Fig. 5-23A&B) , chondrosarcoma, osteosarcoma, rhabdomyosarcoma, and rhabdomyoma

---

TABLE 5-3 Comparative Diagnostic Features of Cytologically Similar Laryngeal Tumors

Characteristics	Rhabdomyoma	Oncocytoma	Granular cell tumor
Cell of origin	Muscle	Oncocyte. Speculate origin from transformed duct or glandular epithelium.	Unknown. Speculate neural tissue, possibly Schwann cells or meningeal cells.
Behavior	Benign	Benign	Unclear
Signalment	Younger, middle-aged	Younger, middle-aged	Dogs > cats
Clinical presentation	Solitary, fleshy, well-circumscribed mass. Originates from submucosa, projects into laryngeal lumen.	Solitary, fleshy, well-circumscribed mass. Originates from submucosa, projects into laryngeal lumen.	Oral cavity is predominant site but cutaneous and CNS forms also reported.
Cytology	Large cells with abundant granular or foamy cytoplasm with large, central to eccentric nuclei with finely clumped chromatin and a single, indistinct nucleolus. Multinucleate cells may be seen.	Large, pale-staining, epithelial cells with abundant foamy cytoplasm, large, centrally located, round nuclei with finely clumped chromatin, and single, indistinct nucleolus.	Variably sized round to polygonal cells with small, eccentric nucleus and abundant granular eosinophilic cytoplasm
Pleomorphism	Moderate	Moderate	Slight to moderate
Histology	Large polygonal cells with abundant eosinophilic granular cytoplasm arranged in sheets, cords, and acinar structures with fine fibrovascular stroma. Striations may be seen.	Large polygonal cells with abundant eosinophilic granular cytoplasm arranged in sheets, cords, and acinar structures with fine fibrovascular stroma. Nuclei may be basally oriented.	Variably sized oval to polygonal cells with abundant, pale, eosinophilic cytoplasm, distinct intracytoplasmic granules, distinct cell margins, and small nuclei.
EM	Abundant mitochondria, myofibrils, Z-bands	Abundant mitochondria	Large numbers of membrane-bound lysosomal vacuoles
Diagnostic Markers	Desmin* Myoglobin Actin PTAH	Cytokeratin* PTAH	All variably reported, no marker is consistent PAS (diastase resistant)* S-100 NSE Vimentin

*Most reliable

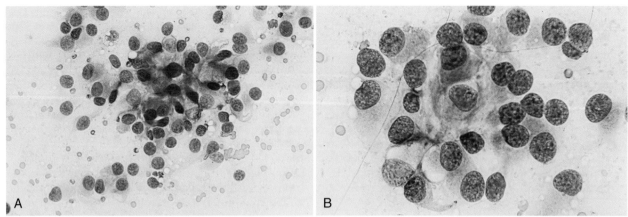

■ FIGURE 5-23. Laryngeal fibrosarcoma. Same case A-B. A, Mass imprint. Cat. Aggregate of mesenchymal-appearing cells in an animal with monthlong-duration dysphonia and recent dyspnea. (Aqueous-based Wright; HP oil.) **B,** An eosinophilic intercellular matrix is associated with the neoplastic cells. Nuclei are oval to round with granular chromatin and small nucleoli. Cytoplasmic borders are wispy and indistinct. Immunohistochemistry was negative for muscle markers. (Aqueous-based Wright; HP oil.) (A and B, Courtesy of Rose Raskin, University of Florida.)

(Figs. 5-24 and 5-25A&B). Malignant melanoma and granular cell tumors may also arise from the laryngeal region in dogs. In general, these tumors resemble their counterparts arising in more common sites, although oncocytomas and rhabdomyomas may be difficult to differentiate without the use of additional diagnostics such as electron microscopy or immunohistochemical staining for desmin, myoglobin, or actin (see Table 5-3). Laryngeal rhabdomyomas (Fig. 5-25A&B) have plump, large cells with abundant granular or foamy to vacuolated cytoplasm. Nuclei are large, round to oval, and centrally located with finely clumped chromatin and

typically contain a single, indistinct nucleolus. Aniso-cytosis and anisokaryosis are common. The tumor frequently contains large areas of hemorrhage, which may result in hemodiluted specimens with few neoplastic cells. Rhabdomyomas are similar cytologically to oncocytomas in other sites. Ultrastructurally, oncocytomas and rhabdomyomas or rhabdomyosarcomas contain numerous mitochondria and may be distinguished by finding myofibrils and Z-bands as evidence of muscle origin (Tang et al., 1994). Definitive diagnosis of muscle origin tumors is best accomplished with immunohistochemical staining for desmin, myoglobin, or actin (Barnhart and Lewis, 2000; Meuten et al., 1985).

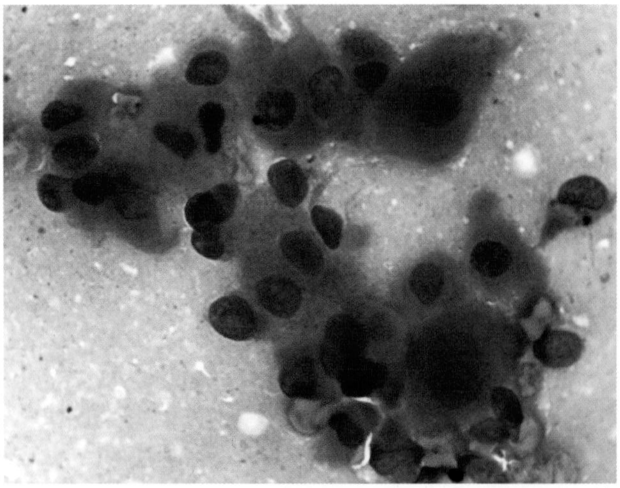

Laryngeal Cysts and Mucoceles

Laryngeal cysts and salivary mucoceles are uncommon findings in the larynx. Fluid aspirated from the cyst is typically of low cellularity and ranges from clear to milky in appearance. Mucoceles will contain macrophages, nondegenerate neutrophils, and perhaps vacuolated salivary epithelial cells. In the single case report of a laryngeal mucocele, variably sized basophilic amorphous, anuclear structures were present and were thought to represent inspissated saliva (Wiedmeyer et al., 2003).

TRACHEA, BRONCHI, AND LUNGS

Normal Anatomy and Histology of the Airways and Lung

The anatomic components of the remaining air passages include the trachea, bronchi, bronchioli, and alveoli. The trachea extends from the base of the larynx to the corina and is composed of incomplete cartilaginous rings supported by connective tissue and smooth muscle lined by ciliated, pseudostratified epithelium. The transition to pseudostratified epithelium begins as the larynx merges with the trachea and extends to the bronchi. Goblet cells are commonly found within the tracheal epithelium.

■ FIGURE 5-24. Laryngeal mass imprint. Dog. Variably sized, cuboidal to polygonal cells with moderate amounts of amphophilic, foamy, to granular cytoplasm. Oncocytoma and rhabdomyoma would be differentials for this cytologic appearance and additional diagnostic tests would be necessary to differentiate the two neoplasms. Electron microscopy and immunohistochemistry indicated that this mass was of muscle origin (Wright-Giemsa; HP oil.) (Glass slide material courtesy of Shawn P. Clark et al, Purdue University; presented at the 2002 ASVCP case review session.)

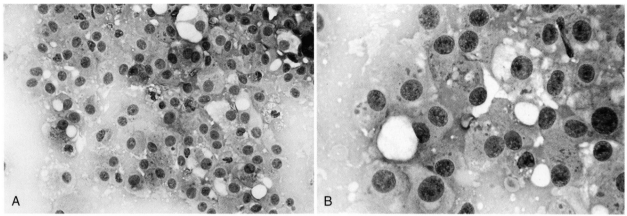

■ **FIGURE 5-25. Laryngeal rhabdomyoma. Mass imprint. Dog. Same case A-B. A,** Highly cellular sample with a monomorphic population of large epithelioid-appearing cells having abundant eosinophilic cytoplasm. Large, distinct, clear vacuoles are present within the cytoplasm of several cells. (Aqueous-based Wright; HP oil.) **B,** Nuclei are generally round with coarse chromatin and small, prominent, single or multiple nucleoli. The cytoplasm may contain large vacuoles that displace the nucleus or large pink granules. Vacuoles were negative for lipid or glycogen. The neoplastic cells were positive for sarcomeric actin, confirming its muscle origin. (Aqueous-based Wright; HP oil.) (A and B, Courtesy of Rose Raskin, University of Florida.)

Bronchi are similar in structure to the trachea; however, bronchial cartilaginous rings are complete rather than C-shaped. Smaller airways, or bronchioles, have no cartilaginous support, are composed of smooth muscle, and are lined by ciliated and nonciliated cuboidal epithelium. Terminal bronchioles branch into respiratory bronchioles that further divide into alveolar ducts, alveolar sacs, and alveoli. Alveoli are lined by flattened epithelium (type I pneumocytes) with lesser numbers of more cuboidal epithelial cells (type II pneumocytes). Type I pneumocytes typically cover more than 90% of the alveolar surface. Type II pneumocytes are responsible for synthesizing pulmonary surfactant. There is a support network of connective tissue underlying the epithelium consisting of fine reticular, collagenous, and elastic fibers with occasional fibroblasts. Intermingling between the alveoli are a large number of capillaries. The lung has a resident population of macrophages that exist primarily in the alveoli. When activated, alveolar macrophages become large, highly vacuolated, and highly phagocytic. Airways contain foci of bronchus-associated lymphoid tissue (BALT) as well as serous and mucous secreting submucosal glands located in the submucosa and lamina propria. These may be sampled during evaluation of the respiratory tract if the overlying epithelium is damaged.

Collection Techniques

Transtracheal wash (TTW) and bronchoalveolar lavage (BAL) are relatively straightforward, inexpensive procedures with high diagnostic potential. The samples can be used for cytologic examination of airway disease as well as for culture and sensitivity. In animals with respiratory disease, it is important to obtain a cytologic sample in a manner that will yield a large number of well-preserved cells. Indications for sampling the airways are clinical and/or radiographic evidence of respiratory disease. Tracheal washes are helpful for examining the larger airways, whereas bronchoalveolar lavage focuses on the smaller

airways and alveoli. It is important to note that studies have shown that 68% of cases have different cytologic characteristics in the TTW fluid versus BAL fluid; therefore, it is essential to interpret results based on the technique that is used (Hawkins et al, 1995). These techniques allow identification of inflammatory processes in the lungs without the risk of lung biopsy. While complications are minimal, appropriate sample handling, transport, and preparation are essential for an accurate and complete diagnosis. There are multiple techniques for collection from the tracheobronchial tract, several of which will be reviewed.

Transtracheal Wash

The purpose of a transtracheal wash is to collect fluid and/or cells from the trachea in a sterile fashion. Airway sampling can be achieved by direct penetration through the tracheal wall or via an endotracheal tube. The former technique is usually reserved for larger dogs, and the latter is performed in smaller dogs and cats.

Direct aspiration of the tracheal lumen can be performed by entering through the cricothyroid ligament or between tracheal rings. The animal should be placed in sternal recumbency for either technique. Sedation is optional depending on the demeanor of the patient. General anesthesia impairs the cough reflex necessary to retrieve an adequate sample and is typically not used for TTW procedures. Sterility should be maintained; therefore, the area of the cricothyroid ligament should be clipped and surgically prepared and sterile gloves should be worn during the procedure. The cricothyroid ligament is palpable as an indentation between the thyroid and cricoid cartilage of the larynx. Lidocaine should be injected in the skin and underlying subcutaneous tissue of this area. A 16- to 19-gauge jugular catheter is used for the wash depending on the size of the animal. Generally, a 16-gauge catheter is recommended for dogs weighing more than 50 lbs, an 18- or 19-gauge catheter is used in dogs weighing 20 to 50 lbs, and a 19-gauge catheter is recommended for cats and dogs weighing less than

20 lbs. The needle of the catheter should be inserted, bevel down, through the area of skin where the lidocaine has been injected. The needle is passed through the ligament at a downward angle to avoid laceration of the larynx and to decrease risk of oropharyngeal contamination. The catheter is passed over the needle, approximately to the level of the corina (4th intercostal space). At this time, the needle is removed, leaving the catheter in place. Approximately 0.1 to 0.2 ml/kg of warm, sterile, nonbacteriostatic saline is used for the wash. Half of the volume is injected rapidly to induce coughing. The syringe is disconnected and replaced with an empty syringe for aspiration (Fig. 5-26). Aspiration is repeated until no more fluid is obtained. The procedure is then repeated with the remainder of the saline.

This method has the advantage that general anesthesia is not required. Also, the chance of oropharyngeal contamination is low, although still possible if the catheter goes cranially and through the vocal folds of the larynx. Complications with this technique are uncommon but may include subcutaneous emphysema, tracheal laceration, hemorrhage, hemoptysis, pneumomediastinum, and/or pneumothorax (Rakich and Latimer, 1989).

An alternative method is to perform the TTW by way of an endotracheal tube. General anesthesia is required for this procedure as an endotracheal tube must be placed. Care must be taken not to contaminate the tip of the endotracheal tube in the oropharynx. After intubation, the cuff is inflated and the animal is placed in lateral recumbency. A jugular catheter or sterile polypropylene urinary catheter is then inserted into the endotracheal tube and extended to the corina. A red rubber feeding tube should not be used since these easily collapse during aspiration of viscous material such as mucus (Smallwood and Zenoble, 1993). Once the catheter is placed, saline is instilled and collected as described above.

Bronchoalveolar Lavage

Bronchoalveolar lavage is used to sample the smaller airways and alveoli and is therefore more effective than TTW at sampling the lower respiratory tract. As for tracheal washes, there are multiple techniques for BAL, each with variable advantages. All techniques yield highly diagnostic samples. The two techniques that will be described are bronchoscopy and BAL via an endotracheal tube.

Bronchoscopy is an excellent method for obtaining a BAL sample. Specific equipment is necessary to utilize this method, and the animal must be of adequate size to allow placement of the bronchoscope beyond the mainstem bronchus. The use of flexible endoscopes that are less than 5 mm in outer diameter for bronchoscopy in cats has been reported to yield highly diagnostic BAL samples with minimal complications (Johnson and Drazenovich, 2007). The animal must be maintained under general anesthesia. After placement of the endotracheal tube, the fiberoptic bronchoscope is passed through the endotracheal tube to allow visualization of the trachea and mainstem bronchi (Fig. 5-27). If radiographs have been taken prior to bronchoscopy, specific lobes of the lung may be selected based on localization or severity of the lesion. Warmed, sterile saline is injected through the biopsy channel in a volume equaling 5 ml/kg and can be aspirated in the same syringe by applying gentle suction (Hawkins and DeNicola, 1995). Saline can be injected as one large bolus or in 2 to 3 aliquots (Rakich and Latimer, 1989). Multiple lung lobes should be lavaged to increase the opportunity of identifying etiologic agents or cells with criteria of malignancy. It is advisable to keep animals on supplemental oxygen after the procedure, if not during, to decrease the risk of hypoxia. Advantages of this technique include the ability to visualize the airway, choose the lobe to be lavaged, and biopsy masses, if observed (McCauley et al., 1998).

If a bronchoscope is unavailable or the patient is too small for the scope to pass through the endotracheal tube or beyond the main stem bronchus, a BAL may be performed via an endotracheal tube (Hawkins et al., 1994). The procedure has been well described in cats but may also be performed in dogs. Again, general anesthesia is required. After intubation, the animal should be placed in lateral recumbency, with the most severely affected

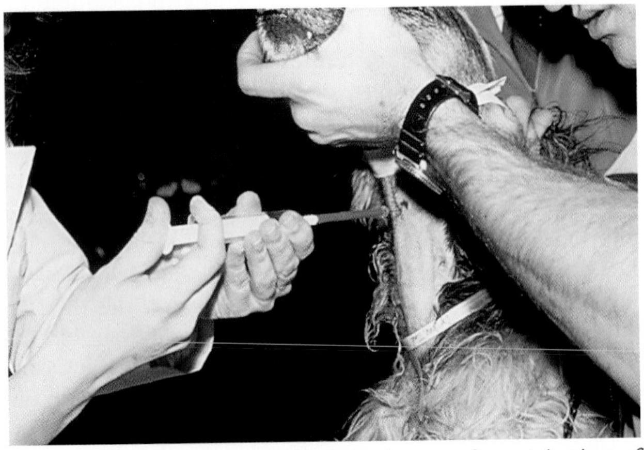

■ **FIGURE 5-26. Transtracheal wash procedure.** Injection of saline fluid following proper placement of catheter through the cricoid ligament in a dog. (Courtesy of Robert King, University of Florida.)

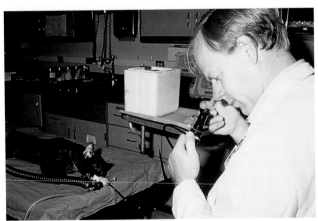

■ **FIGURE 5-27. BAL procedure.** Placement of the fiberoptic scope through the endotracheal tube followed by injection of a saline fluid. (Courtesy of Robert King, University of Florida.)

side down. Following inflation of the endotracheal tube cuff, a syringe adapter is attached to the end of the tube. Three separate aliquots of fluid (warm, sterile saline) should be used totaling 5 ml/kg. The first aliquot should be injected rapidly and followed immediately by application of suction using the same syringe until no more fluid is obtained. This procedure is repeated for the second and third aliquots. The rear of the animal may be elevated to assist with fluid retrieval.

BAL results in localized edema, alveolar distention, mild to moderate congestion, and alveolar collapse. The primary complication of BAL techniques is a transient hypoxia that is associated with decreased compliance and ventilation/perfusion mismatch (Hawkins et al., 1995). The patient should be supplemented with oxygen for 5 to 20 minutes after the BAL and monitored with a pulse oximeter if available.

The sample should immediately be placed on ice and cytocentrifuged within 30 to 60 minutes of collection for optimal results (Hawkins et al., 1990; Latimer, 1993). It is advisable to divide the samples from a BAL into two portions: one portion being placed into an EDTA tube to preserve cellular morphology, and the other portion being placed into a sterile container that does not have anticoagulant for possible microbiologic culture. Neutrophils and macrophages may phagocytize RBCs, extracellular bacteria, and other debris if the sample is not prepared within the recommended time period, thus leading to erroneous interpretation of the sample.

Cell counts can be performed on a standard hemacytometer or by an automated cell counter. The accuracy of these counts may be questionable due to increased mucus and lack of standardization of techniques; however, cell counts are crucial following a BAL to establish adequacy of the sample (Hawkins and DeNicola, 1989). If less than 250 cells/μl are observed, the procedure should be repeated. Recent studies have suggested the use of urea dilution to standardize the cellular and noncellular components of BAL fluid samples for more adequate analysis of nucleated cell counts in epithelial lining fluid (Mills and Litster, 2006). A standardized procedure for sampling needs to be implemented in the hospital to ensure accurate interpretation of all BAL samples.

The sample should be examined grossly and if large mucus plugs are observed, squash preparations should be made as cells and organisms are frequently embedded within mucus. The cellular component of the fluid should be concentrated. Cytocentrifugation is the preferred technique, if available. Alternatively, the sample may be centrifuged at 450 *g* (1000 RPM) for 10 minutes and the supernatant removed, reserving 50 to 100 μl to resuspend the cell pellet. A concentrated direct smear can be made from this sample.

Bronchial Brushing

Bronchial brushings are obtained by use of bronchoscopy. Cytologic findings may be similar to those seen for BAL; however, in dogs with chronic coughs bronchial brushings are more sensitive for detecting the presence of neutrophils and suppurative inflammation (Hawkins et al., 2006). Therefore, obtaining both lavage and brushing samples may be useful in certain cases.

Transthoracic Fine-Needle Aspiration

Transthoracic FNA is an excellent diagnostic method for obtaining material from the lung parenchyma for cytologic evaluation. This technique is most useful when diffuse parenchymal disease or discrete mass or masses are identified via imaging techniques, with discrete lesions yielding higher-quality specimens than those with diffuse interstitial involvement. While a specific diagnosis may not be established in all cases, FNA is useful to categorize the lesion as inflammatory or neoplastic (Wood et al., 1998).

While aspiration of the lung parenchyma is not without the potential for complications, especially in moribund patients or those in severe respiratory distress, these complications are fewer than with thoracotomy or transthoracic biopsy and are typically minimal if a mass lesion is located closely adjacent to the thoracic wall (Teske et al., 1991). Coagulation screening should be performed before transthoracic FNA, including a platelet count, prothrombin time (PT), and activated partial thromboplastin time (APTT). Patients with abnormal hemostasis have a significantly increased risk of severe hemorrhage following FNA of the lung.

The patient may be placed in sternal recumbency or allowed to stand; however, proper restraint is critical. If the patient is distressed or struggling, sedation may be necessary to minimize risks. Local anesthetic may be injected into the anterior edge of the intercostal space as the intercostal vessels and nerves are located just posterior to each rib. Visualizing the mass or site to be aspirated by ultrasound is ideal as imaging guidance allows direct placement of the needle into the lesion, enhancing the likelihood that a diagnostic sample is obtained. Echoendoscopy is a useful technique when traditional ultrasound usage is not possible due to the presence of intervening bone or when an area to be scanned is beyond normal penetration depths. The echoendoscope is unique in that it has an ultrasound transducer at the end of a traditional endoscope. FNA samples of lung masses can be obtained using this technique (Gaschen et al., 2003). If ultrasound is not available, careful localization of the lesion using at least two radiographic views is essential. The right caudal lung lobe is typically sampled with diffuse disease; the standard sampling site is the seventh to ninth intercostal space, one third the distance from the spinal column to the costochondral junction. The most common mistake is to enter the chest too far caudally and aspirate the liver.

If the lesion to be sampled is close to the body wall, a 22- to 25-gauge, 2-inch needle attached to a 3-ml syringe can be used. If the lesion is deeper, a 22-gauge human spinal needle may be required to reach the site. In either case, the needle is introduced through the skin and intercostal muscles at a 90-degree angle to the chest wall in one controlled thrust. Once the chest cavity has been entered, negative pressure is applied to the syringe by pulling back on the plunger slightly. The needle tip is advanced to the appropriate depth as estimated by examination of radiographs or by ultrasonographic visualization. The needle should be advanced, withdrawn slightly, and readvanced through the lesion while maintaining negative pressure. Advancing at slightly different angles will enhance the likelihood of obtaining a representative and diagnostic sample; however, it also increases the potential for complications. After sampling the lesion, the syringe is withdrawn, releasing the negative pressure in the syringe just before the needle leaves the chest cavity. Aspiration should be performed quickly, but in a controlled manner. Because the risk of complications increases with the length of time the needle is in the chest cavity, it is usually safer to perform multiple aspirations than to aspirate continuously from a single needle placement.

Typically, only a small amount of material is aspirated into the needle with little or no material seen in the hub of the needle. The syringe is detached from the needle, filled with air, then reattached to the needle. The air is used to expel the aspirated material within the needle hub onto slides for preparation and staining. If fluid is aspirated, it should be transferred into an EDTA-anticoagulated tube for fluid analysis, including protein concentration and cell counts, as well as cytologic evaluation. If blood or hemorrhagic fluid is aspirated, the procedure should be halted and reattempted at another site. Aspiration of air alone may occur in cases of significant small airway disease. In this instance, aspiration should be repeated with caution as there is an increased risk of pneumothorax.

The patient should be checked frequently for the first few hours following aspiration to assess respiratory and cardiac function. A chest radiograph should be examined one hour after lung aspiration, or at any time following aspiration if the patient's respiration worsens, to evaluate for the presence of pneumothorax, particularly tension pneumothorax.

Normal Cytologic Features

Normal Cytology of the Trachea and Bronchial Tree

The trachea and bronchi are lined by pseudostratified, ciliated epithelial cells that are customarily observed in fluid from tracheal but not bronchoalveolar samples (Box 5-1). These cells are elongate with a round, prominent nucleus and basophilic cytoplasm with cilia at the apical surface (Fig. 5-28). Cilia often detach from these cells if sample preparation is delayed and are visualized free in the background. It is, therefore, important to not confuse these cilia with bacterial rods (Andreasen, 2003). Cuboidal epithelium lines the bronchioles; therefore, these cells may be seen in both TTW and BAL samples. Bronchiolar epithelium appears individually or in sheets. These cells are round to cuboidal, have moderate amounts of basophilic cytoplasm, and contain a round, centrally placed nucleus.

BAL and TTW samples from normal cats and dogs are of low cellularity. TTW samples tend to be hypocellular when compared to BAL samples (Hawkins et al., 1995). Alveolar macrophages are the primary cell type observed in normal TTW and BAL samples (Table 5-4). These cells often appear "activated" and contain numerous small, discrete vacuoles in the cytoplasm filled with phagocytized debris (Fig. 5-29A&B). Other leukocytes may be seen less frequently. Neutrophils typically represent less than 5% to 10% of the nucleated cell population (Hawkins and DeNicola, 1990; Rebar et al., 1980; Vail et al., 1995) although neutrophil populations greater than 20% have been reported (Lécuyer et al., 1995; Padrid et al., 1991). Other cell types observed in lesser numbers include, lymphocytes (5% to 14%), eosinophils in species other than cats (< 5%), and mast cells (< 2%) (Lecuyer et al., 1995; Padrid et al., 1991; Hawkins and DeNicola, 1990; Rebar et al., 1980; Vail et al., 1995). Rare goblet cells may be observed and are not considered an abnormal finding unless numbers are markedly increased. Goblet cells are approximately the size of macrophages but contain abundant cytoplasm filled with distinctive, deeply basophilic, uniform granules (Fig. 5-30). Immunophenotypic studies of canine lymphocytes found in BAL fluid determined the lymphocyte subpopulations were primarily T cells with a greater proportion of CD8 cells as compared to blood resulting in a CD4/CD8 ratio closer to 1:1 (Dirscherl et al., 1995; Vail et al., 1995).

Eosinophil numbers vary markedly between the dog and the cat. Less than 5% is typical for samples from dogs

---

BOX 5-1   Comparison of Normal and Inflammatory Airway Cytology

Normal Cytology of the Airway
Ciliated columnar epithelial cells
Cuboidal epithelial cells
Macrophages, often activated
Mucus
Rare goblet cells
Common Changes with Inflammation
Deeply basophilic, hyperplastic epithelial cells, frequently in sheets
Goblet cell hyperplasia
Inflammatory cells (e.g., neutrophils, macrophages)
Increased mucus and Curschmann's spirals

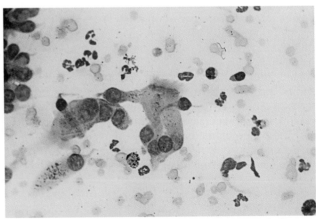

■ **FIGURE 5-28. Normal epithelium. TTW.** Several elongate columnar epithelial cells with eosinophilic cilia at the apical surface. (Wright-Giemsa; HP oil.)

TABLE 5-4 Expected Total Cell Count and Percent Range for Cell Types Seen in Bronchoalveolar Lavage Samples from Clinically Healthy Dogs and Cats[*]

	Total Cells/μl	Macrophage	Lymphocyte	Eosinophil	Neutrophil	Mast Cell
Dog	<500	70%–80%	6%–14%	<5%	<5%	1%–2%
Cat	<400	70%–80%	<5%	up to 25%	<6%	<2%

[*]Actual values may differ between techniques. These counts were compiled from the mean values of several references to be used as a general guide.

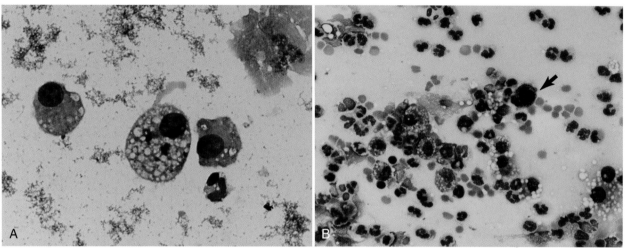

■ **FIGURE 5-29. Macrophages. TTW. A,** The phagocytic cells have abundant cytoplasm with numerous small, discrete vacuoles. Mononuclear cells compose the majority of cells in the tracheal and bronchiolar washes. (Wright-Giemsa; HP oil.) **B,** Numerous macrophages are present in this sample, including one with phagocytized material consistent with hemosiderin *(arrow)*. Also present in the sample are neutrophils and erythrocytes. (Wright-Giemsa; HP oil.)

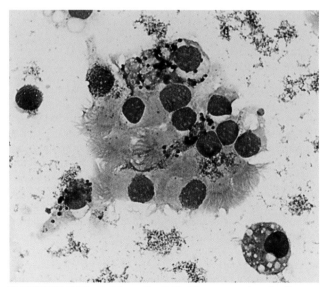

■ **FIGURE 5-30. Goblet cells. BAL.** These granulated cells may be observed along with respiratory epithelial cells. Note the distinct large purple intracytoplasmic globules of goblet cells. (Wright-Giemsa; HP oil.)

(Rebar et al., 1980), whereas a range of 5% to 28% eosinophils may be seen in BAL samples from healthy cats (Dye et al., 1996; Hawkins et al., 1994; Lecuyer et al., 1995; Padrid et al., 1991). The percentages of eosinophils in the airways of apparently healthy cats are extremely variable and thus should be interpreted carefully and in correlation with clinical signs and other diagnostic results. Eosinophils are often overlooked in samples because they can appear differently than the typical eosinophil observed in blood. It is not uncommon for the nucleus to be nonsegmented (Baldwin and Becker, 1993). Eosinophils frequently become entrapped in aggregates of mucus and are unable to completely flatten resulting in dark-red– to brown-staining granules rather than the expected bright-pink to red granules (Rakich and Latimer, 1989) (Fig. 5-31A&B). In samples that have dried slowly (these are usually the samples with thick clumps of mucus), the granules also darken.

Normal Cytology of the Lung

Samples from healthy pulmonary tissue are sparsely cellular and contain primarily respiratory epithelial cells. Respiratory epithelial cells are lightly basophilic, columnar

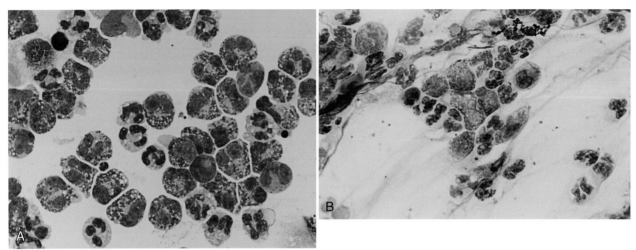

■ **FIGURE 5-31. Eosinophils. TTW. A,** Abundant canine eosinophils from a tracheal wash. Note that some eosinophils have reduced nuclear lobularity resulting in cells with bean-shaped or round nuclei. (Wright-Giemsa; HP oil.) **B,** When eosinophils become trapped in mucus they do not stain well. Note dark granules of these canine eosinophils as compared to A. (Wright-Giemsa; HP oil.)

to cuboidal cells containing oval nuclei with granular chromatin situated towards the basilar aspect of the cell (Fig. 5-32). Cilia are commonly seen on the apical surface. Goblet cells may contain pink to purple granules. A small number of alveolar macrophages, erythrocytes, and white blood cells may also be seen. Mucus is often present in respiratory samples as ribbons of eosinophilic material but is typically sparse in aspirates from normal lung tissue. Obtaining a sample that is cytologically "normal" does not preclude the possibility of pulmonary disease but instead suggests that the lesion was not sampled. Reaspiration should be considered.

Oropharyngeal Contamination

Oropharyngeal contamination is a complication associated with several procedures for sampling the airways. Cytologically, this is observed as the presence of mature,

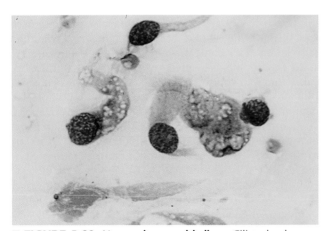

■ **FIGURE 5-32. Upper airway epithelium.** Ciliated columnar epithelium and goblet cells shown here are representative of those found in the trachea, bronchi, or large bronchioles. Epithelium becomes cuboidal in the small bronchioles. Two mucus-secreting cells with gray-blue foamy cytoplasm are shown. (Wright-Giemsa; HP oil.)

keratinized, squamous epithelial cells, often coated with a mixed population of bacteria, including colonies of *Simonsiella* sp., which are considered normal flora of the oropharyngeal cavity (see Fig. 5-4A&B). Neutrophils are a common inhabitant of the oral cavity, particularly associated with dental disease. Airway samples with evidence of oropharyngeal contamination cannot be properly interpreted, as it is impossible to determine the source of the inflammation. Rarely, a sample that appears to contain oropharyngeal contamination may represent a true biologic process such as in the case of recurrent aspiration of pharyngeal material or a bronchoesophageal fistula (Burton et al., 1992). To differentiate these processes, the procedure should be repeated with increased effort to minimize the potential for oropharyngeal contamination.

Inflammation of the Tracheobronchial Tract and Lungs

Inflammation can be classified as acute neutrophilic, chronic active (mixed), chronic, eosinophilic, hemorrhagic, or neoplastic inflammation (Hawkins and DeNicola, 1990). Inflammatory cell populations change dramatically depending on the inciting cause of the inflammation. Neutrophils and eosinophils are observed in more acute processes, whereas increasing numbers of macrophages and lymphocytes, in addition to the neutrophils or eosinophils, are more consistent with chronic inflammation. Inflammation of the lung parenchyma consists predominantly of neutrophils, eosinophils, alveolar macrophages, epithelioid macrophages, or mixed cell population. The type of inflammation may suggest a specific disease process (e.g., large numbers of eosinophils are seen with allergic disease) or cause (e.g., granulomatous inflammation with fungal infection). Increased mucus is a nonspecific finding and may be associated with many pathologic processes of both infectious and noninfectious etiologies.

Chronic Inflammation

There are multiple causes of chronic bronchitis in dogs and cats, including congenital abnormality in structure of the airway, abnormal function of cilia, parasitic infestation, viral or bacterial infection, and inhalation of noxious substances that include smoke (Padrid and Amis, 1992). In chronic inflammation, macrophages become activated and may be bi- or multinucleated with highly vacuolated cytoplasm. Inflammation is commensurate with the underlying cause; however, suppurative inflammation is the most typical finding. Additional changes are consistent with chronic inflammation such as hyperplastic epithelial cells, goblet cell hyperplasia, and increased mucus.

Epithelial hyperplasia is a nonspecific change associated with inflammation that results in variably sized, deeply basophilic epithelial cells. Goblet cell hyperplasia may also be seen in inflammatory disease of the respiratory tract. Increased mucus is common and may present cytologically as inspissated mucus in a tight spiral coil, also known as a Curschmann's spiral, that resembles a bottle washer brush (Fig. 5-33A&B). These

are designative of small airway disease (see Box 5-1) (Rebar et al., 1992).

Suppurative Inflammation

Neutrophils are the primary cell seen as part of a suppurative inflammatory process. Neutrophils are commonly associated with both acute and chronic inflammation. When neutrophils are the predominant cell type, the sample should be examined closely for infectious agents, particularly if the neutrophils are degenerate (Fig. 5-34A&B). Degenerate neutrophils, or karyolytic

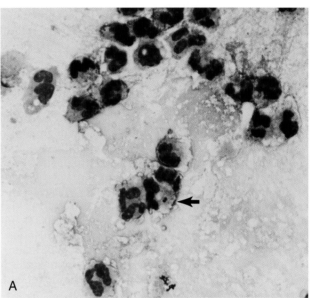

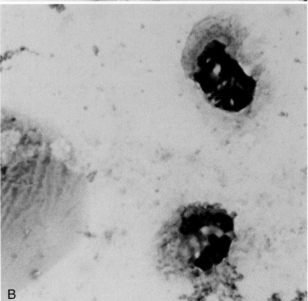

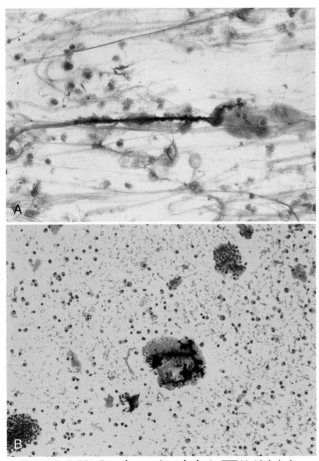

■ **FIGURE 5-33. Curschmann's spiral. A, TTW.** Lightly basophilic mucus strands and mononuclear cells appear in the background. Inspissated mucus forms a distinct filamentous appearance resembling a bottle washer brush. These spirals are prominent in cases of chronic inflammation such as chronic bronchitis. (Wright-Giemsa; HP oil.) **B, BAL.** Densely wound, deeply basophilic mucus strands in a background of streaming eosinophilic mucus and cells. (Wright-Giemsa; HP oil.)

■ **FIGURE 5-34. Suppurative inflammation. BAL. A,** Sample from a dog with infectious tracheobronchitis. Numerous well-preserved, primarily nondegenerate neutrophils that rarely contain intracellular cocci *(arrow)*. Abundant streaming eosinophilic mucus in the background. (Wright-Giemsa; LP.) **B,** Sample from a dog with infectious tracheobronchitis. Low cellularity sample; however, degenerate neutrophils contain intracellular bacteria. (Wright-Giemsa; LP.)

neutrophils, have a swollen, paler-staining nucleus that has lost the discrete segmentation of healthy neutrophils. Karyolysis is induced by toxic substances or internal enzyme release. If a sample is not processed immediately, neutrophils can begin to degenerate due to enzyme release caused by cell degeneration. These neutrophils will appear karyolytic even in the absence of bacteria. However, it is still recommended to culture any sample that contains karyolytic neutrophils.

Increased neutrophils may also be observed with noninfectious causes. Examples include neoplasia or foreign body pneumonia due to inhaled or aspirated substances (Fig. 5-35A&B). Increased numbers of neutrophils are present in the first aliquot from a BAL. This is thought to be due to the relative adhesiveness of cells to the epithelial lining (Hawkins et al., 1994). The absolute and relative numbers of neutrophils increase with subsequent BAL or TTW procedures.

Macrophagic and Mixed Inflammation

Alveolar macrophages are often seen in either acute or chronic forms of inflammation and may be the predominant cell type (Fig. 5-36). These cells are large, have abundant blue-gray foamy cytoplasm, and are frequently vacuolated and contain phagocytized material. A key feature to aid in the identification of alveolar macrophages is the eccentric position of the nucleus, which is usually round to oval. In chronic disease, binucleate and multinucleate forms may be seen. A mixed inflammatory response composed of nondegenerate neutrophils and macrophages is frequently seen in noninfectious pulmonary disease such as inhalation pneumonia, lung lobe torsion, or necrosis secondary to a neoplastic lesion.

Lipid pneumonia is a rarely reported disease in dogs and cats. This disease is classified as either exogenous lipid pneumonia due to inhalation of fat or oil, or as endogenous lipid pneumonia that is not associated with inhalation of external material (Dungworth, 1993; Lopez, 2000). Endogenous lipid pneumonia has been reported, albeit rarely, in both cats (Jerram et al., 1998; Jones et al., 2000)

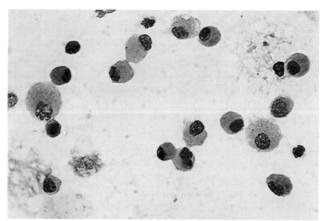

■ **FIGURE 5-36. Macrophagic inflammation. BAL. Cat.** This diagnostic procedure was performed to rule out an active inflammatory condition in the lungs. The cell population consists primarily of alveolar macrophages distinguished by their eccentrically placed nuclei. The cytoplasm is blue-gray with distinct granules noted in some cells. These were later identified as Prussian blue positive for iron and consistent for chronic hemorrhage (see Figure 5-50 B&C). (Wright-Giemsa; HP oil.) (Courtesy of Rose Raskin, University of Florida.)

and dogs (Raya et al., 2006). Clinical signs of endogenous lipid pneumonia include dyspnea, cough, and mucus expectoration, but patients may be asymptomatic as well (Raya et al., 2006). Diagnosis of this disease is facilitated by radiography, sputum examination, lung aspiration, computed tomography, and/or BAL. Sudan IV stain will create intense staining of the abundant lipid-rich vacuoles present in the macrophages. Histology of the lungs reveals multifocal interstitial pneumonia, characterized by interstitial fibrosis, accumulation of macrophages, lymphocytes, and small numbers of neutrophils in alveolar spaces, presence of multinucleated giant cells, and proliferation of type II pneumocytes (Raya et al., 2006). The exact etiology of this disease is uncertain; however, it is suspected to be related to diseases that incite airway obstruction. Chronic

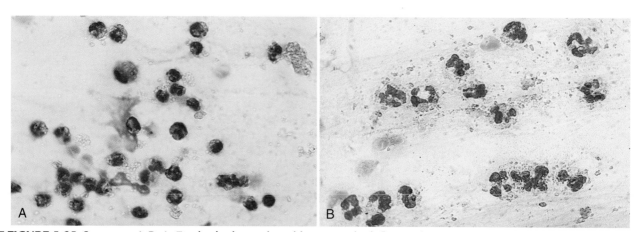

■ **FIGURE 5-35. Same case A-B. A, Foreign body reaction with suppurative inflammation. Sputum smear. Dog.** Aspiration pneumonia occurred following a barium study of the digestive tract. Numerous cells contain yellow-green refractile crystals and similar material is found in the background, consistent with the contrast dye. (Wright-Giemsa; HP oil.) **B, Barium aspiration.** Fine yellow-green crystals are seen within degenerate neutrophils. (Wright-Giemsa; HP oil.) (A and B, Courtesy of Rose Raskin, University of Florida.)

bronchitis, bronchogenic carcinoma, and *Dirofilaria immitis* have been coexistent with endogenous lipid pneumonia in both dogs and cats (Jerram et al., 1998; Jones et al., 2000; Raya et al., 2006).

Granulomatous Inflammation

Granulomatous inflammation is characterized cytologically by the presence of epithelioid macrophages and multinucleate giant cells. Epithelioid macrophages are blue-gray to pale pink with plump, round, well-defined cytoplasmic borders (Fig. 5-37A). Cells are frequently seen in small aggregates and are therefore termed *epithelioid*. Neutrophils may also be present (pyogranulomatous inflammation) as well as lesser numbers of plasma cells, lymphocytes, and eosinophils. Granulomatous or pyogranulomatous inflammation is seen in fungal infections such as blastomycosis (Fig. 5-37B), coccidioidomycosis, and aspergillosis. A foreign body or material such as barium sulfate present within the pulmonary parenchyma may provoke the same reaction. Barium sulfate can be detected as a phagocytized, refractile, greenish material in the cytoplasm of macrophages (Nunez-Ochoa et al., 1993).

Eosinophilic Inflammation

Clinical signs of allergic bronchitis include coughing, increased tracheal sensitivity, and crackles and wheezes on auscultation of the lung. Cytologically, this syndrome is characterized by increased mucus, Curschmann's spirals, and increased numbers of eosinophils with varying numbers of macrophages, neutrophils, and mast cells in TTW and BAL fluids (Fig. 5-38A). Other causes of increased eosinophils in BAL/TTW include eosinophilic granulomas, aspergillosis, paraneoplastic syndromes, and rarely, bacterial pneumonia.

Eosinophils are typically sparse in lung samples (< 5%). When eosinophils represent more than 10% of the nucleated cells, one should consider a hypersensitivity, parasitic, or infiltrative process (Fig. 5-38B). Eosinophilia in the lung may be seen with or without blood eosinophilia. Other inflammatory cell types may be seen, including small numbers of mast cells, lymphocytes, and plasma cells. Tumor-associated tissue eosinophilia is occasionally seen in dogs and cats, most reports of which are associated with malignant neoplasia.

Pulmonary eosinophilic granulomatosis is a syndrome identified in dogs characterized by infiltration of the pulmonary parenchyma by eosinophils (Calvert et al., 1988). The cause is unknown but pulmonary eosinophilic granulomatosis is inconsistently associated with *Dirofilaria immitis* infection. Dogs may present with either a diffuse interstitial infiltrate or discrete masses. Cytology is similar in both instances and includes large numbers of eosinophils admixed with variable numbers of macrophages, neutrophils, plasma cells, and basophils (Fig. 5-38C). This condition may be confused cytologically with lymphomatoid granulomatosis, a T-cell lymphoid neoplasm of the lung composed of a similar pleocellular population that is distinguished histologically.

Infectious Causes of Disease of the Tracheobronchial Tract and Lungs

Neutrophils typically predominate in bacterial, protozoal, viral, and many fungal infections. In addition, macrophages, lymphocytes, and plasma cells may also be present.

Bacterial Pneumonia

Degenerate neutrophils are the most common cell type observed with bacterial pneumonia. Mucus and numbers of macrophages are also frequently increased. The presence of intracellular bacteria, in the absence of oropharyngeal contamination, is diagnostic for bacterial pneumonia. Extracellular bacteria are also observed with pneumonia but may also be present due to contamination; therefore, identification of intracellular bacteria is necessary to confirm the diagnosis. Usually a uniform bacterial population is present; however, a mixed population can be seen with aspiration pneumonia (Rakich and Latimer, 1989). If mycobacterial pneumonia is suspected,

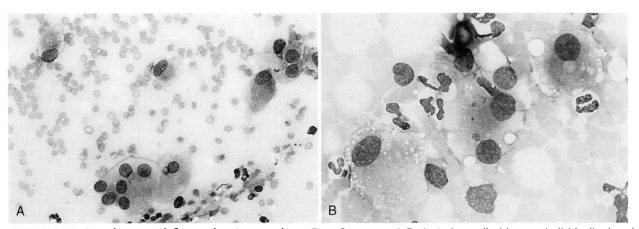

■ **FIGURE 5-37. Granulomatous inflammation. Lung aspirate. Dog. Same case A-B. A,** A giant cell with many individualized nuclei is present along with several epithelioid macrophages that have abundant blue-gray cytoplasm and a distinct cytoplasmic outline. (Wright-Giemsa; HP oil.) **B,** A tissue aspirate contains epithelioid macrophages along with extracellular yeast forms consistent with *Blastomyces*. (Wright-Giemsa; HP oil.) (A and B, Courtesy of Rose Raskin, University of Florida.)

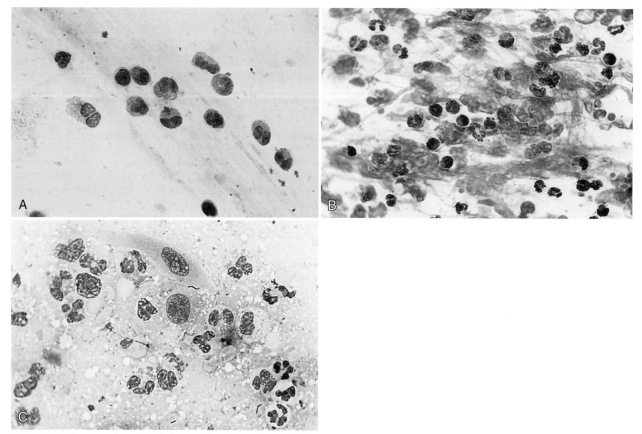

■ **FIGURE 5-38. A, Eosinophilic inflammation. BAL. Cat.** Numerous eosinophils accounting for 95% of the cell population were found in this animal with a chronic cough suspected to arise from a hypersensitivity reaction. Eosinophilic amorphous strands consistent with mucus are present in the background. Note the orange to blue-gray color of the eosinophilic granules resulting from altered staining. (Wright-Giemsa; HP oil.) **B, Eosinophilic inflammation. Sputum smear. Dog.** Numerous eosinophils are enmeshed in mucus from an animal with heartworm disease that exhibited frequent coughing. (Wright-Giemsa; HP oil.) **C, Eosinophilic granulomatosis. Bronchus exudate smear. Dog.** Mixed inflammatory cell population consisting of numerous eosinophils and low numbers of neutrophils and mononuclear cells is shown along with a fibroblast (top center). Histopathology of the pulmonary mass confirmed the diagnosis. (Aqueous-based Wright; HP oil.) (A and B, Courtesy of Rose Raskin, University of Florida. C, Glass slide material courtesy of Ruanna Gossett and Jennifer Thomas, Texas A&M University; presented at the 1992 ASVCP case review session.)

macrophages should be examined closely for thin, negative-staining, filamentous bacteria (Fig. 5-39A).

Bacterial infections may be a primary disease of the lung but are also commonly seen secondary to viral infections, mucosal irritation, and decreased mucociliary clearance (Anderton et al., 2004) such as occurs in *Bordetella bronchiseptica* infection (Fig 5-39B), fungal infections, and neoplasia. Microbiologic culture and sensitivity is suggested if bacteria are seen since cytologic classification of bacteria based on morphology is frequently unreliable. The presence of filamentous rods suggests infection with either *Nocardia* or *Actinomyces* spp., or rarely *Fusobacterium*. Since these species require special culture techniques, the lab should be alerted if such organisms are suspected.

Mycoplasma sp. has been described in a transtracheal wash from a 4-month-old dog. Small basophilic coccoid structures (0.3 to 0.9 μm in diameter) were observed in low to moderate numbers within neutrophils and adherent to epithelial cells in a direct smear using Wright-Giemsa stain (Williams et al., 2006). One report of *Mycobacterium bovis* infection in a dog describes the

presence of calcospherite-like bodies and caseous necrotic debris in tracheal mucus from this patient (Bauer et al., 2004). These findings are similar to what is seen in human patients with tuberculosis and are described as globular, lipid-like material and round, concentrically laminated crystalline structures intermixed with proteinaceous mucus.

Infectious pneumonia has been shown to be uncommon in cats. Cats that have infectious pneumonia may not exhibit clinical signs, and this disease has been associated with varied etiologies. Bacterial infection was the most common at 50%, viral causes were 25%, and the remainder was due to fungal, protozoal, parasitic, or mixed causes. CBC and thoracic radiographs may be normal even though systemic infection exists. Due to this, clinicians should evaluate the respiratory tract with other techniques such as a BAL when infection is detected in other organ systems (Macdonald et al., 2003).

While *Yersinia pestis* is an uncommon inhabitant of the respiratory tract, the pneumonic form of plague in cats has a high zoonotic potential, thus making identification of the organism crucial. *Yersinia pestis* is a

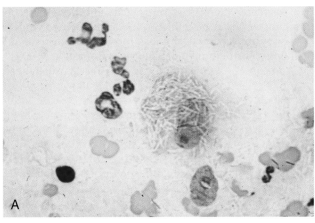
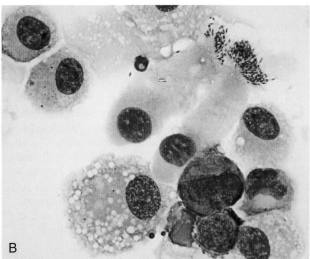

■ **FIGURE 5-39. A, Mycobacterial infection.** Negative–staining, rod-shaped bacteria located intra- and extracellularly consistent with *Mycobacterium* sp. (Wright-Giemsa; HP oil.) **B, Bordetella infection. BAL. Dog.** Columnar epithelium with dark-staining bacterial rods of *Bordetella bronchiseptica* tightly adhered to cilia. (Wright; HP oil.) (B, Courtesy of Michael Scott, Michigan State University.)

gram-negative bacillus cytologically recognizable as bipolar coccobacilli present both intra- and extracellularly with large numbers of degenerate neutrophils. Pneumonic plague accounts for approximately 10% of feline cases and can be seen with or without the classic bubonic presentation (Eidson et al., 1991).

While most bacterial pneumonias are associated with suppurative inflammation, mycobacteriosis is typically associated with granulomatous or pyogranulomatous inflammation. In addition to neutrophils, Langhans' multinucleate giant cells and large epithelioid macrophages with ill-defined cytoplasmic borders are seen along with variable numbers of neutrophils. *Mycobacteria* do not stain with routine cytologic stains and can be difficult to visualize. However, careful examination of the cells and background material reveals the presence of distinctive negatively stained thin rods present both intra- and extracellularly (see Fig. 5-39A). The organisms can be confirmed by acid-fast staining. Siamese cats are suggested to have increased susceptibility to mycobacteriosis (Jordan et al., 1994).

Viral Pneumonia

Viral infections are accompanied by neutrophilic inflammation. Although this is often due to secondary bacterial infection, viral infections alone may induce an increase in absolute and relative neutrophil counts. Cats with FIV infection have significantly higher total cell counts and higher relative neutrophil numbers in BAL fluid (Hawkins et al., 1996). Canine distemper and adenovirus are the most common viral pathogens in dogs. Samples from suspected cases should be examined closely for viral inclusions. When seen, viral inclusions will be found in respiratory epithelial cells coincident with clinical signs. Distemper inclusions are eosinophilic, vary in size, and can be intranuclear or intracytoplasmic (Fig. 5-40). Inclusions may be observed in multiple cell types, including macrophages,

lymphocytes, red blood cells, and epithelial cells. They can persist in lung tissue for more than 6 weeks. Infection with canine adenovirus type-2 results in the presence of large, amphophilic or basophilic intranuclear inclusions that are most commonly seen in bronchiolar epithelial cells. Acidophilic intranuclear viral inclusions in lung tissue may be seen during the acute infection period in dogs infected with canine herpesvirus; however, these are more commonly demonstrated in nasal respiratory epithelium.

Experimental and natural infection with strains of the influenza virus has been reported in both dogs and cats (Crawford et al., 2005; Kuiken et al., 2004); however, the cytologic features have yet to be described.

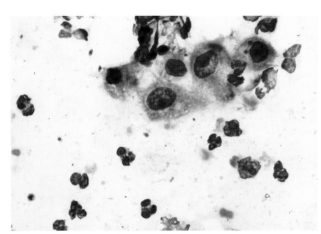

■ **FIGURE 5-40. Distemper inclusions. Lung imprint. Dog.** Eosinophilic viral inclusions compatible with canine distemper are present in the macrophage *(arrow)*. In the background are several loose, crescent-shaped *Toxoplasma* tachyzoites. (Romanowsky stain; HP oil.) (Glass slide material courtesy of Ron Tyler and Rick Cowell, Oklahoma State University; presented at the 1982 ASVCP case review session.)

Protozoal Pneumonia

Toxoplasma gondii is a protozoal organism that can cause interstitial pneumonia in the dog and cat. Cytologic examination of TTW or BAL samples reveals an increase in the numbers of nondegenerate neutrophils. *Toxoplasma gondii* tachyzoites are 1- to 4-μm, crescent-shaped bodies with lightly basophilic cytoplasm and a central metachromatic nucleus (Fig. 5-41A&B) (see Table 5-1). Organisms may be found intracellularly (primarily within macrophages) and extracellularly. These organisms may occasionally be retrieved by BAL and rarely by TTW samples (Bernsteen et al., 1999; Hawkins et al., 1997). However, because toxoplasmosis causes an interstitial pneumonia and these procedures focus on the airways, it may be difficult to retrieve these organisms unless disease is marked. Absence of organisms in a suspect patient does not negate the possibility of infection. A case of feline toxoplasmosis involving lung aspiration reported the use of immunohistochemical staining for definitive diagnosis (Poitout et al., 1998).

Neospora caninum infection of dogs is usually seen in animals less than 1 year of age and results in progressive, frequently fatal, ascending paralysis. The disease in older dogs is diverse but characterized by systemic involvement, including marked pulmonary infiltration with associated pneumonia (Greig et al., 1995; Ruehlmann et al., 1995). Examination of aspirated samples reveals a mixed inflammatory response composed of neutrophils, macrophages, lymphocytes, plasma cells, and eosinophils with intra- and extracellular tachyzoites indistinguishable from those of *T. gondii* (Fig. 5-41C&D). Tachyzoites are 1 to 5 μm by 5 to 7 μm, oval to crescent-shaped structures

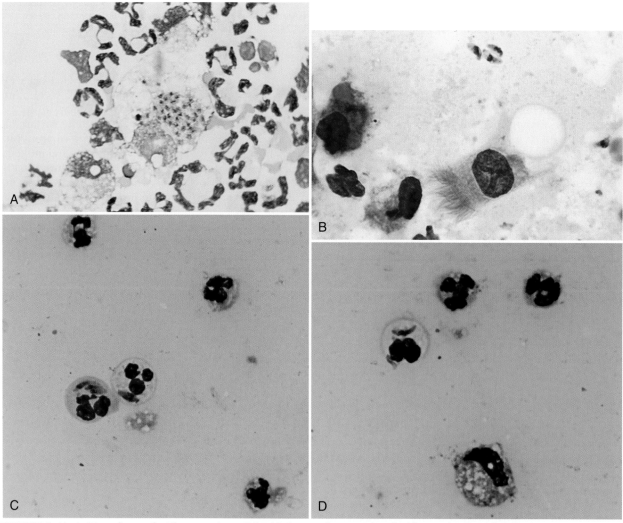

■ **FIGURE 5-41. A, Toxoplasmosis. Tissue aspirate.** Mixed inflammation associated with *Toxoplasma gondii* infection. Numerous organisms are seen within the macrophage. Neutrophils show minimal signs of degeneration. (Wright-Giemsa; HP oil.) **B, Toxoplasmosis.** Same case as in Figure 5-40. Banana-shaped organisms with a metachromatic central nucleus are typical of the tachyzoites of *Toxoplasma gondii*. Similar appearance is found with *Neospora*, which can be distinguished by immunohistochemistry. (Romanowsky stain; HP oil.) **C, Neospora.** Compare banana-shaped morphology of *Neospora* organisms with those of *Toxoplasma gondii* seen in B. (Wright-Giemsa; HP oil.) **D, Neospora.** *Neospora* organism within neutrophil, compare with *Toxoplasma* in B (Wright-Giemsa; HP oil.) (C, Glass slide material courtesy of Tara Holmberg et al., University of California, Davis; presented at the 2004 ASVCP case review session. D, Glass slide material courtesy of Tara Holmberg et al, University of California, Davis; presented at the 2004 ASVCP case review session.)

with a central metachromatic nucleus and lightly baso-philic cytoplasm (see Table 5-1).

Fungal Pneumonia

Systemic mycoses spreading to the lungs are more likely to be found in the pulmonary interstitium than in the airways or alveoli. Thus, while mycotic agents may be detected by airway washes (Fig. 5-42A&B) (Hawkins and DeNicola, 1990), FNA of the pulmonary parenchyma has increased sensitivity for detection of these organisms (see Table 5-1).

Blastomyces dermatiditis is a dimorphic fungus that can infect numerous tissues, but the lung is the most frequently involved organ in primary infection. Pulmo-nary lesions consist of multiple, variably sized nodules dispersed through all lung fields. Infection usually occurs in young, large-breed dogs. The prevalence is less in cats compared to dogs; however, Siamese seem especially susceptible. Organisms can be readily retrieved via TTW/BAL in animals with radiographic evidence of disease (see Table 5-1). Usually, the yeast form of the organism is observed; however, the rare hyphal stage may be seen. The extracellular yeast forms are dark blue, round, and 5 to 20 μm in diameter, with a thick, biconcave wall hav-ing a granular internal structure (Fig. 5-43; see Fig. 5-37B). Broad-based budding may be seen. The organisms are likely found in aggregates of mucus and necrotic debris, so that squash preparations are vital for organism identi-fication. Pyogranulomatous or granulomatous inflamma-tion is the rule.

Histoplasma capsulatum is also a dimorphic fungus that infects both cats and dogs. Pulmonary disease is common in affected cats. In addition to systemic histo-plasmosis seen in both species, a self-limiting syndrome of pulmonary histoplasmosis is also seen in dogs. The small, yeastlike organisms are round to oval and 1 to 4 μm in diameter with a purple nucleus and lightly baso-philic protoplasm surrounded by a thin, clear halo (Fig. 5-44). Organisms are seen within macrophages and neutrophils as well as extracellularly. Macrophages may be packed with organisms. *Histoplasma* infection in-duces a mixed to pyogranulomatous reaction.

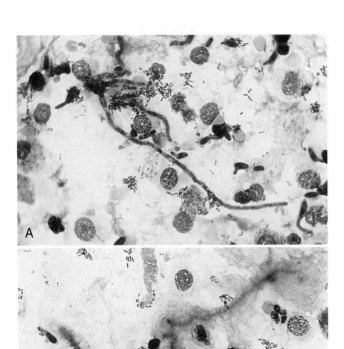

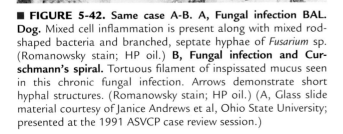

■ **FIGURE 5-42. Same case A-B. A, Fungal infection BAL. Dog.** Mixed cell inflammation is present along with mixed rod-shaped bacteria and branched, septate hyphae of *Fusarium* sp. (Romanowsky stain; HP oil.) **B, Fungal infection and Cur-schmann's spiral.** Tortuous filament of inspissated mucus seen in this chronic fungal infection. Arrows demonstrate short hyphal structures. (Romanowsky stain; HP oil.) (A, Glass slide material courtesy of Janice Andrews et al, Ohio State University; presented at the 1991 ASVCP case review session.)

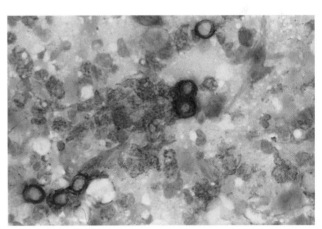

■ **FIGURE 5-43. Blastomycosis. Tissue aspirate.** Several large, thick-walled, deeply basophilic yeast forms of *Blastomyces derma-titidis* are present against a necrotic cellular background. (Wright-Giemsa; HP oil.)

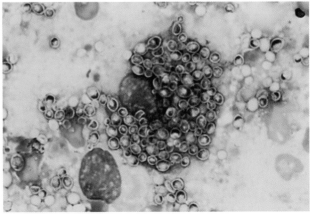

■ **FIGURE 5-44. Histoplasmosis. Tissue aspirate.** One macro-phage is filled with numerous *Histoplasma capsulatum* organisms as well as many found loose in the background. Note the small size and thin capsule of the yeast form. (Wright-Giemsa; HP oil.)

Coccidioides immitis is primarily a respiratory pathogen found in arid regions. Animals within endemic areas are frequently infected but development of clinical signs is relatively uncommon. Disseminated disease occurs after primary lung infection, especially in dogs. Boxers and Doberman pinschers may be predisposed to disseminated disease. Until recently, cats were thought to be resistant to infection with *Coccidioides,* but more recent cases indicate both susceptibility to infection and development of clinical signs in endemic areas, with respiratory involvement noted in approximately 25% of infected cats (Greene and Troy, 1995). Coccidioidomycosis is associated with pyogranulomatous or granulomatous inflammation. *Coccidioides immitis* spherules (sporangium) are large organisms seen extracellularly (Fig. 5-45). Spherules range in size from 10 to 100 μm in Romanowsky-stained preparations and contain a thick, double-contoured wall with finely granular, blue-green protoplasm. Occasionally internal endospores of 2 to 5 μm may be seen. The organism's size and internal structure is easier to appreciate on wet-mount preparations as the fixing and staining process results in shrinkage and distortion of the organism. Organisms are scarce in cytologic preparations and multiple slides may need to be examined to find the organism. TTW or BAL rarely reveals these organisms. Due to the organism's large size, scanning is best done with a scanning objective (e.g., 10×). Mycelia may rarely be seen in tissue.

Cryptococcosis is frequently associated with the nasal cavity; however, approximately 30% of affected cats also have pulmonary lesions. The capsule material of *Cryptococcus neoformans* can give the sample a mucinous texture. The presence of an inflammatory response varies seemingly related to the thickness of the capsule. See Figure 5-10 and the section on nasal cryptococcosis for additional information.

Pneumocystis carinii is most commonly reported in young dogs, primarily miniature dachshunds (Lobetti, 2001) but has also been reported in Cavalier King Charles spaniels (Watson et al., 2006; Sukura et al., 1996) and a Yorkshire terrier (Cabanes et al., 2000). Several immune defects have been identified that may predispose some dogs to *Pneumocystis carinii* including hypogammaglobulinemia, decreased lymphocyte proliferation, and reduced numbers of B lymphocytes (Lobetti, 2000; Watson et al., 2006). Infection results in a diffuse interstitial pneumonia. The abundant foamy fluid present in the alveoli often contains trophozoite and cyst forms. Cysts are extracellular, 5 to 10 μm in diameter and contain 4 to 8 round, 1- to 2-μm basophilic bodies (Fig. 5-46A&B). Trophozoites are pleomorphic, ranging from 2 to 7 μm in length (Fig. 5-46B&C). Diagnosis may be confirmed by organism morphology, staining (Grocott's methenamine silver), and a polymerase chain reaction assay (Hagiwara et al., 2001).

Sporothrix schenckii are uncommonly identified in the pulmonary parenchyma of dogs and cats. When present, large numbers of organisms are seen in infected cats, whereas organisms are relatively rare in other species. Round to oval to cigar-shaped 2 × 7-μm organisms with a thin, clear halo, slightly eccentric purple nucleus, and lightly basophilic cytoplasm are observed both within macrophages and extracellularly. The presence of cigar-shaped organisms differentiates sporotrichosis from histoplasmosis.

Parasitic Infestations

There are numerous parasites capable of infestation of the respiratory tract of dogs and cats. TTW and BAL can be helpful in identifying either the larvae or the egg; however, the etiologic agent is not always present in the sample. An increase in airway eosinophils should be accompanied by heartworm and fecal testing.

Aleurostrongylus abstrusus is a feline metastrongylid lungworm that is generally considered asymptomatic but may induce coughing. Adults live in respiratory bronchioles and alveoli and lay eggs in alveolar spaces, which hatch to release larvae. The ova (Fig. 5-47A) and larvae, not the adults, induce the inflammatory reaction (Rakich and Latimer, 1989). Similar to conditions found in *Filaroides* sp. infection, parasitic nodules are more commonly seen in the peripheral lung fields. Eosinophils and neutrophils found in TTW or BAL samples characterize the early infection associated with the nodules (Fig. 5-47B). With time, however, fibromuscular hyperplasia occurs and the reaction appears more fibroblastic. Most typically, the larval stage is seen but occasionally ova may also be identified (Table 5-5). The pale or unstained larvae are usually coiled on themselves; the tail has a double bend and a dorsal spine.

Paragonimus kellicotti is a trematode primarily seen in cats in North America, while *Paragonimus westermanii* is more common in the orient (see Table 5-5). The caudal lung lobes, particularly those of the right side, are frequently affected by this lung fluke. This focal location within the caudal lung lobe makes cytologic visualization of the ova via TTW or BAL difficult (Fig. 5-48); however, the eggs can be readily identified by fecal examination, using either Baermann's apparatus or flotation. Cytologic examination of the inflammatory cysts demonstrates numerous eosinophils with concurrent granulomatous inflammation.

Eucoleus (formerly *Capillaria*) *aerophila* is a parasite of dogs and cats that lives in the trachea and bronchi

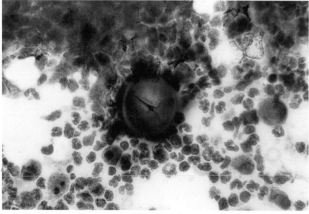

■ **FIGURE 5-45. Coccidioidomycosis. Tissue aspirate.** *Coccidioides immitis* spherule with thick, double-contoured wall. (Wright-Giemsa; HP oil.)

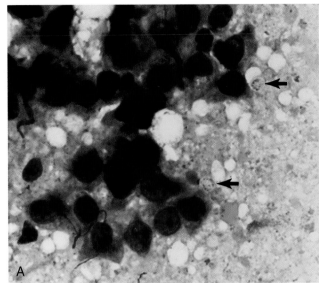

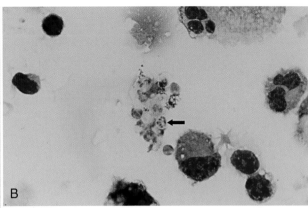

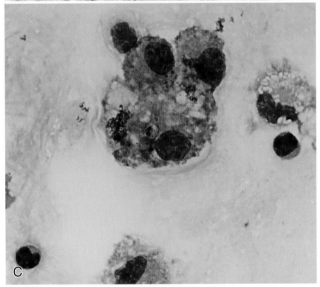

■ **FIGURE 5-46. Pneumocystis. A, Lung imprint. Dog.** Clusters of deeply basophilic respiratory epithelial cells are seen admixed with necrotic tissue debris and small (1-2 μm) trophozoites. Adjacent to the cell cluster are several extracellular cysts of *Pneumocystis carinii.* Cysts are 5-10 μm in diameter and contain 4 to 8 basophilic bodies arranged in a circle. (Wright-Giemsa; HP oil.) **Same case B-C. BAL. Horse. B,** Several *Pneumocystis carinii* trophozoites and one cyst form are seen extracellularly. (Wright-Giemsa; HP oil.) **C,** A single clearly defined trophozoite is present within the macrophage. The foamy cytoplasm likely contains several less visible organisms. (Wright-Giemsa; HP oil.) (A, Glass slide material courtesy of Tara Holmberg et al, University of California, Davis & IDEXX Laboratories; presented at the 2005 ASVCP case review session. B and C, Glass slide material courtesy of Amy MacNeill et al, University of Florida; presented at the 2001 ASVCP case review session.

but also can be found in the nasal passages. Parasite eggs may be observed in bronchial washings (see Table 5-5).

The canine lungworm, *Filaroides hirthi,* lives in the alveoli and bronchioles (Rebar et al., 1992). Both embryonated ova and larvae (Fig. 5-49) can be retrieved by TTW/BAL (see Table 5-5) (Rakich and Latimer, 1989). *Filaroides hirthi* and *milksi* can be found in subpleural nodules within the pulmonary parenchyma of dogs (in contrast to *Oslerus [Filaroides] osleri,* in tracheal nodules). The adults live in alveoli and respiratory bronchioles. While live worms tend not to generate a significant immune response, dead or dying worms are associated with an eosinophilic granulomatous reaction characterized by variable numbers of eosinophils, macrophages, and fibroblasts. *Filaroides* larvae are more likely to incite a suppurative reaction than an eosinophilic reaction. Cytologic identification of adults or larvae is rare in samples obtained by FNA (Andreasen and Carmichael, 1992). Embryonated ova and larvae are more commonly detected by airway samples (see Table 5-5). The ova of

O. osleri are identical to those of *F. hirthi.* The former parasite is uncommon and causes formation of firm nodules at the tracheal bifurcation (see Table 5-5).

Crenosoma vulpis infection can be identified using BAL (Unterer et al., 2002). Inflammation with a predominance of eosinophils is most commonly found; however, eosinophils with neutrophils as well as primarily neutrophilic inflammations are found rarely. The larval stage of *C. vulpis* can be identified in BAL fluid. Fecal examination using the Baermann technique is the most sensitive method for diagnosis (Unterer et al., 2002).

Tissue Injury

Hemorrhage

Hemorrhage is characterized cytologically by one or more of several criteria, including erythrophagocytosis, hemosiderin-laden macrophages, and hematoidin crystals (Fig. 5-50A-C). Hemorrhage is a complication of many of the methods used to sample the respiratory tree,

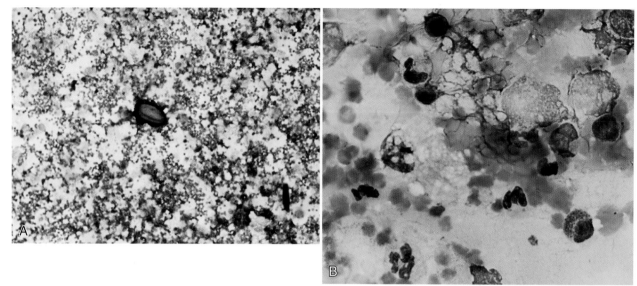

■ **FIGURE 5-47. A, *Aleurostrongylus*. Cat.** A single *Aleurostrongylus* ovum is present in the center of the slide. Numerous erythrocytes, leukocytes, and necrotic debris are present in the background. (Wright-Giemsa; LP.) **B, Eosinophilia induced by *Aleurostrongylus*. Cat.** Mixed inflammatory response containing neutrophils, eosinophils, and macrophages. The inflammatory response is directed against the ova and larva, not the adults. (Wright-Giemsa; HP oil.)

TABLE 5-5   Parasites Found in Airway Samples from Dogs and Cats

Parasite	Species	Location	Adult	Larva	Ova
Filaroides hirthi	Dog	Alveoli	2-3 mm (M)	240-290 μm	80 × 50 μm
		Bronchioles	6-13 mm (F)		Hatch prior to passing in feces
Oslerus (Filaroides) osleri	Dog	Trachea	5 mm (M)	232-266 μm	80 × 50 μm
		Bronchi	9-15 mm (F)	S-shaped tail	Identical to *F. hirthi*
Aleurostrongylus abstrusus	Cat	Terminal bronchiole	7 mm (M)	360 μm	80 × 70 μm
		Deep lung	10 mm (F)	Notched tail	
Paragonimus kellicoti	Cat	Lung parenchyma	7-16 × 4-8 μm red-brown	NA	75-118 × 42-67 μm Single operculum
Eucoleus aerophilus	Dog, Cat	Trachea	15-44 mm	—	58-80 × 30-40 μm
		Bronchi			Bipolar operculum
Dirofilaria immitis	Dog, Cat	Ectopic in lung parenchyma	12-16 cm (M)	290-330 μm	—
			25-30 cm (F)	No cephalic hook	

so the presence of erythrophagia, preferably with hemosiderin, is important to distinguish pathologic from iatrogenic hemorrhage or blood contamination. Hemorrhage is a common sequela to FNA of the pulmonary parenchyma. Increased red blood cells in TTW/BAL are observed with congestive heart failure, neoplasia, heartworm emboli, and coagulopathy. A high percentage of cats with respiratory inflammatory disease such as rhinitis and asthma had mild to moderate numbers of hemosiderophages in TTW fluid (DeHeer and McManus, 2005). Prussian blue stain can be used to distinguish hemosiderophages.

Pulmonary Alveolar Proteinosis

This is an uncommon condition with prominent cytologic findings in lung aspirates or bronchoalveolar lavages (Silverstein et al., 2000). Dogs present with a chronic history of exercise intolerance and coughing, Cytology reveals abundant amounts of basophilic homogenous structures or globules suggestive of inspissated mucus or degenerate cells. This may be accompanied by bronchial epithelial cells, cholesterol clefts, and low numbers of inflammatory cells. Pulmonary lavage may be therapeutic to reduce this excess accumulation of surfactant proteins.

Pulmonary Atelectasis or Collapse

Finding large numbers of respiratory epithelial cells is atypical and suggests pulmonary atelectasis, collapse, or hyperplasia. Respiratory epithelial cells may undergo dysplastic changes (see hyperplasia/dysplasia below) but typically lack sufficient criteria of malignancy to confirm a diagnosis of neoplasia. Numerous macrophages may also be present.

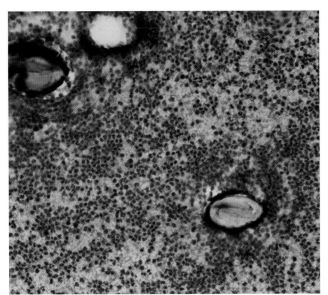

■ **FIGURE 5-48.** *Paragonimus.* **Cat.** Two *Paragonimus* ova are seen in a background of marked cellularity containing leukocytes, erythrocytes, and necrotic debris. This organism typically induces a strong eosinophilic and granulomatous inflammation. (Wright-Giemsa; IP.) (Glass slide material courtesy of Linda Berent et al, University of Illinois; presented at the 2001 ASVCP case review session.)

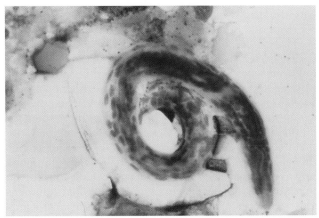

■ **FIGURE 5-49. Lungworm. BAL. Dog.** Larva of *Filaroides hirthi* present in an animal with verminous pneumonia. (Wright-Giemsa; HP oil.)

Necrosis

Necrotic material is frequently aspirated from lungs affected by either inflammatory or neoplastic changes. Necrosis is characterized cytologically by abundant amounts of basophilic granular to amorphous background material. Usually inflammatory or neoplastic cells are admixed within the necrotic debris; however, acellular aspirates or those with only remnant cell membranes or "ghost cells" may occasionally be obtained. In these cases, reaspiration is indicated and particular care should be taken to obtain samples from the periphery of the lesion while avoiding the necrotic center.

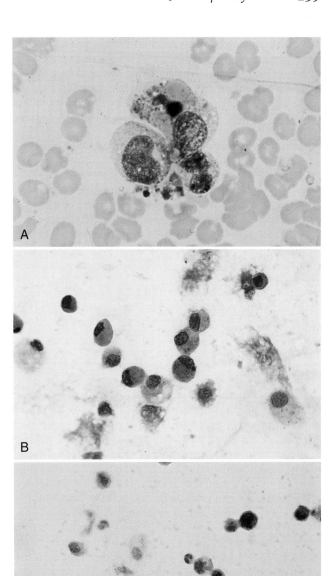

■ **FIGURE 5-50. A, Hemorrhage.** Note the macrophage, which has red blood cells as well as hemosiderin within its cytoplasm. Observation of erythrophagia and hemosiderin-laden macrophages is indicative of acute and chronic hemorrhage, respectively. (Wright-Giemsa; HP oil.) **Same case B-C. Chronic hemorrhage. BAL. B,** Same case as in Figure 5-36. Alveolar macrophages stain blue-gray and finely granular owing to the presence of hemosiderin, verified in C. (Wright-Giemsa; HP oil.) **C,** Dense blue-black accumulations of iron within the cytoplasm of alveolar macrophages. Nuclear counterstain is red. (Prussian blue; HP oil.) (B and C, Courtesy of Rose Raskin, University of Florida.)

Hyperplasia and Dysplasia of the Lung

Respiratory epithelial cells may undergo hyperplastic or dysplastic changes in non-neoplastic pulmonary disease. Hyperplasia of bronchiolar and alveolar type II pneumocytes is frequently associated with chronic inflammation.

Epithelial cells appear atypical and share some features with malignant cells but lack sufficient criteria of malignancy to diagnose neoplasia. Normal columnar epithelial cells become more cuboidal and, when seen individually, may appear round. Nuclei assume a central instead of basilar form, are larger, and contain clumped nuclear chromatin and prominent nucleoli. The cytoplasm stains with an increased basophilia and may contain punctate vacuoles.

Increased cell proliferation *(hyperplasia)* or asynchronous cytoplasmic and nuclear maturation *(dysplasia)* may occur secondary to chronic inflammation or tissue necrosis. These conditions can be difficult to differentiate cytologically from neoplasia. As a further complication, these cytologic changes may also be seen with preneoplastic changes that can progress to overt neoplasia. Reaspiration at a site more or less affected may be warranted to help characterize the degree of involvement or identify an underlying cause. If insufficient criteria of malignancy are present cytologically, a lung biopsy is indicated.

Metaplasia of the Lung

Metaplasia is the replacement of normal cells with a secondary, but non-neoplastic, population. Metaplasia can occur in response to hormonal or growth factor alterations or as part of an adaptive response to protect against chronic irritation. Aspirates from areas of squamous metaplasia are moderately cellular, yielding large, round to polygonal squamous epithelial cells that may be seen in sheets or individually (Fig. 5-51). Nuclei are relatively small in comparison to the cell size (low nuclear-to-cytoplasmic ratio). Occasional cells may contain pyknotic nuclei as part of the keratinization process. Lightly basophilic cytoplasm is abundant and may become folded or angular as the cells become keratinized. Anuclear superficial cells and keratin flakes may also be seen depending on the degree of keratinization. Squamous metaplasia can be difficult to differentiate from squamous neoplasia. In addition, squamous cell

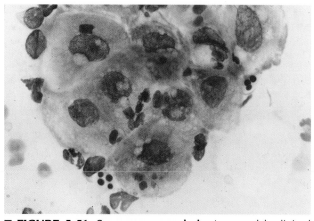

■ **FIGURE 5-51. Squamous metaplasia.** Increased hyalinized cytoplasm associated with squamous metaplasia secondary to chronic inflammation. (Wright-Giemsa; HP oil.)

carcinoma of the lung typically originates from areas of squamous metaplasia.

Neoplasia

Primary neoplasia of the lung and respiratory tree as well as metastatic neoplasia can be diagnosed through bronchial washings and lung aspiration. In dogs and cats, especially young animals, the lung is more often affected by metastatic neoplasia than by primary lung tumors. Both carcinomas and sarcomas may spread to the lung via the blood or lymphatics. Metastatic tumors are more likely to present as multiple nodules scattered throughout all lung lobes, particularly the periphery, whereas a solitary lesion is more typical of primary pulmonary neoplasia. In a study of cats with primary lung tumors, 38 of 45 were identified from cytologic samples (Hahn and McEntee, 1997). Similarly, cytologic examinations of fine-needle aspirates were helpful in the diagnosis of primary lung tumors in dogs (Oglivie et al., 1989). The most common neoplasia diagnosed by BAL or TTW is carcinoma, either primary or metastatic (Rebar et al., 1992). Epithelial cells exfoliate readily and can be identified in these samples. It is important to examine cells for criteria of malignancy, specifically variation in cell and nuclear size, prominent nucleoli, multiple nuclei and/or nucleoli, and nuclear molding (Fig. 5-52A–D). Dysplastic or metaplastic changes to epithelial cells secondary to inflammation can complicate the diagnosis, so the sample should be scrutinized for evidence of inflammation.

Carcinoma

Multiple types of lung carcinomas have been identified in dogs and cats. Adenocarcinomas of bronchogenic or bronchiolar/alveolar origin are most prevalent; however, carcinomas can arise from any level of the respiratory epithelium (Fig. 5-53A–C). Cytologic differentiation is not possible. Lung carcinomas most typically present as multifocal nodules seen in the periphery of the lung lobes; however, they may involve the entire lung lobe or be present only in the hilar region. Eosinophilic infiltrates may occur in association with bronchoalveolar carcinoma in dogs (Fig. 5-53D).

Numerous carcinomas metastasize to the pulmonary parenchyma, such as mammary carcinomas and carcinomas of the urinary bladder, prostate, and endocrine glands. Cytologic preparations from primary and metastatic carcinomas are similar, and the two cannot be definitively differentiated by cytologic evaluation alone (Figs. 5-54, 5-55A&B).

Aspirates contain moderate numbers of epithelial cells in sheets, aggregates, and clusters with lesser numbers of individualized cells. Individual cells may appear round and can be confused with discrete cell neoplasia, but they are typically larger than those from discrete cell tumors and can be distinguished by finding cell-to-cell association. Acinar formation indicates glandular origin suggesting an adenocarcinoma. Moderate to marked pleomorphism between clumps of cells, as well as within cells of

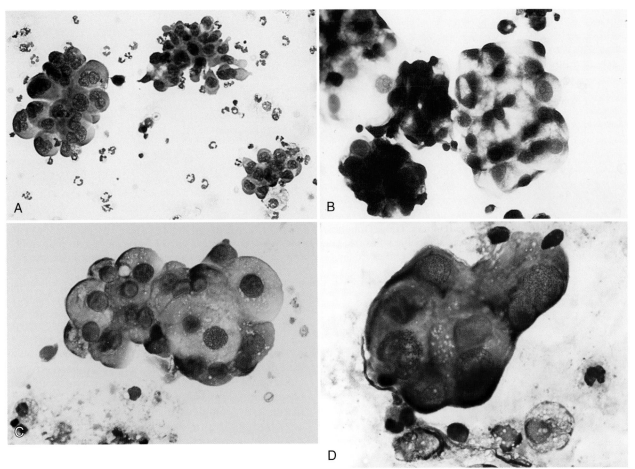

■ **FIGURE 5-52. A, Pulmonary carcinoma. BAL. Dog.** Large clusters of pleomorphic epithelium are present along with nonseptic suppurative inflammation. Multinucleated forms are noted. (Romanowsky stain; IP.) **B, Carcinoma. TTW. Dog.** Clusters of epithelial cells with pale, abundant cytoplasm suggest a secretory function. (Wright-Giemsa; IP.) **C, Carcinoma. TTW. Dog.** Clusters of very large, lightly basophilic epithelial cells with finely stippled chromatin and indistinct nucleoli. Compare size of cells to macrophage in lower left-hand corner. (Wright-Giemsa; HP oil.) **D, Carcinoma. TTW. Dog.** In contrast to carcinoma cells of B and C, these cells have more deeply basophilic cytoplasm and marked pleomorphism. Note punctate vacuolation in center cells. A neutrophil and macrophage are present in the lower right for size comparison. (Wright-Giemsa; HP oil.) (A, Courtesy of Robert King, University of Florida.)

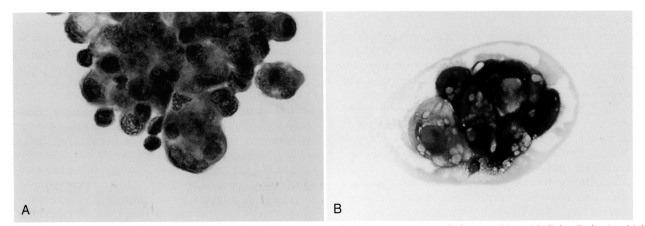

■ **FIGURE 5-53. A, Bronchogenic carcinoma.** Note the strongly cohesive arrangement of pleomorphic epithelial cells having high nuclear-to-cytoplasmic ratios. (Wright-Giemsa; IP.) **B, Bronchogenic carcinoma. Dog.** Cells from bronchogenic carcinomas that exfoliate into the thoracic fluid may have prominent vacuolation due to the fluid environment. (Wright-Giemsa; HP oil.)

Continued

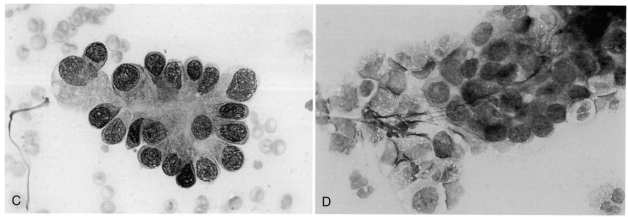

■ **FIGURE 5-53, cont'd. C, Adenocarcinoma. Lung. Dog.** Acinar formation suggesting glandular origin. (Wright-Giemsa; HP oil.) **D, Bronchoalveolar carcinoma with eosinophilic infiltrate. Lung mass imprint. Dog.** Malignant features present in an epithelial cell cluster along with numerous eosinophils that infiltrate the neoplasm. Suspect a tumor-associated eosinophilic infiltrate. Peripheral eosinophilia was not noted in this case. (Wright-Giemsa; HP oil.) (C, Courtesy of Rose Raskin, University of Florida. D, Glass slide material courtesy of Karen Young and Richard Meadows, University of Wisconsin; presented at the 1992 ASVCP case review session.)

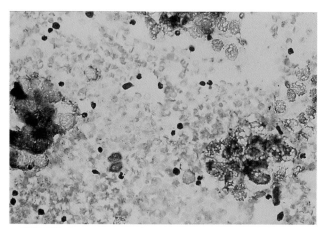

■ **FIGURE 5-54. Metastasis. Lung. Dog.** Metastatic lesion suspected to originate from carcinoma affecting the urethra. (Wright-Giemsa; HP oil.) (Courtesy of Rose Raskin, University of Florida.)

the same cluster, is common in pulmonary carcinomas. Nuclei are round and frequently eccentrically placed, and contain coarsely clumped chromatin and prominent, single to multiple nucleoli. Anisokaryosis is common. The cytoplasm is deeply basophilic and punctate vacuolation, particularly in the perinuclear region, is frequently prominent. Other criteria of malignancy that may be seen include nuclear molding, signet ring cell formation, cell or nuclear gigantism, and the presence of binucleate and multinucleate cells.

Only squamous cell carcinoma has distinguishing features that allow for identification during cytologic evaluation (Fig. 5-56A&B). Aspiration of a squamous cell carcinoma tends to yield moderately cellular samples for cytologic evaluation. Cells occur individually, in sheets, and in clusters with moderate to marked variation in cell size, nuclear size, nuclear-to-cytoplasmic ratios, amount of cytoplasm, and degree of keratinization. Individual cell

morphology ranges from basal squamous cells with little or no keratinization to fully keratinized squamous cells. The basal cells are cuboidal to round with deeply basophilic cytoplasm, large central nuclei, coarse chromatin, and prominent nucleoli. Mature squamous cells are large with abundant homogenous cytoplasm and pyknotic or karyorrhectic nuclei. Dysynchrony of cytoplasmic and nuclear maturation is common in squamous cell carcinoma.

Squamous metaplasia may occur with chronic inflammation and caution should be taken when differentiating squamous metaplasia from neoplasia (see Fig. 5-51). However, SCC of the lung typically originates from areas of squamous metaplasia of the bronchial epithelium, suggesting that metaplasia may readily proceed to neoplasia in the lower respiratory tract. Bronchogenic tumors frequently contain both glandular and squamous components.

Hemolymphatic Neoplasia

Hemolymphatic neoplasia may disseminate throughout the parenchyma, resulting in diffuse infiltrative disease or as discrete nodules. Several presentations have been identified, including lymphoma, malignant histiocytosis, and lymphomatoid granulomatosis. These are more commonly reported in dogs than in cats.

BAL samples have been shown to be more sensitive than radiographs in diagnosing malignant multicentric lymphoma (Fig. 5-57A&B) (Hawkins et al., 1995; Hawkins et al., 1993; Yohn et al., 1994). However, BAL is likely only important for staging this neoplasm, since primary lung lymphoma has not been reported to occur in animals, as it has in humans. The degree of involvement by a monomorphic population of lymphoid cells is helpful in distinguishing between a reactive population of lymphocytes, especially when malignant features are minimal (Fig. 5-58A&B). Histopathology with immunophenotyping may be helpful in establishing the malignant nature of the lymphoid population (Fig. 5-58C–E).

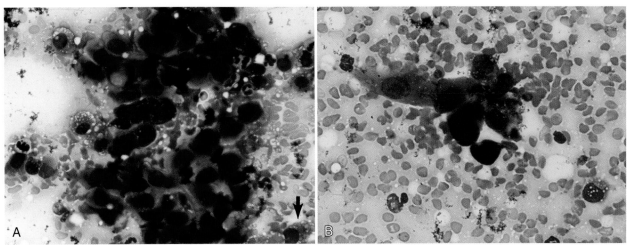

■ **FIGURE 5-55. Anaplastic carcinoma. Dog. Same case A-B. A,** Dense clusters of epithelial cells with moderate to marked pleomorphism. Some cells appear cohesive, while others have wispy, spindled borders and others appear round in shape. The origin of this neoplasia was not determined. A large secretory vacuole is seen in the upper cluster of cells. Note abundant punctate perinuclear vacuolation in several cells. Identification of individualized cells as neoplastic cells or macrophages can be difficult, particularly in this case as the number of neutrophils appears to be increased suggesting an inflammatory response. Erythrophagia is noted *(arrow)*. (Wright-Giemsa; HP oil.) **B,** Note the spindled appearance of several of the cells. (Wright-Giemsa; HP oil.)

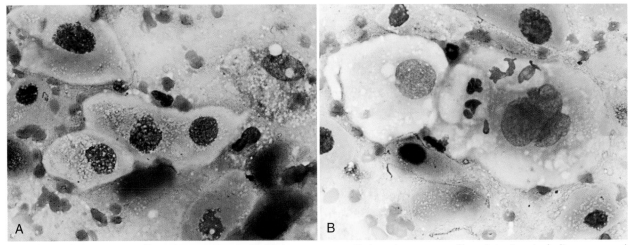

■ **FIGURE 5-56. Squamous cell carcinoma. Cat. A,** Multiple squamous cells in various stages of keratinization, including two anuclear keratin flakes. (Wright-Giemsa; HP oil.) **B,** Very large squamous epithelial cells. The cell on the right has multiple nucleoli and neutrophils exhibiting emperiopolesis. (Wright-Giemsa; HP oil.)

The lung is one of the primary sites of infiltration in malignant histiocytosis of both dogs and cats. In dogs, malignant histiocytosis and malignant fibrous histiocytoma have been proposed to be related tumors either through alternative differentiation of the same precursor cell or by differentiation of different precursors to a similar phenotype (Kerlin and Hendrick, 1996). Early reports suggested a predisposition in Bernese mountain dogs, Rottweilers, Golden Retrievers, and Flat-Coated Retrievers for both tumor types: however, the disease has since been reported in numerous breeds and likely any breed can be affected. More recently, histiocytic neoplasia in

the dog has been defined as a spectrum of diseases characterized by proliferation of Langerhans dendritic cells, interstitial dendritic cells, or macrophages (Affolter and Moore, 2000; Affolter and Moore, 2002; Moore et al., 2006). Malignant histiocytosis has also been identified in cats, primarily affecting the liver, spleen, and bone marrow more commonly than the lung (Kraje et al., 2001; Walton et al., 1997). The cell of origin in cat is unclear; however, a recent report suggests that at least in some cases, malignant histiocytic neoplasia in the cat may originate in the skin (Affolter and Moore, 2006). Malignant histiocytes are large, often markedly pleomorphic

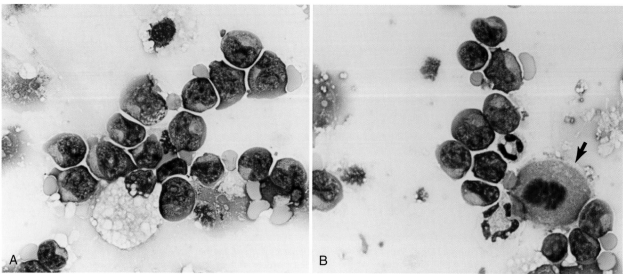

■ **FIGURE 5-57. Lymphoma, BAL. Dog. Same case A-B. A,** Increased numbers of medium to large lymphocytes. Nuclei are often cleaved or clover-leaf shaped and contain prominent nucleoli. A perinuclear clearing area is apparent in many cells that contain faint azurophilic granules. (Wright-Giemsa; HP oil.) **B,** Mitotic figure is present in the field *(arrow).* (Wright-Giemsa; HP oil.) (A and B, Glass slide material courtesy of Michel Desnoyers et al., University of Montreal; presented at the 2001 ASVCP case review session.)

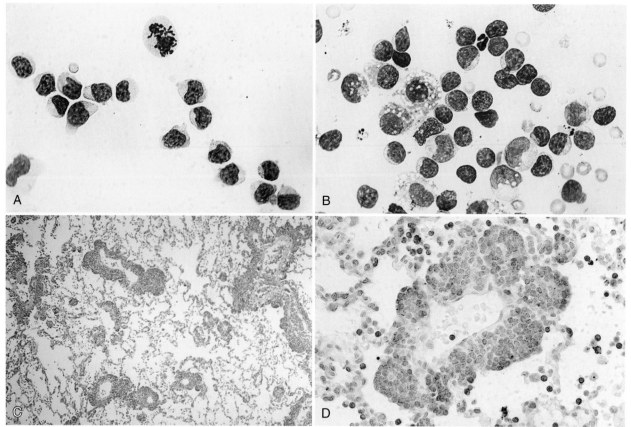

■ **FIGURE 5-58. Same case A-E. Pulmonary lymphoma. Dog. A, BAL.** Increased fluid cell count (945 cells/µl) with 79% medium-sized lymphocytes having a uniform appearance. Note the atypical mitotic figure in top center. (Wright-Giemsa; HP oil.) **B, Lung imprint.** Mixed cell population consisting of activated macrophages and numerous uniform-appearing, medium-sized lymphocytes with indistinct nucleoli. Morphology is compatible with the lymphoblastic subtype of lymphoma. (Wright-Giemsa; HP oil.) **C, Lung section.** Neoplastic lymphocytes were present as a cuff around blood vessels and bronchioles primarily. Evidence for vascular invasion and destruction was absent, ruling out lymphomatoid granulomatosis. Dog initially presented with only respiratory signs, suggesting a possible primary pulmonary lymphoma. (H&E; LP.) **Same case D-E. D, Lung section.** Positive immunohistochemical staining for T-lymphocytes present around a blood vessel and occasionally within alveolar septa. (CD3 antibody; HP oil.)

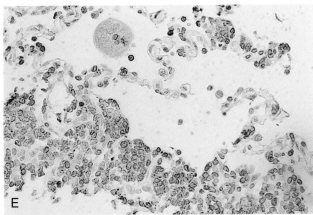

■ **FIGURE 5-58, cont'd. E, Pulmonary lymphoma. Lung section.** Dense staining with T-cell markers of cuffed lymphoid cells. Note the negative-stained giant cell with engulfed, positive-stained lymphocytes at left of center. (CD3 antibody; HP oil.) (A-E, Courtesy of Rose Raskin, University of Florida.)

discrete cells that contain abundant, often vacuolated, deeply basophilic cytoplasm. Nuclei are oval to reniform and contain lacy chromatin and prominent nucleoli (Fig. 5-59A–C). A continuum between discrete histiocytic cells and spindled mesenchymal cells may be seen; the appearance frequently varies in masses from the same animal and may even vary from different sites of the same mass. Multinucleated cells are frequently present but the

number seen is variable. Cells may also exhibit phagocytosis of erythrocytes and leukocytes, which helps to suggest a histiocytic origin; however, phagocytosis is not a consistent feature. Malignant histiocytosis can be cytologically difficult to differentiate from granulomatous inflammation, large cell anaplastic carcinoma, large cell T-cell lymphoma, pulmonary lymphomatoid granulomatosis, and plasmacytoma or extramedullary myeloma. Positive immunoreactivity to lysozyme can aid in this differentiation (Brown et al., 1994).

Pulmonary lymphomatoid granulomatosis is an uncommon pleocellular T-cell lymphoid neoplasia that has been recognized primarily in young to middle-aged dogs (Postorino et al., 1989; Bain et al., 1997; Fitzgerald et al., 1991). Typically, extensive infiltration of one or more lung lobes is seen. Pulmonary lymphomatoid granulomatosis is characterized by variable numbers of large, pleomorphic, mononuclear cells that range from lymphoid to plasmacytoid to histiocytic in appearance; binucleate cells and mitoses are common (Fig. 5-60A–D). Neoplastic cells may actually compose the minority of the cell population present and are admixed with numerous small lymphocytes, eosinophils, and plasma cells. Peripheral basophilia and canine dirofilariasis have been inconsistently associated with lymphomatoid granulomatous. Grossly and cytologically, this condition may be confused with eosinophilic granulomatosis, which consists of a pleocellular population of epithelioid cells, macrophages, eosinophils, and lymphocytes. What distinguishes them is the presence histologically of vascular

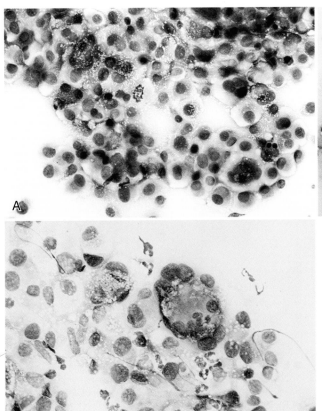

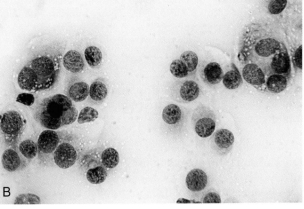

■ **FIGURE 5-59. Malignant histiocytosis. Same case A-B. A, Lung imprint. Dog.** Highly cellular collection of atypical round cells, many with numerous punctate vacuoles. Note the mitotic figure in the center. (Modified Wright; HP oil.) **B,** Binucleate and multinucleate forms are frequent. Cytoplasmic borders range from distinct to indistinct. Immunostaining (not shown) for a histiocytic marker (CD 18) was positive. (Modified Wright; HP oil.) **C, Tissue imprint.** Numerous vacuolated, pleomorphic histiocytes, including bi-, tri-, and multinucleate cells consistent with malignant histiocytosis. (Wright-Giemsa; HP oil.) (A, Glass slide material courtesy of Elizabeth Besteman et al., VA-MD Regional CVM; presented at the 1999 ASVCP case review session.)

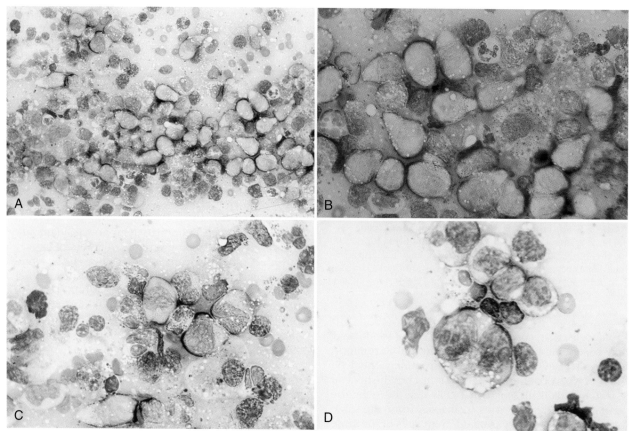

■ **FIGURE 5-60. Lymphomatoid granulomatosis. Dog. Same case A-C. A, Lung imprint.** Highly cellular sample with many large, poorly differentiated mononuclear cells. (Wright-Giemsa; HP oil.) **B,** Intermixed between the large mononuclear cells are eosinophils, neutrophils, and small lymphocytes. (Wright-Giemsa; HP oil.) **C,** In some areas, eosinophils are the predominant cell type and normal histiocytes may be found. A malignant T-cell lymphoid population is considered responsible for this neoplasm, as supported by antibody markers. (Wright-Giemsa; HP oil.) **D, Tissue imprint.** Pulmonary lymphomatoid granulomatosis is characterized by the presence of large, discrete, pleomorphic cells such as the one shown here admixed with lymphocytes and eosinophils. (Wright-Giemsa; HP oil.) (A-C, Courtesy of Rose Raskin, University of Florida.)

and airway invasion and destruction in lymphomatoid granulomatosis, a feature that is lacking in eosinophilic granulomatosis.

Mesenchymal Neoplasia

Tumors arising from the pulmonary connective tissue are relatively rare in dogs and cats. These include osteosarcoma, chondrosarcoma, hemangiosarcoma, fibrosarcoma, rhabdomyoma, rhabdomyosarcoma, and schwannoma. When reported, the neoplastic cell population resembles those seen in the more common sites (Fig. 5-61).

Nonrespiratory Aspirate

Occasionally samples are obtained that are not consistent with the lung parenchyma. The two most common nonrespiratory cells seen with lung aspirates are mesothelial cells and hepatocytes. It is important to recognize these cells so as not to mistake them for a neoplastic population. Sheets of mesothelial cells are seen if the lung surface is scraped during the aspiration process. The sheets are comprised of bland, monomorphic cells with angular, cohesive borders resembling fish

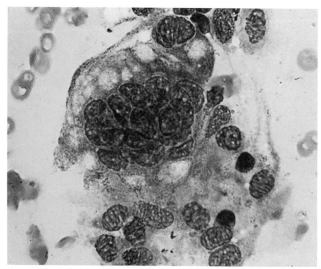

■ **FIGURE 5-61. Giant cell sarcoma. Lung mass. Dog.** Multinucleate giant cell and pleomorphic mesenchymal cells from a possible metastatic sarcoma. (Wright-Giemsa; HP oil.) (Courtesy of Rick Alleman, University of Florida.)

scales, pale cytoplasm, and small, round central nuclei (Fig. 5-62). As the cells begin to exfoliate from the sheets, they round up, become more basophilic, and begin to demonstrate the glycocalyx halo (eosinophilic fringe) associated with more classical mesothelial cells seen commonly in thoracic and abdominal fluids. Aspiration of the liver occurs when the chest is entered too far caudally (Fig. 5-63).

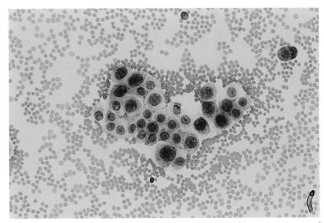

■ **FIGURE 5-62. Mesothelial cells. Lung aspirate.** A sheet of mildly pleomorphic mesothelial cells. Presence of mesothelial cells from a lung biopsy indicates sampling of the surface lining only. (Wright-Giemsa; IP.)

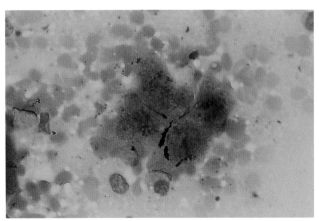

■ **FIGURE 5-63. Accidental liver aspirate.** Presence of hepatocytes with prominent canaliculi containing bile, consistent with cholestasis. Liver may be aspirated if the needle is placed too caudally when attempting to sample the lung. (Wright-Giemsa; HP oil.)

REFERENCES

Affolter VK, Moore PF: Canine cutaneous and systemic histiocytosis: reactive histiocytosis of dermal dendritic cells, *Am J Dermatopathol* 22:40-48, 2000.

Affolter VK, Moore PF: Localized and disseminated histiocytic sarcoma of dendritic cell origin in dogs, *Vet Pathol* 39:74-83, 2002.

Affolter VK, Moore PF: Feline progressive histiocytosis, *Vet Pathol* 43:646-655, 2006.

Anderton TL, Makell DJ, Preston A: Ciliostasis is a key early event during colonization of canine tracheal tissue by Bordetella bronchiseptica, *Microbiol* 150:2843-2855, 2004.

Andreasen CB: Bronchoalveolar lavage, *Vet Clin North Am Small Anim Pract* 33:69-88, 2003.

Andreasen CB, Carmichael P: What is your diagnosis? Lung aspirate and transtracheal wash from a 1-year-old dog with dyspnea, *Vet Clin Pathol* 21:77-78, 1992.

Bain PJ, Alleman AR, Sheppard BJ, et al: What is your diagnosis? Lung mass from an 18-month-old Boxer, *Vet Clin Pathol* 26:55, 91-92, 1997.

Baldwin F, Becker AB: Bronchoalveolar eosinophilic cells in a canine model of asthma: two distinctive populations, *Vet Pathol* 30:97-103, 1993.

Barnhart K, Lewis B: Laryngopharyngeal mass in a dog with upper airway obstruction, *Vet Clin Pathol* 29:47-50, 2000.

Bauer NB, O'Neill E, Sheahan BJ, et al: Calcospherite-like bodies and caseous necrosis in tracheal mucus from a dog with tuberculosis, *Vet Clin Pathol* 33:168-172, 2004.

Bernsteen L, Gregory CR, Aronson LR, et al: Acute toxoplasmosis following renal transplantation in three cats and a dog, *J Am Vet Med Assoc* 215:1123-1126, 1999.

Bright RM, Gorman NT, Goring RL et al: Laryngeal oncocytoma in two dogs, *J Am Vet Med Assoc* 184: 738-740, 1994.

Brown DE, Thrall MA, Getzy DM, et al: Cytology of canine malignant histiocytosis, *Vet Clin Pathol* 23:118-123, 1994.

Burgener DC, Slocombe RF, Zerbe CA: Lymphoplasmacytic rhinitis in five dogs, *J Am Anim Hosp Assoc* 23:565-568, 1987.

Burton SA, Honor DJ, Horney BS, et al: What is your diagnosis? Transtracheal aspirate from a dog, *Vet Clin Pathol* 21:112-113, 1992.

Cabanes FJ, Roura X, Majo N, et al: Pneumocystis carinii pneumonia in a Yorkshire terrier dog, *Med Mycol* 38:451-453, 2000.

Cafarchia C, Sasanelli M, Lia RP, et al: Lymphocutaneous and nasal sporotrichosis in a dog from southern Italy: case report, *Mycopathologia* 163:75-79, 2007.

Calvert CA, Mahaffey MB, Lappin MR, et al: Pulmonary and disseminated eosinophilic granulomatosis in dogs, *J Am Anim Hosp Assoc* 24:311-320, 1988.

Caniatti M, Roccabianca P, Scanziani E, et al: Nasal rhinosporidiosis in dogs: four cases from Europe and a review of the literature, *Vet Rec* 142:334-338, 1998.

Carswell JL, Williams KJ: Respiratory system. In Maxie MG, editor: *Jubb, Kennedy, and Palmer's pathology of domestic animals*, Philadelphia, Saunders, 2007, pp 523-653.

Clercx C, Wallon J, Gilbert S, et al: Imprint and brush cytology in the diagnosis of canine intranasal tumours, *J Small Anim Pract* 37:423-427, 1996.

Crawford PC, Dubovi EJ, Castleman WL, et al: Transmission of equine influenza virus to dogs, *Science* 310:482-485, 2005.

Day MJ, Henderson SM, Belshaw Z, et al: An immunohistochemical investigation of 18 cases of feline nasal lymphoma, *J Comp Pathol* 130:152-161, 2004.

De Lorenzi D, Bonfanti U, Masserdotti C, et al: Diagnosis of canine nasal aspergillosis by cytological examination: a comparison of four different collection techniques, *J Small Anim Pract* 47:316-319, 2006a.

De Lorenzi D, Bonfanti U, Masserdotti C, et al: Nasal melanosis in three dogs, *J Small Anim Pract* 47:682-685, 2006b.

DeHeer HL, McManus P: Frequency and severity of tracheal wash hemosiderosis and association with underlying disease in 96 cats: 2002-2003, *Vet Clin Pathol* 34:17-22, 2005.

Dennis JC, Allgier JG, Desouza LS, et al: Immunohistochemistry of the canine vomeronasal organ, *J Anat* 203:329-338, 2003.

Dirscherl P, Beisker W, Kremmer E, et al: Immunophenotyping of canine bronchoalveolar and peripheral blood lymphocytes, *Vet Immunol Immunopathol* 48:1-10, 1995.

Doughty RW, Brockman D, Neiger R, et al: Nasal oncocytoma in a domestic shorthair cat, *Vet Pathol* 43:751-754, 2006.

Duncan C, Stephen C, Lester S, et al: Sub-clinical infection and asymptomatic carriage of *Cryptococcus gattii* in dogs and cats during an outbreak of cryptococcosis, *Med Mycol* 43:511-516, 2005.

Dungworth DL: The respiratory system. In Jubb KVF, Kennedy PC, Palmer N, editors: *Pathology of domestic animals*, San Diego, Academic Press, 1993, pp 610-613.

Dye JA, McKiernan BC, Rozanski EA, et al: Bronchopulmonary disease in the cat: historical, physical, radiographic, clinicopathologic, and pulmonary functional evaluation of 24 affected and 15 healthy cats, *J Vet Intern Med* 10: 385-400, 1996.

Eidson M, Thilsted JP, Rollag OJ: Clinical, clinicopathologic, and pathologic features of plague in cats: 119 cases (1977-1988), *J Am Vet Med Assoc* 199:1191-1197, 1991.

Elie M, Sabo M: Basics in canine and feline rhinoscopy, *Clin Tech Small Anim Pract* 21:60-63, 2006.

Fitzgerald SD, Wolf DC, Carlton WW: Eight cases of canine lymphomatoid granulomatosis, *Vet Pathol* 28:241-245, 1991.

Flatland B, Greene RT, Lappin MR: Clinical and serologic evaluation of cats with cryptococcosis, *J Am Vet Med Assoc* 209:1110-1113, 1996.

French TW: The use of cytology in the diagnosis of chronic nasal disorders, *Compend Contin Educ Pract Vet* 9:115-121, 1987.

Gaschen L, Kircher P, Lang J: Endoscopic ultrasound instrumentation, applications in humans, and potential veterinary applications, *Vet Radiol Ultrasound* 44:665-680, 2003.

Ginel PJ, Molleda JM, Novales M, et al: Primary transmissible venereal tumour in the nasal cavity of a dog, *Vet Rec* 136:222-223, 1995.

Gori S, Scasso A: Cytologic and differential diagnosis of rhinosporidiosis, *Acta Cytol* 38:361-366, 1994.

Greene RT: Cryptococcosis. In Greene CE, ed: *Infectious diseases of the dog and cat*, WB Saunders, Philadelphia, 1998, pp 383-390.

Greene RT, Troy GC: Coccidioidomycosis in 48 cats: a retrospective study (1984-1993), *J Vet Intern Med* 9:86-91, 1995.

Greig B, Rossow KD, Collins JE, et al: Neospora caninum pneumonia in an adult dog, *J Am Vet Med Assoc* 206:1000-1001, 1995.

Hagiwara Y, Fujiwara S, Takai H, et al: Pneumocystis carinii pneumonia in a Cavalier King Charles Spaniel, *J Vet Med Sci* 63:349-351, 2001.

Hahn KA, McEntee MF: Primary lung tumors in cats: 86 cases (1979-1994), *J Am Vet Med Assoc* 211:1257-1260, 1997.

Hawkins EC, Davidson MG, Meuten DJ, et al: Cytologic identification of Toxoplasma gondii in bronchoalveolar lavage fluid of experimentally infected cats, *J Am Vet Med Assoc* 210:648-650, 1997.

Hawkins EC, DeNicola DB: Collection of bronchoalveolar lavage fluid in cats, using an endotracheal tube, *Am J Vet Res* 50:855-859, 1989.

Hawkins EC, DeNicola DB: Cytologic analysis of tracheal wash specimens and bronchoalveolar lavage fluid in the diagnosis of mycotic infections in dogs, *J Am Vet Med Assoc* 197:79-83, 1990.

Hawkins EC, DeNicola DB, Kuehn NF: Bronchoalveolar lavage in the evaluation of pulmonary disease in the dog and cat. State of the art, *J Vet Intern Med* 4:267-274, 1990.

Hawkins EC, DeNicola DB, Plier ML: Cytological analysis of bronchoalveolar lavage fluid in the diagnosis of spontaneous respiratory tract disease in dogs: a retrospective study, *J Vet Intern Med* 9:386-392, 1995.

Hawkins EC, Kennedy-Stoskopf S, Levy J, et al: Cytologic characterization of bronchoalveolar lavage fluid collected through an endotracheal tube in cats, *Am J Vet Res* 55:795-802, 1994.

Hawkins EC, Kennedy-Stoskopf S, Levy JK, et al: Effect of FIV infection on lung inflammatory cell populations recovered by bronchoalveolar lavage, *Vet Immunol Immunopathol* 51:21-28, 1996.

Hawkins EC, Morrison WB, DeNicola DB, et al: Cytologic analysis of bronchoalveolar lavage fluid from 47 dogs with multicentric malignant lymphoma, *J Am Vet Med Assoc* 203:1418-1425, 1993.

Hawkins EC, Rogala AR, Large EE, et al: Cellular composition of bronchial brushings obtained from healthy dogs and dogs with chronic cough and cytologic composition of bronchoalveolar lavage fluid obtained from dogs with chronic cough, *Am J Vet Res* 67:160-167, 2006.

Hicks DG, Fidel JL: Intranasal malignant melanoma in a dog, *J Am Anim Hosp Assoc* 42:472-476, 2006.

Jerram RM, Guyer CL, Braniecki A, et al: Endogenous lipid (cholesterol) pneumonia associated with bronchogenic carcinoma in a cat, *J Am Anim Hosp Assoc* 34:275-280, 1998.

Johnson LR, Clarke HE, Bannasch MJ, et al: Correlation of rhinoscopic signs of inflammation with histologic findings in nasal biopsy specimens of cats with or without upper respiratory tract disease, *J Am Vet Med Assoc* 225:395-400, 2004.

Johnson LR, De Cock HE, Sykes JE, et al: Cytokine gene transcription in feline nasal tissue with histologic evidence of inflammation, *Am J Vet Res* 66:996-1001, 2005.

Johnson LR, Drazenovich TL: Flexible bronchoscopy and bronchoalveolar lavage in 68 cats (2001-2006), *J Vet Intern Med* 21:219-225, 2007.

Johnson LR, Drazenovich TL, Herrera MA, et al: Results of rhinoscopy alone or in conjunction with sinuscopy in dogs with aspergillosis: 46 cases (2001-2004), *J Am Vet Med Assoc* 228:738-742, 2006.

Jones DJ, Norris CR, Samii VF, et al: Endogenous lipid pneumonia in cats: 24 cases (1985-1998), *J Am Vet Med Assoc* 216: 1437-1440, 2000.

Jones JC, Ober CP: Computed tomographic diagnosis of nongastrointestinal foreign bodies in dogs, *J Am Anim Hosp Assoc* 43:99-111, 2007.

Jordan HL, Cohn LA, Armstrong PJ: Disseminated Mycobacterium avium complex infection in three Siamese cats, *J Am Vet Med Assoc* 204:90-93, 1994.

Kerlin RL, Hendrick MJ: Malignant fibrous histiocytoma and malignant histiocytosis in the dog-convergent or divergent phenotypic differentiation? *Vet Pathol* 33:713-716, 1996.

King RR, Greiner EC, Ackerman N, et al: Nasal capillariasis in a dog, *J Am Anim Hosp Assoc* 26:381-385, 1990.

Kraje AC, Patton CS, Edwards DF: Malignant histiocytosis in 3 cats, *J Vet Intern Med* 15:252-256, 2001.

Kuehn NF: Nasal computed tomography, *Clin Tech Small Anim Pract* 21:55-59, 2006.

Kuiken T, Rimmelzwaan G, van Riel D, et al: Avian H5N1 influenza in cats, *Science* 306:241, 2004.

Lana SE, Withrow SJ: Tumors of the respiratory system—nasal tumors. In Withrow SJ, MacEwen EG, editors: *Small animal clinical oncology*, Saunders, Philadelphia, 2001 pp 370-377.

Latimer KS: Cytology examination of the respiratory tract—part 2, The 11th Annual ACVIM Forum, Washington, DC, 1993.

Lécuyer M, Dube PG, DiFruscia R, et al: Bronchoalveolar lavage in normal cats, *Can Vet J* 36:771-773, 1995.

Leme LR, Schubach TM, Santos IB, et al: Mycological evaluation of bronchoalveolar lavage in cats with respiratory signs from Rio de Janeiro, Brazil, *Mycoses* 50:210-214, 2007.

Llanos-Cuentas EA, Roncal N, Villaseca P, et al: Natural infections of Leishmania peruviana in animals in the Peruvian Andes, *Trans R Soc Trop Med Hyg* 93:15-20, 1999.

Lobetti R: Common variable immunodeficiency in miniature dachshunds affected with Pneumocystis carinii pneumonia, *J Vet Diagn Invest* 12:39-45, 2000.

Lobetti RG: Pneumocystis carinii infection in miniature dachshunds, *Compend Contin Educ Pract Vet* 23:320-324, 2001.

Lopez A: Respiratory system, thoracic cavity, and pleura. In Thomson RG, McGavin MD, Carlton WW, et al, editors: *Thomson's special veterinary pathology*, Philadelphia, Mosby, 2000, pp 125-195.

Macdonald ES, Norris CR, Berghaus RB, et al: Clinicopathologic and radiographic features and etiologic agents in cats with histologically confirmed infectious pneumonia: 39 cases (1991-2000), *J Am Vet Med Assoc* 223:1142-1150, 2003.

Malik R, Martin P, Wigney DI, et al: Nasopharyngeal cryptococcosis, *Aust Vet J* 75:483-488, 1997.

McCauley M, Atwell RB, Sutton RH, et al: Unguided bronchoalveolar lavage techniques and residual effects in dogs, *Aust Vet J* 76:161-165, 1998.

McKay JS, Cox CL, Foster AP: Cutaneous alternariosis in a cat, *J Small Anim Pract* 42:75-78, 2001.

Medleau L, Barsanti JB: Cryptococcosis. In Greene CE, editor: *Infectious diseases of the dog and cat*, WB Saunders, Philadelphia, 1990, pp 687-695.

Meier WA, Meinkoth JH, Brunker J, et al: Cytologic identification of immature endospores in a dog with rhinosporidiosis, *Vet Clin Pathol* 35:348-352, 2006.

Meuten DJ, Calderwood-Mays MB, Dillman RC, et al: Canine laryngeal rhabdomyoma, *Vet Pathol* 22:533-539, 1985.

Michiels L, Day MJ, Snaps F, et al: A retrospective study of non-specific rhinitis in 22 cats and the value of nasal cytology and histopathology, *J Feline Med Surg* 5:279-285, 2003.

Mills PC, Litster A: Using urea dilution to standardise cellular and non-cellular components of pleural and bronchoalveolar lavage (BAL) fluids in the cat, *J Feline Med Surg* 8:105-110, 2006.

Moore AS, Ogilvie GK: Tumors of the respiratory tract. In Moore AS, Ogilvie GK, editors: *Feline oncology: a comprehensive guide to compassionate care*, Veterinary Learning Systems, Trenton, NJ, 2001, pp 368-384.

Moore PF, Affolter VK, Vernau W: Canine hemophagocytic histiocytic sarcoma: a proliferative disorder of CD11d+ macrophages, *Vet Pathol* 43:632-645, 2006.

Mukaratirwa S, van der Linde-Sipman JS, Gruys E: Feline nasal and paranasal sinus tumours: clinicopathological study, histomorphological description and diagnostic immunohistochemistry of 123 cases, *J Feline Med Surg* 3:235-245, 2001.

Nunez-Ochoa L, Desnoyers M, Lecuyer M: What is your diagnosis? Transtracheal wash from a 2-year-old dog, *Vet Clin Pathol* 22:122, 1993.

Oakes MG, McCarthy RJ: What is your diagnosis? Soft-tissue mass within the lumen of the larynx, caudal to the epiglottis, *J Am Vet Med Assoc* 204:1891-1892, 1994.

Ogilvie GK, Haschek WM, Withrow SJ, et al: Classification of primary lung tumors in dogs: 210 cases (1975-1985), *J Am Vet Med Assoc* 195:106-108, 1989.

Padrid P, Amis TC: Chronic tracheobronchial disease in the dog, *Vet Clin North Am Small Anim Pract* 22:1203-1229, 1992.

Padrid PA, Feldman BF, Funk K, et al: Cytologic, microbiologic, and biochemical analysis of bronchoalveolar lavage fluid obtained from 24 healthy cats, *Am J Vet Res* 52:1300-1307, 1991.

Papazoglou LG, Koutinas AF, Plevraki AG, et al: Primary intranasal transmissible venereal tumour in the dog: a retrospective study of six spontaneous cases, *J Vet Med A Physiol Pathol Clin Med* 48:391-400, 2001.

Pass DA, Huxtable CR, Cooper BJ, et al: Canine laryngeal oncocytomas, *Vet Pathol* 17:672-677, 1980.

Patnaik AK: Histologic and immunohistochemical studies of granular cell tumors in seven dogs, three cats, one horse, and one bird, *Vet Pathol* 30:176-185, 1993.

Patnaik AK, Ludwig LL, Erlandson RA: Neuroendocrine carcinoma of the nasopharynx in a dog, *Vet Pathol* 39:496-500, 2002.

Peeters D, Peters IR, Helps CR, et al: Distinct tissue cytokine and chemokine mRNA expression in canine sino-nasal aspergillosis and idiopathic lymphoplasmacytic rhinitis, *Vet Immunol Immunopathol* 117:95-105, 2007.

Perez J, Bautista MJ, Carrasco L, et al: Primary extragenital occurrence of transmissible venereal tumors: three case reports, *Can Pract* 19:7-10, 1994.

Petite AF, Dennis R: Comparison of radiography and magnetic resonance imaging for evaluating the extent of nasal neoplasia in dogs, *J Small Anim Pract* 47:529-536, 2006.

Poitout F, Weiss DJ, Dubey JP: Lung aspirate from a cat with respiratory distress, *Vet Clin Pathol* 27:10, 1998.

Postorino NC, Wheeler SL, Park RD, et al: A syndrome resembling lymphomatoid granulomatosis in the dog, *J Vet Intern Med* 3:15-19, 1989.

Rakich PM, Latimer KS: Cytology of the respiratory tract, *Vet Clin North Am Small Anim Pract* 19:823-850, 1989.

Raya AI, Fernandez-de Marco M, Nunez A, et al: Endogenous lipid pneumonia in a dog, *J Comp Pathol* 135:153-155, 2006.

Rebar AH, DeNicola DB, Muggenburg BA: Bronchopulmonary lavage cytology in the dog: normal findings, *Vet Pathol* 17:294-304, 1980.

Rebar AH, Hawkins EC, DeNicola DB: Cytologic evaluation of the respiratory tract, *Vet Clin North Am Small Anim Pract* 22:1065-1085, 1992.

Rudorf H, Brown P: Ultrasonography of laryngeal masses in six cats and one dog, *Vet Radiol Ultrasound* 39:430-434, 1998.

Ruehlmann D, Podell M, Oglesbee M, et al: Canine neosporosis: a case report and literature review, *J Am Anim Hosp Assoc* 31:174-183, 1995.

Sako T, Shimoyama Y, Akihara Y, et al: Neuroendocrine carcinoma in the nasal cavity of ten dogs, *J Comp Pathol* 133:155-163, 2005.

Salazar I, Sanchez Quinteiro P, Cifuentes JM, et al: The vomeronasal organ of the cat, *J Anat* 188 (Pt 2):445-454, 1996.

Silverstein D, Greene C, Gregory E, et al: Pulmonary alveolar proteinosis in a dog, *J Vet Intern Med* 14:546-551, 2000.

Smallwood LJ, Zenoble RD: Biopsy and cytological sampling of the respiratory tract, *Semin Vet Med Surg (Small Anim)* 8(4):250-257, 1993.

Sukura A, Saari S, Järvinen AK, et al: Pneumocystis carinii pneumonia in dogs-a diagnostic challenge, *J Vet Diagn Invest* 8:124-130, 1996.

Tang KN, Mansell JL, Herron AJ, et al: The histologic, ultrastructural, and immunohistochemical characteristics of a thyroid oncocytoma in a dog, *Vet Pathol* 31:269-271, 1994.

Tasker S, Foster DJ, Corcoran BM, et al: Obstructive inflammatory laryngeal disease in three cats, *J Feline Med Surg* 1:53-59, 1999a.

Tasker S, Knottenbelt CM, Munro EA, et al: Aetiology and diagnosis of persistent nasal disease in the dog: a retrospective study of 42 cases, *J Small Anim Pract* 40:473-478, 1999b.

Tennant K, Patterson-Kane J, Boag AK, et al: Nasal mycosis in two cats caused by Alternaria species, *Vet Rec* 155:368-370, 2004.

Teske E, Stokhof AA, van den Ingh TSGAM, et al: Transthoracic needle aspiration biopsy of the lung in dogs with pulmonic diseases, *J Am Anim Hosp Assoc* 27:289-294, 1991.

Unterer S, Deplazes P, Arnold P, et al: Spontaneous Crenosoma vulpis infection in 10 dogs: laboratory, radiographic and endoscopic findings, *Schweiz Arch Tierheilkd* 144:174-179, 2002.

Vail DM, Mahler PA, Soergel SA: Differential cell analysis and phenotypic subtyping of lymphocytes in bronchoalveolar lavage fluid from clinically normal dogs, *Am J Vet Res* 56:282-285, 1995.

Walton RM, Brown DE, Burkhard MJ, et al: Malignant histiocytosis in a domestic cat: cytomorphologic and immunohistochemical features, *Vet Clin Pathol* 26:56-60, 1997.

Watson PJ, Wotton P, Eastwood J, et al: Immunoglobulin deficiency in Cavalier King Charles Spaniels with Pneumocystis pneumonia, *J Vet Intern Med* 20:523-527, 2006.

Whittemore JC, Webb CB: Successful treatment of nasal sporotrichosis in a dog, *Can Vet J* 48:411-414, 2007.

Wiedmeyer CE, Whitney MS, Dvorak LD, et al: Mass in the laryngeal region of a dog, *Vet Clin Pathol* 32(1):37-39, 2003.

Williams M, Olver C, Thrall MA: Transtracheal wash from a puppy with respiratory disease, *Vet Clin Pathol* 35: 471-473, 2006.

Windsor RC, Johnson LR, Herrgesell EJ, et al: Idiopathic lymphoplasmacytic rhinitis in dogs: 37 cases (1997-2002), *J Am Vet Med Assoc* 224:1952-1957, 2004.

Wood EF, O'Brien RT, Young KM: Ultrasound-guided fine-needle aspiration of focal parenchymal lesions of the lung in dogs and cats, *J Vet Intern Med* 12:338-342, 1998.

Yohn SE, Hawkins EC, Morrison WB, et al: Confirmation of a pulmonary component of multicentric lymphosarcoma with bronchoalveolar lavage in two dogs, *J Am Vet Med Assoc* 204:97-101, 1994.

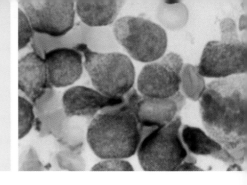

CHAPTER 6

Body Cavity Fluids

Alan H. Rebar and Craig A. Thompson

Typically there is little fluid present in the peritoneal, pleural, and pericardial cavities, and thus they are considered potential spaces. Detailed physiologic descriptions of serous body cavity homeostasis are available (Bouvy et al., 1991; Forrester, 1988; Kirby, 2003). These serous body cavities are lined by specialized cells, termed *mesothelial cells*. Clinical signs of the presence of increased amounts of fluid include abdominal distension, abdominal pain, dyspnea, muffled heart sounds, and cardiac arrhythmia. Collection and evaluation of fluid from these sites may be therapeutic as well as diagnostic for the presence of inflammatory, hemorrhagic, neoplastic, lymphatic, or bilious conditions. Additionally, further diagnostic tests may be indicated by the cytologic characteristics. Removal and examination of fluid is highly recommended unless anesthetic risks or bleeding diathesis are present or further injury is likely.

COLLECTION TECHNIQUES

Abdominal Fluid

Place the patient in left lateral recumbency and restrain. Clip and surgically prepare an area (e.g., 4 to 6 inches square) with the umbilicus in the center. The urinary bladder should be emptied before performing paracentesis. Infiltrate a small area with local anesthetic, if desired. Use a 20-to 22-gauge needle or over-the-needle catheter to penetrate the abdomen. Attempt to obtain fluid in four quadrants, allowing the fluid to flow freely by gravity and capillary action. If needed, gentle suction with a 3- or 6-ml syringe can be employed. For a complete description of the technique, the reader is referred elsewhere (Ford and Mazzaferro, 2006). Allow the animal to rest quietly while fluid is being removed. Moving the animal or allowing the patient to move while the needle is in the abdomen can result in laceration of the organs. Some investigators prefer to have the patient standing for fluid removal; however, it is more likely that the omentum will occlude the needle if the patient is in a standing position.

Pleural Fluid

For removal of fluid from the thorax, the patient should be in a standing or in ventral /sternal recumbency. Clip the hair and surgically prepare the thoracic wall from the 5th to the 11th intercostal space. Infiltrate a small area at the 7th to 8th intercostal space at the level of the costochondral junction with local anesthetic. It is best to attach extension tubing to the hub of the needle or over-the-needle catheter and a three-way stopcock for removal of pleural fluid. Insert the needle or catheter into the chest wall at the surgically prepared site taking care to avoid the intercostal vessels located just caudal to each rib. For a complete description of this technique, the reader is referred elsewhere (Ford and Mazzaferro, 2006).

Pericardial Fluid

For removal of fluid from the pericardial sac, sedate the patient if necessary. Surgically prepare an area over the lower to mid 5th to 7th intercostal space bilaterally. Place the patient in lateral or sternal recumbency. Attach ECG leads to monitor for dysrhythmias during the procedure. Infiltrate an area at the costochondral junction, or approximately where the lower and mid thorax meet, with local anesthetic. Use an over-the-needle catheter or Intrafusor system with a three-way valve to which a 30-ml syringe is attached. Always maintain negative pressure on the syringe as the chest wall is punctured. Carefully advance the needle into the 4th intercostal space through a nick incision in the direction of the heart. Advance the needle until resistance is met (from the pericardium). A release will be felt as the needle enters the pericardial sac and a flash of blood is often seen. Thread the tubing or catheter so that it is securely within the pericardial sac. For a complete description of this technique, the reader is referred elsewhere (Ford and Mazzaferro, 2006).

SAMPLE HANDLING

Note the color and character of the fluid initially upon removal (Fig. 6-1). If the fluid is clear initially then turns red, iatrogenic blood contamination is likely. The fluid should be collected into both a lavender-top tube (EDTA anticoagulant) for cytology and a red-top tube (or any sterile tube without additives) for potential bacterial culture. Also at collection, make both direct unconcentrated smears by a squash or blood smear technique and smears from spun samples. Romanowsky-type stains such as Wright stain or an aqueous-based Wright (quick) stain can be applied to a few slides for immediate in-house evaluation. The remaining unstained smears, as well as an EDTA and serum tube filled with fluid, should be submitted to the laboratory. This will allow the clinical pathologist evaluating the sample to compare the cellularity of the sample and the appearance of the cells at the time of collection with that which was submitted in the tube.

LABORATORY EVALUATION

Protein Quantitation

Protein quantitation is typically done via refractometry; however, some institutions will determine protein via spectrophotometry or automated analysis. Both methods offer accurate readings in a wide range of protein concentrations (George, 2001; George and O'Neill, 2001). It has been shown with canine effusions that refractometry underestimates the protein content when < 2.0 g/dl and that the spectrophotometry using the biuret method is more accurate when there is high protein content (Braun et al., 2001). Others have found that refractometry can be used accurately down to 1.0 g/dl (George and O'Neill, 2001). A similar finding of underestimating protein content in feline effusions with refractometry may

occur (Papasouliotis et al., 2002). In that same study, a dry chemistry analyzer produced increased globulin concentration and therefore lower Albumin:Globulin (A:G) ratios when compared with a reference wet analyzer using the same biuret and bromocresol green methodologies (Papasouliotis et al., 2002). This finding is particularly important since decreased A:G ratios support a diagnosis of feline infectious peritonitis (Hartmann et al., 2003).

For cloudy or turbid samples and bloody samples, the fluid should be centrifuged and the protein measured on the supernatant. Turbidity may interfere with evaluation of protein by either refractometry or spectrophotometry. The protein content is used with the nucleated cell count to classify the effusion and help formulate a list of possible causes.

Red Blood Cell and Total Nucleated Cell Count

Although an initial impression of the cellularity and amount of blood can usually be made by visual inspection of the sample (see Fig. 6-1), knowledge of the actual cell counts for erythrocytes and nucleated cells is important for further classification of the type of fluid. With this information, one can begin to narrow down the list of possible causes for the abnormal fluid accumulation. For samples being submitted to a reference laboratory, placing some of the sample in a lavender-top tube (EDTA) and some in a red-top tube is recommended. The lavender-top tube contains anticoagulant, which prevents the sample from clotting if there is a high protein content. EDTA is bactericidal, however, and is contraindicated if a sample is to be cultured (Songer and Post, 2005). Thus, some of the fluid should also be put into a red-top tube or sterile tube without additives. The cell counts will be done either with a hemocytometer or an automated cell-counting instrument. If the amount of fibrinogen in the fluid sample is high, then the sample in the red-top tube is likely to clot, producing erroneous results.

Note: **Do not use gel-containing serum separator tubes (SST) for submission of fluid to a reference laboratory. Cells may bind to the gel in these tubes and result in an artifactually lowered cell count.**

Nucleated Cell Differential

Standard procedures for performing a differential of the nucleated cells vary among laboratories. Some laboratories do no differential, others a three-part differential of 100 cells (large mononuclear cells, small mononuclear cells, and neutrophils), while others will provide a 100-cell differential of all cell types observed. The differential provides a relative picture of the types and numbers of cells and aids in establishing a list of potential causes for the fluid accumulation. A differential is not a substitute for a cytologic evaluation. The cytologic evaluation is performed in an attempt to determine a specific diagnosis.

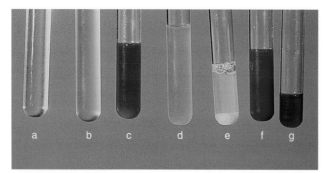

■ **FIGURE 6-1. Effusion color and character.** Gross appearance of various effusions. From left to right these are: (a) clear and colorless—transudate; (b) yellow and slightly turbid—modified transudate; (c) red and slightly turbid (likely hemolyzed red blood cells)—hemorrhage; (d) orange and turbid—likely inflammatory fluid with blood; (e) sedimented fluid—note thick pellet of cells on the bottom of the tube; (f) red and turbid—bloody as a result of either hemorrhage or iatrogenic blood contamination; (g) brown and slightly turbid—possible bile or red blood cell breakdown.

NORMAL CYTOLOGY AND HYPERPLASIA

Normally, only a very small amount of fluid is found in the peritoneal, pleural, and pericardial spaces; thus cytologic evaluation is generally not typically performed unless an increased amount of fluid accumulates. Normal fluid is clear and colorless (see Fig. 6-1). Several types of cells may be found in body cavity effusions and their relative proportions vary depending on the cause of the fluid accumulation. Cells expected to be in normal fluid include mesothelial, mononuclear phagocytes, lymphocytes, and rare neutrophils. Mesothelium will easily become hyperplastic or reactive when increased body cavity fluid or inflammation is present.

Mesothelial Cells

In most cases, the cytologist will find reactive mesothelial cells in body cavity fluids. These are considered as large mononuclear cells for the purpose of the three-part cell differential. Mesothelial cells may be seen as individualized cells or in variably sized clusters. They contain a moderate amount of medium-blue cytoplasm (Fig. 6-2). Hyperplastic mesothelial cells are large (12 to 30 μm) with deep-blue cytoplasm and may display a pink to red "fringed" cytoplasmic border (Fig. 6-3A&B). This feature helps identify these cells as mesothelial cells. These cells may contain one or more nuclei of equal size (see Fig. 6-3B). Nucleoli may be visible and occasional mitotic figures may be evident.

Macrophages

Macrophages are large mononuclear cells with abundant pale-gray to light-blue cytoplasm and a round to kidney bean–shaped nucleus (Figs. 6-3A and 6-4). The chromatin may be fine and nucleoli may be visible. Macrophages often contain vacuoles or previously phagocytosed cells

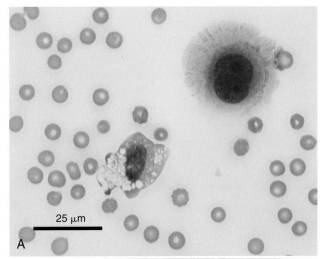

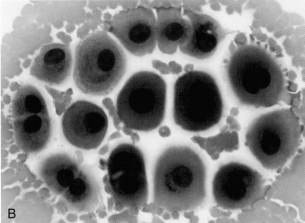

■ **FIGURE 6-3. Reactive mesothelial cell. A,** Exfoliated binucleate mesothelial cell (upper right) and mildly vacuolated and basophilic macrophage in an effusion. The mesothelial cell has a characteristic pink fringe along the cytoplasmic border. (Modified Wright; HP oil.) **B,** A loose group of variably reactive mesothlelial cells at the feathered edge of a smear made from an effusion. These cells may contain one or more nuclei. Note the presence of the "fringe" (glycocalyx) on the mesothelial cells. Several cells contain paranuclear dark granules, the significance of which is unknown. (Modified Wright; HP oil.)

and/or debris if there is inflammation or if the fluid has been present for a long time (Fig. 6-5). Macrophages are considered as large mononuclear cells for the purpose of the three-part cell differential.

Lymphoid Cells

Small and medium lymphocytes found in effusions appear similar to those found in peripheral blood. These nucleated cells often have a thin rim of lightly basophilic cytoplasm and a round nucleus. Lymphocytes are considered as small, mononuclear cells for the purpose of the three-part cell differential. In normal fluids they are present in higher proportions in cats and cattle than in dogs and horses. The nucleus nearly fills the cell, producing a uniformly high nuclear-to-cytoplasmic (N:C) ratio. The chromatin is finely stippled to evenly clumped; nucleoli are not visible (Fig. 6-6A&B).

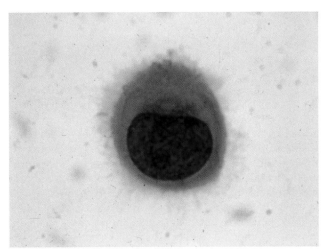

■ **FIGURE 6-2. Normal mesothelial cell.** Exfoliated cell in an effusion with its characteristic pink fringe along the cytoplasmic border. (Wright-Giemsa; HP oil.) (From Meyer DJ, Franks PT: Classification and cytologic examination, *Compend Contin Educ Pract Vet* 9:123-29, 1987.)

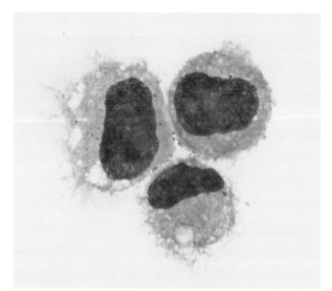

■ **FIGURE 6-4. Macrophages.** Three unremarkable to mildly basophilic and vacuolated macrophages from an effusion are present. (Modified Wright; HP oil.)

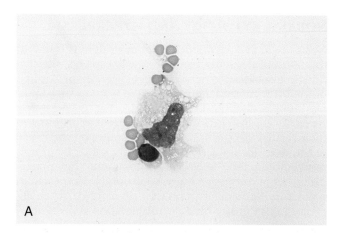

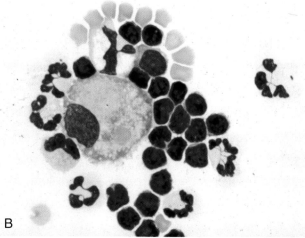

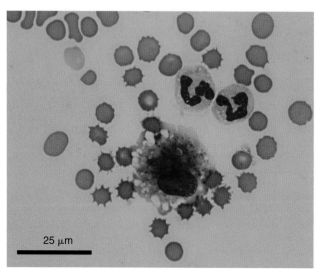

■ **FIGURE 6-5. Macrophage. Neutrophils.** Shown are a moderately vacuolated and basophilic macrophage and two nondegenerate neutrophils. (Modified Wright; HP oil.)

■ **FIGURE 6-6. A, Normal fluid/transudate.** Note the macrophage and small lymphocyte with several erythrocytes. Normal fluid and transudates contain very low nucleated cell counts (<1000/µl) and low protein content (<2.5 g/dl). (Romanowsky; HP oil.) **B, Modified transudate. Pleural. Cat.** The effusion cells have been concentrated in this animal with cardiomyopathy. Note a large macrophage, many small lymphocytes, and nondegenerate neutrophils. This fluid had a protein of 2.5g/dl and an increased nucleated cell count of 4000 cells/µl. The macrophage has phagocytized a red blood cell. (Romanowsky; HP oil.)

Neutrophils

Neutrophils appear similar to those found in peripheral blood. They are medium-sized cells with pale to clear cytoplasm and a segmented nucleus. Neutrophils should be absent or present in very low numbers in normal fluid but they will be found in increased numbers with chronic fluid accumulation or with inflammation (see Figs. 6-5 and 6-6B).

GENERAL CLASSIFICATION OF EFFUSIONS

Effusions are usually classified as transudates, modified transudates, and exudates, related to the protein concentration, nucleated cell count, and cell types present (Table 6-1).

Transudate

Fluids are classified as transudates when they have a low protein content and a low cell count (protein < 2.5 g/dl and cells < 1000/µl). These fluids increase in volume in response to physiologic mechanisms, such as increased hydrostatic vascular pressure or decreased colloidal osmotic pressure, that cause the normal homeostatic mechanisms of fluid production and resorption to be overwhelmed. Some causes for transudate accumulation include severe hypoalbuminemia, portal hypertension, hepatic insufficiency, portosystemic shunt, and early myocardial insufficiency. The cells commonly found in transudates are similar to those in normal fluid, which are mostly mononuclear cells consisting of macrophages, small lymphocytes, and mesothelial cells (see Fig. 6-6A). Neutrophils may compose a small proportion of the population.

TABLE 6-1   Classification of Common Body Cavity Effusions Based on Fluid Characteristics

Effusion Type	Color/Turbidity	Total Protein (g/dl)	Specific Gravity*	WBC (# per μl)	Predominant Cell Type (s)
General Conditions					
Transudate	Colorless/clear	<2.5	<1.017	<1000	Mesothelial Mononuclear phagocytes
Modified transudate	Light yellow to apricot/ clear to cloudy	≥2.5	1.017–1.025	>1000	Mononuclear cells
Exudate	Apricot to tan/cloudy	>3.0	>1.025	>5000	Neutrophils *Nonseptic* (nondegenerate) *Septic* (degenerate)
Specific Conditions					
Chylous	White/opaque	>2.5	>1.017	Variable	Acute: Small lymphocytes *Chronic:* Mixed population
Neoplastic	Light yellow to apricot/ clear to cloudy	>2.5	>1.017	Variable	Reactive mesothelium Neoplastic cells
Hemorrhagic	Pink to red/cloudy	>3.0	>1.025	>1000	Erythrocytes Leukocytes similar to blood Macrophages display erythrophagocytosis
Bilious	Dark yellow or brown or green/opaque	>3.0	>1.025	>5000	Mixed population with blue-green, brown, or yellow material phagocytized by macrophages

* Note that measurement of specific gravity using a standard refractometer has not been validated for use with body cavity fluids, only urine. Therefore, values should be regarded with caution (George, 2001).

Modified Transudate

A fluid is classified as a modified transudate when a transudate changes its physical features. The accumulation of transudative fluid in a body cavity causes increased pressure, which is irritating to the mesothelial cells lining the space. They respond by proliferating and sloughing into the effusion. With time, the sloughed mesothelial cells die and in so doing release chemoattractants that draw small numbers of phagocytes into the effusion to remove cellular debris. The result is a mild increase in both total protein (≥2.5 g/dl) and nucleated cell count (less than 5,000/µl). Thus, modified transudates are generally transudates that have been present long enough to elicit a mild inflammatory reaction (see Fig. 6-6B). It is most often associated with cardiovascular disease or neoplastic conditions.

In cases of extended duration, modified transudates can have a cloudy to almost milky gross appearance. Such fluids strongly resemble chyle and, in fact, have in the past been called "pseudochylous effusions" (a term no longer used). The gross appearance of these fluids is the result of high lipid content (due to higher cholesterol content than serum) but is in no way related to a true chylous effusion, as there are no triglycerides or chylomicrons present (Hillerdal, 1997; Tyler and Cowell, 1989). The phagocytes attracted to remove cellular debris from transudates are rich in enzymes that digest protein but are virtually devoid of enzymes that will break down complex lipids. Consequently,

while most of the constituents of dying cells are removed by phagocytosis, lipid content of the cells simply accumulates in the effusion. Effusions formed in this manner are easily distinguished cytologically from true chylous effusions.

The principle cellular constituent of the modified transudate is the reactive mesothelial cell (see Fig. 6-3A). Because of the ability of mesothelial cells to respond to irritation by proliferation, the presence of increased numbers of mesothelial cell clusters and rafts is a common finding in reactivity (see Fig. 6-3B). Mitoses are increased and occasional multinucleated reactive mesothelial cells are seen. Reactive mesothelial cells in clusters are capable of imbibing lipid from the effusion fluid and when they do, they take on the characteristics of secretory cells. In this form they must be differentiated from metastatic adenocarcinoma or mesothelioma. This may be done by critically evaluating the cell populations for criteria of malignancy.

As modified transudates mature, the proportion of inflammatory cells they contain will increase. In most cases the principal inflammatory cell is the nondegenerate neutrophil, but neutrophils rarely account for more than 30% of the total cell population. Over time, modified transudates gradually become cytologically indistinguishable from nonspecific exudates. One method used to distinguish modified transudates from exudates or transudates from exudates is measurement of C-reactive protein concentration in canine effusions (Parra et al., 2006).

Exudate

Exudates are the result of either increased vascular permeability secondary to inflammation or vessel injury/leakage (hemorrhagic effusion, chylous effusion). An exudative fluid usually contains both increased protein and an increased nucleated cell count. The total protein concentration is usually greater than 3.0 g/dl along with cell counts greater than 5,000/μl. Infectious causes for exudates include bacteria (Fig. 6-7A&B), fungi, viruses, protozoa such as *Toxoplasma* (Toomey et al., 1995), or helminthes such as *Mesocestoides* sp. (Caruso et al., 2003). Noninfectious causes involve organ inflammation such as pancreatitis, steatitis, inflammatory neoplasia

and irritants such as bile or urine. Cytologic evaluation is useful to determine an underlying cause in cases of exudative effusions.

Inflammatory effusions are classified according to the standard rules for inflammation as neutrophilic, mixed, or macrophagic. In neutrophilic reactions, neutrophils (either nondegenerate or degenerate) comprise >70% of the inflammatory cells seen. Mixed reactions are characterized by a mixture of neutrophils and macrophages. In histiocytic inflammation, macrophages are the prevalent cell seen.

Most inflammatory effusions are cytologically nonspecific in terms of etiologic diagnosis. However, as with inflammatory responses elsewhere, cytomorphology provides significant clues as to the underlying cause. Neutrophilic inflammatory effusions indicate severe active irritation (Fig. 6-8). If neutrophils are degenerate, an effort should be made to identify bacterial organisms within phagocytes (primarily neutrophils). This is generally easiest at the feathered edge of the smear. If organisms are not seen, the fluid should still be cultured. Mixed and macrophagic inflammatory effusions reflect less severe irritation and are found with resolving acute effusions or in association with less irritating etiologic agents than bacteria (e.g., fungal organisms or foreign bodies). Chemical evaluation of effusion fluid is also useful in recognizing sepsis.

Septic effusions may be diagnosed by use of biochemical parameters in dogs and cats. It was shown that effusion fluid in dogs and cats with a pH <7.2, pCO_2 >55 mm Hg, glucose concentration <50 mg/dl, and lactate concentration >5.5 mmol/L is highly likely to have bacterial infection (Swann et al., 1996). A study involving peritoneal fluid in dogs and cats evaluated blood and effusion fluid glucose concentrations. This study found that a difference of blood-effusion glucose >20 mg/dl provides a rapid and reliable means to differentiate septic and nonseptic effusion fluid (Bonczynski et al., 2003). In this

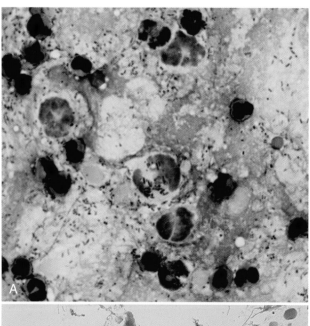

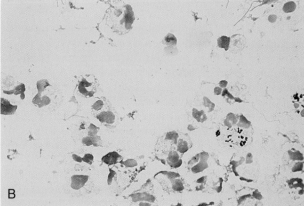

■ **FIGURE 6-7. A, Septic peritonitis, dog.** Numerous degenerate neutrophils are noted with a large number of pleomorphic bacteria seen, both in the background and within neutrophils. This concentrated smear was made from a dog with a ruptured pancreatic abscess. (Modified Wright; HP oil.) **B, Septic exudate. Pleural. Cat.** Degenerate neutrophils are bloated, with foamy or vacuolated cytoplasm and also swollen lytic nuclei. Note presence of small gram-positive, pleomorphic bacterial rods. Aerobic and anaerobic cultures are recommended in cases of pyothorax. This sample contains many nucleated cells (>100,000 cells/μl) and >3.0 g/dl protein. (Gram; HP oil.)

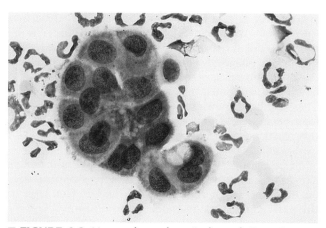

■ **FIGURE 6-8. Nonseptic exudate. Peritoneal. Dog.** Concentrated fluid from an animal with pancreatitis showing one cluster of reactive mesothelial cells and neutrophils. The protein content in this sample was 3.0 g/dl with a cell count of 8000 cells/μl. Most of the cells are neutrophils, suggesting an underlying inflammatory condition. Further testing (e.g., fluid and serum lipase or ultrasonography) is required to determine the specific cause for the fluid accumulation. (Romanowsky; HP oil.)

study, a difference of blood-effusion lactate concentration in dogs <−2.0 mmol/L was 100% sensitive and 100% specific for the diagnosis of septic peritonitis.

SPECIFIC TYPES OF EFFUSIONS

While most inflammatory effusions are cytologically nonspecific, some etiologies cause reactions with characteristic diagnostic features. These effusions are discussed below.

Feline Infectious Peritonitis

Feline infectious peritonitis (FIP) is unique among the causes of inflammatory effusion in that the fluid that accumulates is usually high in protein, yet has a low cellularity (McReynolds et al., 1997). Classification as an inflammatory effusion is based primarily on the presence of high total protein (often >4.5 g/dl) which is a reflection of a similar elevation in serum protein. Electrophoresis of either the effusion fluid or the serum reveals a polyclonal gammopathy. An albumin-to-globulin ratio of less than 0.8 on the fluid is very suggestive for FIP. It has been reported that if gamma globulin is greater than 32% of the protein in the effusion fluid, this is suggestive of FIP (Shelly et al., 1988). An additional test that can help rule in or rule out FIP is the Rivalta test. To perform this relatively simple test, place one drop of 98% acetic acid into 5 ml distilled water and mix well in a reagent tube. Then add slowly one drop of the effusion fluid to the surface of the acetic acid solution. A positive test requires that the drop of effusion retain its form on the surface or slowly sink to the bottom as a droplet or jellyfish-like shape (Fig. 6-9A). This test indicates a high protein content as well as fibrin and inflammatory mediators. This test has a positive predictive value of 86% and a negative predictive value of 97% (Hartmann et al., 2003). A more specific cytologic test for FIP involves immunofluorescence of intracellular feline coronavirus (FCo V) within effusion macrophages. When positive (Fig 6-9B), this test is diagnostic for FIP; however, the negative predictive value is 57%, so a negative test may miss cases of FIP (Hartmann et al., 2003).

Cytologically these fluids are usually relative low in cell number (1000 to 30,000/µl) and inconsistent with regard to the cell types present. In a majority of cases the predominant cell is the nondegenerate neutrophil (Fig. 6-9C). However, mixed to macrophagic reactions may be seen (Fig. 6-9D). In rare cases, the lymphocyte is prevalent. Regardless of the predominant cell type, slides in all cases have a purple granular background that results from the high protein content (see Fig. 6-9C).

Nocardial/Actinomycotic Effusions

Complex bacteria such as *Nocardia asteroides* and *Actinomyces* sp. are important causes of both peritoneal and pleural effusions in dogs and cats. Grossly, these effusions are turbid and yellow to blood-tinged "tomato soup." Even when collected in EDTA they typically contain visible particulates or granules (the so-called "sulfur granules") (Songer and Post, 2005).

On the basis of physical parameters, these effusions are typical exudates, with high total protein and markedly high cellularity. Because of the high cellularity, direct smears are generally adequate for cytologic examination. If particles are observed in the fluid, it is important to make squash preparations of these particles in addition to making smears of the fluid alone.

Microscopically, nocardial and actinomycotic infections are characterized by neutrophilic to mixed inflammation, probably dependent on the duration of the disease. In the more chronic reactions, there is generally a significant reactive mesothelial cell component to the response. A striking feature of the inflammatory response is the morphology of the neutrophils. Whereas most cases of septic pleuritis and peritonitis are signaled by the presence of predominantly degenerating neutrophils, in nocardial and actinomycotic effusions the majority of the neutrophils away from the organisms are nondegenerate. Degenerating neutrophils are only seen immediately in the vicinity of the bacterial organisms because these agents, in contrast to most other bacteria, produce only weak local toxins. The net effect of this phenomenon is that smears in these cases may be easily misinterpreted as noninfectious, particularly if the organisms are not widespread. Because the particles seen grossly often are composed of bacterial colonies, it is extremely important that squash preparations of these particles be examined to ensure that the diagnosis is not missed (Fig. 6-10A&B).

Morphology of the organisms microscopically is quite characteristic. Colonies are composed of delicate filamentous, often beaded, organisms and are often found at the feathered edge of smears (Fig. 6-10C). The most significant diagnostic feature of these organisms is that the filaments are branching. Using standard hematologic stains, Nocardia organisms cannot be differentiated from Actinomyces. However, *Nocardia* sp. is gram positive and are variably acid-fast positive whereas *Actinomyces* sp. are gram positive and acid-fast negative (Songer and Post, 2005).

Cytologic diagnosis should be confirmed by bacterial culture of the effusion and/or sulfur granules. Because these species have special culture requirements, it is important that the bacteriology laboratory be fully aware of the provisional diagnosis at the time of sample submission.

Systemic Histoplasmosis

Systemic histoplasmosis caused by *Histoplasma capsulatum* is a moderately frequent cause of peritoneal effusion in dogs living in the Ohio River Valley (United States). Because the fungus is ubiquitous in the area, serology cannot be relied upon for diagnosis. In many cases, cytologic identification of the organism is essential.

The effusion fluid of histoplasmosis is relatively unique. The fluid is usually clear and colorless. On the basis of physical characteristics, the fluid is a modified transudate; however, cytologically, it is clearly inflammatory

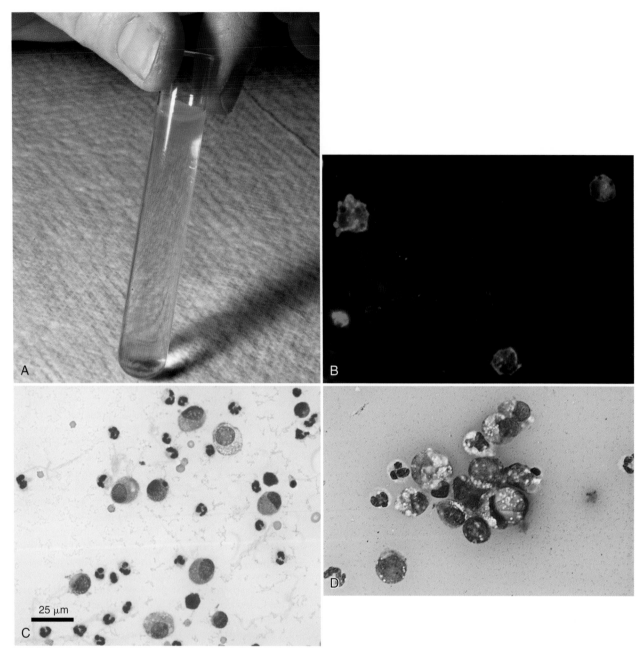

■ **FIGURE 6-9. A-C, Abdominal effusion, cat. A, Rivalta test**. Positive test results are indicated by a layer of gel on top of the acetic acid solution. Fluid is from a cat with PCR confirmed FIP. The cat was moderately icteric. Note the yellow streaks of gel in the middle of the tube from partially floating material. **B, FCo V immunofluorescence test**. A specific cytologic test for FIP involves immunofluorescence of intracellular feline coronavirus (FCo V). Shown are three infected and intact macrophages *(green)* present in abdominal fluid from a cat with FIP. (FCo V; HP oil.) **C,** This concentrated smear comes from a cat diagnosed with FIP. Note the moderately basophilic macrophages and nondegenerate neutrophils. The background contains basophilic, coarsely granular protein as well as basophilic protein crescents and strands of fibrin. (Modified Wright; HP oil.) **D, Nonseptic exudate. Peritoneal. Cat.** This animal was diagnosed with FIP. Fluid contains foamy, vacuolated macrophages, mildly degenerate neutrophils, and intermediate to large lymphoid cells. Lymphocytes may be intermediate in size and appear reactive in some cases of FIP. Also note the granular precipitated protein throughout the slide. (Romanowsky; HP oil.) (A, Photo by Sam Royer, Purdue University. B, Courtesy of Jacqueline Norris, University of Sydney, Australia.)

with significantly more neutrophils than are seen in the typical canine modified transudate. Whenever inflammatory modified transudates are seen in dogs, the possibility of histoplasmosis should be considered in the differential diagnosis. If seen in an effusion, the disease is considered disseminated and can be found elsewhere such as the liver, spleen, bone marrow, rectal wall, and peripheral blood.

Demonstration of the organism is best done in macrophages (Fig. 6-11) at the feathered edge of sediment smears. Histoplasma organisms measure approximately 2 to 3 μm in diameter, are round to ovoid in shape, and

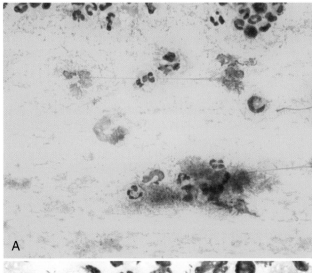

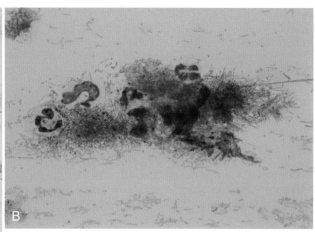

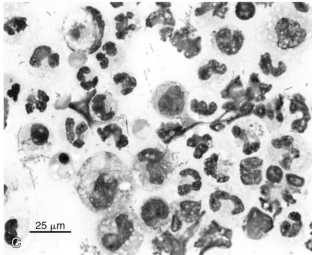

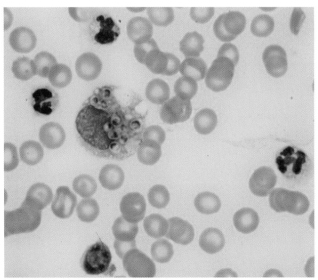

■ **FIGURE 6-10. Septic exudate, actinomycosis. Pleural. Dog. Same case A-C. A,** Direct smear from a pleural effusion demonstrates a dense colony (i.e., sulfur granule) along with many lysed cells and nuclear streaks. These granules often are dragged to the feathered edge, as was the case with this smear. (Modified Wright; IP.) **B,** Higher magnification of the colony in A. (Modified Wright; HP oil.) **C,** The fluid has marked suppurative inflammation with many degenerate neutrophils and several foamy macrophages. Short and long filamentous organisms and lysed cells are seen throughout the background. In areas of the smear lacking bacteria (not shown), the neutrophils were only mildly degenerate. (Modified Wright; HP oil.)

■ **FIGURE 6-11. Histoplasmosis. Dog.** A macrophage containing numerous oval 2-3 µm yeast organisms of *Histoplasma capsulatum* is seen at left center. There are numerous red cells in the background of the smear. (Modified Wright; HP oil.)

have a single basophilic nucleus surrounded by a thick, colorless cell wall. In fluids, it is common to see individual organisms free in the background. The only other organisms of similar cytologic morphology are Leishmania. However, Leishmanial protozoans are distinguished by the presence of an internal kinetoplast, which gives them the appearance of having two nuclei.

Bilious Effusion

Rupture of the gall bladder or common bile duct may occur in any species secondary to direct trauma or disease of the biliary tree. In addition, it is an infrequent accompaniment to diaphragmatic hernia from any cause in the dog and cat. When the results of direct trauma are mainly to the biliary system, leakage of bile is virtually always restricted to the peritoneal cavity, with a resulting peritonitis. When associated with diaphragmatic hernia, leakage of bile occurs when liver is trapped in the diaphragmatic rent and there is necrosis of the gall bladder or common bile duct. In this circumstance, both peritonitis and pleuritis can result. Bile is a very irritative substance; its presence quickly elicits an inflammatory response. Grossly, the fluid may be initially brown (see Fig. 6-1G) to yellow to greenish; however, as the response becomes more and more cellular, this discoloration may become masked. Large volumes of fluid can usually be obtained.

Cytologically, the striking feature of bilious effusion is the presence of bile on the slide. Frequently, bile is seen as yellow to green to blue-black granular material scattered in the slide background (Fig. 6-12A–C) and in the cytoplasm of neutrophils, reactive mesothelial cells, and macrophages. In reactions of greater duration, bile granules may have all been converted to rhomboidal to amorphous golden crystals of bile pigment. When such crystals are found in the cytoplasm of effusion phagocytes in the absence of evidence of prior hemorrhage (e.g., erythrophagocytosis), the possibility of bilious effusion should be strongly considered. In addition to the typical appearance of bilious effusions, acellular, amorphous, fibrillar blue-grey mucinous material (Fig. 6-13A) has been associated with biliary tree rupture, particularly of the common bile duct in dogs (Owens et al., 2003). Instead of the green or yellow bile granules present, lakes of extracellular material are the predominant

cytologic finding. It is suspected that this bile-free material is produced by biliary and gallbladder epithelium as a consequence to extrahepatic biliary obstruction with regurgitation of normal bile into hepatic lymph and venous blood.

The cellular response to bile is generally mixed with large numbers of neutrophils nearly always present (Fig. 6-13B&C). The degree of degeneration of neutrophils is variable. In addition, bile causes severe irritation to the mesothelial lining of the body cavities, resulting in marked reactive mesothelial cell hyperplasia.

Fluid bilirubin levels that are markedly elevated and several times than levels in serum also give support for a diagnosis of bilious effusion (Owens et al., 2003).

Eosinophilic Effusion

Effusions with more than 10% eosinophils are termed *eosinophilic effusions* regardless of the protein content or cell count. This condition is uncommonly seen in veterinary medicine. With large numbers of eosinophils, the fluid grossly may have a green tint. The presence of

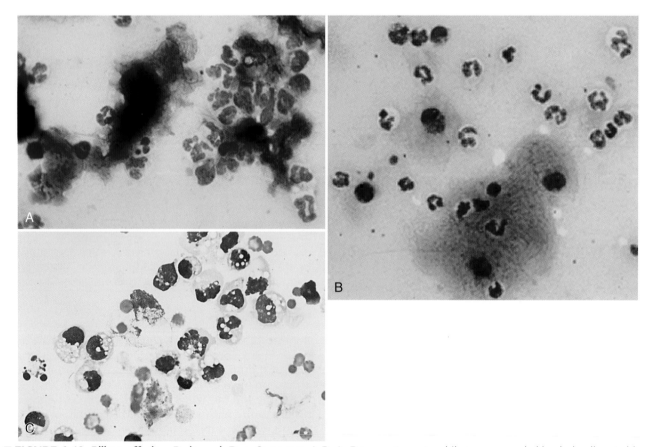

■ **FIGURE 6-12. Bilious effusion. Peritoneal. Dog. Same case A-B. A,** Degenerate neutrophils are surrounded by dark yellow to black amorphous bile material that is free in the background. (Wright-Giemsa; HP oil.) **B,** Large numbers of mostly nondegenerate neutrophils accompany the presence of amorphous material. The basophilic bile material is coated by stain precipitate producing a pink, granular appearance. This greenish, flocculent fluid had a protein level of 3.0 g/dl and an estimated nucleated cell count of greater than 60,000/μl. (Wright-Giemsa; HP oil.) **C,** Note extracellular gold-brown crystalline material, vacuolated neutrophils, and macrophages. Some of the neutrophils contain pyknotic nuclei and others contain karyolytic nuclei. (Romanowsky; HP oil.) (A and B, Courtesy of Rose Raskin, University of Florida.)

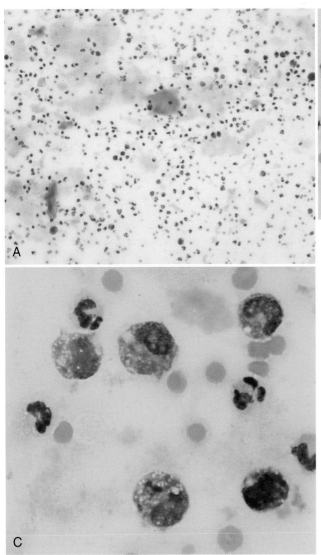

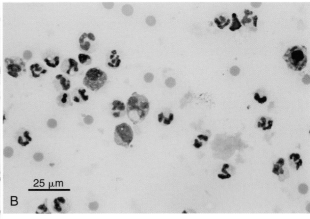

■ **FIGURE 6-13. Bile peritonitis. Dog. Same case A-C. A,** This is a concentrated smear of fluid from a dog with a ruptured gall bladder. Note the numerous neutrophils and lakes of blue-grey amorphous mucinous material that are present throughout the background. (Modified Wright; IP.) **B,** Note the suppurative inflammation with variably degenerate neutrophils as well as basophilic and foamy macrophages. Amorphous blue-gray material, likely mucin, is seen in the background. (Modified Wright; HP oil.) **C,** Note the suppurative inflammation and foamy macrophages that contain blue-grey to dark blue granular material. The background contains mucinous and finely granular protein. (Modified Wright; HP oil.)

eosinophils does not provide a specific diagnosis and the cause is often unknown in these cases. Neoplasia such as lymphoma or mastocytosis involved half of the cases in one study (Fossum et al., 1993). Heartworm disease, systemic mastocytosis, interstitial pneumonia, disseminated eosinophilic granulomatosis, and lymphomatoid granulomatosis are other possibilities in dogs (Mertens et al., 2005; Bounous et al., 2000).

Uroperitoneum

Urine in the peritoneal space results in chemical irritation. The protein content may be markedly low as a result of dilution from the urine but the cell count and predominant cell type is usually indicative of inflammation or an exudate (see Table 6-1). Early in the condition, a mononuclear cell population may predominate, suggestive of a modified transudate. Bacteria may or may not be present. Neutrophils exposed to the irritant material may show karyolysis with ragged nuclear borders (Fig. 6-14). In some cases, urinary crystals are found on cytologic examination, which leads to a diagnosis of uroperitoneum. In one study in cats, creatinine or potassium was increased in fluid and served as a useful predictor for uroperitoneum, generally in a ratio of 2:1 compared with that in serum (Aumann et al., 1998). Simultaneous evaluation of fluid and serum creatinine should show a higher creatinine in the fluid, as it equilibrates much slower than urea nitrogen (BUN). In addition, the serum Na:K also tends to depress in cases of uroabdomen (Aumann et al., 1998; Burrows and Bovee, 1974).

Parasitic Ascites (Abdominal Cestodiasis)

In a small number of dogs with ascites, often from western North America, the etiology is aberrant cestodiasis from *Mesocestoides* infection (Stern et al., 1987; Crosbie et al., 1998; Caruso et al., 2003). Rare reports of infection involve cats. Peritoneal aspirates from anorexic, ascitic dogs are macrophagic with the appearance of tapioca pudding or cream of wheat (Fig. 6-15).

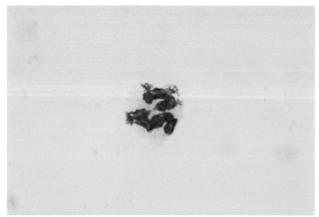

■ **FIGURE 6-14. Uroperitoneum. Dog.** The fluid contained a high number of neutrophils, many of which appeared similar to this "ragged" cell. Urine acts as a chemical irritant causing karyolytic changes to cells. (Wright-Giemsa; HP oil.) (Courtesy of Rose Raskin, University of Florida.)

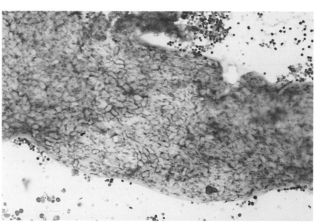

■ **FIGURE 6-16. Cestodiasis.** Acoelomic metacestode tissue with amorphous degenerate debris and calcareous corpuscles. Inflammatory cells are also present surrounding the structure. (Romanowsky; LP.)

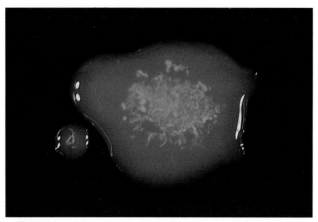

■ **FIGURE 6-15. Cestodiasis. Peritoneal. Dog.** The ascitic fluid had a tapioca pudding appearance grossly. Motility of these granules may be observed with the unaided eye. (Courtesy of Jocelyn Johnsrude, IDEXX, West Sacramento, CA.)

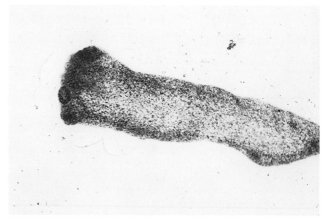

■ **FIGURE 6-17. Cestodiasis. Tetrathyridia larval stage.** Same case as in Figure 6-15. Note the oval structures at one end that represent suckers and identify the parasite as *Mesocestoides* spp. (Romanowsky; LP.)

Motile cestodes can be seen in fluid with the unaided eye. Microscopic examination may show acephalic metacestodes or acoelomic tissue with calcareous corpuscles (Fig. 6-16), which may be seen in nonspecific cestode infections. Less often seen microscopically are metacestodes with visible tetrathyridia, a unique larval form having four suckers that represents the asexual reproductive form of *Mesocestoides* spp. infection (Fig. 6-17). Cestode ova are not usually found in the feces (Crosbie et al., 1998).

Chylous Effusions

Chylous effusions contain chyle, which is a mixture of lymph and chylomicrons. Chylomicrons, derived from dietary lipids processed in the intestine and transported via lymphatics, are primarily composed of triglycerides. Historically, chylous effusions were thought to be primarily a result of thoracic duct rupture. It is now

known that there are a variety of causes for chylous effusions and that rupture of the thoracic duct is uncommon. Causes for chylous effusions in the thoracic cavity include cardiovascular disease, neoplasia (e.g., lymphoma, thymoma, and lymphangiosarcoma), heartworm disease, diaphragmatic hernia, lung torsion, mediastinal fungal granulomas, chronic coughing, vomiting, or idiopathic (Fossum, 1993; Fossum et al., 1986a; Forrester et al., 1991; Waddle and Giger, 1990). In one study (Fossum et al., 1986a). Afghan hounds appeared to have a higher incidence of chylothorax compared to other breeds of dogs. It seems that chylous pleural effusions are more common in cats than dogs, presumably because their lymphatics are more easily damaged by trauma or obstruction.

Chylous ascites is less common. Causes for chyloperitoneum include intra-abdominal neoplasia, steatitis, biliary cirrhosis, lymphatic rupture or leakage, postoperative accumulation following ligation of the thoracic duct, congenital lymphatic abnormalities, and other causes (Fossum et al., 1992; Gores et al., 1994).

Grossly, chylous effusions are described as "milky" white to pink-white fluids, depending on dietary fat content and the presence or absence of hemorrhage (Fig. 6-18A&B). Some cases of chylous effusion may have fluid that is clear to serosanguineous. Chylous effusions contain triglycerides at a level higher than that found in serum in a ratio often greater than 3:1 (Meadows and MacWilliams, 1994). A cholesterol-to-triglyceride (C/T) ratio of less than 1 is generally considered characteristic of a chylous effusion (Fossum et al., 1986b). Based on lipoprotein electrophoretic studies, pleural chylous effusions can be better identified by fluid triglyceride concentrations greater than 100 mg/dl and nonchylous effusions by concentrations less than 100 mg/dl (Waddle and Giger, 1990). In those same studies, C/T ratios were less reliable.

Cell counts and protein concentrations are elevated over pure transudate levels and therefore chylous effusions generally fit into modified transudate or exudate (most commonly) categories depending on the degree of chronicity. The total protein evaluated by refractometry can be spurious due to interference by the lipid in the solution (George, 2001).

Cytologically, they are characterized by the presence of large numbers of morphologically normal small lymphocytes (Figs. 6-19 and 6-20A). Lesser numbers of reactive lymphocytes are also usually present. Because these fluids are mildly irritating, long-standing chylous effusions also may contain moderate numbers of reactive mesothelial cells and other inflammatory cells that may contain phagocytized lipid. This lipid generally appears as multiple discrete, colorless vacuoles within the cytoplasm (Fig. 6-20B). Some cases of chronic chylous effusion present with significant numbers of eosinophils. The presence of lipid in the background of the slide, visualized as small, unstained droplets at the periphery of the nucleated cells, is variable.

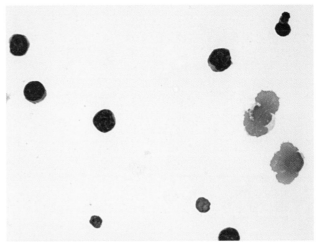

■ **FIGURE 6-19. Chylous effusion. Peritoneum. Dog.** This direct smear is characteristic of the entire smear. It is composed of essentially all small lymphocytes. Numerous lysed cells are present, as the lipid in the solution acts as a detergent, making the cells particularly fragile. (Modified Wright; HP oil.)

Hemorrhagic Effusions

True hemorrhagic effusions can occur in any of the major body cavities. Grossly, these effusions are red to serosanguineous depending on the age of the exudate and the extent of the hemorrhage. Physical evaluation reveals a protein level reflective of, but somewhat less than, that of peripheral blood. Both nucleated cell counts and red blood cell counts are usually elevated.

Cytology is needed to differentiate true hemorrhagic effusions from sample contamination at the time of collection. Hemorrhagic effusions contain predominantly red blood cells with lesser numbers of nucleated cells. The most significant indicator of true hemorrhage is the presence of macrophages containing phagocytized red cells (erythrophagocytosis) and/or hemosiderin (Figs 6-21 and 6-22A). Hemosiderin in macrophages

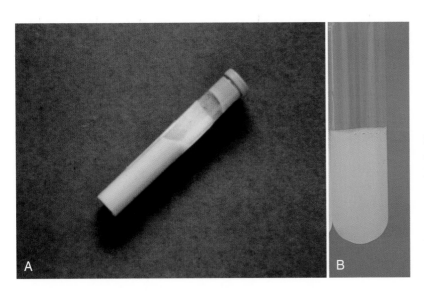

■ **FIGURE 6-18. Chylous effusion. Pleural. Cat. A,** A pink tint is found in this chylous effusion, indicating some degree of hemorrhage is present. The fluid had 13,000/µl nucleated cell count, 267 mg/dl triglycerides, and 169 mg/dl cholesterol. **B,** Turbid "milky" fluid in most cases, due to the presence of chyle. Measurement of high fluid triglyceride levels confirms the diagnosis. The cell count of this sample is <10,000 cells/µl and the protein is 4.0 g/dl. (A, Courtesy of Rose Raskin, University of Florida.)

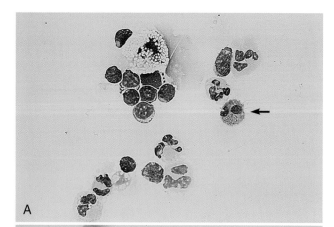

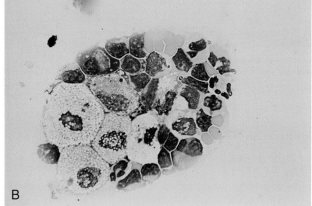

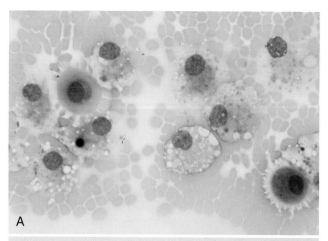

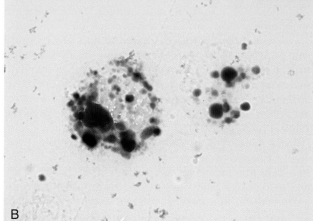

■ **FIGURE 6-20. Chylous effusion. Pleural. Cat. A-B same case as in Figure 6-18B. A,** Note small lymphocytes, neutrophils, one eosinophil *(arrow),* and one large macrophage. Initially chylous effusions contain predominantly small lymphocytes and macrophages. As the duration of fluid presence increases, neutrophils and eosinophils will increase in number. (Romanowsky; HP oil.) **B,** Concentrated preparation. Note the punctate lipid vacuoles within macrophages along with small lymphocytes, neutrophils, and low number of red blood cells. (Romanowsky; HP oil.)

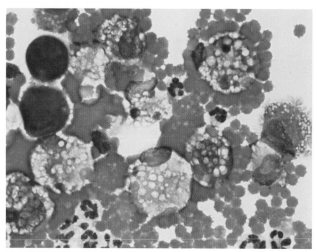

■ **FIGURE 6-21. Hemorrhagic effusion. Pleura. Dog.** This direct smear shows numerous enlarged and vacuolated macrophages, a few nondegenerate neutrophils, and two deeply basophilic reactive mesothelial cells (left). Many macrophages contain varying amounts of hemosiderin and erythrophagia is occurring in several cells. (Modified Wright; HP oil.)

■ **FIGURE 6-22. Hemorrhagic effusion. Cat. Same case A-B. A,** Several moderately foamy macrophages contain variable amounts of blue-grey, finely granular pigment, presumed to be hemosiderin. Also noted are two mildly basophilic and granular mesothelial cells, likely reactive. (Modified Wright; HP oil.) **B,** Two hemosiderophages are noted filled with Prussian blue positive material, confirming it as hemosiderin. (Prussian Blue; HP oil.)

indicates that the hemorrhage occurred more than two days before collection. These cells are best observed at the feathered edge of sediment smears. Erythrophagocytosis is not seen if hemorrhage is strictly a collection artifact. A second significant observation is whether platelets are seen. True hemorrhagic exudates are devoid of platelets but they are commonly observed in contaminated samples. If uncertainty exists whether the pigment is hemosiderin, in contrast to bile, melanin, or carbon, Prussian blue staining can indicate the presence of iron in hemosiderin (Fig. 6-22B).

Neoplastic Effusions

Neoplastic processes, both primary and metastatic, are relatively common causes of both abdominal and thoracic effusions in dogs and cats. Neoplastic effusions may be accompanied by significant hemorrhage and/or inflammation but generally they are noninflammatory. Grossly, the fluid may be clear to cloudy and hemorrhagic. Total protein levels are often elevated but nucleated cell counts are highly variable.

In dogs and cats, the common causes of neoplastic effusions are lymphoma (pleural), and adenocarcinoma or carcinoma (either pleural or peritoneal). Sarcomas may cause effusions but neoplastic cells of mesenchymal origin seldom shed cells into the effusion fluid. Mesothelioma can be a rare cause of effusion in any species.

Regardless of the type of neoplasia present, diagnostic cells may or may not be evident in an effusion. If a mass is known to be present, fluid analysis a well as fine-needle aspiration of the mass may be necessary for definitive diagnosis. In one study of the detection of malignant tumors in abdominal and thoracic fluids, sensitivity was low at 64% for dogs and 61% for cats; however, specificity was high at 99% for dogs and 100% for cats (Hirschberger et al., 1999). In the following paragraphs the cytologic features of the principal neoplastic effusions are summarized and illustrated.

Lymphoma

Lymphomatous effusions are generally highly cellular and contain a pleomorphic population of discrete round cells that are morphologically consistent with lymphocytes. The neoplastic cells have high nuclear-to-cytoplasmic ratios, scant to moderate amounts of cytoplasm, and often scattered, small cytoplasmic vacuoles. Occasionally granular lymphocytes are the predominant neoplastic cell (Fig. 6-23). Moderate numbers of mitoses are seen.

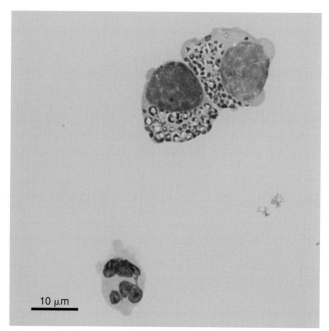

10 μm

■ **FIGURE 6-23. Neoplastic effusion. Granular lymphoma. Pleural. Cat.** This fluid was light yellow, hazy with a protein of 4.2 g/dl and WBC of 5600/μl. 63% of nucleated cells were granulated; two are shown. Granules varied from fine to coarse (as shown) and were frequently eccentrically placed to one side of the cell. Nondegenerate neutrophils (one shown), small lymphocytes, and occasional phagocytes were also present. (Wright-Giemsa; HP oil.) (Courtesy of Rose Raskin, University of Florida.)

Scattered among the neoplastic cells are red blood cells, reactive mesothelial cells, and inflammatory cells.

The principle differential diagnosis for lymphomatous effusion is chylous effusion. In truth, lymphomatous invasion of lymphatics often causes a concomitant chylous effusion. However, recognizing the presence of lymphoma is generally not a major problem. Most cases of lymphoma consist of malignant cells that are much larger and more pleomorphic than normal lymphocytes with nuclei containing prominent, often bizarre and angular nucleoli (Fig. 6-24A&B). Only rare cases of lymphoma have cells that are morphologically the same as normal small lymphocytes. In these cases the principal differentiating feature of the neoplastic disease is a much greater cellularity than what is generally seen with chylous effusion alone.

Evaluation of the types of lymphoid cells found within the fluid by immunocytochemistry or flow cytometry may provide significant information related to the origin of these lymphoid cells. A monotypic population of medium and/or large lymphocytes is more likely associated with neoplasia (Figs. 6-24C, 6-25, and 6-26) than with a reactive process. Immunocytochemistry with antibodies against the molecules CD3 (T-cell) and CD79a (B-cell) is helpful in these cases.

Carcinoma and Adenocarcinoma

Carcinomatous effusions in dogs and cats may be the result of either a primary or secondary neoplastic process. In the chest, the principal primary neoplasm is pulmonary adenocarcinoma. In order for neoplastic cells from this tumor to be present in pleural effusions, the neoplasm must have invaded either into pulmonary vessels and lymphatics or directly through the pleural surface of the lung and into the pleural cavity.

Pulmonary adenocarcinoma is a relatively uncommon tumor that rarely extends into the pleural cavity. As a consequence, most carcinomatous pleural effusions are the result of metastatic disease. In females, by far the most common cause of such effusions is metastatic mammary carcinoma; in males, the two most common metastatic carcinomas seen are prostatic carcinoma and transitional cell carcinoma.

In the peritoneal cavity the principal causes of carcinomatous effusions are those neoplasms which spread by implantation on the peritoneal surface. Significant among these are cholangiocarcinoma, pancreatic adenocarcinoma, ovarian adenocarcinoma in females, and prostatic carcinoma in males. Metastatic mammary carcinoma is also a common cause of peritoneal carcinomatosis.

Cytologically, all of these tumors are morphologically similar and cannot be readily differentiated (Clinkenbeard, 1992). Carcinomatous effusions are characterized by the presence of rafts and acinar arrays (adenocarcinoma) of round to polygonal cells with variable amounts of often extremely basophilic cytoplasm. Cytoplasmic basophilia may be so intense as to obscure nuclear detail. Inflammation may or may not be present, but reactive mesothelial cell hyperplasia is a constant feature (Figs. 6-27A&B and 6-28A&B).

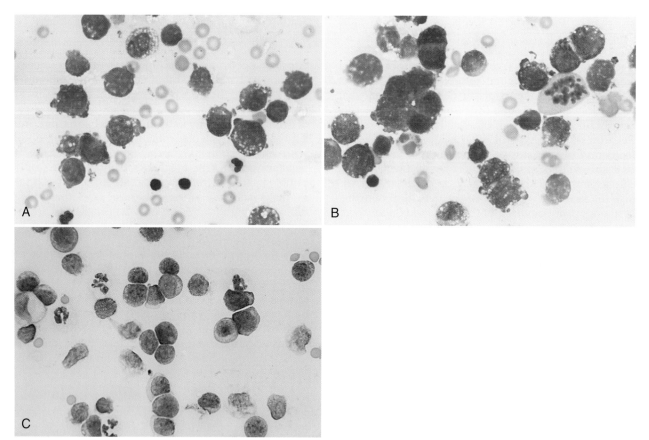

■ FIGURE 6-24. Neoplastic effusion. Lymphoma. Pleural. A, Dog. Note the individual large round cells with high nuclear-to-cytoplasmic ratio and mildly vacuolated cytoplasm. Also evident are two small lymphocytes and one neutrophil. Light-purple, round structures are free nuclei from lysed cells. These cells cannot be evaluated. The cellularity of this sample is 15,000 cells/μl with a protein of 3.4 g/dl. (Romanowsky.) **B, Dog.** Note individual lymphoblasts, one mitotic figure, two intermediate-size lymphocytes, and one small lymphocyte. A few lysed cells and red blood cells are also present. (Romanowsky.) **C, Cat.** Note the monomorphic population of large lymphoblasts, few neutrophils, and few lysed cells. The lymphoblasts are larger than neutrophils and contain a small rim of cytoplasm with a large, round nucleus. The nuclear chromatin is fine and nucleoli are visible in many of the cells. The nucleated cell count of this fluid is 14,000 cells/μl with increased protein (4.0 g/dl). (Romanowsky; ×200.)

Establishing a diagnosis of pleural or peritoneal carcinomatosis is probably the most difficult challenge in diagnostic fluid cytology. Carcinoma cells strongly resemble reactive mesothelial cells and cytoplasmic basophilia in both of these populations makes evaluation of nuclear criteria of malignancy particularly difficult. The problems become even more exaggerated when significant inflammation is present because reactive mesothelial cells can become quite dysplastic. For these reasons it is particularly important to search diligently for nuclear criteria of malignancy in suspect populations of cells. Areas where nuclear detail can be seen must be found (see Figs. 6-27B and 6-28B). Whereas in most circumstances four nuclear criteria are sufficient to allow a diagnosis of malignancy, in the case of pleural or peritoneal carcinomatosis, at least five distinct nuclear criteria should be demonstrated.

Once the diagnosis of malignancy has been established, differentiation of carcinoma from adenocarcinoma is much easier. Adenocarcinomas are secretory

tumors; as such, most instances of these vacuoles are unstained. In some cells the amount of secretory product is sufficient to displace the nucleus peripherally. Simple carcinomas are devoid of secretory vacuoles.

Mesothelioma

Mesothelioma is a rare tumor that can occur in any species. The neoplasm arises from the mesothelial lining of the serous body cavities. Cytologically, the tumor is very difficult to differentiate from carcinoma and reactive mesothelial hyperplasia. Tumor cells are round to polygonal and are arranged primarily in clusters. Nuclei are hyperchromic and located centrally. Often nuclei of adjacent cells within a cluster appear to press against each other resulting in triangulation of nuclei (nuclear molding). Because of the difficulty of differentiating mesothelioma from reactive mesothelial hyperplasia, caution must be used when evaluating suspect populations for criteria of malignancy. As with carcinomatous effusions, at least five definite nuclear criteria

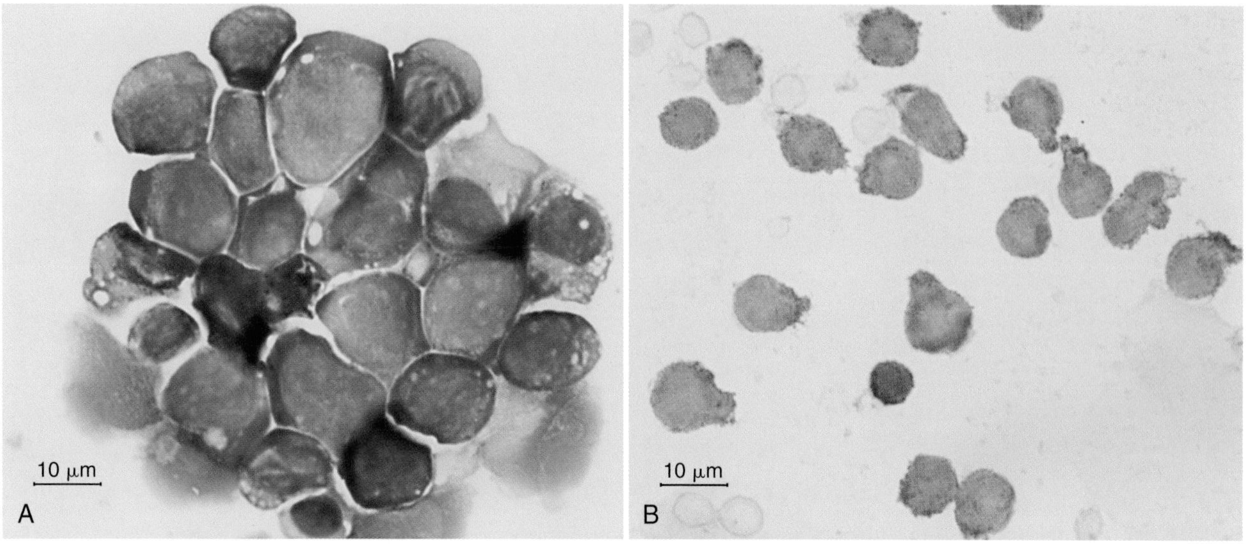

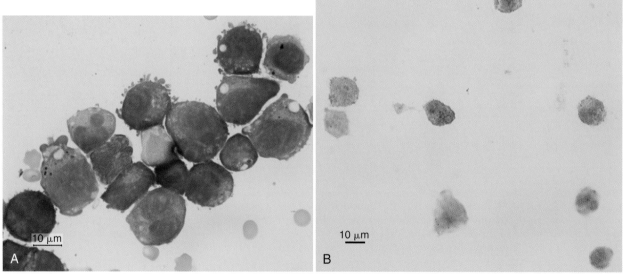

■ **FIGURE 6-25. Neoplastic effusion. Pleural. T-cell lymphoma. Dog. Same case A-B. A,** Cytocentrifugated specimen demonstrating a variably sized round cell population having scant to moderate amounts of basophilic cytoplasm, fine to moderately coarse chromatin with occasional prominent nucleoli, and variable N:C. (Modified Wright; HP oil.) **B,** Sediment smear displays positive cell surface staining in all lymphoid cells for the CD3 antigen, which supports a clonal population of T-lymphocytes. Note the small, likely normal, lymphocyte below center. Red cells are barely visible beneath the size bar. Rare small normal lymphocyte reacted with CD79a antibody (not shown). (CD3 antibody; HP oil.) (A and B, Courtesy of Rose Raskin, Purdue University.)

■ **FIGURE 6-26. Neoplastic effusion. Pleural. B-cell lymphoma. Cat. Same case A-B. A,** Cytocentrifuged specimen demonstrating marked pleomorphism of round cells. Some cells have multiple nuclei and irregularly shaped nuclei. Nucleoli are usually large and multiple. There is surface blebbing on several cells, which may be mesothelial in origin. (Modified Wright; HP oil.) **B,** All large round cells are positively stained for the CD79a antigen in this sediment smear of pleural fluid supporting a B-cell neoplasm. CD3 antigen was absent on all cells (not shown). (CD79a antibody; HP oil.) (A and B, Courtesy of Rose Raskin, Purdue University.)

of malignancy must be seen before a presumptive diagnosis is made (Fig. 6-29A–C).

Once the diagnosis of malignancy has been established, an attempt to differentiate mesothelioma from carcinoma can be made. There are no well-established morphologic criteria for differentiating these tumors; consequently, such attempts are often an exercise in

futility. Based on relative frequency of occurrence, most of these effusions are simply considered to be carcinomatous until proven otherwise. A case of mesothelioma has been recognized by the use of the immunohistochemical marker calretinin in a horse (Stoica et al., 2004); it is possible that this marker can be used to differentiate mesothelioma and carcinoma in other species.

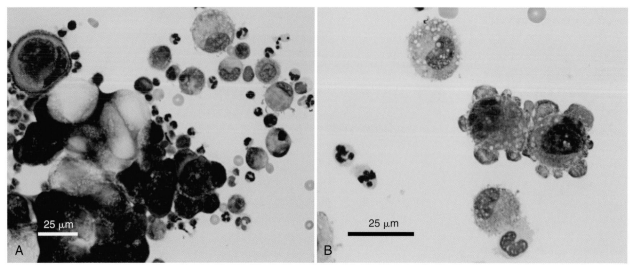

■ **FIGURE 6-27. Neoplastic effusion. Adenocarcinoma. Pleural. Dog. Same case A-B. A,** Note the cohesive cluster of neoplastic epithelial cells. The large, distorting vacuoles suggest a secretory nature to the tissue of origin. Prominent nuclear molding is seen in the upper left side of the image. The background contains a mixture of inflammatory cells. (Modified Wright; HP oil.) **B,** Note the two neoplastic cells that exhibit marked pleomorphism of their nucleoli. Compare the neoplastic cells to the nearby macrophages. (Modified Wright; HP oil.)

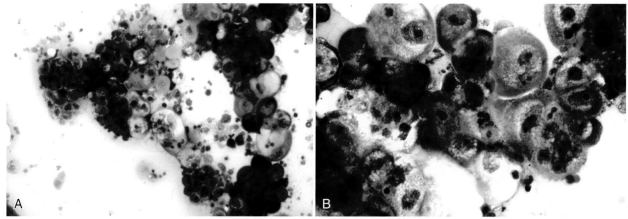

■ **FIGURE 6-28. Neoplastic effusion. Adenocarcinoma. Pleural. Cat. Same case A-B. A,** Note the presence of clusters and sheets of large cells. This fluid is highly cellular (23,000 cells/μl) and has an increased protein content (3.6 g/dl). Inflammatory cells are often found in effusions associated with neoplasia. (Romanowsky; IP.) **B,** Note that the cells are large with abundant basophilic, lightly vacuolated cytoplasm. The nuclei are round with granular coarse chromatin and a large prominent nucleolus. Neutrophils can be seen within the cytoplasm of some of the neoplastic cells. (Romanowsky; HP oil.)

PERICARDIAL EFFUSIONS

Pericardial effusions may also be classified as transudates, modified transudates, or exudates. Because they are somewhat unique in their presentation, they are considered separately.

In many cases, pericardial effusion fluid is hemorrhagic (Figs. 6-30 and 6-31). Causes of pericardial effusions include neoplasia, which involves 41% (Kerstetter et al., 1997) to 58% (Dunning, 2001) of canine cases examined. Benign idiopathic pericardial hemorrhage accounted for up to 45% of cases in dogs in one study (Kerstetter et al., 1997). A variety of other infrequently seen causes, including infection, cardiac insufficiency, uremia, trauma,

foreign body, coagulopathy, pericarditis, hernia, or left atrial rupture, have been reported (Bouvy and Bjorling, 1991; Petrus and Henik, 1999; Shubitz et al., 2001; Peterson et al., 2003). Pericardial effusions in cats are most often related to congestive heart failure (28%). FIP, which accounted for 17%, is the second most frequent disease causing pericardial effusion in cats (Bouvy and Bjorling, 1991).

Cytologic evaluation of pericardial effusion is challenging, but is most valuable in ruling out infection and inflammation. The pericardium is notorious for eliciting mesothelial hyperplasia. These mesothelial cells become very large and basophilic, often binuclate with prominent nucleoli (see Fig. 6-3B) and mitotic figures.

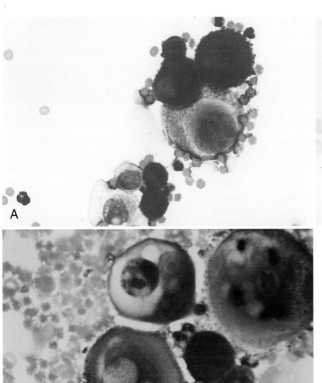

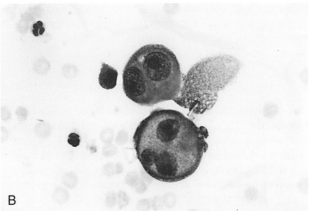

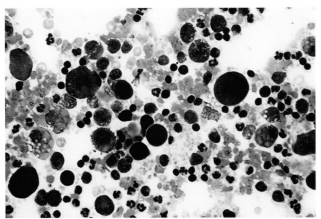

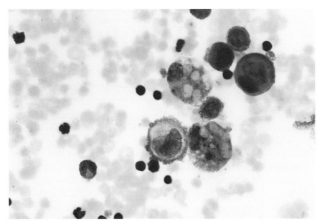

■ FIGURE 6-29. Neoplastic effusion. Mesothelioma. Same case A-C. A, Pleural. Dog. The neoplastic cells are present as individual cells and in small clusters. The nucleoli are variably shaped and very prominent. (Romanowsky; HP oil.) **B,** These cells contain a variable amount of cytoplasm with one or more nuclei. The nuclei may be of odd number and variable size. (Romanowsky; HP oil.) **C,** The nuclear chromatin is coarsely granular and irregularly clumped with large prominent nucleoli. Many cells retain the fringed glycocalyx border. Also present are low numbers of small lymphocytes, neutrophils, and red blood cells. (Romanowsky; HP oil.)

■ FIGURE 6-30. Hemorrhagic effusion. Pericardial. Dog. Buffy-coat preparation. Note the variety of cells, including neutrophils, lymphocytes, erythrophages, and reactive mesothelial cells. This fluid was red and turbid with 5,000,000 red blood cells/μl, 7000 nucleated cells/μl, and protein of 4.0 g/dl. (Romanowsky; HP oil.)

■ FIGURE 6-31. Hemorrhagic effusion. Pericardial. Dog. Observe the erythrophagia, reactive mesothelial cells, macrophage, and small lymphocytes with many red blood cells. Also note that one macrophage contains brown hemosiderin pigment. One mesothelial cell contains two nuclei. Cytologic evaluation of pericardial fluid is important to rule out infection and some types of neoplasia. Often additional testing is required to determine the cause of hemorrhagic pericardial effusion. (Romanowsky; HP oil.)

It is often not possible to distinguish these reactive mesothelial cells from possible neoplastic cells. In addition, hemangiosarcoma may cause pericardial hemorrhage, but neoplasia of mesenchymal origin typically will not shed neoplastic cells into effusions. In one study (Sisson et al., 1984), 74% of 19 neoplastic effusions were not detected on the basis of cytologic findings and 13% of

31 non-neoplastic effusions were falsely reported as positive, leading the authors to conclude that pericardial fluid analysis did not reliably distinguish neoplastic from non-neoplastic disorders. More recently, cardiac troponins I (cTnI) and T (cTnT) have been evaluated in

pericardial fluid. Results from this study involving 37 dogs suggest that cTNI may be useful in differentiating idiopathic pericardial effusions from those caused by hemangiosarcoma (Shaw et al., 2004).

Further testing is often required (e.g., ultrasonography, coagulation testing, pericardiectomy, finding other evidence of trauma) to determine the underlying cause for the effusion. In a study of 51 dogs with pericardial effusions, the pH of the fluid was examined and compared with a final diagnosis (Edwards, 1996). When measured by precise instrumentation, the pH indicated that a reading greater than 7.3 was likely due to noninflammatory conditions, usually neoplasia. Using a less accurate urinary dipstick, pericardial fluid pH = 7.0 was associated with neoplasia in 93% of the cases, while <7.0 suggested benign or non-neoplastic conditions. The pH of the fluid needs to be measured shortly after obtaining the sample. A recent study found similar results; however, considerable overlap was detected, thus limiting the usefulness of pH to differentiate the etiology of pericardial effusions (Fine et al., 2003).

ANCILLARY TESTS

In some instances, other laboratory tests on an effusion may be indicated to help determine a specific cause for the fluid accumulation. A summary of previously described tests is shown in Table 6-2.

TABLE 6-2 Biochemical and Electrophoretic Tests Used to Evaluate Effusions

Test	Use/Expected Result	Effusion
Creatinine/potassium	Fluid values are higher than those of serum creatinine and/or potassium	Uroperitoneum
Triglycerides	Fluids often contain triglycerides that exceed 100 mg/dl	Chylous
Cholesterol	Fluid level that is higher than that of serum cholesterol	Nonchylous
Bilirubin	Fluid level that is higher than serum bilirubin	Bile peritonitis/pleuritis
Lipase/amylase	Fluid values are higher than those of serum lipase and/or amylase	Pancreatitis
Protein electrophoresis	A:G ratio of <0.8 on the fluid is very suggestive for FIP	FIP infection
Lipoprotein electrophoresis	Presence of chylomicrons in fluid when triglyceride levels are equivocal	Chylous
pH	pH <7.0 may suggest benign or non-neoplastic conditions	Pericardial
pH, pCO$_2$, glucose, lactate	Fluids with pH <7.2, pCO$_2$ >55 mm Hg, glucose <50 mg/dl, or lactate >5.5 mmol/L are likely to have bacterial infection	Septic
Serum-effusion glucose	A difference of serum-effusion glucose of >20 mg/dl indicates bacterial infection	Septic peritonitis
Serum-effusion lactate	A difference in serum-effusion lactate of <−2.0 mmol/L (in dogs) indicates bacterial infection	Septic peritonitis

REFERENCES

Aumann M, Worth LT, Drobatz KJ: Uroperitoneum in cats: 26 cases (1986-1995), *J Am Anim Hosp Assoc* 34:315-324, 1998.

Bonczynski, JJ, et al: Comparison of peritoneal fluid and peripheral blood pH, bicarbonate, glucose, and lactate concentrations as a diagnostic tool for septic peritonitis in dogs and cats, *Vet Surg* 32:161, 2003.

Bounous DI, Bienzle D, Miller-Liebl D: Pleural effusion in a dog, *Vet Clin Pathol* 29:55-58, 2000.

Bouvy BM, Bjorling DE: Peritoneal effusion in dogs and cats. Part I. Normal pericardium and causes and pathophysiology of pericardial effusion, *Compend Contin Educ Pract Vet* 13:417-424, 1991.

Braun JP, et al: Comparison of four methods for determination of total protein concentrations in pleural and peritoneal fluid from dogs, *Am J Vet Res* 62:294, 2001.

Burrows CF, Bovee KC: Metabolic changes due to experimentally induced rupture of the canine urinary bladder, *Am J Vet Res* 35(8)1083-1088, 1974.

Caruso KJ, James MP, Fisher D, et al: Cytologic diagnosis of peritoneal cestodiasis in dogs caused by *Mesocestoides sp.*, *Vet Clin Pathol* 32(1):50-60, 2003.

Clinkenbeard KD: Diagnostic cytology: carcinomas in pleural effusions, *Compend Contin Educ Pract Vet* 14(2): 187-194, 1992.

Crosbie PR, Boyce WM, Platzer EG, et al: Diagnostic procedures and treatment of eleven dogs with peritoneal infections caused by *Mesocestoides* spp., *J Am Vet Med Assoc* 213: 1578-1583, 1998.

Dunning D: Pericardial effusion. In Wingfield WE (ed): *Veterinary emergency medicine secrets*, ed 2, Hanley and Belfus, Philadelphia, 2001, pp 219-23.

Edwards NJ: The diagnostic value of pericardial fluid pH determination, *J Am Anim Hosp Assoc* 32:63-67, 1996.

Fine DM, Tobias AH, Jacob KA: Use of pericardial fluid pH to distinguish between idiopathic and neoplastic effusions, *J Vet Intern Med* 17(4): 525-529, 2003.

Ford RB, Mazzaferro EM: *Handbook of veterinary procedures and emergency treatment*, ed 8, Saunders, Philadelphia, 2006, pp. 6-7, 52-53, 132-33.

Forrester SD, Fossum TW, Rogers KS: Diagnosis and treatment of chylothorax associated with lymphoblastic lymphosarcoma in four cats, *J Am Vet Med Assoc* 198:291-294, 1991.

Forrester SD, Troy GC, Fossum TW. Pleural effusions: pathophysiology and diagnostic considerations, *Compend Contin Educ Pract Vet* 10:121-136, 1988.

Fossum TW: Feline chylothorax, *Compend Contin Educ Pract Vet* 15:549-567, 1993.

Fossum TW, Birchard SJ, Jacobs RM: Chylothorax in 34 dogs, *J Am Vet Med Assoc* 188:1315-1318, 1986a.

Fossum TW, Hay WH, Boothe HW, et al: Chylous ascites in three dogs, *J Am Vet Med Assoc* 200:70-76, 1992.

Fossum TW, Jacobs RM, Birchard SJ: Evaluation of cholesterol and triglyceride concentrations in differentiating chylous and nonchylous pleural effusions in dogs and cats, *J Am Vet Med Assoc* 188:49-51, 1986b.

Fossum TW, Wellman M, Relford RL, et al: Eosinophilic pleural or peritoneal effusions in dogs and cats: 14 cases (1986-1992), *J Am Vet Med Assoc* 202:1873-1876, 1993.

George JW: The usefulness and limitations of hand-held refractometers in veterinary laboratory medicine: an historical and technical review, *Vet Clin Pathol* 30(4):201-210, 2001.

George JW, O'Neill SL: Comparison of refractometer and biuret methods for total protein measurement in body cavity fluids, *Vet Clin Pathol* 30(1):16-18, 2001.

Gores BR, Berg J, Carpenter JL, et al: Chylous ascites in cats: Nine cases (1978-1993), *J Am Vet Med Assoc* 205:1161-1164, 1994.

Hartmann K, Binder C, Hirschberger J, et al: Comparison of different tests to diagnose feline infectious peritonitis, *J Vet Intern Med* 17:781-790, 2003.

Hillerdal G: Chylothorax and pseudochylothorax, *Euro Resp J* 10(5):1157-1162, 1997.

Hirschberger J, DeNicola DB, Hermanns W, et al: Sensitivity and specificity of cytologic evaluation in the diagnosis of neoplasia in body fluids from dogs and cats, *Vet Clin Pathol* 28:142-146, 1999.

Kerstetter KK, Krahwinkel DJ, Millis DL, et al: Pericardiectomy in dogs: 22 cases (1978-1994), *J Am Vet Med Assoc* 211:736-740, 1997.

Kirby BM: Peritoneum and Peritoneal Cavity. In Slatter D (ed): *Textbook of small animal surgery*, ed 3, Saunders, Philadelphia, 2003, pp 414-418.

McReynolds C, Macy D: Feline infectious peritonitis. Part I: Etiology and diagnosis, *Compend Contin Educ Pract Vet* 19(9):1007-1016, 1997.

Meadows RL, MacWilliams PS: Chylous effusions revisited, *Vet Clin Pathol* 23:54-62, 1994.

Mertens MM, Fossum TW, MacDonalds KA: Pleural and extrapleural diseases. In Ettinger EJ, Feldman EC (eds): *Textbook of veterinary internal medicine*, ed 6, Saunders, Philadelphia, 2005, pp 1272-1283.

Meyer DJ, Franks PT: Effusion: classification and cytologic examination, *Compend Contin Educ Pract Vet* 9:123-129, 1987.

Owens SD, Gossett R, McElhaney MR, et al: Three cases of canine bile peritonitis with mucinous material in abdominal fluid as the prominent cytologic finding, *Vet Clin Pathol* 32:114-120, 2003.

Papasouliotis K, et al: Use of the Vettest 8009 and refractometry for determination of total protein, albumin, and globulin concentrations in feline effusions, *Vet Clin Pathol* 31:162, 2002.

Parra MD, Papasouliotis K, Ceron JJ: Concentrations of C-reactive protein in effusions in dogs, *Vet Rec* 158:753-757, 2006.

Peterson PB, Miller MW, Hansen EK, et al: Septic pericarditis, aortic endarteritis, and osteomyelitis in a dog, *J Am Anim Hosp Assoc* 39(6):528-532, 2003.

Petrus DJ, Henik RA: Pericardial effusion and cardiac tamponade secondary to brodifacoum toxicosis in a dog, *J Am Vet Med Assoc* 215:647-648, 1999.

Shaw SP, Rozanski EA, Rush JE: Cardiac troponins I and T in dogs with pericardial effusion, *J Vet Intern Med* 18(3):322-324, 2004.

Shelly SM, Scarlett-Kranz J, Blue JT: Protein electrophoresis on effusions from cats as a diagnostic test for feline infectious peritonitis, *J Am Anim Hosp Assoc* 24:495-500, 1988.

Shubitz LF, Matz ME, Noon TH, et al: Constrictive pericarditis secondary to *Coccidioides immitis* infection in a dog, *J Am Vet Med Assoc* 218(4):537-540, 2001.

Sisson D, Thomas WP, Ruehl WW, et al: Diagnostic value of pericardial fluid analysis in the dog, *J Am Vet Med Assoc* 184:51-55, 1984.

Songer JG, Post KW: *Veterinary microbiology: bacterial and fungal agents of animal disease*, Saunders, St. Louis, 2005, pp 10-12, 55-59, 83-86.

Stern A, Walder EJ, Zontine WJ, et al: Canine *Mesocestoides* infections, *Compend Contin Educ Pract Vet* 9:223-231, 1987.

Stoica G, Cohen N, Mendes O, et al: Use of immunohistochemical marker calretinin in the diagnosis of a diffuse malignant metastatic mesothelioma in an equine, *J Vet Diagn Invest* 16(3):240-243, 2004.

Swann H, et al: Use of abdominal fluid pH, pCO$_2$, [glucose] and [lactate] to differentiate bacterial peritonitis from nonbacterial causes of abdominal effusion in dogs and cats, *J Vet Emerg Crit Care* 6:114, 1996.

Toomey JM, Carlisle-Nowak MM, Barr SC, et al: Concurrent toxoplasmosis and feline infectious peritonitis in a cat, *J Am Anim Hosp Assoc* 31:425-428, 1995.

Tyler RD, Cowell Rl: Evaluation of pleural and peritoneal effusions, *Veterinary Clinics of North America: Small Animal Practice* 19(4):743-768, 1989.

Waddle JR, Giger U: Lipoprotein electrophoresis differentiation of chylous and nonchylous pleural effusions in dogs and cats and its correlation with pleural effusion triglyceride concentration, *Vet Clin Pathol* 19:80-85, 1990.

7

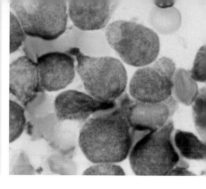

Oral Cavity, Gastrointestinal Tract, and Associated Structures

Claire B. Andreasen, Albert E. Jergens, and Denny J. Meyer

Endoscopy has facilitated increased access to the mucosal surface of the gastrointestinal tract and enhanced the application of diagnostic cytology for its evaluation. It is an especially useful adjunct procedure when combined with the histologic examination of tissue for the complete assessment of gastrointestinal tract. The cytologic and histologic findings tend to be disparate when: (1) the specimens are obtained from different sites, (2) the lesion is deeply located in the lamina propria or submucosa precluding exfoliation, (3) surface-associated findings are lost during processing of the histologic sample, and (4) cell or tissue distortion (artifact) is present in either the cytologic or the histologic specimen.

In our experience, both touch imprint and brush cytologic preparations can provide useful information when concurrently examined with the histologic specimen (Jergens et al., 1998). Brush cytology tends to exfoliate more cells but also has the potential to induce hemorrhage and introduce leukocytes that may be mistaken for inflammation. Brush cytology often represents pathology of the deeper lamina propria compared to touch imprints, which reflect the surface and mucosal changes. The criteria that differentiate benignity and malignancy must be carefully evaluated when examining esophageal and gastrointestinal cytologic specimens since the cellular atypia associated with epithelial hyperplasia and regeneration as a consequence of inflammation can mimic epithelial neoplasia.

ORAL CAVITY

The most common reason for the cytologic examination of the oral cavity is for the evaluation of a mass or an ulcerative lesion. Radiographic findings will indicate if there is bone involvement.

Normal Cytology

Superficial and intermediate squamous epithelial cells are the commonly exfoliated cell type for the buccal cavity and the surface of the tongue (Fig. 7-1A). A variety of oropharyngeal bacteria can be seen in samples from the oral cavity. Noteworthy is *Simonsiella* sp. (Fig. 7-1B&C). Neutrophils are normally lost via transmigration through the mucous membranes into the oral cavity and may be observed in low numbers.

Inflammation

Inflammatory diseases that can affect the oral cavity include immune-mediated diseases such as bullous disease, foreign bodies, dental disease, systemic manifestation of uremia, and bacterial, viral, and fungal infections (Guilford, 1996a). The inflammatory exudate can be composed of leukocytes, necrotic debris, and bacterial flora. Some raised plaque-like oral lesions with ulcerated surface will contain a pure eosinophilic population or mixed with eosinophils and neutrophils. Reports of an ulcerative eosinophilic stomatitis in the Cavalier King Charles spaniels (Fig. 7-2A&B) suggest this eosinophilic inflammatory response may occur concurrent with other affected systems and represent a hypersensitivity response in this breed (Joffe and Allen, 1995; German et al., 2002). In another condition, the undersides of the tongue may occasionally display a raised white mass which cytologically in addition to normal epithelium contains variable amounts of fine to coarse crystalline material. Most often it is extracellular but many crystals can be found within macrophages (Fig. 7-3A&B). This macrophagic or granulomatous (if giant cells are observed) inflammation is typical of a lingual calcinosis circumscripta. While urates may be considered, calcium is typical and can

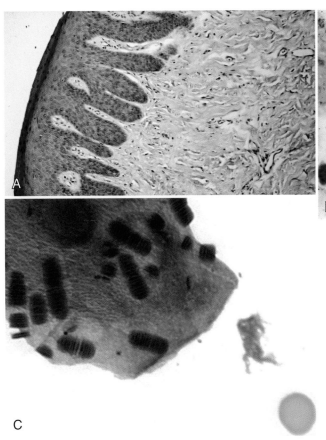

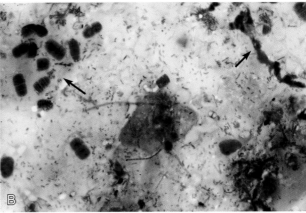

■ **FIGURE 7-1. A, Oral cavity. Normal gingival epithelium. Dog.** Keratinized stratified squamous epithelium forms papillary projections of the lamina propria (connective tissue). (H&E; LP.) **B, Oral cavity. Normal cytologic findings.** An angular squamous epithelial cell is covered with *Simonsiella* sp. (*long arrow*); an angular, partially keratinized squamous epithelial cell is located in the center, and the background is composed of numerous bacteria of varying size and shapes set in a lightly basophilic proteinaceous background. A stream of free nuclear protein from a ruptured cell is present (*short arrow*). (Wright; HP oil.) **C, Oral cavity. Normal epithelium with flora. Dog.** One intermediate squamous epithelial cell is covered with *Simonsiella* sp. (rounded rectangular structures with cross striations). A single erythrocyte is present in the lower right corner for size comparison. (Wright; HP oil.) (A and C, Courtesy of Rose Raskin, Purdue University.)

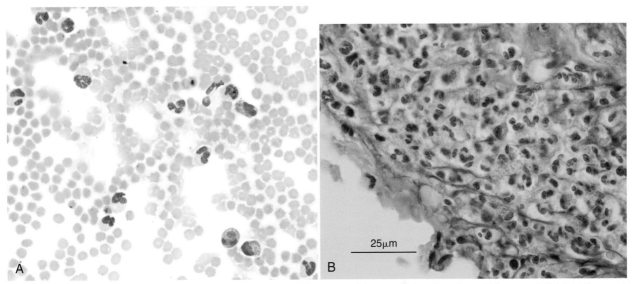

■ **FIGURE 7-2. Same case A-B. A, Eosinophilic and neutrophilic stomatitis. Touch imprint. Dog.** This nonpainful 2 × 2 cm raised plaque-like lesion with ulcerated surface appeared on the soft palate of a Cavalier King Charles spaniel. A mixed population of mostly nondegenerate neutrophils and eosinophils appear against a hemodiluted background. Both cell types were within normal reference ranges in circulation. (Wright; HP oil.) **B, Ulcerative eosinophilic stomatitis. Histology.** The ulcerated surface is densely infiltrated with a mixture of neutrophils and eosinophils. Adjacent to this area (not shown) was granulation tissue. However, granuloma formation was not observed. (H&E; IP.) (A and B, Courtesy of Rose Raskin, Purdue University.)

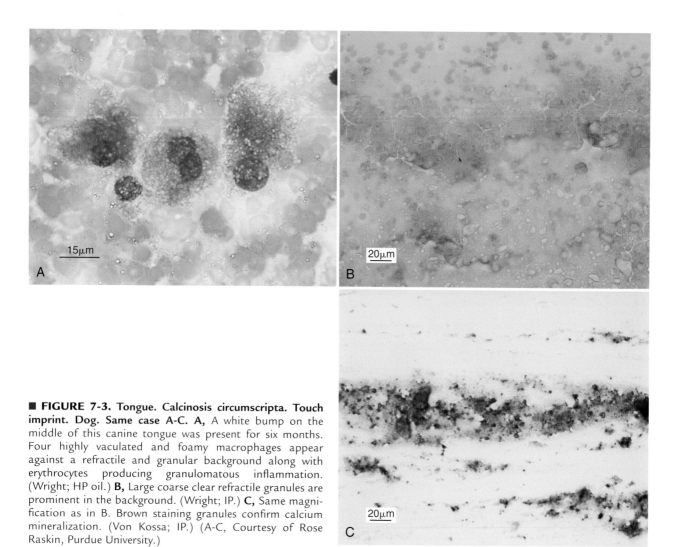

■ **FIGURE 7-3. Tongue. Calcinosis circumscripta. Touch imprint. Dog. Same case A-C. A,** A white bump on the middle of this canine tongue was present for six months. Four highly vaculated and foamy macrophages appear against a refractile and granular background along with erythrocytes producing granulomatous inflammation. (Wright; HP oil.) **B,** Large coarse clear refractile granules are prominent in the background. (Wright; IP.) **C,** Same magnification as in B. Brown staining granules confirm calcium mineralization. (Von Kossa; IP.) (A-C, Courtesy of Rose Raskin, Purdue University.)

be confirmed with Von Kossa stain (Fig. 7-3C) or Alizarin red S (Marcos et al., 2006).

Neoplasia

Epithelial, mesenchymal, and discrete (round) cell neoplasia can involve the oral cavity. As in other organ systems, the diagnostic sensitivity of cytology is highest for discrete cell neoplasia and lowest for mesenchymal tumors. This is due to reduced exfoliation and the difficulty differentiating neoplastic mesenchymal cells from reactive fibrocytes/fibroblasts that compose inflammatory/reparative lesions. Discrete cell neoplasia includes lymphoma, mast cell tumor, plasmacytoma, transmissible venereal tumor, and histiocytoma. The plasmacytoma can involve the oral mucous membranes, tongue, or mucosa of the digestive tract and be difficult to diagnose definitively without immunocytochemical or immunohistochemical characterization (Rakich et al., 1989). The most common epithelial neoplasm is squamous cell carcinoma (Fig. 7-4A&B). Less common is epithelial odontogenic neoplasia (Poulet et al., 1992) (Fig. 7-5A–C). Squamous cell carcinoma can occur anywhere in the oral cavity but in cats it often occurs in the frenulum of the tongue with early metastasis to the regional lymph nodes. An epulis is a common gingival mass of dogs or cats that can be a developmental, hyperplastic, inflammatory (Fig. 7-6A&B), or neoplastic lesion. A study of feline epulides (de Bruijn et al., 2007) determined the multinucleate cells of the giant cell epulis likely reflect an inflammatory response through osteoclast formation from mononuclear macrophages. These can be confusing lesions to evaluate cytologically because they can be composed of dental epithelial nests enrobed in stromal fibrous tissue. When the diagnosis is in doubt cytologically, it is prudent to pursue an excisional biopsy. Oral melanomas often are malignant and infiltrative, may contain abundant or only minimal pigment (amelanotic melanomas), and rapidly metastasize to the regional lymph nodes (Head et al., 2002) (Fig. 7-7A–C). Fibrosarcoma, chondrosarcoma, and osteosarcoma (Fig. 7-8) are the mesenchymal tumors that more commonly involve the oral cavity. Fibroma, hemangiosarcoma, and liposarcoma are less frequent (Bernreuter, 2008). Fibrosarcomas of the mandible and maxilla occasionally can have cytologic and histologic benign morphologic features but

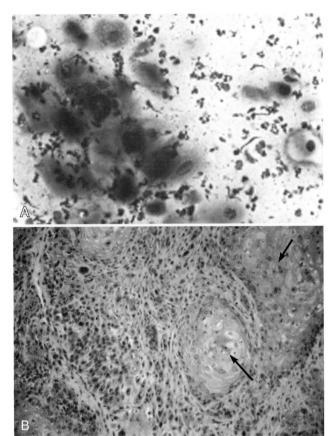

■ **FIGURE 7-4. Oral squamous cell carcinoma. A, Touch imprint.** This specimen is from a mass that extended from the frenulum of the tongue into the mandible of a cat. There are numerous squamous epithelial cells of varying immaturity with shapes that vary from oval to angular. Some of the cells show dyskeratosis (far left). Other abnormal morphologic features include variable nuclear-to-cytoplasmic (N:C) ratios and variable staining. Numerous neutrophils are scattered amongst the neoplastic cells. Many show nuclear degeneration or are ruptured resulting in streaks of free nuclear protein. Squamous cells and keratin often induce neutrophilic inflammation. (Wright; HP oil.) **B, Histology.** Cords of pleomorphic squamous cells are separated by a fine fibrous stroma. Central cores of keratinocytes (*arrows*) demonstrate dyskeratosis (premature or abnormal keratinization of epithelial cells that have not reached the surface) and stain more intensively eosinophilic. (H&E; IP.)

demonstrate aggressive biologic behavior (Ciekot et al., 1994). Neoplasia detected in the soft or hard palate may be extensions from the nasal cavity. In a study of lingual lesions (Dennis et al, 2006), about 4% of the cases in dogs involved the granular cell tumor, tumor of varied histogenesis (Head et al., 2002). Granular cell tumors (Fig. 7-9A–C) are mostly associated with the tongue than elsewhere in the oral cavity of older dogs and may occur in the cat as well. It is thought the majority of granular cell tumors arise from neuroectodermal origin and are set within reticulin fibers. Tumors appear as a sessile raised firm white mass which act benign. Cytologically, cells are individualized with eccentric nucleus with abundant eosinophilic or strongly periodic acid-Schiff-positive cytoplasmic phagolysosomal granules.

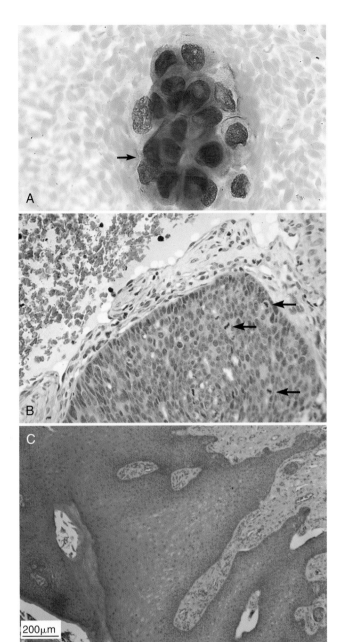

■ **FIGURE 7-5. A, Oral epithelial odontogenic tumor. Touch imprint.** A cytologic impression of an epithelial cell neoplasm can be made based on the general morphology of the clustered interdigitating neoplastic epithelial cells. They show mild to moderate anisocytosis and anisokaryosis and the nuclei show mild to moderate shape variation. The lower group appears to be forming a disorganized acinar structure with a central lumen (*arrow*). The morphologic features are suggestive of an epithelial cell malignancy. The cytoplasm contains fine eosinophilic granules. Numerous erythrocytes surround the neoplastic cell clump. (Wright; HP oil.) **B, Oral epithelial odontogenic malignancy. Histology.** The dense neoplastic epithelial cell population shows mild central swirling with palisading cuboidal to columnar epithelial cells located at the periphery. Mitotic figures are present (*arrows*). The neoplastic cells are surrounded by a less-dense (pale pink) fibrovascular stroma. (H&E; IP.) **C, Gingiva. Acanthomatous ameloblastoma. Histology. Dog.** A layer of keratinizing epithelium (thin outer pink near size marker) covers the thick acanthomatous epithelium characteristic of this malignant neoplasm. This is an infiltrative tumor which forms cords of epithelium into the submucosa. (H&E; LP.) (C, Courtesy of Rose Raskin, Purdue University.)

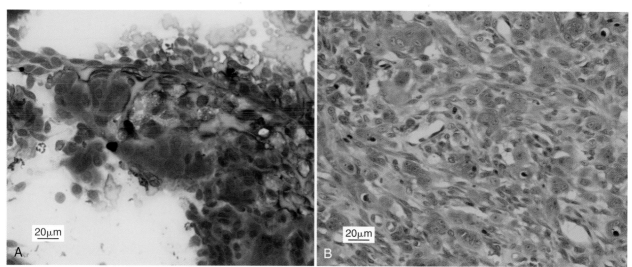

■ **FIGURE 7-6. Gingiva. Giant cell epulis. Dog. Same case A-B. A, Aspirate.** Aggregates of inflammatory cells composed of multinucleate histiocytes and individualized macrophages are prominent. Fibrovascular stroma creates a linear form (upper half) (Wright-Giemsa; IP.) **B, Histology.** Frequent anaplastic nuclear features are present in this solid mass of multinucleate cells with minimal stroma. (H&E; LP.) (A and B, Courtesy of Rose Raskin, Purdue University.)

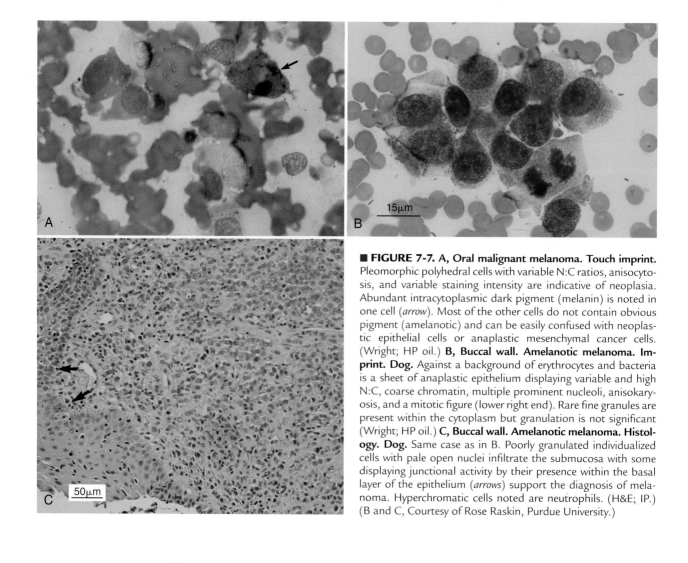

■ **FIGURE 7-7. A, Oral malignant melanoma. Touch imprint.** Pleomorphic polyhedral cells with variable N:C ratios, anisocytosis, and variable staining intensity are indicative of neoplasia. Abundant intracytoplasmic dark pigment (melanin) is noted in one cell (*arrow*). Most of the other cells do not contain obvious pigment (amelanotic) and can be easily confused with neoplastic epithelial cells or anaplastic mesenchymal cancer cells. (Wright; HP oil.) **B, Buccal wall. Amelanotic melanoma. Imprint. Dog.** Against a background of erythrocytes and bacteria is a sheet of anaplastic epithelium displaying variable and high N:C, coarse chromatin, multiple prominent nucleoli, anisokaryosis, and a mitotic figure (lower right end). Rare fine granules are present within the cytoplasm but granulation is not significant (Wright; HP oil.) **C, Buccal wall. Amelanotic melanoma. Histology. Dog.** Same case as in B. Poorly granulated individualized cells with pale open nuclei infiltrate the submucosa with some displaying junctional activity by their presence within the basal layer of the epithelium (*arrows*) support the diagnosis of melanoma. Hyperchromatic cells noted are neutrophils. (H&E; IP.) (B and C, Courtesy of Rose Raskin, Purdue University.)

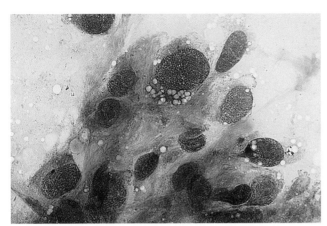

■ **FIGURE 7-8. Oral osteosarcoma. Touch imprint.** Pleomorphic mesenchymal cells show marked anisocytosis and anisokaryosis. The nuclei have stippled nuclear chromatin that contains multiple faintly stained variably sized nucleoli and are surrounded by moderately abundant basophilic cytoplasm with indistinct cell borders. The swirls of intercellular eosinophilic matrix produced by the neoplastic cells supports the cytologic impression of a malignant bone tumor. (Wright; HP oil.)

SALIVARY GLAND

Normal Cytology

Cytologic evaluation of salivary gland disease is diagnostically rewarding. The salivary gland also may be sampled accidentally when attempting to aspirate the submandibular lymph node. Cytologically, the salivary gland contains uniform secretory epithelial cells that are clustered and/or individual with eccentric, dark basophilic nuclei, and clear, vacuolated to foamy cytoplasm (Fig. 7-10). The cytoplasmic staining of the cells differs between serous cells (distinguishable) and mucous cells (may appear clear). Individual epithelial cells can be difficult to differentiate from macrophages, however, they have uniformly clear to finely vacuolated cytoplasm and do not contain phagocytic material. Eosinophilic-staining mucus is commonly observed and when present may cause erythrocytes to "stream" or line up in parallel rows (Fig. 7-11).

Hyperplasia

Hyperplasia is suspected when there is glandular enlargement and the epithelial cells appear relatively normal cytologically. The cells may be surrounded by abundant mucus. A differential consideration would be a sialocele.

Inflammation

The most common inflammatory lesion is caused by a salivary mucocele (sialocele) or ranula. A ranula is a cystic distension of an epithelial lined duct in the floor of the mouth. A sialocele is an accumulation of salivary secretions in nonepithelial lined cavities adjacent to the duct. While the cause is not known, trauma plus a developmental predisposition is proposed. The accumulated saliva stimulates an inflammatory reaction that changes over time. The initial inflammatory influx is composed of

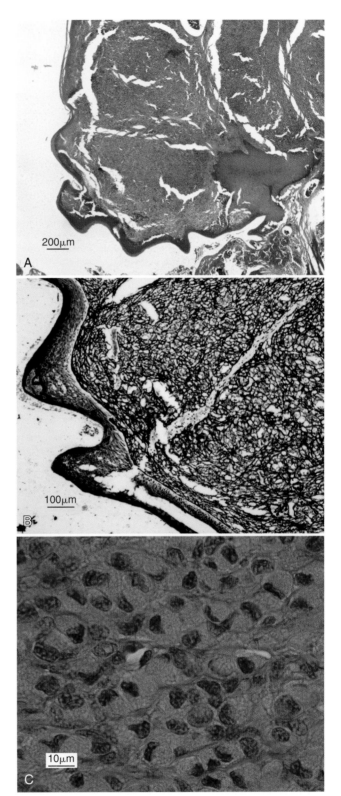

■ **FIGURE 7-9. Tongue. Granular cell tumor. Histology. Cat. Same case A-C. A,** Low magnification of a small raised lingual mass. (H&E; LP.) **B,** Dense network of stromal fibers separate the cells into small aggregates. (Reticulin; LP.) **C,** Stromal fibers create cords of individualized cells with abundant granular eosinophilic cytoplasm and hyperchromatic eccentric nucleus. (H&E; HP oil.) (A-C, Courtesy of Rose Raskin, Purdue University.)

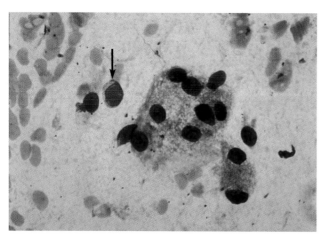

■ **FIGURE 7-10. Salivary gland epithelial cells, normal. Touch imprint.** The epithelial cells that compose this small cluster have abundant basophilic, granular-appearing cytoplasm that surrounds a dense, often eccentric nucleus. The morphologic features are consistent with normal secretory epithelium such as salivary gland. A large lymphocyte with a small rim of lightly basophilic cytoplasm (*arrow*) and a free round nucleus are located to the left of center. The surrounding erythrocytes can be used to judge the size of the cells. (Wright; HP oil.)

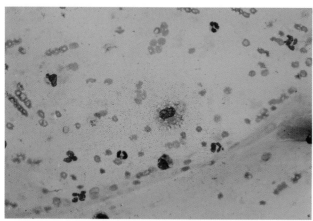

■ **FIGURE 7-11. Sialocele (salivary mucocele). Aspirate.** This specimen is an aspirate from a fluctuant submandibular swelling. The pinkish-blue mucus and occasional foamy macrophage along with a low number of neutrophils and erythrocytes are indicative of a sialocele. The rowing of erythrocytes (linear arrangement) suggests the presence of mucus. (Wright; HP oil.)

neutrophils and macrophages along with secretory epithelial cells set in an eosinophilic to basophilic mucus background (see Fig. 7-11). Lymphocytes replace the neutrophilic component and can become a prominent feature. Although the foamy macrophages can appear morphologically similar to the plump secretory epithelial cells, differentiation is not necessary when formulating the cytologic impression.

Neoplasia

The salivary adenocarcinoma is uncommon and demonstrates the general characteristics of epithelial malignancy that range from relatively well-differentiated to marked

pleomorphism (Fig. 7-12A&B) (Spangler and Culbertson, 1991). The neoplastic epithelial cells can form acinar structures and some of the cells can have abundant retained cytoplasmic secretions that displace the nucleus to the periphery, forming a cell that appears similar to a signet ring. Mixed salivary neoplasms are rare and contain both neoplastic epithelial cell and mesenchymal cell components that can include bone and cartilage.

PANCREAS

Normal and Hyperplasia Cytology

The pancreas is not usually sampled unless a mass is detected. Cellular characteristics can rapidly deteriorate owing to extracellular pancreatic enzyme activity associated with pancreatitis. Hyperplastic nodules

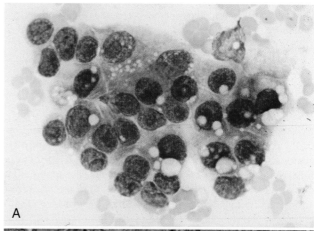

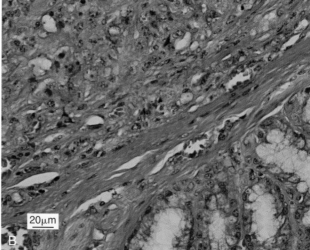

■ **FIGURE 7-12. A, Parotid salivary gland. Adenocarcinoma. Aspirate. Cat.** A cluster of immature cells display moderate anisokaryosis, coarse chromatin, prominent nucleolus and high N:C. Histopathology confirmed the malignant appearance. (Wright; HP oil.) **B, Salivary gland. Adenocarcinoma. Histology.** Salivary gland tissue from the tonsillar region demonstrates marked distortion of architecture (above pink connective tissue line) compared with the normal glandular structure (lower right) (H&E; IP.) (A, Courtesy of Rick Alleman, University of Florida. B, Courtesy of Rose Raskin, Purdue University)

(see Fig. 2-4) can appear cytologically similar to normal epithelium. In these cases, the nuclear-to-cytoplasmic ratio is higher and nucleoli may be prominent.

Inflammation

Pancreatitis may cause focal abdominal fluid accumulations or effusions with the characteristics of either a modified transudate or a sterile purulent exudate (Fig. 7-13). If a proteinaceous background is present, it can have a "dirty," moderately basophilic appearance that corresponds to saponified fat observed histologically. A hemorrhagic effusion is occasionally noted. Pancreatic cysts or abscesses can be detected as intra-abdominal masses and sampled by ultrasound-guided aspiration. The samples are often sterile and composed of neutrophils embedded in a proteinaceous background (Salisbury et al., 1988).

Neoplasia-Exocrine Pancreas

Pancreatic adenocarcinoma can be diagnosed directly via ultrasound-guided cytology/biopsy. It is a diagnostic consideration when carcinoma cells are observed in an abdominal effusion or in a thoracic effusion secondary to their metastasis via the diaphragmatic lymphatics. The pancreatic adenocarcinoma has characteristics similar to those of other adenocarcinomas, including a high nuclear-to-cytoplasmic ratio, prominent nucleolus, fine cytoplasmic vacuolization, cytoplasmic hyperchromatic basophilia, and a tendency to form acinar structures (Fig. 7-14A–C).

ESOPHAGUS

Normal Cytology

The mucosal layer of the esophagus has a stratified squamous epithelium that contains openings for the ducts of the esophageal mucous glands. Exfoliated stratified squamous epithelial cells can either appear angular or

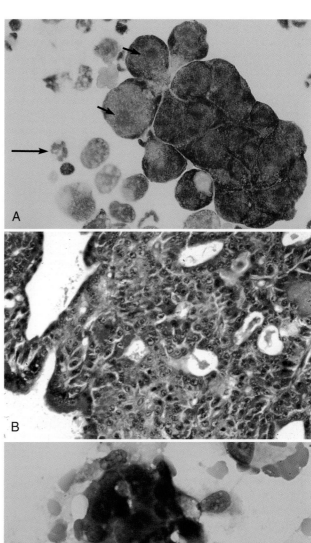

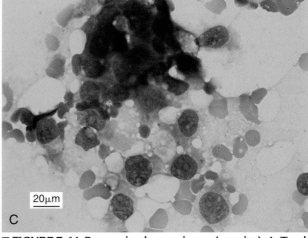

■ **FIGURE 7-14. Pancreatic adenocarcinoma (exocrine). A, Touch imprint.** This specimen was taken from a pancreatic mass. There is a dense, slightly elongated basophilic epithelial cell cluster that shows marked anisocytosis and anisokaryosis. The cytoplasm is not easily observed but the N:C ratio is markedly increased. Gigantic nucleoli are observed in some of the cells (*short arrows*). The cells at the upper end of the cluster appear to be forming a disorganized acinar structure. The inappropriately large size of the neoplastic cells can be appreciated by comparison to a neutrophil (*long arrow*). (Wright; HP oil.) **B, Histology. Papillary** (elongated clump) and cluster formation of pancreatic exocrine epithelial cells that are forming disorganized glandular and ductular structures. (H&E; IP.) **C, Imprint. Dog.** Cell cluster of pancreatic secretory epithelium with acinar formation is present along with individualized cells having prominent nucleoli and open chromatin pattern. (Wright-Giemsa; HP oil.) (C, Courtesy of Rose Raskin, Purdue University)

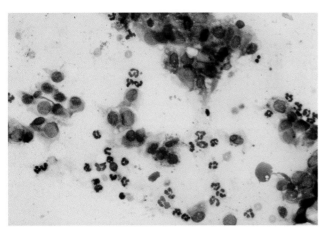

■ **FIGURE 7-13. Pancreas. Neutrophilic inflammation. Aspirate. Dog.** There are small clusters of round epithelial cells with foamy pale cytoplasm and small punctuate vacuoles. Moderate numbers of nondegenerate and pyknotic neutrophils surround the pancreatic epithelium. There is no evidence of sepsis. (Wright-Giemsa; IP.) (Courtesy of Rose Raskin, Purdue University)

have the rounded shape of intermediate epithelial cells and basal cells with eccentric nuclei. Large numbers of basal epithelial cells can indicate trauma, inflammation, or erosion (Green, 1992). The stromal cells and glandular cells usually do not exfoliate. Samples from the gastroesophageal region may contain squamous epithelium mixed with gastric columnar epithelium. Ingesta with oropharyngeal flora consisting of a mixed bacterial population of rods, cocci, and *Simonsiella* sp. may be noted in esophageal samples (see Fig. 7-1).

Inflammation

Reflux esophagitis most commonly involves the distal esophagus. It is caused by the action of regurgitated gastric (pepsin and acid) and possibly duodenal (bile acids and pancreatic enzymes) secretions that have a corrosive effect on the stratified squamous epithelium. Esophageal inflammation has a prominent neutrophilic component (Fig. 7-15) and the epithelial cells show reactive hyperchromasia, or nuclear and cytoplasmic degenerative changes. Esophageal inflammation is suggested if oropharyngeal contamination is not present and the site sampled appears inflamed endoscopically.

Neoplasia

The differential considerations for esophageal masses include the neoplasia and parasitic granuloma. Squamous cell carcinoma has neoplastic features that vary from relatively well differentiated to anaplastic. Well-differentiated squamous cell carcinomas can be difficult to differentiate from hyperplasia, but the presence of bizarre cell forms along with variable nuclear-to-cytoplasmic ratios, variable cytoplasmic basophilia, and fine cytoplasmic vacuolization support a neoplastic cell population. An adenocarcinoma of the esophageal glands is a less common epithelial neoplasm. Its location and cytologic features can be similar to a thyroid carcinoma. *Spirocerca lupi* is a spirurid nematode that parasitizes the esophageal wall of dogs in

warm climates where the dung beetle serves as the intermediate host. Endoscopically, the mass appears as a smooth, nonulcerated firm tumor. It can be diagnosed by finding embryonated eggs in a fecal flotation. Pleomorphic spindle-shaped cells exfoliated from the granuloma are easily mistaken for sarcoma. In fact, esophageal sarcomas are usually associated with the presence of the parasite (Fox et al., 1988). Another spindle-shape sarcoma is an esophageal leiomyosarcoma in which the cells may contain eosinophilic cytoplasmic granules as well as nuclear glycogen vacuoles and pleomorphism (Fig. 7-16A&B).

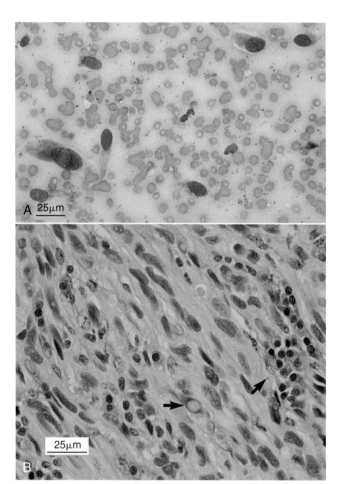

■ **FIGURE 7-16. Esophagus. Leiomyosarcoma. Dog. Same case A-B. A, Imprint.** Several spindle-shaped cells with indistinct cell borders of variable cell size, variable N:C, and anisokaryosis are present along with hemodilution. Eosinophilic granulation is prominent ranging from fine to coarse in the cytoplasm of some of the mesenchymal cells as well as within the background. Intranuclear glycogen appears as single or multiple vacuoles, a finding usually associated with hepatocytes but may be found in neoplastic cells with glycogen synthetase activity. (Wright; IP.) **B, Histology.** This esophageal mass is composed of haphazardly arranged spindle cells with multifocal perivascular aggregates of lymphocytes and plasma cells (*long arrow*). Neoplastic cells have marked variation in nuclear shape and size with oval or spindloid or bizarre shaped nuclei with clumped chromatin, vacuolar inclusions (*short arrow*) and frequent mitotic figures. The cell margins are indistinct and cell cytoplasm and/or intercellular matrix is sparse to abundant, eosinophilic and slightly fibrillar. Smooth muscle actin was present on immunohistology supporting the diagnosis. (H&E; HP oil.) (A and B, Courtesy of Rose Raskin, Purdue University.)

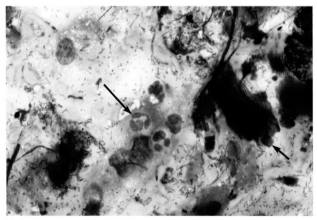

■ **FIGURE 7-15. Esophagitis. Brushing.** This specimen was obtained endoscopically from an inflamed site in the esophagus. Esophagitis is indicated by the presence of neutrophils (*long arrow*). Other findings include angular squamous epithelial cells, keratin bar (*short arrow*), and numerous bacteria (oral flora). (Wright; HP oil.)

CRITERIA FOR GASTROINTESTINAL CYTOLOGY

Cytologic grading criteria provide guidelines for the uniform evaluation of the gastrointestinal specimen, in which the frequent presence of bacterial flora and cell debris complicates the cytologic interpretation. These criteria ensure that a consistent and quantifiable assessment of the gastrointestinal cytologic specimen is achieved. Fibrosis and lesions deep to the lamina propria usually will not be detected with endoscopic cytology.

Box 7-1 lists the categories developed by Jergens et al. (1998) that compose the grading system. A scale of 0 to 7 was applied to all categories. The one used for epithelial cell clusters differs from the others. Boxes 7-2

and 7-3 list the definitions of the grading system for the microscopic findings (Jergens et al., 1998). Depending on the location, some categories would be present normally, such as bacterial rods and cocci in colonic or rectal scrapings, yet the complete absence of bacteria may indicate an alteration in flora due to prolonged antibiotic use or sampling technique. Even though bacterial flora is categorized, bacterial overgrowth cannot be diagnosed cytologically.

Knowledge of the patient's history, endoscopic appearance of the lesion, and endoscopic site sampled is vital for formulating an accurate interpretation of gastrointestinal cytologic specimens. Adequate assessment of these cytologic specimens is relatively time consuming and labor intensive. Cytology and histology are complementary processes for the evaluation of gastrointestinal disease. However, one should not be discouraged if pathology is not detected either cytologically or histologically. In one study, the majority of gastric specimens, 25% of intestinal samples, and 33% of colonic samples were classified as normal even though gastrointestinal disease was suspected (Jergens et al., 1998).

BOX 7-1   Cytologic Findings That Comprise the Grading System of the Cytologic Specimen of the Gastrointestinal Tract

Inflammatory cells: Neutrophils, lymphocytes, plasma cells, eosinophils, macrophages
Atypical cells
Epithelial cell clusters
Spiral bacteria that resemble gastric spiral organisms
Bacterial flora consisting of rods and cocci
Hemorrhage (recent)
Debris or ingesta consisting of plant or food fiber and dark particulate material
Mucous consisting of diffusely stained secretory product or mucin granules (globules)

BOX 7-2   Definition of Grades Used for the Microscopic Findings Listed in Box 7-1

Inflammatory Cells
Grades 0 to 7 denote the corresponding total number of inflammatory cells per 50x-oil objective (e. g., finding 3 inflammatory cells per 50x-oil objective is assigned a grade 3; finding 7 or more inflammatory cells per 50x-oil objective is assigned grade 7)
Grades 0 to 7 denote the corresponding total number of atypical cells per 50x-oil objective
Atypical Cells
Spiral bacteria that resemble gastric spiral organisms, bacterial flora, hemorrhage, debris or ingesta, and mucus or mucin granules were each graded as follows:
Grade 0 = none present
Grades 1 to 2 = slight
Grades 3 to 4 = moderate
Grades 5 to 7 = marked
A minimum of 10 fields should be examined since there often is exfoliation variability among the tissue imprint areas. Because of sampling and exposure to digestive contents, neutrophils may appear slightly degenerate and lymphocytes may exhibit cellular swelling, both morphologic changes resulting in reduced chromatin clumping and staining intensity. For the inflammatory and atypical cell categories, grades of 2 or less are considered of questionable diagnostic importance (i. e., considered within normal variation).

STOMACH

Normal Cytology

Gastric mucosal epithelial cells are columnar and appear as uniform cell clusters with oval to round nuclei and moderate amounts of lightly basophilic to light eosinophilic cytoplasm (Fig. 7-17A&B). There can be a mucin vacuole at the luminal surface of the columnar cells. The columnar morphology is more obvious in large cell clusters. The variable amount of mucus in the cytologic specimen has variable staining characteristics. Fundic glandular epithelium consists of rounded parietal cells (lightly eosinophilic cytoplasm) and chief cells (granular lightly basophilic cytoplasm) and may be seen in oval to elliptical clusters (Fig. 7-18A&B). Mucous neck cells also may be seen in association with parietal cells (Fig. 7-19). The tinctorial characteristic of the cell appears to be affected by the amount of mucus present. Cardiac glands and pyloric glands also secrete mucus, but do not contain parietal and chief cells.

BOX 7-3   Definition of Grades Used for Epithelial Cell Clusters per 10x-Objective*

Grade 0 = 0 cell clusters
Grade 1 = 1 to 2 cell clusters
Grade 2 = 3 to 4 cell clusters
Grade 3 = 4 to 5 cell clusters
Grade 4 = 6 to 7 cell clusters
Grade 5 = 7 to 8 cell clusters
Grade 6 = 9 to 10 cell clusters
Grade 7 = greater than 10 cell clusters

*Adequate cell clusters are needed for a representative sample. Samples with epithelial clusters of grade 2 or less are not likely to yield diagnostic information.

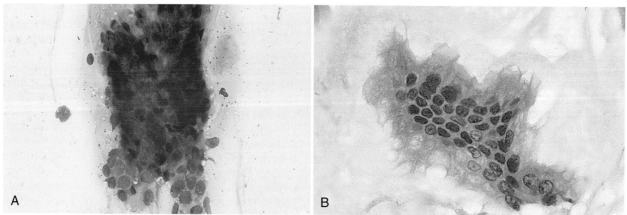

■ **FIGURE 7-17. Gastric mucosal epithelial cells. A, Normal. Touch imprint.** The epithelial cells in this touch imprint are relatively uniform with round to oval nuclei containing dispersed chromatin and moderate amounts of basophilic cytoplasm. The features can be observed at the periphery of the cell cluster where the cells are in a monolayer, emphasizing the importance of proper sample management. (Wright; HP oil.) **B, Histology.** Note the relatively uniform morphologic features and the absence of leukocytes and bacteria. The jagged border of the tissue is an artifact. (H&E; HP oil.)

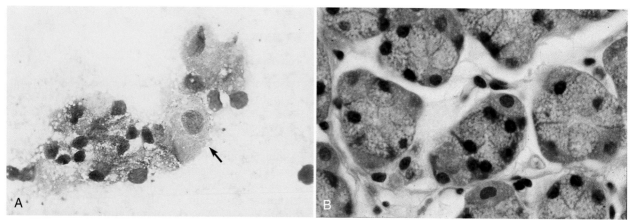

■ **FIGURE 7-18. A, Gastric fundic glandular epithelial cells. Touch imprint.** Two epithelial cell populations are present. The larger epithelial cells (*arrow*) with abundant, homogeneous, lightly eosinophilic cytoplasm are consistent with parietal cells. The smaller epithelial cells with granular-like or microvesicular basophilic cytoplasm are consistent with chief cells. Both cell types compose the fundic glands of the stomach. (Wright; HP oil.) **B, Gastric fundic glands. Histology.** The oval-shaped fundic glands are composed of two epithelial cell types. The parietal cells stain intensively eosinophilic and the pale-staining chief cells have microvesicular cytoplasm. (H&E; HP oil.)

The presence of oropharyngeal flora such as *Simonsiella* sp., along with mucus, pyknotic neutrophils, mixed bacterial flora, and digesta debris, is a common finding in gastric samples from a nondiseased stomach. These neutrophils probably represent those blood cells that are continually lost through the mucous membranes of the gastrointestinal tract. Neutrophils that are not associated with oropharyngeal or esophageal digesta may represent true gastritis (Fig. 7-20). Again, the endoscopic visualization of an inflamed area corroborates the cytologic impression of gastritis.

Gastric spiral bacteria often are associated with the mucus (Fig. 7-21A&B) and are more consistently observed in brush cytology specimens. The organisms may not be observed histologically owing to the loss of the mucous biolayer (Happonen et al., 1996). *Helicobacter*

felis-like bacteria and *Gastrospirillum*-like bacteria cannot be differentiated by light microscopy (Fig. 7-21C). The experienced cytopathologist can potentially differentiate them from *Helicobacter pylori*-like bacteria because of their smaller size. In 96 gastric samples, 48% contained gastric spiral organisms (Jergens et al., 1998). The Warthin-Starry stain accentuates the identification of the organism. Culture is needed to identify specific types of spiral bacteria. The importance of spiral bacteria as a cause of gastric disease in dogs and cats requires additional clarification since these organisms are common in animals without clinical disease or histologic abnormalities and do not alter gastric function experimentally (Eaton, 1999; Jenkins and Bassett, 1997; Happonen et al., 1996; Hermanns et al., 1995; Simpson et al., 1999a, 1999b).

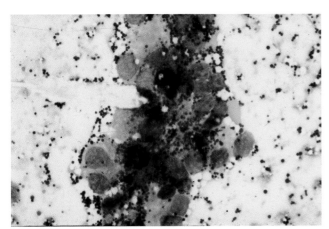

■ FIGURE 7-19. Gastric biopsy with mucin granules. Touch imprint. There is a dense cluster of mucin-producing epithelial cells that are identified by the presence of numerous purplish mucin granules (globules) located in their cytoplasm. Many extracellular mucin granules from ruptured cells are observed. The size and morphology of the mucin granules appear similar to bacterial cocci. These cells should not be confused with mast cells that have smaller metachromatic cytoplasmic granules. Contrast to Figure 9-30A. (Wright; HP oil.)

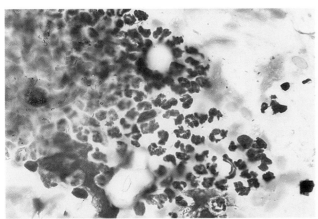

■ FIGURE 7-20. Neutrophilic gastritis. Brushing. Marked numbers of neutrophils are observed. Ulcerative and erosive lesions were observed endoscopically. (Wright; HP oil.)

Hyperplasia

The cytologic impression of mucosal and secretory hyperplasia is subjective. Increased numbers of mucosal secretory cells or goblet cells with attendant diffuse mucin granules (globules) may indicate mucosal secretory hyperplasia. A definitive diagnosis requires histology.

Inflammation

Neutrophils along with other inflammatory cells are associated with gastric ulcers (see Fig. 7-20). As indicated above, the presence of oropharyngeal flora or digesta admixed with neutrophils tempers the cytologic impression of true inflammation. Mucosal inflammation, per se, is devoid of mixed bacterial flora and digesta. The presence of lymphocytes with or without plasma cells along

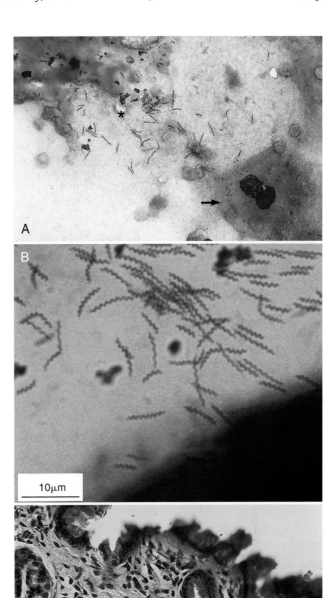

■ FIGURE 7-21. A-B, Spiral-shaped bacteria. Touch imprint. A, Numerous *Helicobacter*-like or *Gastrospirillium*-like spiral-shaped bacteria are embedded in the mucus (*asterisk*). Spiral-shaped organisms are commonly observed cytologically in both nondiseased and diseased stomachs of dogs and cats. An angular squamous epithelial cell is present (*arrow*). (Wright; HP oil.) **B, Dog.** Close up of spiral organisms from another case. (Wright; HP oil.) **C, Lymphocytic gastritis. Histology.** Although no inflammatory cells were observed in the cytologic specimen, there was mild increase in lymphocytes, stromal fibrosis, and edema around the gastric glands (*asterisk*). Microscopic examination of a biopsy is generally required to determine the presence or absence of inflammation. Only a rare spiral-shaped organism was observed (not shown) on the mucosal surface, probably due to the absence of the mucous layer. A Warthin-Starry stain can be used to identify the organism in tissue. (H&E; HP oil.) (B, Courtesy of Rose Raskin, Purdue University.)

with macrophages defines chronic inflammation. Lymphocytic or lymphoplasmacytic inflammation is associated with chronic gastritis (Fig. 7-22A&B). *Physaloptera* sp. is one specific cause of chronic inflammation that can be observed endoscopically (Fig. 7-23). Other parasites that cause gastritis, especially in cats, are *Ollulanus* and *Gnathostoma* (Brown et al., 2007; Guilford and Strombeck, 1996b). Parasites or parasite fragments are rarely seen on cytology (Jergens et al., 1998). Gastric nodular lymphocytic inflammation can be associated with *Helicobacter* sp.

Gastric phycomycosis or zygomycosis can be associated with severe gastric inflammation (Miller, 1985). Prolonged treatment with antibiotics or immunosuppression may lead to gastric candidasis (Fig. 7-24A). The oral and esophageal mucous membranes are additional sites for candidiasis. Periodic acid-Schiff or Gomori's methenamine silver stains can be used to highlight yeast, true fungal, and oomycetal (*Pythium*) organisms (Fig. 7-24B&C).

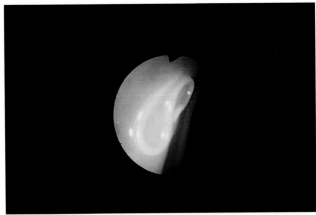

■ **FIGURE 7-23.** ***Physaloptera.*** Gastric endoscopic view. An approximately 2-cm-long white nematode consistent with *Physaloptera* was endoscopically observed in the fundus of a dog with recurrent vomiting. It is one cause (uncommon) of chronic gastritis. (Courtesy of Colin Burrows and Denny Meyer, University of Florida.)

A discussion of additional organisms that may be found throughout the intestinal tract, including the stomach, is present in the section on inflammation in the colon.

Neoplasia

Gastric neoplasms are uncommon and most are malignant. The relatively more common carcinoma/adenocarcinoma is difficult to diagnose cytologically when it is located in the submucosa or muscularis. In addition, the occasional development of reactive fibrosis adds an additional barrier that precludes exfoliation of the neoplastic cells. Malignant cells usually exfoliate readily when gastric ulceration is present.

More commonly, infiltrative lymphoma can be diagnosed on gastric cytology (refer to Figs. 7-35 and 7-43 for examples). Unless there are large numbers of predominantly immature lymphocytes present cytologically, lymphoma can be difficult to differentiate from severe lymphocytic inflammation. Small cell lymphoma (well-differentiated lymphocytes) usually cannot be confidently diagnosed with cytology and requires histology.

INTESTINE

Normal Cytology

The intestinal mucosal epithelium is columnar and glands are present. The duodenum is the region most commonly sampled endoscopically. Mucosal cell types that can be observed in cytologic specimens include columnar epithelial cells, mucus-producing goblet cells, and globule leukocytes (Figs. 7-25 to 7-27). Although controversial, it is probably derived from the mast cell based on cytochemical and ultrastructural findings, may be associated with type-1 hypersensitivity reactions, and is also found in the respiratory tract (Murray et al., 1968; Huntley, 1992; Narama et al., 1999; Breeze and Wheeldon, 1977; Baldwin and Becker, 1993). Intestinal globule leukocyte

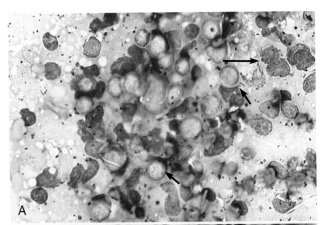

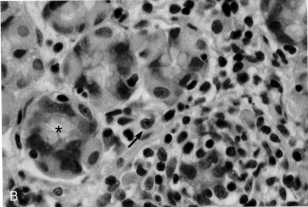

■ **FIGURE 7-22. Lymphocytic gastritis. A, Touch imprint.** A dense population of lymphocytes is a notable feature. The predominant cell type is a medium to large lymphocyte with a nucleus that is composed of bland chromatin surrounded by minimal cytoplasm (*short arrows*). There are frequent irregular formations of free nuclear protein from ruptured cells (*long arrow*) and numerous granules that represent mucin granules. The differential considerations include lymphocytic gastritis or gastric lymphoma. (Wright; HP oil.) **B, Histology.** A heterogeneous population of lymphocytes (*arrow*) surrounds the gastric glands (*asterisk*). A small number of plasma cells were admixed (not shown) resulting in a morphologic diagnosis of lymphoplasmacytic gastritis. (H&E; HP oil.)

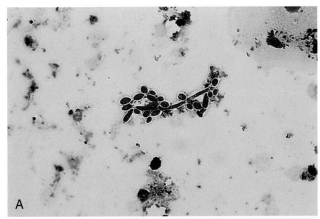

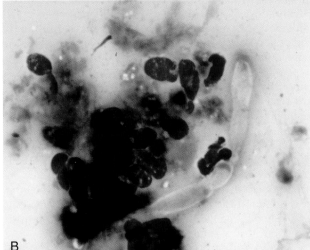

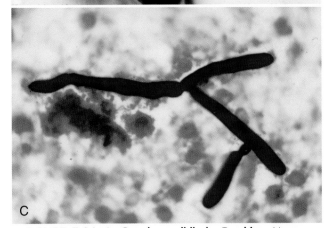

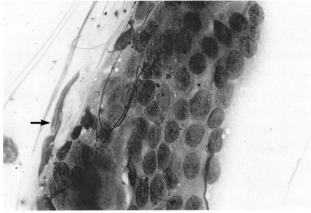

■ **FIGURE 7-25. Intestinal epithelial cells, normal. Touch imprint.** Cluster of uniform epithelial cells with round to oval nuclei and confluent basophilic cytoplasm. Streaks of free nuclear protein are noted on the left (*arrow*). (Wright; HP oil.)

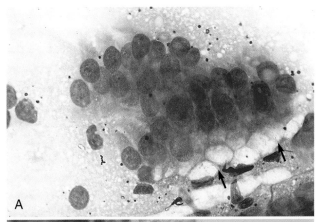

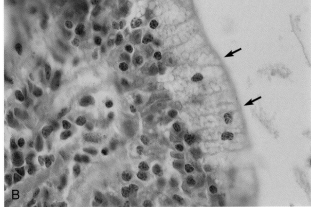

■ **FIGURE 7-24. A, Gastric candidiasis. Brushing.** Numerous basophilic pseudohyphae and blastospores of *Candida* sp. A silver stain (Gomori's methenamine stain) can be used to highlight the organism in tissue. (Wright; HP oil.) **B-C, Gastric pythiosis. Touch imprint. Dog. B,** Inflammatory cells aggregate around a barely visible hyphal structure that is highlighted by the basophilic proteinaceous background. (Wright-Giemsa; HP oil.) **C,** Same case as in B. Use of silver stain demonstrates the presence of this water mold. (GMS; HP oil.) (B and C, Courtesy of Rose Raskin, Purdue University.)

■ **FIGURE 7-26. Intestinal mucosal epithelial cells, normal. A, Touch imprint.** The columnar epithelial cells have large clear cytoplasmic vacuoles (*arrows*) that represent apical mucous vacuoles. The cells have indistinct cell borders and a few mucin granules are scattered around them. (Wright; HP oil.) **B, Histology.** The columnar epithelial cells contain basilar nuclei and show cytoplasmic rarefaction (increased lucency) in the apical end (*arrows*) due to their cytoplasmic mucus content. (H&E; HP oil.)

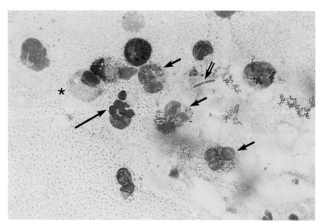

■ **FIGURE 7-27. Globule leukocyte, eosinophilic colitis. Fecal smear.** The mononuclear cell left of center (*long arrow*) has a round to oval eccentric nucleus composed of homogeneous chromatin and the light bluish-gray cytoplasm is packed with large, distinct metachromatic cytoplasmic granules. The globule leukocyte is located in the intestinal epithelium of the crypt and lower villus and in the lamina propria. Also present are three eosinophils (*three short arrows*) with poorly stained brownish cytoplasmic granules, a plasma cell with its notable darkly basophilic cytoplasm (top), and an other globular leukocyte with an eccentric oval nucleus surrounded by abundant bluish-gray cytoplasm that contains the spherical outlines of globules that did not stain (*asterisk*). A large bacterial rod-shaped bacterium is located to the right of center (*double arrow*). The granules of eosinophils often do not stain intensely in fecal smears. The presence of abundant eosinophils is suggestive of eosinophilic colitis. The morphologic diagnosis from a colonic biopsy was eosinophilic colitis. (Wright; HP oil.)

tumors have been described (Honor et al., 1986). The mucosal epithelial cells contain basophilic round to oval nuclei with moderate amounts of light basophilic cytoplasm and chromatin that is smooth to finely stippled (less aggregated than that observed in lymphocytes) and indistinct nucleoli. Mucus may be diffuse or

seen as distinct basophilic to purple granules (Fig. 7-28). These structures should not be confused with the irregularly shaped granular magenta-stained particles of gel-type products that are used for lubrication and are common contaminants (Fig. 7-29). Paneth cells contain coarse eosinophilic granular cytoplasm and can be difficult to distinguish from mucus-producing cells.

Aggregated lymphoid follicles (Peyer's patches) are scattered in the mucosa of the antimesenteric wall of the small intestine. Endoscopically they appear as oval to elongated thickenings that are a few millimeters to several centimeters in diameter. They may project slightly above the mucosal surface or appear as slight depressions and be mistaken for an ulcerlike lesion. The follicular aggregate of B-lymphocytes is covered by a mixed population of T- and B-lymphocytes extending into the lamina propria in rounded mucosal projections. An erroneous cytologic impression of lymphocytic inflammation or even lymphoma is possible if a follicle is unknowingly sampled or if the endoscopist does not communicate with the cytopathologist (Fig. 7-30). A heterogeneous lymphocyte population generally comprises a lymphoid follicle or inflammatory reaction and that variability aids in differentiation from the homogeneous lymphocyte population characteristic of lymphoma. Small numbers of lymphocytes and plasma cells may be seen (grade 0–1) cytologically but they are less frequent than one might anticipate based on the number present histologically in tissue without pathology. Granulated (large granular) lymphocytes may be normally observed in low numbers, especially in cats (Fig. 7-31). Bacteria are usually not normally observed or are only present in low numbers (Baker and Lumsden, 2000).

Hyperplasia

A cytologic impression of hyperplasia is based on prominent numbers of mucus-secreting epithelial cells and/or a marked increase in goblet cells. It is important

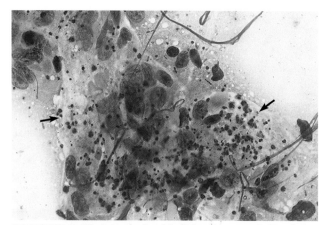

■ **FIGURE 7-28. Intestinal epithelial cells, normal. Touch imprint.** Numerous mucin secretory granules cover a dense cluster of uniform intestinal epithelial cells (*arrows*). The cellular distortion is an artifact of the preparation. Streaks of free nuclear protein are present (top). (Wright; HP oil.)

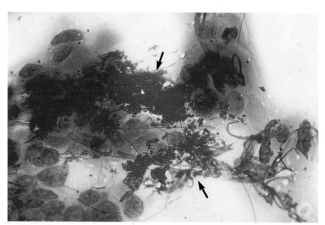

■ **FIGURE 7-29. Intestinal epithelial cells, normal, gel lubricant. Touch imprint.** In the center of these dense clumps of intestinal epithelial cells are irregularly shaped homogeneous islands of magenta-stained material that represent the gel used for lubrication of the endoscope (*arrows*). (Wright; HP oil.)

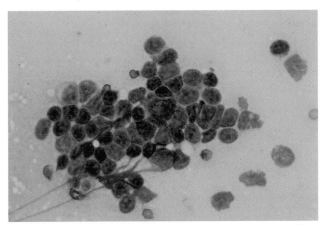

■ **FIGURE 7-30. Intestinal aggregated lymphoid follicle (Peyer's patch). Brushing.** This densely packed cluster of lymphocytes is composed of small (darkest stained), medium, and large lymphocytes (lightest stained with visible rim of lightly basophilic cytoplasm). Four free nuclei are located to the far right. (Wright; HP oil.)

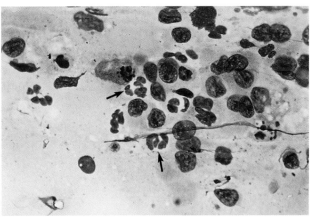

■ **FIGURE 7-32. Purulent enteritis. Grade 5/6. Touch imprint.** Numerous neutrophils (*arrows*) are intimately admixed with lightly basophilic-stained intestinal epithelial cells. An occasional eosinophil (not visible) was noted and is a common finding that has no added diagnostic importance. Karyorrhectic debris is located to the lower right. (Wright; HP oil.)

to differentiate changes of epithelial hyperplasia or metaplasia due to reparative lesions from relatively well-differentiated neoplasia. Criteria for hyperplasia include preservation of polarity, uniformity of cell size with minimal anisocytosis, and cohesiveness of cells. Correlation with the histologic findings is recommended when there are problematic cytologic findings.

Inflammation

Inflammatory cells are categorized according to the grading system, with a grade of 2 or more indicating the corresponding degree of significant inflammation (see Box 7-2). The grading system is used to express the presence and magnitude of the neutrophilic (Fig. 7-32) or lymphocytic-plasmacytic inflammatory constituents

(see Fig. 7-31). Severe lymphocytic enteritis may be difficult to differentiate from malignant lymphoma when medium to large lymphocytes are prominent (see Neoplasia, below). Comparative correlation with the histologic findings is imperative. An increase in the number of granulated lymphocytes appears to be a nonspecific component of enteritis, especially in the cat. Eosinophils, mast cells, Paneth cells, and mucus-secreting cells may be difficult to confidently differentiate cytologically because of altered staining characteristics (Figs. 7-27 and 7-33), moderate to marked cell

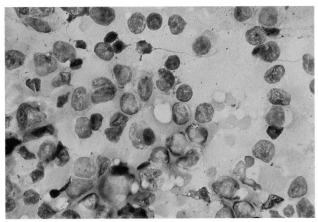

■ **FIGURE 7-31. Lymphocytic enteritis. Grade 6/7, granular lymphocyte. Touch imprint.** Medium and large lymphocytes are prominent with scattered small lymphocytes admixed. A granular lymphocyte is located slightly to the right of center (*arrow*). In other areas, occasional neutrophils and macrophages contributed to the inflammatory reaction. (Wright; HP oil.)

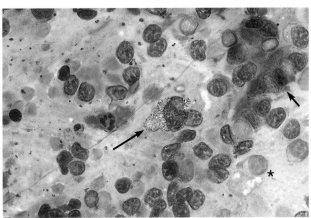

■ **FIGURE 7-33. Intestinal epithelial cells, normal, mast cell. Touch imprint.** In the center is a mast cell composed of a distorted oval nucleus with ropy chromatin surrounded by moderately abundant cytoplasm with faintstaining metachromatic granules (*long arrow*). An occasional mast cell is a normal finding in an intestinal cytologic specimen. Basophilic epithelial cells (*short arrow*) and lightly stained medium-sized lymphocytes with round nuclei composed of diffuse chromatin surrounded by a moderate rim of lightly basophilic cytoplasm are present (*asterisk*). Free nuclei that retain moderate chromatin clumping are scattered throughout the specimen. (Wright; HP oil.)

distortion, rupture, and lysis that accompanies the general reaction to inflammation. When inflammation is present, periodic acid-Schiff or Gomori's methenamine silver stains can be used to highlight fungal and protozoal agents. Giardiasis can be diagnosed by finding the trophozoites in duodenal specimens. They appear as binucleate, pear-shaped organisms with four pairs of flagella (Fig. 7-34). A variety of infectious agents can be found in the intestine, as well as the colon, and these are discussed under the section on inflammation of the colon.

Neoplasia

The ability to detect intestinal neoplasia cytologically depends on the extent of infiltration and the presence of ulceration. Lymphoma readily exfoliates, which facilitates a cytologic diagnosis (Fig. 7-35A&B). Franks et al. (1986) published the clinical, histologic, and ultrastructural findings of this case (see Fig. 7-35B). The neoplasm often involves the intestinal tract and jejunal lymph nodes. (Darbes et al., 1998). One study suggested that these "granulated round cell tumors"

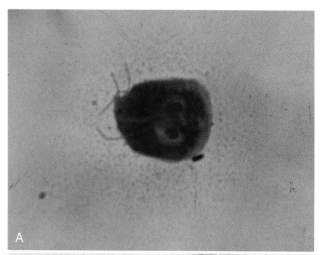

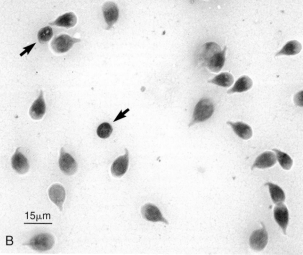

■ **FIGURE 7-34. Giardiasis. A, Duodenal aspirate.** *Giardia intestinalis (lamblia* or *duodenalis)* is recognized by its paired metachromatically stained nuclei and multiple eight flagella (two located to the left). A rod-shaped bacterium is on its lower right surface. The diagnosis also can be made by zinc sulfate fecal flotation or ELISA or immunofluoresence fecal tests. (Wright; ×250.) **B, Duodenal imprint. Dog.** The duodenal mucosa appeared endoscopically normal in this dog presenting with hypoproteinemia. Numerous trophozoites were present in association with epithelium (not shown). Compare size of giardial trophozoites to two small lymphocytes *(arrows).* (Wright; HP oil.) (A, Courtesy of Denny Meyer. B, Courtesy of Rose Raskin, Purdue University.)

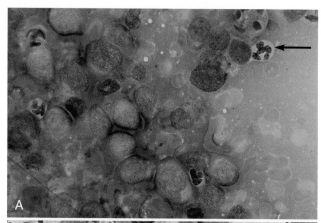

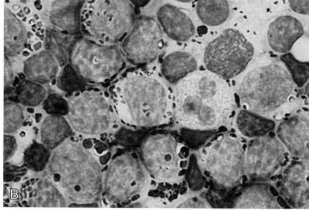

■ **FIGURE 7-35. A, Intestinal lymphoma. Touch imprint.** Numerous lymphoblasts are embedded in basophilically stained mucus. The large immature lymphocytes have an oval to irregularly shaped nucleus composed of homogeneous, pale-staining chromatin surrounded by minimal to moderately abundant lightly basophilic cytoplasm. Their large size can be appreciated by comparison to the neutrophil *(long arrow).* Karyorrhectic debris is located above the neutrophil. (Wright; HP oil.) **B, Large granular lymphoma. Fine-needle aspirate of abdominal mass. Cat.** This monomorphic population of cells has a round to oval nucleus with ropy chromatin surrounded by a minimal to moderate amount of lightly basophilic cytoplasm and contains prominent variably-sized metachromatically stained granules. Some of the cells have smaller granules that formed a packet in one location of the cytoplasm (not shown). Darkly stained normal small lymphocytes are sandwiched amongst the neoplastic cells and a segmented eosinophil with faintly stained granules is centrally located. At surgery, the confluent mass involved the lymph nodes and small intestine. (Wright; HP oil.) (A, Courtesy of Denny Meyer.)

have a common cellular origin that may involve cells in transition between mucosal mast cells and globule leukocytes (see Fig. 7-27) (McEntee et al., 1993). However, it can be missed cytologically because neoplastic lymphocytes often stain less intensively and easily rupture. Occasionally, the differentiation of severe lymphocytic enteritis from lymphoma is problematic. Also, the reader is referred to the discussion under Normal Cytology, above, regarding the potential misimpression that can occur if an aggregated lymphoid follicle is sampled. Correlation with the histologic findings is imperative when there are problematic cytologic findings.

The intestinal adenocarcinoma has the general characteristics of neoplastic epithelial cells (Fig. 7-36A&B). In our experience, other intestinal neoplasms (e.g., leiomyosarcomas, leiomyomas, and fibrosarcomas) are difficult to diagnose cytologically because of their deeper location and decreased tendency to exfoliate.

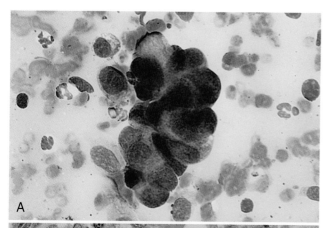

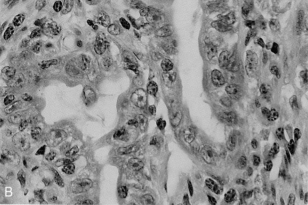

■ **FIGURE 7-36. Intestinal adenocarcinoma. A, Touch imprint.** Epithelial cells in this dense cluster demonstrate increased basophilia, marked anisocytosis and anisokaryosis, variable N: C ratios, and overgrowth of neighboring cells. Their abnormally large size is appreciated by comparison to the neutrophils. (Wright; HP oil.) **B, Histology.** Disorganized epithelial tubules are formed by cells that demonstrate moderate to marked anisocytosis and anisokaryosis, variable nuclear chromatin patterns, prominent nucleoli, variable N: C ratios. (H&E; HP oil.)

COLON/RECTUM/FECAL

Normal Cytology

Colonic cytologic specimens consist of groups or sheets of uniform columnar epithelial cells with goblet cells that contain mucin and basilar nuclei (Fig. 7-37). A prominent mixed bacterial flora is a common finding. Rectal scrapings contain columnar epithelial clusters and fecal material. Aggregated lymphoid follicles are present in the colon and a mixture of small, medium, and large lymphocytes are observed cytologically. Again the reader is referred to the discussion under Normal Cytology, above, regarding the potential misimpression that can occur if an aggregated lymphoid follicle is sampled. Fecal cytology is covered more in detail in Chapter 8.

Hyperplasia

Observing a relatively normal-appearing mucosa endoscopically combined with a cytologic finding of a uniform population of epithelial cells supports a diagnosis of mucosal hyperplasia. Hyperplastic epithelial cells can have mild cellular atypia and distinct nucleoli, especially associated with rectal mucosal hyperplasia (Fig. 7-38A&B).

Inflammation

The finding of neutrophils indicates active inflammation involving the colon and/or rectum because neutrophils entering the more proximal intestinal lumen would be rapidly destroyed (Fig. 7-39A). Possible infectious causes of neutrophilic colitis include bacteria (*Clostridium perfringens* (Fig. 7-39B), *Campylobacter jejuni*, *Salmonella* sp., an enterotoxic strain of *Escherichia coli*) and parasites (*Trichuris vulpis*) (Fig. 7-39C). The presence of small to medium lymphocytes with or without plasma cells is consistent with a generic morphologic impression of chronic colitis (Fig. 7-40A&B). Hemorrhage induced by sampling is common in colonic and rectal

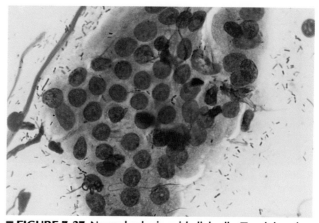

■ **FIGURE 7-37. Normal colonic epithelial cells. Touch imprint.** The sheet of epithelial cells demonstrates uniform cytomorphologic features and staining. Numerous bacteria of varying size and shapes are a normal finding. (Wright; HP oil.)

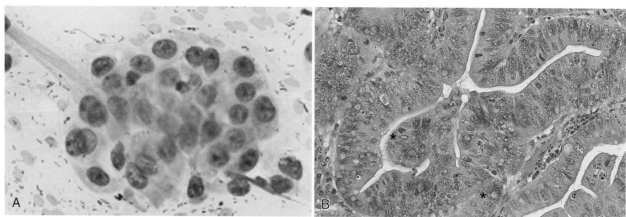

■ **FIGURE 7-38. Hyperplastic colonic epithelial cells. A, Touch imprint.** The slightly understained sheet of epithelial cells have nuclei composed of stippled chromatin, contain one to two prominent nucleoli, and show minimal variation in nuclear size and shape. Cytologic differential considerations for this mass lesion are polyp, adenoma, or well-differentiated carcinoma. Numerous bacteria in the background are normal colonic flora. (Wright; HP oil.) **B, Histology.** Papillary projections (*asterisks*) are covered by hyperplastic columnar mucosal epithelial cells with basilar nuclei, coarse chromatin, and prominent nucleoli. The tissue architecture is consistent with a benign lesion. (H&E; IP.)

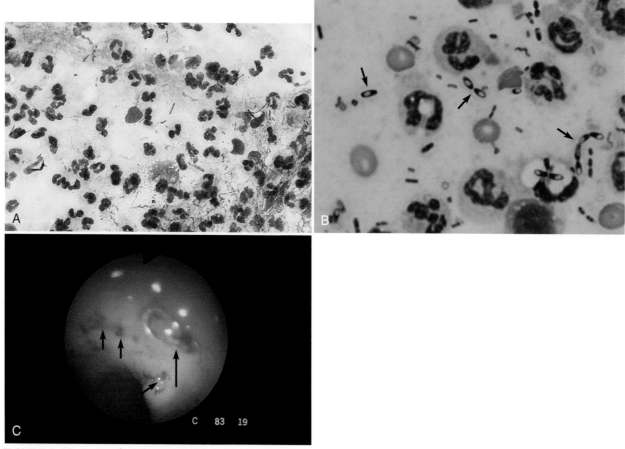

■ **FIGURE 7-39. A, Purulent (neutrophilic) colitis. Scraping.** Neutrophils are the prominent abnormal microscopic feature. Colonic bacterial flora is admixed. Differential diagnostic considerations include infections by *Campylobacter, Salmonella, Clostridium,* and *Trichuris.* A cause was not determined in this case. (Wright; HP oil.) **B, Clostridial colitis. Rectal smear.** Numerous neutrophils were present upon scanning of this direct fecal smear. An increased number of large rod-shaped bacterial endospores with a clear center and an increased density predominantly on one end ("safety pin" appearance) are the notable feature (*short arrows*). The bacterial morphology is consistent with *Clostridium perfringens.* Occasional organisms can be normally seen but greater than 5 organisms per 1000X oil field is considered abnormal. (Wright; HP oil.) **C, *Trichuris vulpis*-induced colitis. Endoscopic view.** *Trichuris vulpis* is attached to a hemorrhagic colonic mucosal site (*long arrow*). Several other areas of mucosal inflammation/hemorrhage are present (*short arrows*). A moderate number of neutrophils were observed in a fecal smear. (B, Courtesy of Rose Raskin, Purdue University. C, Courtesy of Colin Burrows and Denny Meyer.)

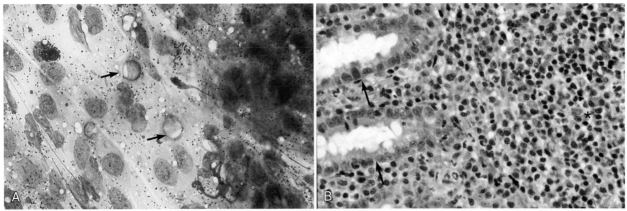

■ **FIGURE 7-40. Lymphocytic colitis. A, Touch imprint.** An increased number of small to medium-sized lymphocytes composed of a round to oval nucleus with homogeneous chromatin and a small rim of clear to lightly basophilic cytoplasm are present (*arrows*). Dense basophilic clusters of epithelial cells (far right) and abundant mucin granules suggestive of mucosal hyperplasia are set in a lightly basophilic background of mucus. (Wright; HP oil.) **B, Histology.** There is a moderate to marked increase in small to medium-sized lymphocytes that invade the deeper mucosal region (*asterisk*). Hypertrophic mucosal glands are lined by prominent goblet cells with large clear mucus-filled vacuoles (*arrows*). (H&E; HP oil.)

sampling. Leukocytes in the blood can confound the cytologic interpretation, especially if there is a concurrent leukocytosis.

Colonic samples can be used to detect *Prototheca* sp. (rectum), *Histoplasma capsulatum* (intestine, rectum), *Balantidium coli* (rectum), and *Cryptococcus neoformans* (intestine) (Rakich and Latimer, 1999). *Prototheca* sp. is a colorless algae (1.3-13.4 μm wide and 1.3-16.1 μm long) with basophilic granular cytoplasm, a clear cell wall, and a small nucleus (Rakich and

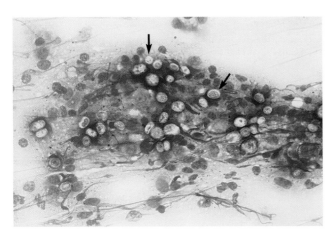

■ **FIGURE 7-41.** *Prototheca* **sp. Colonic touch imprint.** The algae appear as variably sized, oval clear structures with eosinophilic to basophilic stippling (*arrows*). The organisms are embedded in a dense sheet of epithelial cells. (Wright; HP oil.)

Latimer, 1999) (Fig. 7-41). Endosporulation may be noted. Systemic fungal infections can be initially detected by a rectal scraping. These include *H. capsulatum* (2-4 μm) that is often located within macrophages (Fig. 7-42A) and *C. neoformans* (yeast, 3.5-7 μm) with its microscopic hallmark of a prominent clear, nonstaining capsule. *B. coli* (40-80 μm X 25-45 μm to 30-300 μm X 30-100 μm) is a ciliated protozoan that infects dogs ingesting pig feces. It is thought that damage to the colonic mucosa by trichuriasis may predispose to *B. coli* infection. Less commonly, *Blastomyces dermatitidis* (yeast, 7-15 μm) may be found as a refractile, deeply basophilic yeast with a thick cell wall in the stomach, intestine, and/or colon (Fig. 7-42B).

Recently, there are reports of a yeast, *Cyniclomyces guttulatus (Saccharomycopsis guttulata)* occurring as a nonpathogen in canine gastric, intestinal and colonic samples, and we have observed this as well (Fig. 7-42C). This is an organism that occurs in rabbit feces in high numbers (Neel et al., 2006; Zierdt et al., 1988), and may be seen in dogs after consuming rabbit fecal pellets.

Neoplasia

Colonic carcinoma/adenocarcinoma and lymphoma (Fig. 7-43) are most commonly diagnosed and appear cytologically similar to those described in other parts of the intestinal tract. Plasmacytomas can occur in the colon, as well as other areas of the digestive tract, including the oral cavity (Fig. 7-44).

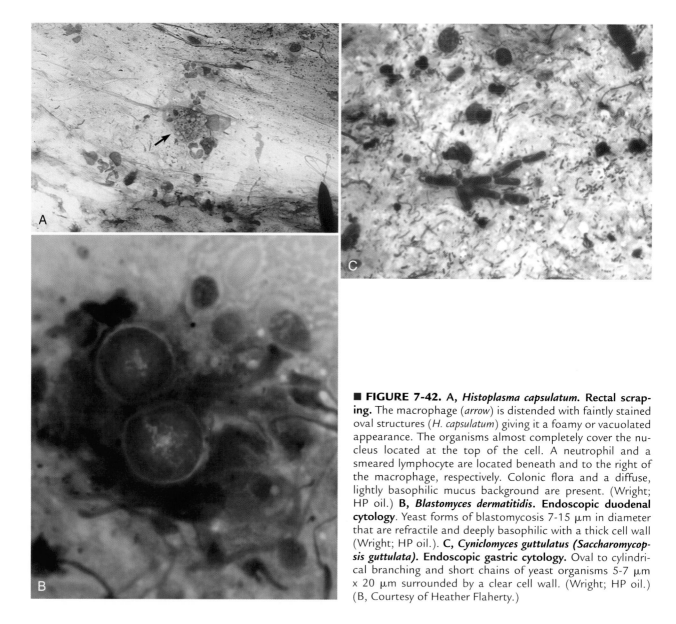

■ **FIGURE 7-42. A,** *Histoplasma capsulatum.* **Rectal scraping.** The macrophage (*arrow*) is distended with faintly stained oval structures (*H. capsulatum*) giving it a foamy or vacuolated appearance. The organisms almost completely cover the nucleus located at the top of the cell. A neutrophil and a smeared lymphocyte are located beneath and to the right of the macrophage, respectively. Colonic flora and a diffuse, lightly basophilic mucus background are present. (Wright; HP oil.) **B,** *Blastomyces dermatitidis.* **Endoscopic duodenal cytology.** Yeast forms of blastomycosis 7-15 μm in diameter that are refractile and deeply basophilic with a thick cell wall (Wright; HP oil.). **C,** *Cyniclomyces guttulatus (Saccharomycopsis guttulata).* **Endoscopic gastric cytology.** Oval to cylindrical branching and short chains of yeast organisms 5-7 μm x 20 μm surrounded by a clear cell wall. (Wright; HP oil.) (B, Courtesy of Heather Flaherty.)

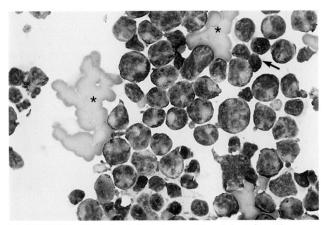

■ **FIGURE 7-43. Colonic lymphoma. Touch imprint.** Pleomorphic lymphoblasts composed of irregularly shaped to reniform to convoluted nuclei surrounded by moderately abundant dark basophilic cytoplasm are the notable abnormal microscopic finding. Their anaplastic morphology makes them difficult to recognize as a lymphoid cell type. A few small lymphocytes with dense nuclei and minimal cytoplasm are admixed (*arrow*). Two small islands of yellowish-green erythrocytes are present (*asterisks*). (Wright; HP oil.)

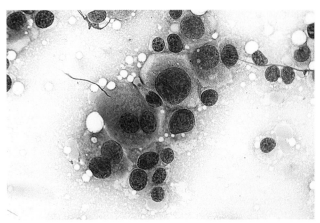

■ **FIGURE 7-44. Colonic plasmacytoma. Touch imprint.** These cells demonstrate characteristics of malignancy that include marked anisocytosis and anisokaryosis and variable N:C ratio. While they have morphologic features that are consistent with an anaplastic carcinoma, the eccentric nucleus and basophilic cytoplasm is also suggestive of a plasma cell derivation. Histology along with immunohistochemical staining of the biopsy confirmed a plasmacytoma. (Wright; HP oil.)

REFERENCES

Baker R, Lumsden JH: The gastrointestinal tract. In Baker R, Lumsden JH (eds): *Color atlas of cytology of the dog and cat*, Mosby, St. Louis, 2000, pp 177-183.

Baldwin F, Becker AB: Bronchoalveolar eosinophilic cells in a canine model of asthma: two distinctive populations, *Vet Pathol* 30:97-103, 1993.

Bernreuter DC: The oropharynx and tonsils. In Cowell RL, Tyler RD, Meinkoth JH, et al (eds): *Diagnostic cytology and hematology of the dog and cat*, ed 3, Mosby, St. Louis, 2008, pp 138-148.

Breeze RB, Wheeldon EB: The cells of the pulmonary airways: state of the art, *Am Rev Resp Dis* 116:705-721, 1977.

Brown CC, Baker DC, Barker IK: Alimentary system. In Maxie MG (ed): *Jubb, Kennedy, and Palmer's pathology of domestic animals*, ed 5, Saunders/Elsevier, Philadelphia, 2007, pp 1-296.

Ciekot PA, Powers BE, Withrow SJ, et al: Histologically low-grade, yet biologically high-grade, fibrosarcomas of the mandible and maxilla in dogs: 25 cases (1982-1991), *J Am Vet Med Assoc* 204(4):610-615, 1994.

Darbes J, Majoub M, Breuer W, Hermanns W: Large granular lymphocyte leukemia/lymphoma in six cats, *Vet Pathol* 35:370-379, 1998.

de Bruijn ND, Kirpensteijn J, Neyens IJS, et al: A clinicopathological study of 52 feline epulides, *Vet Pathol* 44:161-169, 2007.

Dennis MM, Ehrhart N, Duncan CG, et al: Frequency of and risk factors associated with lingual lesions in dogs: 1,196 cases (1995-2004), *J Am Vet Med Assoc* 228:1533-1537, 2006.

Eaton KA: Editorial: Man bites dog: Helicobacter in the new millennium, *J Vet Int Med* 13:505-596, 1999.

Fox SM, Burns J, Hawkins J: Spirocercosis in dogs, *Comp Cont Educ Pract Vet* 10:807-822, 1988.

Franks PT, Harvey JW, Calderwood-Mays M, et al: Feline large granular lymphoma, *Vet Pathol* 23:200-202, 1986.

German AJ, Hall EJ, Day MJ: Immune cell populations within the duodenal mucosa of dogs with enteropathies, *J Vet Intern Med* 15(1):14-25, 2001.

Green L: Gastrointestinal cytology. In Atkinson BF (ed): *Atlas of diagnostic cytopathology*, WB Saunders, Philadelphia, 1992, pp 283-316.

Guilford WG: Diseases of the oral cavity and pharynx. In Guilford WG, Center SA, Strombeck DR, Williams DA, Meyer DJ (eds): *Strombeck's small animal gastroenterology*, ed 3, WB Saunders, Philadelphia, 1996a, pp 189-201.

Guilford WG, Strombeck DR: Chronic gastric diseases. In Guilford WG, Center SA, Strombeck DR, Williams DA, Meyer DJ (eds): *Strombeck's small animal gastroenterology*, ed 3, WB Saunders, Philadelphia, 1996b, pp 275-302.

Happonen I, Saari S, Castren L, et al: Comparison of diagnostic methods for detecting gastric *Helicobacter*-like organisms in dogs and cats, *J Comp Pathol* 115(2):117-127, 1996.

Head KW, Else RW, Dubielzig RR: Tumors of the alimentary tract. In Meuten DJ (ed): *Tumors in domestic animals*, ed 4, Iowa State Press, Ames, 2002, pp 401-481.

Hermanns W, Kregel K, Breuer W, Lechner J: *Helicobacter*-like organisms: histopathological examination of gastric biopsies from dogs and cats, *J Comp Pathol* 112(3): 307-318, 1995.

Honor DJ, DeNicola DB, Turek JJ, et al: A neoplasm of globule leukocytes in a cat, *Vet Pathol* 23:287-292, 1986.

Huntley JF: Mast cells and basophils: a review of their heterogeneity and function, *J Comp Pathol* 107:349-372, 1992.

Jenkins CC, Bassett JR: *Helicobacter* infection, *Comp Cont Educ Pract Vet* 19(3):267-279, 1997.

Jergens AE, Andreasen CB, Hagemoser WA, et al: Cytologic examination of exfoliative specimens obtained during endoscopy for diagnosis of gastrointestinal tract disease in dogs and cats, *J Am Vet Med Assoc* 213:1755-1759, 1998.

Joffe DJ, Allen AL: Ulcerative eosinophilic stomatitis in three Cavalier King Charles spaniels, *J Am Anim Hosp Assoc* 31(1):34-37, 1995.

Marcos R, Santos M, Oliveira J, et al: Cytochemical detection of calcium in a case of calcinosis circumscripta in a dog, *Vet Clin Pathol* 35:239-242, 2006.

McEntee MF, Horton S, Blue J, Meuten DJ: Granulated round cell tumor of cats, *Vet Pathol* 30:195-203, 1993.

Miller RI: Gastrointestinal phycomycosis in 63 dogs, *J Am Vet Med Assoc* 186(5):473-478, 1985.

Murray M, Miller HRP, Jarrett WFH: The globule leukocyte and its derivation from the subepithelial mast cell, *Lab Invest* 19:222-234, 1968.

Narama I, Ozaki K, Matsushima S, Matsuura T: Eosinophilic gastroenterocolitis in iron lactate overload rats, *Toxicol Pathol* 27:318-324, 1999.

Neel JA, Tarigo J, Grindem CB: Gallbladder aspirate from a dog, *Vet Clin Pathol* 35(4):467-470, 2006.

Poulet FM, Valentine BA, Summers BA: A survey of epithelial odontogenic tumors and cysts in dogs and cats, *Vet Pathol* 29(5):369-380, 1992.

Rakich PM, Latimer KS: Rectal mucosal scrapings. In Cowell RL, Tyler RD, Meinkoth JH (eds): *Diagnostic cytology and hematology of the dog and cat*, Mosby, St. Louis, 1999, pp 249-253.

Rakich PM, Latimer KS, Weiss R, et al: Mucocutaneous plasmacytomas in dogs: 75 cases (1980-1987), *J Am Vet Med Assoc* 194(6):803-810, 1989.

Salisbury SK, Lantz GC, Nelson RW, et al: Pancreatic abscess in dogs: six cases (1978-1986), *J Am Vet Med Assoc* 193(9):1104-1108, 1988.

Simpson KW, Strauss-Ayali D, McDonough PL, et al: Gastric function in dogs with naturally acquired gastric *Helicobacter* spp. infection, *J Vet Int Med* 13:507-515, 1999a.

Simpson KW, McDonough PL, Strauss-Ayali D, et al: *Helicobacter felis* infection in dogs: effects on gastric structure and function, *Vet Pathol* 36:237-248, 1999b.

Spangler WL, Culbertson MR: Salivary gland disease in dogs and cats: 245 cases (1985-1988), *J Vet Med Assoc* 198(3):465-469, 1991.

Zierdt CH, Detlefson C, Muller J, Waggie KS: *Cyniclomyces guttulatus (Saccharomycopsis guttulata)*-culture, ultrastructure, and physiology, *Antonie Van Leeuwenhoek* 54(4):357-366, 1988.

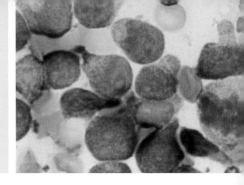

8

Dry-Mount Fecal Cytology

Heather L. Wamsley

There are several diagnostic tests of feces that may be necessary during complete evaluation of patients with clinical signs referable to the gastrointestinal tract. Optimal fecal assessment, including potential tests (e.g., wet-mount fecal cytology, dry-mount fecal cytology, bacterial culture, fecal antigen detection methods, fecal flotation, fecal sedimentation, Baermann technique) and their required sample handling, diagnostic indications, and interpretations, have been compiled elsewhere (Broussard, 2003). Dry-mount fecal cytology (air-dried smear) is one component of a thorough diagnostic evaluation of patients with gastrointestinal signs. Since some fecal pathogens can be morphologically indistinguishable from incidental nonpathogens, results of dry-mount fecal cytology should be interpreted in the context of the patient's clinical presentation and results of other diagnostic tests, such as wet-mount fecal cytology, bacterial culture, and fecal antigen detection methods.

When evaluating dry-mount fecal cytology, it may be useful to apply a systematic approach aimed at evaluation of attendant background cells and detection of abnormal eucaryotic cells and pathogenic microorganisms (Box 8-1).

SAMPLE COLLECTION AND PROCESSING

The method of fecal sample collection can affect which portion of the rectum is represented (luminal vs. mucosal) and the cellular (eucaryotic and procaryotic) content of the sample. The ideal sampling method, desired amount to collect, and subsequent sample handling depends upon the intended fecal testing (Broussard, 2003). Important goals of sampling for fecal cytology include examination of a fresh sample (less than 5 minutes old) that is representative of the mucosal surface and preparation of a fecal thin film preparation that is not excessively dense. Excessively dense areas of fecal thin film preparations are prone to detach during staining or, if they do not fall off during staining, obscure cytologic details. Because the cellular content of fecal material is dynamic and will likely continue to change after sample

collection, immediate examination following collection is recommended.

> **KEY POINT** Preparation of thin fecal film of fresh material is preferred over a densely packed smear. Results of dry-mount fecal cytology should be interpreted in view of the patient's clinical presentation and results of other diagnostic tests.

> **KEY POINT** As fecal material readily falls off during staining, it is important to stain fecal slides at the end of a batch as well as change the stain solution if a dip technique is used. These precautions will help avoid bacterial contamination to subsequent specimens being stained.

For fecal cytology, there are a few possible sampling methods, including collection of unadulterated fecal material, rectal saline lavage, and rectal scraping. A small amount of fresh fecal material may be obtained during digital rectal examination or using a moistened, cotton-tipped applicator or fecal loop if digital rectal exam is not possible. Immediately collected, voided feces may also be used; however, voided samples may be more representative of the luminal portion of the rectum, which is not ideal for fecal cytology. Voided fecal material is a preferred sample for other diagnostic tests, such as fecal flotation, fecal sedimentation, or the Baermann technique, since it is more copious and may be rich in parasitic eggs and cysts (Broussard, 2003). Usually, if a small amount of fecal material is obtained using a moistened, cotton-tipped applicator, the cotton tip of the applicator can be gently rolled on the slide to prepare a direct thin film. Otherwise, slight dilution of the feces may be used to prepare a thin film preparation by placing a drop of sterile, normal saline on a clean, glass microscope slide, adding a very small amount of fecal material (no larger than a match-head), mixing with a sterile, wooden applicator, and spreading as for other fluid thin film preparations. Prior to

---

and after spreading, newsprint should be legible though the preparation.

Rectal saline lavage enriches for mucosal material, including mucus, motile protozoa, and bacteria. Lavage fluid contains relatively less luminal fecal material and is ideal for fecal cytology (Broussard, 2003). Properly collected lavage fluid should have a mudlike consistency, and a single drop can be used to prepare a thin film preparation.

Material obtained by rectal scraping is often submitted as a sample for dry-mount fecal cytology, though feces and rectal scrape material are not synonymous. Rectal scraping with a swab or blunt spatula is a somewhat more invasive method of sampling the rectal mucosa by direct scraping of its surface. Rectal scraping is typically required to identify some infections that localize to the deeper portion of the mucosa (e.g., histoplasmosis, protothecosis) or to characterize deep mucosal cellular infiltrates.

Dry-mount fecal cytology can be useful to examine the microorganism flora and any host cells that may be present (e.g., epithelial, inflammatory) and to detect other pathogens that may be present (e.g., bacterial, fungal, algal, oomycetal, or protozoal). Occasionally, evaluation of dry-mount fecal cytology is diagnostic. More often it aids in ruling selected causes of diarrhea to be less likely.

KEY POINT Many abnormalities, particularly those involving the background flora, are nonspecific, representing incidental findings associated with other underlying diseases, physiologic processes, or previous antimicrobial treatments.

NORMAL OR INCIDENTAL MICROSCOPIC FINDINGS

The background microbial flora should be predominantly comprised of an extremely polymorphic population of several different bacterial bacilli (Fig. 8-1). There should be fewer than 5 spore-forming bacilli per 100× objective field (Broussard, 2003). Cocci should be absent or only rarely observed. A low number of extracellular, circular or ovoid, 5 to 10 μm diameter, stippled, variably basophilic yeast with a thin, colorless capsule may occasionally be seen (Figs. 8-2, 8-3, 8-4). While these yeast structures are frequently found in diarrheal stools, it is not certain whether there is a direct causal relationship.

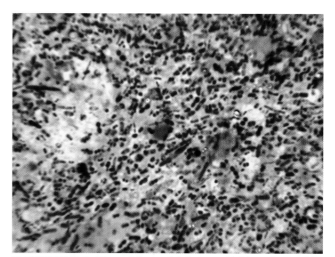

■ **FIGURE 8-1. Normal bacterial flora.** A highly polymorphic, mixed bacterial flora that is comprised predominantly of several different bacilli is expected to be observed in feces and is typically found on an amorphous, pale basophilic background that contains either none or few host cells. (Wright-Giemsa; HP oil.)

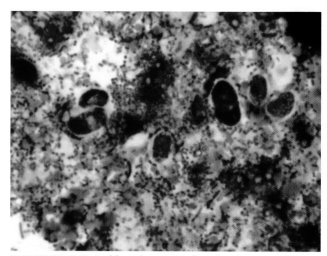

■ **FIGURE 8-2. Incidental yeast.** A few circular or ovoid, 5 to 10 μm diameter, stippled, basophilic yeast with a thin, colorless capsule may occasionally be incidentally observed extracellularly within fecal smears. (Wright-Giemsa; HP oil.)

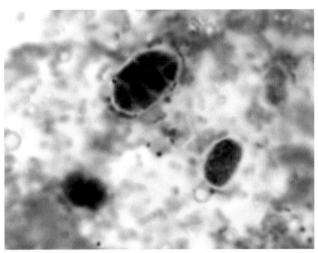

■ **FIGURE 8-3. Incidental yeast.** Closer magnification extracellular fecal yeast that can be observed incidentally in fecal smears. (Wright-Giemsa; HP oil.)

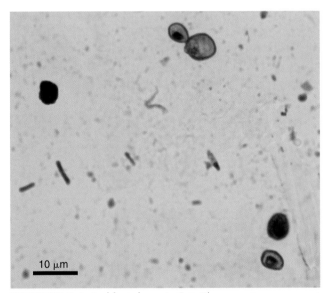

■ **FIGURE 8-4. Incidental yeast. Cat.** These yeast were present in an adult cat with diarrhea. They appear both as single and budding forms with both clear and focally dense staining areas within the structure. The significance of the yeast is unknown in causing the diarrhea; however, they occur more commonly in watery stools possibly by producing a wash effect that releases the organisms more readily. (Wright; HP oil.) (Courtesy of Rose Raskin, Purdue University.)

Cyniclomyces guttulatus (formerly *Saccharomycopsis guttulata*) is part of the normal flora of some rodents and lagomorphs (rabbits, guinea pigs, and chinchillas) (Zierdt, 1988). Occasionally, a low number of individual or doublet *Cyniclomyces* may be observed as an incidental finding in canine feces and are thought to represent a nonpathogenic result of coprophagia (Fig. 8-5). However, there is uncertainty about whether this yeast is entirely nonpathogenic in dogs. A few preliminary research or anecdotal reports have associated

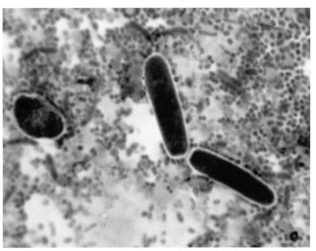

■ **FIGURE 8-5. Yeast.** An abnormal bacterial flora, containing numerous diplococci, is present on a pale basophilic background that contains a small amount of irregularly shaped, refractile, amber material and a single incidental, extracellular fecal yeast (left) and two *Cyniclomyces guttulatus* organisms. (Wright-Giemsa; HP oil.)

this yeast with clinical cases of chronic diarrhea (Houwers and Blankenstein, 2001; Mandigers, 2007; Saito et al., 2000). During evaluation of some patients with chronic diarrhea, the only abnormality detected in dry-mount fecal cytology may be the presence of an extremely large number of *Cyniclomyces* both individually and in large mats of numerous budding organisms (Figs. 8-6, 8-7). The observation of many apparently replicating organisms in a fresh fecal sample may represent a factor contributing to the ongoing diarrhea or may simply represent abnormal flora due to underlying disease, physiologic processes, or prior antimicrobial treatments. At this time, the pathogenicity of this yeast is unproven, though it is occasionally observed in

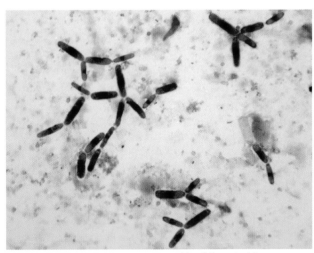

■ **FIGURE 8-6. Yeast. Dog.** Several budding *Cyniclomyces guttulatus* organisms observed in the feces of a dog with chronic diarrhea. (Wright-Giemsa; IP.)

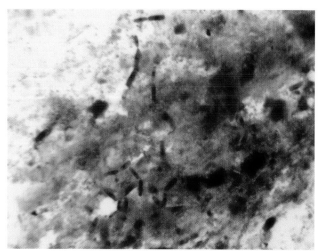

■ **FIGURE 8-7. Yeast.** Large mat of budding *Cyniclomyces guttulatus* associated with amorphous grey-brown ingesta and squamous epithelial cells. (Wright-Giemsa; IP.)

large number in the feces of dogs with chronic diarrhea; in such cases, this observation should be reported as an abnormal finding.

It is common to see a variable amount of irregularly shaped, colorless or amber material and green-blue material with parallel cell walls, representing digesta and ingested plant matter, respectively (Fig. 8-8). The background also commonly contains a variable amount of amorphous basophilic material consistent with mucus. The amount of mucus observed depends on whether the underlying disease is associated with rectal oversecretion of mucus and whether the sampling method is more representative of the rectal mucosa or the rectal lumen. Being more representative of the rectal mucosa, samples obtained by rectal saline lavage or rectal scraping may contain more mucus than samples collected by other means.

Well-differentiated epithelial cells, including squamous or low columnar epithelial cells, may be present in variable numbers depending on sample collection method and underlying disease (Figs. 8-9, 8-10). With atraumatic sample collection methods, low numbers of well-differentiated epithelial cells may be present individually or in small sheets. With more invasive collection methods that may abrade the mucosa (i.e., rectal scrape or catheterization for saline lavage), the numbers of epithelial cells are expected to be increased and the sheets of cells will likely be larger. In a sample that has been collected atraumatically, observation of a large number of epithelial cells in large, multicellular sheets should not be considered normal and

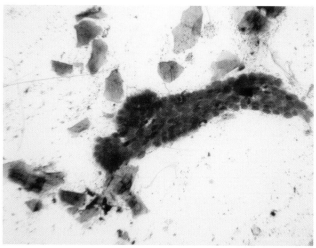

■ **FIGURE 8-9. Rectal epithelium.** A single large, tightly cohesive, multicellular sheet of low columnar epithelial cells is present in a rectal scrape direct smear, surrounded by a few individualized anucleate, keratinized squamous epithelial cells and scant streaming nuclear material from lysed cells. (Wright-Giemsa; IP.)

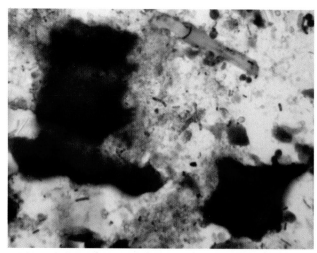

■ **FIGURE 8-8. Plant material.** Green-blue ingested plant matter with parallel cell walls is commonly seen in canine and feline fecal smears. (Wright-Giemsa; HP oil.)

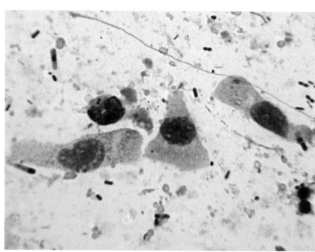

■ **FIGURE 8-10. Columnar epithelium.** A single small lymphocyte (left) is present in the fecal smear of a dog with diarrhea along with three well-differentiated low columnar epithelial cells on a pale basophilic background that contains a pleomorphic bacterial population comprised predominantly of small bacilli. (Wright-Giemsa; HP oil.)

should raise concern for underlying mucosal pathology with sloughing of apical epithelial cells.

ABNORMAL MICROSCOPIC FINDINGS

Abnormal Flora

Overgrowth of microorganisms typically is a secondary, nonspecific finding associated with other underlying diseases, recent enteric surgical procedures, abnormal physiologic processes, or recent antimicrobial administration; however, microbial overgrowth may exacerbate underlying pathology. Primary overgrowth can uncommonly be the primary cause of gastrointestinal disease. There is no way to distinguish between secondary or primary microbial overgrowth using dry-mount fecal cytology, which may reveal the presence of a bacterial population that consists of monomorphic or oligomorphic bacilli, an increased number of cocci, or an increased number of yeast (e.g., *Candida, Cyniclomyces*) (Figs. 8-5, 8-11, 8-12, 8-13, 8-14, 8-15).

Fecal Leukocytes

The presence of fecal neutrophils should be considered an abnormal finding that suggests distal colitis or proctitis (Figs. 8-11, 8-16). Fecal neutrophils should prompt diagnostic consideration of causes of bacterial enteritis, such as salmonellosis, clostridial colitis, enteric colibacillosis, campylobacteriosis, and infection by other invasive or enterotoxigenic bacteria (Broussard, 2003). Other considerations for fecal neutrophils include whipworm infestation, which is usually associated with hemorrhagic, mucoid diarrhea; primary inflammatory bowel disease, which is associated with other infiltrating leukocytes (i.e., lymphoplasmacytic

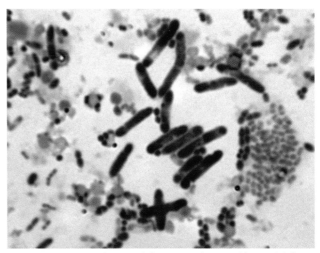

■ **FIGURE 8-12. Abnormal flora.** An abnormal bacterial flora, exhibiting overgrowth of a single large, plump bacillus and an increased number of diplococci, is present on a pale basophilic background. (Wright-Giemsa; HP oil.)

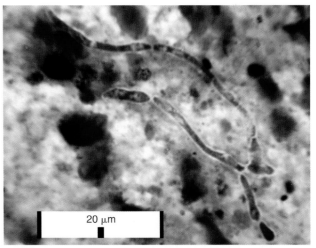

20 μm

■ **FIGURE 8-13. Candidiasis. Dog.** *Candida* pseudohyphae are present in fecal material collected from a dog with chronic gastrointestinal signs after recent exploratory laparotomy. The pale basophilic background, devoid of the usual bacterial flora, contains a moderate amount of incidental irregularly shaped, refractile, amber material and deeply basophilic mucus. (Wright-Giemsa; HP oil.)

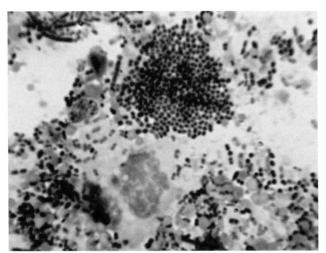

■ **FIGURE 8-11. Abnormal flora.** An abnormal bacterial flora, containing numerous diplococci and a microcolony (top center) of diplococci, is present on a pale basophilic background that contains a small amount of irregularly shaped, refractile, amber material and a single poorly preserved, karyolytic neutrophil. (Wright-Giemsa; HP oil.)

or eosinophilic inflammation); or inflammation associated with primary structural disease associated with inflammation and/or necrosis, such as neoplasia.

Eosinophilic inflammation (see Chapter 7) may be observed with primary inflammatory bowel disease (e.g., eosinophilic gastroenterocolitis or eosinophilic colitis), a condition in which the number of mast cells are also expected to be increased relative to normal animals (Kleinschmidt et al., 2007). Eosinophilic inflammatory bowel disease may occur in dogs or cats of any breed or age; however, it is more common in young adult animals, and the Boxer, Doberman Pinscher, and

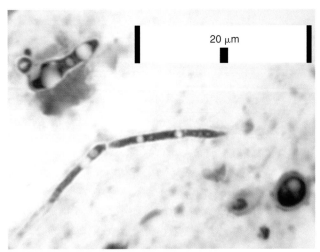

■ **FIGURE 8-14. Candidiasis. Dog.** Same case as in Figure 8-12. *Candida* pseudohyphae and blastospore (dark round structure at lower right) in a fecal smear that is devoid of normal background bacterial flora. (Wright-Giemsa; HP oil.)

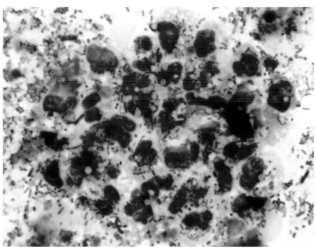

■ **FIGURE 8-16. Neutrophilic inflammation. Dog.** A large aggregate of several neutrophils is present amongst the microbial flora in a dog with diarrhea. (Wright-Giemsa; HP oil.)

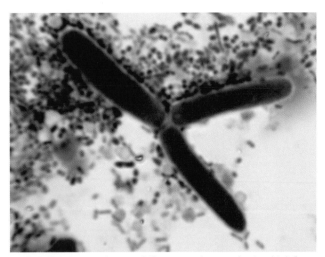

■ **FIGURE 8-15. Abnormal flora.** An abnormal microbial flora, exhibiting reduced bacterial polymorphism, an increased number of diplococci, and numerous budding *Cyniclomyces guttulatus* is present on a pale basophilic background. (Wright-Giemsa; HP oil.)

German Shepherd appear to be predisposed. The diagnosis of eosinophilic inflammatory bowel disease is possible after other causes of eosinophilic inflammation have been excluded (Hall and German, 2005). Eosinophilic inflammation is also likely to be observed as a component of the mixed inflammatory response to certain infections (e.g., fungal, oomycetal, algal, or nematode parasites) or a foreign body. Eosinophils may also infiltrate certain neoplasms (e.g., lymphoma).

Small and intermediate lymphocytes (see Chapter 7) with or without plasma cells may be observed with any cause of chronic inflammation (e.g., infectious) or with primary inflammatory bowel disease (e.g., lymphocytic-plasmacytic enterocolitis or lymphocytic-plasmacytic colitis). Lymphoplasmacytic inflammatory bowel disease typically occurs in older animals with increased incidence in German Shepherds, Chinese Shar-Peis, and

purebred cats. Unique forms of inflammatory bowel disease also affect Basenjis and Soft Coated Wheaten Terriers (Hall and German, 2005). The morphology of neoplastic lymphocytes is similar to those observed in other tissues. However, in cats, lymphocyte morphology may not be useful to distinguish lymphocytic inflammation from feline small cell lymphoma. A full thickness enteric biopsy is needed to confirm the diagnosis (Evans et al., 2006; Kleinschmidt et al., 2006).

Macrophagic inflammation (see Chapter 7) may be observed with various causes of chronic inflammation or with infectious causes of inflammation (e.g., fungal, oomycetal, or algal) with which intracellular microorganisms may be identified. Another specific consideration, given the anatomic location, is histiocytic ulcerative colitis. Histiocytic ulcerative colitis is an inflammatory disease that primarily affects young Boxers and other brachycephalic breeds (e.g., French Bulldogs and Bulldogs) and requires histology for diagnosis. This disease has also rarely been reported in other dog breeds and in cats. The presence of large macrophages that are strongly periodic acid-Schiff–positive is a characteristic of histiocytic ulcerative colitis that is considered a distinctive feature compared to other types of inflammatory bowel disease (German et al., 2000; Hostutler et al., 2004).

Other Nucleated Mammalian Cells

The number of epithelial cells observed in a sample depends on the collection method. In a sample that has been collected atraumatically, observation of a large number of epithelial cells in multicellular sheets should raise concern for underlying mucosal pathology with sloughing of apical epithelial cells (Fig. 8-17). If inflammation is absent, epithelial cells should be cytologically well differentiated. Criteria for assessment of atypia in epithelial cells are similar to those in other tissues; inflammation can induce a hyperplastic response associated with cytoplasmic and/or nuclear

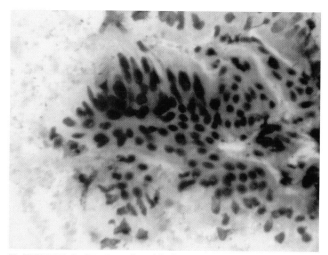

■ **FIGURE 8-17. Rectal epithelium via traumatic scraping. Dog.** A very large, tightly cohesive, multicellular sheet of low columnar epithelial cells is present in the rectal scrape of a dog with chronic diarrhea. A few *Cyniclomyces guttulatus* organisms that stain pale basophilic are also visible in the left portion of the image. (Wright-Giemsa; IP.)

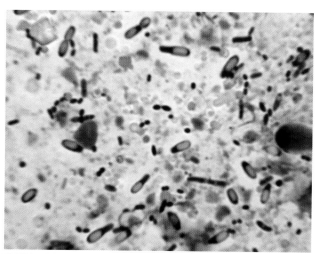

■ **FIGURE 8-18. Sporulating bacilli. Dog.** An increased number of spore-forming bacilli (>5 per 100× objective field) are present in the feces of a dog with diarrhea. These bacilli may either be *Bacillus* spp. or *Clostridium* spp. Individualized spores are visible along with the sporulated bacilli, which, in this field, often contain a terminally located spore that renders a tennis racket–like appearance. When the spores are centrally located, sporulated bacilli may have a safety pin–like appearance. (Wright-Giemsa; HP oil.)

changes that can be cytologically indistinguishable from those observed with neoplasia. In such cases, histopathology may provide definitive diagnosis. In samples obtained by rectal scrape, other neoplastic cell types may also be observed, such as those from lymphoma, mast cell tumor, or gastrointestinal mesenchymal tumor (see Chapter 7).

Potential Microbial Pathogens

In addition to the microbial flora that is expected in feces, potential pathogens may also be present. In some instances, definitive cytologic diagnosis of infectious disease underlying a patient's gastrointestinal signs is possible (e.g., fungal, algal, oomycetal, or protozoal). However, by dry-mount fecal cytology alone, pathogenic bacteria are morphologically indistinguishable from nonpathogens that may be incidentally observed. For bacterial culture of feces, unique sample collection, handling, and culture conditions are essential for enteric pathogen detection (Broussard, 2003).

Spore-forming bacteria can be an incidental finding in feces (Figs. 8-18, 8-19, 8-20). There are typically no more than 5 spore-forming bacteria per 100× objective field. An increased number of spores can be observed in dogs with diarrhea. However, a direct cause-effect relationship remains arguable. There is a poor correlation between the number of fecal spores per 100× objective field and the detection of *Clostridium perfringens* enterotoxin (Broussard, 2003). There are a few potential explanations for this poor correlation. *Clostridia* spp. are not the only bacteria that sporulate; common soil *Bacillus* spp. are also large sporulating bacilli. Not all sporulated *Clostridia* spp. produce *Clostridium perfringens* enterotoxin (Broussard, 2003). Sporulating bacteria may form spores during a delay in sample processing. Also, quantitative culture has revealed

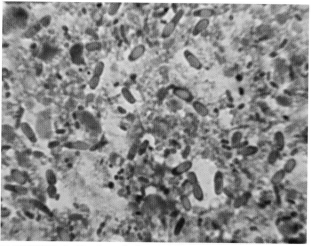

■ **FIGURE 8-19. Sporulating bacilli. Dog.** Same case as in Figure 8-18. Malachite green is a microbiologic stain used to identify the presence of bacterial spores such as *Bacillus* spp. or *Clostridium* spp. Steam is included in the staining process to permeabilize the hard, dehydrated, multilamellar spore walls. A pink safranin counterstain is used to distinguish the spores. (Malachite green/Safranin; HP oil.)

that up to 75% of normal dogs harbor *C. perfringens* without detectable fecal *Clostridium perfringens* enterotoxin (Broussard, 2003). The current recommendation is that greater than 5 spore-forming bacteria per 100× objective field is considered an abnormal finding. Finding fecal neutrophils and/or a positive ELISA for *C. perfringens* or *C. difficile* enterotoxins further supports bacteria-induced diarrhea (Broussard, 2003).

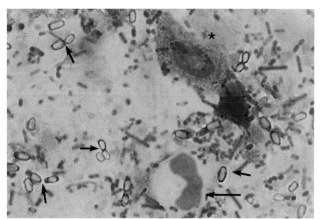

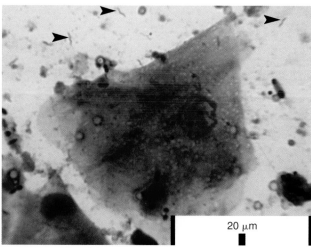

■ **FIGURE 8-20. Clostridial colitis. Fecal smear.** Numerous neutrophils were present upon scanning of this direct fecal smear. An increased number of large, rod-shaped bacterial endospores with a clear center and an increased density predominantly on one end ("safety pin" appearance) are the notable feature *(short arrows)*. The bacterial morphology is consistent with *Clostridium perfringens*. Occasional organisms can normally be seen but greater than 5 organisms per 100× oil field is considered abnormal. (Twedt, 1992) Confirmation was made by measurement of the enterotoxin in the feces. (Twedt, 1992; Marks et al., 1999) A degenerate neutrophil *(long arrow)* and epithelial cell *(asterisk)* are present. (Wright; HP oil.) (Courtesy of Denny Meyer and Dave Twedt, Purdue University.)

Pleomorphic fecal bacteria that exhibit gull-wing and spiral morphology on dry-mount fecal cytology include treponeme-like bacteria, *Serpulina* spp., *Helicobacter* spp., *Anaerobiospirillum* spp., and *Campylobacter* spp. (Figs. 8-21, 8-22, 8-23, 8-24, 8-25). It is unusual to observe pleomorphic gull-wing and spiral-shaped

■ **FIGURE 8-22. Campylobacteriosis. Dog.** Same case as in Figure 8-21. A few miniscule, pleomorphic, gull wing–shaped bacteria *(arrowheads)* are seen near a pigmented, squamous epithelial cell. (Wright-Giemsa; HP oil.)

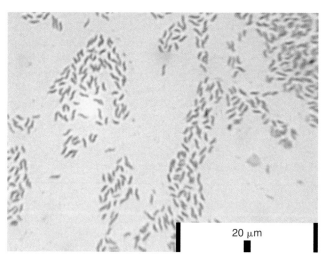

■ **FIGURE 8-23. Campylobacteriosis. Dog.** Same case as in Figure 8-21. Gram stain of *Campylobacter* spp. cultured from the feces indicate the bacteria are gram-negative bacilli. (Gram stain; HP oil.)

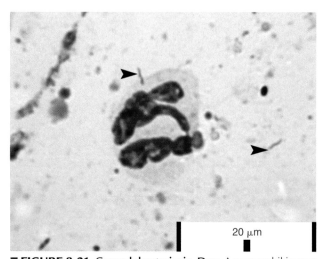

■ **FIGURE 8-21. Campylobacteriosis. Dog.** A neutrophil is seen along with two miniscule, pleomorphic, gull wing–shaped bacteria *(arrowheads)* in a fecal smear from a dog with diarrhea and *Campylobacter* spp. isolated by bacterial culture. The bacteria observed in this fecal smear from a dog with confirmed *Campylobacter* infection are much smaller than those observed in Figures 8-24 and 8-25. (Wright-Giemsa; HP oil.)

bacteria in routine dry-mount fecal cytology and should be reported as an abnormal finding when observed in large numbers. These organisms are quite small (0.5 to 1.0 μm × 5 to 10 μm) and can be easily overlooked during microscopic examination particularly when these organisms are present in low numbers. The likelihood of observing these microorganisms is enhanced by high-power–magnification examination of areas of the preparation that contain a lesser amount of background flora, such as very thin areas of the preparation or areas of the preparation that are mucus-rich since these microorganisms localize to the mucus-rich mucosal surface. Diarrhea has been associated with fecal isolation of bacteria from all of these genera except for the treponeme-like bacteria, and bacteria from all of these genera have also been isolated from the feces of

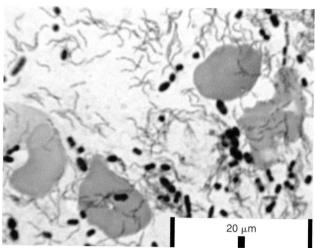

■ **FIGURE 8-24. Spiriliform bacteria. Dog.** Numerous fine, pleomorphic gull wing–shaped and spiriliform fecal bacteria consistent with *Serpulina* spp. are a bit larger than those shown in Figures 8-21 through 8-23. The dog presented with chronic mucoid diarrhea. The large number of spiriliform bacteria in this sample may reflect the mucoid nature of the diarrhea since bacteria with this morphology are found in large numbers within mucoid gastrointestinal tract secretions (Wright-Giemsa; HP oil.).

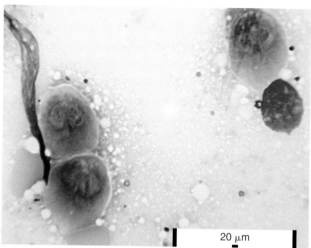

■ **FIGURE 8-26. Giardiasis. Dog.** *Giardia* trophozoites are shown from the feces of a dog with diarrhea. These flagellate protozoan organisms are pyriform with two apical nuclei. It is uncommon to diagnose *Giardia* using dry-mount fecal cytology. *Giardia* trophozoites may be more easily identified in fecal wet-mounts, although care should be taken to distinguish them from trichomonads, which have a single nucleus, prominent central axostyle, and an undulating membrane. As opposed to *Giardia* cysts, trophozoites that are fecally shed are labile and rapidly die after elimination. *Giardia* cysts are usually not detected by dry-mount fecal cytology; fecal flotation is usually required for this purpose. (Wright-Giemsa; HP oil.)

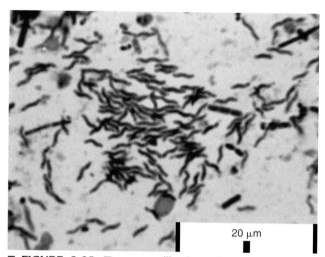

■ **FIGURE 8-25. Treponeme-like bacteria. Dog.** Numerous darkly stained, spiriliform fecal bacteria that exhibit several complete convolutions are seen in the fecal smear of a dog with diarrhea. These bacteria are larger than those shown in Figures 8-21 through 8-23. Examination of a fecal wet-mount may be useful to more conclusively identify these as a nonpathogenic treponeme-like bacterium, which exhibits very rapid forward motility in the fluid medium (Broussard, 2003). (Wright-Giemsa; HP oil.)

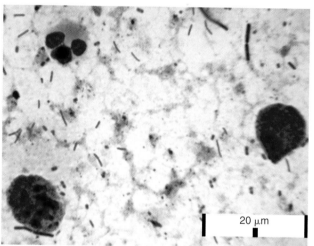

■ **FIGURE 8-27. Entamoebiosis. Dog.** Two *Entamoeba histolytica* protozoal organisms are present along with a single neutrophil (upper left corner) in the feces of a dog with diarrhea. (Wright-Giemsa; HP oil.). (Courtesy of A. Rick Alleman, University of Florida.)

asymptomatic dogs and cats (Bender et al., 2005; Broussard, 2003; De Cock et al., 2004; Malnick et al., 1990; Misawa et al., 2002; Rossi et al., 2008). Concurrent observation of fecal neutrophils would support a bacterial cause of the diarrhea.

Fungal, pseudofungal (algal, oomycetal), or protozoal infections are occasionally diagnosed (Figs. 8-26, 8-27, 8-28, 8-29) using dry-mount fecal cytology (Graves et al., 2005)

or rectal scrape (Chapman et al., 2009). Nonsporulated endospores of the algae *Prototheca* may appear morphologically similar to incidentally observed, round or oval, extracellular fecal yeast described previously (see Figs. 8-2, 8-3, 8-4, 8-5). Incidental yeast should not be observed intracellularly within macrophages, whereas *Prototheca* should be observed both intracellularly within macrophages (Fig. 8-30) and extracellularly.

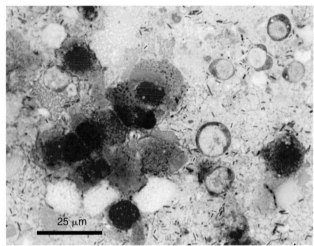

■ **FIGURE 8-28. Blastocystosis. Rectal scraping. Dog.** Several organisms and well-differentiated epithelial cells are present in a background of mixed bacteria in a rectal scrape from a dog with diarrhea. The intestinal organism is most consistent with *Blastocystis* spp, an algal-like protist (stramenopile). The binucleated forms support this identification, rather than *Iodamoeba bütschlii,* which can look similar. (Aqueous-based Wright; HP oil.) (Courtesy of Craig Thompson, Purdue University.)

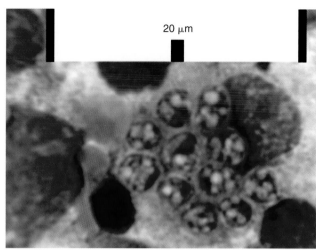

■ **FIGURE 8-30. Protothecosis. Dog.** Several nonendosporulated *Prototheca* are seen intracellularly within a macrophage in the rectal scrape of a dog with diarrhea. When microorganisms with this morphology are observed intracellularly within macrophages concern should be raised for potential *Prototheca* infection. (Wright-Giemsa; HP oil.)

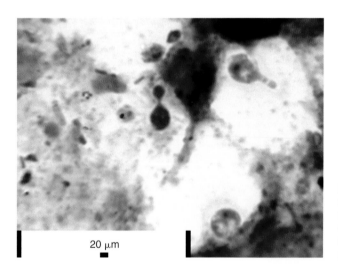

■ **FIGURE 8-29. Cryptococcosis. Dog.** Three budding (top) and one nonbudding (lower right) *Cryptococcus* organisms are present with a few bacilli in the feces of a dog with diarrhea. Most forms of *Cryptococcus* develop a thick, polysaccharide capsule that does not stain and is represented by the wide, colorless area surrounding the narrow-based–budding, purple yeast. (Wright-Giemsa; HP oil.)

REFERENCES

Bender JB, Shulman SA, Averbeck GA, et al: Epidemiologic features of *Campylobacter* infection among cats in the upper Midwestern United States, *J Am Vet Med Assoc* 226(4): 544-547, 2005.

Broussard JD: Optimal fecal assessment, *Clin Tech Small Anim Pract* 18(4):218-230, 2003.

Chapman S, Thompson C, Wilcox A, et al: What is your diagnosis? Rectal scraping from a dog with diarrhea, *Vet Clin Pathol* 38(1):59-62, 2009.

De Cock HE, Marks SL, Stacy BA, et al: Ileocolitis associated with *Anaerobiospirillum* in cats, *J Clin Microbiol* 42(6): 2752-2758, 2004.

Evans SE, Bonczynski JJ, Broussard JD, et al: Comparison of endoscopic and full-thickness biopsy specimens for diagnosis of inflammatory bowel disease and alimentary tract lymphoma in cats, *J Am Vet Med Assoc* 229(9):1447-1450, 2006.

German AJ, Hall EJ, Kelly DF, et al: An immunohistochemical study of histiocytic ulcerative colitis in boxer dogs, *J Comp Pathol* 122(2-3):163-175, 2000.

Graves TK, Barger AM, Adams B, et al: Diagnosis of systemic cryptococcosis by fecal cytology in a dog, *Vet Clin Pathol* 34:409-412, 2005.

Hall EJ, German AJ: Diseases of the small intestine. In: Ettinger SJ, Feldman EC, (eds): *Textbook of veterinary internal medicine*, ed 6, St. Louis, Saunders, 2005, pp 1367-1373.

Hostutler RA, Luria BJ, Johnson SE, et al: Antibiotic-responsive histiocytic ulcerative colitis in 9 dogs, *J Vet Intern Med* 18(4):499-504, 2004.

Houwers DJ, Blankenstein B: *Cyniclomyces guttulatus* and diarrhea in dogs, *Tijdschr Diergeneeskd* 126(14-15):502, 2001.

Kleinschmidt S, Meneses F, Nolte I, et al: Retrospective study on the diagnostic value of full-thickness biopsies from the stomach and intestines of dogs with chronic gastrointestinal disease symptoms, *Vet Pathol* 43(6):1000-1003, 2006.

Kleinschmidt S, Meneses F, Nolte I, et al: Characterization of mast cell numbers and subtypes in biopsies from the gastrointestinal tract of dogs with lymphocytic-plasmacytic or eosinophilic gastroenterocolitis, *Vet Immunol Immunopathol* 120(3-4):80-92, 2007.

Malnick H, Williams K, Phil-Ebosie J, et al: Description of a medium for isolating *Anaerobiospirillum* spp., a possible cause of zoonotic disease, from diarrheal feces and blood of humans and use of the medium in a survey of human, canine, and feline feces, *J Clin Microbiol* 28(6):1380-1384, 1990.

Mandigers PJ: *Cyniclomyces guttulatus,* a differential diagnosis in chronic diarrhea (poster). In *Proceedings 17th ECVIM-CA Congress and 9th ESVCP Congress,* September 2007:Poster 1.

Marks SL, Melli A, Kass PH, et al: Evaluation of methods to diagnose *Clostridium perfringens*-associated diarrhea in dogs, *J Am Vet Med Assoc* 214:357-360, 1999.

Misawa N, Kawashima K, Kondo F, et al: Isolation and characterization of *Campylobacter, Helicobacter,* and *Anaerobiospirillum* strains from a puppy with bloody diarrhea, *Vet Microbiol* 87(4):353-364, 2002.

Rossi M, Hänninen ML, Revez J, et al: Occurrence and species level diagnostics of *Campylobacter* spp., enteric *Helicobacter* spp. and *Anaerobiospirillum* spp. in healthy and diarrheic dogs and cats, *Vet Microbiol* 129(3-4):304-314, 2008.

Saito K, Saito H, Watanabe T, et al: *Cyniclomyces guttulatus:* it can now be clearly observed in canine feces. In *2000/9/2 Second Board of Veterinary Practitioners Proceedings of Japan* 245-246. Available at *http://www33.ocn.ne.jp/~saitoahohp/Cyniclomyces.htm.* Accessed May 23, 2008.

Twedt DC: Clostridium perfringens-associated enterotoxicosis in dogs. In Kirk RW, Bonagura JD (eds): *Current veterinary therapy XI-small animal practice,* WB Saunders, Philadelphia, 1992, pp 602-607.

Zierdt CH, Detlefson C, Muller J, et al: *Cyniclomyces guttulatus (Saccharomycopsis guttulata)*-culture, ultrastructure and physiology, *Antonie Van Leeuwenhoek* 54(4):357-366, 1988.

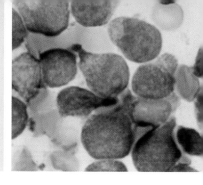

CHAPTER 9

The Liver

Denny J. Meyer

The microscopic examination of hepatic cytology is diagnostically rewarding when applied judiciously. Although fine-needle aspiration biopsy (FNAB) of the liver is practical and economical, it has defined (limited) diagnostic utility and its cavalier use can result in incomplete or inaccurate information. The information cytologically derived from a needle aspirate is often projected to equate with a histologic-based diagnosis (Roth, 2001). For inflammatory liver disease this is often an erroneous assumption since tissue architecture cannot be assessed and histopathologic findings cannot be quantified. These are critical elements for the microscopic assessment of the hepatic pathology (Ishak, 1994; Meyer, 1996). The ultrasonographic examination of the liver has added another dimension of potential "abnormal" findings that contribute to the complexities of working up patients with abnormal liver tests. It has facilitated the "guided" acquisition of cytologic specimens from focal lesions that can be either diagnostic (e.g., metastatic neoplasia) or descriptively nonspecific (e.g., vacuolar change) (Wang et al., 2004). The objective of this chapter is to suggest areas of hepatic pathology for which the cytologic interpretation of a FNAB can be diagnostic (Stockhaus et al., 2004) and to provide histologic comparators that illustrate the limitations of hepatic FNAB as well as provide differential considerations for the descriptive cytologic findings.

SAMPLING THE LIVER

Indications and Contraindications

Hepatic cytology is valuable for the initial evaluation of hepatomegaly. Causes of hepatomegaly include feline hepatic lipidosis syndrome, lymphoma, myeloproliferative neoplasia, mast cell neoplasia, hepatocellular carcinoma, corticosteroid hepatopathy, and amyloidosis. In addition, primary and metastatic neoplasia or a focal infection, identified with ultrasound examination, usually can be further characterized with cytology. However, it is not possible to differentiate benign, focal inflammatory pathology from "chronic" progressive disease or accurately

assess the extent of its pathology. It is not possible to make a definitive cytologic diagnosis of nodular regenerative hyperplasia or differentiate its relatively benign inflammatory reaction and hepatocellular cytoplasmic changes from other diseases that cause similar hepatic pathology. For these types of hepatic pathology, histologic examination is required for determining severity, providing a prognosis (e.g., identify bridging necrosis, bridging fibrosis), and directing (and monitor) therapy.

Abnormal hemostasis is a potential contraindication for FNAB of the liver. Since FNAB utilizes either a "capillary" or suction sampling technique, cutting or laceration of the vascular tissue is a relatively lesser risk compared to the use of a cutting needle or wedge biopsy procedure. If one or more of the coagulation tests are abnormal, their temporary correction often can be attained within 12 hours by the subcutaneous administration of vitamin K_1. A reduced platelet count is a greater concern. A value less than 20,000/µl is a contraindication and the sampling procedure should be preceded by the administration of platelet-rich plasma. A platelet count value between 20,000 to 50,000/µl is a relative contraindication. Depending on the underlying pathology, the sampling procedure can be performed knowing that there is an inherent risk factor with careful monitoring of the patient for 24 hours. Prior to any sampling procedure of a vascular organ, notably liver and spleen, the integrity of platelet function should be assessed. The von Willebrand factor concentration should be measured in breeds at risk (e.g., Doberman Pinscher, Airedale Terrier, German Shepherd Dog, Golden Retriever) and the history should ascertain if drugs have been recently administered that alter platelet function (e.g., nonsteroidal antiinflammatory drugs, synthetic penicillins, cephalosporins).

A large cavitational lesion identified by ultrasound examination in an older dog, notably male German Shepherd Dogs and Golden Retrievers, is a relative contraindication for FNAB. The probability of a hemangiosarcoma is high, obtaining a definitive cytologic diagnosis is unlikely, and the potential of rupturing a necrotic capsule is a possibility. The spleen should be examined with ultrasound since hepatic metastasis is common. Exploratory surgery should be considered as both a diagnostic and treatment option.

Tumor seeding undoubtedly occurs but the frequency has not been determined (Evans et al., 1987; Navarro et al., 1998; Ishii et al., 1998). However, since treatment options are often limited and long-term survival usually has a poor prognosis, the use of FNAB as a diagnostic tool is a reasonable risk noting the aforementioned caveat pertaining to cavitational lesions.

Technique

Sampling the liver is performed with the patient standing on a nonslippery (e.g., rubber-matted) surface, lying with the right lateral side down, or in dorsal recumbency together with imaging assistance. The need for chemical restraint depends on the disposition of the patient. Since the liver moves with the excursions of the diaphragm, the needle is directed generally in a craniodorsad direction to reduce the risk of laceration. Choice of needle size ranges from 1 to 2½ inch 20 to 22 gauge depending on the indication and on size of animal. A longer needle is probably of greater value when attempting to sample a focal lesion in a liver that is not enlarged. If a 2½-inch needle is used, the stylet is left in place until the liver is entered to reduce contamination from skin and mesenteric fat as it is penetrated. A 6- to 12-ml syringe can be attached directly to the needle or via an intravenous infusion extension tube to facilitate greater manipulative flexibility if a suction technique is used (see below).

For hepatomegaly, the site of needle entry into the abdominal cavity is at the "triangle" formed by the union of xiphoid and last left rib. Once the needle is within the hepatic parenchyma of the left lobe, it is directed in two or three different planes using a to-and-fro motion. Acquisition of the specimen can be obtained by either aspiration or by nonaspiration ("capillary" action) procedures (see Chapter 1). Generally, the nonaspiration approach should be tried first since it reduces the amount of blood contamination. If the specimen is nondiagnostic, the aspiration technique can be attempted. After collection of the specimen, the tip of the needle is placed over a glass slide and the contents expelled using a syringe filled with several cubic centimeters of air. Often multiple slide preparations can be made from a single sampling procedure by use of the compression method (see Chapter 1). The cytologic slide preparations are air-dried, fixed, and stained. Protection from formalin fumes is critical to preserve morphologic detail (no open formalin containers can be in the room prior to fixation and staining). At least one unfixed cytologic slide preparation should be saved for potential special stains such as a Gram, copper, iron, Congo red, or immunocytochemical stain.

Occasionally, the gallbladder or large bile duct is penetrated as evidenced by yellow to green to dark-green fluid in the syringe. Aspiration should be continued until no more fluid is obtained. As long as the biliary tissue is healthy, it will heal without side effects, although it is prudent to closely observe the patient for 24 hours for signs of peritonitis. Feeding a small amount of food or the oral administration of corn oil 30 minutes prior to FNAB has been suggested as means of contracting the gallbladder and reducing the risk of penetration. While there is probably no downside, the unpredictability of the canine gallbladder's response to meal-stimulated contraction (Rothuizen et al., 1990) makes the procedure more reassuring for the operator than helpful to the patient in most cases. Light-yellow, acellular fluid also can be obtained from cystic lesions, which are especially prominent in cats. These would have been identified as cavitational lesions with ultrasonography and are probably congenital. Obtaining clear to whitish mucinous fluid from a cavitational lesion is suggestive of a cystadenoma.

NORMAL LIVER AND GALLBLADDER

Hepatocytes constitute the predominant cell type of a normal liver (Fig. 9-1A&B). They are slightly oval to polygonal plump cells 25 to 30 μm in diameter (approximately 3 to 4 erythrocyte diameters). They contain a centrally placed, round to slightly oval nucleus composed of a coarse network of chromatin and a nucleolus that may be prominent. The nucleus is surrounded by abundant, moderately bluish to basophilic cytoplasm that is often granular appearing and punctuated by granular, pinkish hues because of the varying tinctorial properties of the different organelles. Hepatocytes appear to increase in size and number of nuclei per cell in older dogs (Stockhaus et al., 2002). An occasional mast cell is a normal finding within the hepatic parenchyma (Fig. 9-1C). Neutrophils are more frequent in young and older dogs than middle-aged dogs (Stockhaus et al., 2002). Rectangular nuclear crystalloid inclusions (Fig. 9-2) are noted in clinically healthy dogs of all ages with an unknown clinical significance. Dense clumps of biliary epithelial cells can be observed occasionally (Stockhaus et al., 2002). The dense collection of their basilar nuclei give the cells a cuboidal shape (Fig. 9-3A). Larger bile ducts including the common bile duct are lined by ciliated columnar cells (Fig. 9-3B–D). Bile fluid from the gallbladder appears dark green grossly but a shiny golden-,yellow as an unstained smear on a glass slide. With Romanowsky staining the fluid smear appears basophilic and microscopically displays a blue-gray finely granular appearance (Fig 9-3E) that is often referred to as "white bile." Fluid from the gallbladder or common bile duct has been shown to be mucinous in the dog (Owens et al., 2003). Other cells observed during the sampling procedure of the liver are sheets of mesothelial cells that can be mistaken for biliary epithelium or a neoplastic cell population (Fig. 9-4A&B).

NON-NEOPLASTIC DISEASES AND DISORDERS

Nuclear Changes

A nuclear inclusion that is more likely to be observed in chronic liver disease appears as a hollow, globule-like structure (Fig. 9-5A). It represents a membrane-bound cytoplasmic invagination that contains glycogen and mitochondria (Stalker and Hayes, 2007). This should not

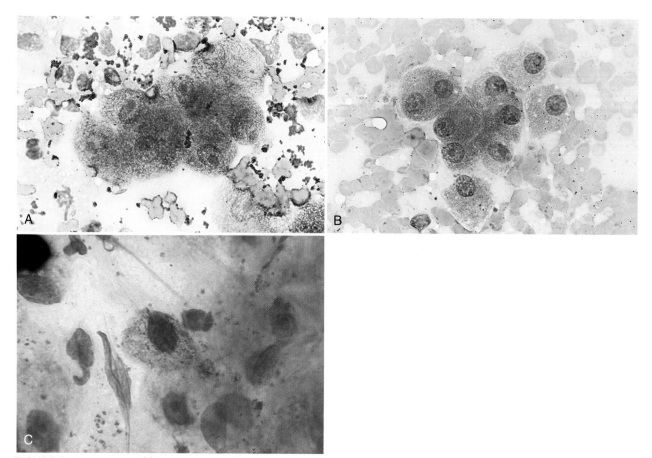

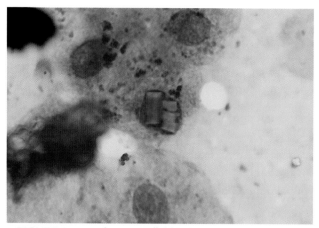

■ **FIGURE 9-1. A-B, Normal hepatocytes. A,** Clumps of greenish-stained erythrocytes and small, irregular clumps of metachromatic-stained gel used for ultrasound examination surround this island of hepatocytes. (Wright-Giemsa; HP oil.) **B,** An occasional binucleated hepatocyte (lower left of center) is a normal finding. (Wright-Giemsa; HP oil.) **C, Hepatic mast cell.** An occasional mast cell is a normal finding. The granules often do not stain intensively. (Wright-Giemsa; HP oil.) Contrast this image to an example of a hepatic mast cell neoplasia (Figures 9-30A&B).

■ **FIGURE 9-2. Nuclear crystalloid inclusion.** One or two crystal-like, rectangular structures are occasionally observed in the nuclei of hepatocytes; an incidental finding of no known diagnostic importance. The cytoplasm contains bluish to bluish black pigment consistent with lipofuscin. (Wright-Giemsa; HP oil.)

be mistaken for a viral inclusion. Canine adenovirus 1 infection produces viral inclusions (Fig. 9-5B&C) that appear as large, magenta, homogenous structures of various sizes in dogs with infectious canine hepatitis. There is associated hepatocellular necrosis and nuclear swelling causing a pale rim around the inclusion and chromatin margination producing the appearance of a thickened nuclear membrane.

Cytoplasmic Changes

Hepatocellular cytoplasmic changes are common in association with metabolic disease and secondary to injury. Discrete small (microvesicular) or large (macrovesicular) vacuoles in the hepatocyte are representative of lipid that has been cleared during the staining process (Fig. 9-6A–E). Excess accumulation of lipid in the liver is referred to as *lipidosis, fatty liver,* or *steatosis.* The feline hepatic lipidosis syndrome is the most common disease associated with this cytoplasmic alteration. One drop of oil red O and one drop of new methylene blue placed together on an unfixed cytologic specimen along with a coverslip helps define the presence of lipid as the stain is readily taken up by lipoid substances (Fig. 9-6F). An

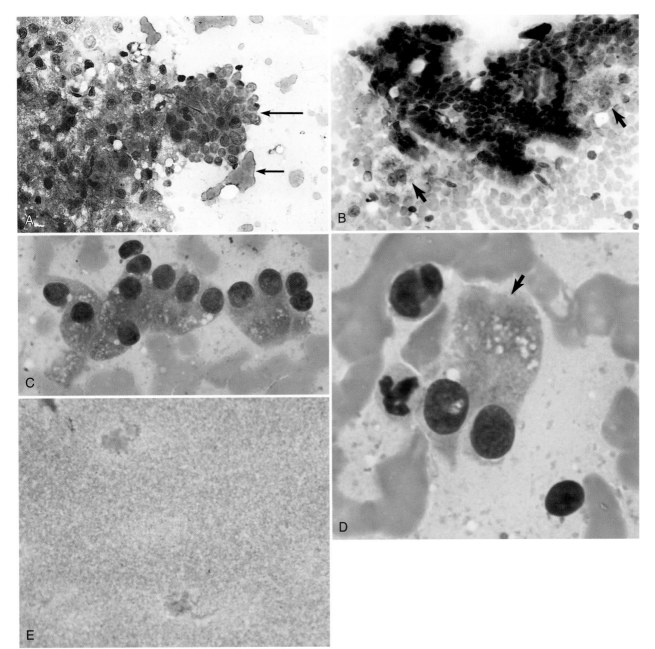

■ **FIGURE 9-3. A-D, Biliary epithelium. A,** A dense cluster of biliary epithelial cells *(long arrow)* is present to the right of a sheet of hepatocytes. The biliary epithelial cells have a scant rim of lightly stained cytoplasm that often appears "invisible." Note that the round nuclei, composed of dense, granular to homogeneous chromatin, are relatively uniform and slightly larger than the nucleus of a hepatocyte. Clumps of greenish-stained erythrocytes are also present *(short arrow)*. (Wright-Giemsa; IP.) **B, Aspirate. Dog.** Dense tubular collections of normal biliary ductal cells are present along with several large pale-staining hepatocytes *(arrows)*. (Wright; IP.) **Same case C-D. C, Imprint. Dog.** A row of columnar epithelium with vacuolated and finely granulated cytoplasm from a case of chronic active hepatitis with thickened gallbladder. Note the basilar location of the nuclei. (Wright; HP oil.) **D,** Two biliary duct cells display a ciliated brush border *(arrow)*. (Wright; HP oil.) **E, Normal bile fluid. Cat.** This aspirated gallbladder fluid was dark green with a protein of 12.8 g/dl. Note the finely granular to amorphous character of mucinous bile that stains blue-gray. (Wright; HP oil.) (B-E, Courtesy of Rose Raskin, Purdue University.)

underlying disease such as cancer and pancreatitis (identified with ultrasound examination and/or feline specific lipase) should be considered before classifying the lipidosis as idiopathic (Ferreri, 2003). Congenital lipid storage diseases are a cause of hepatomegaly in young animals due to diffuse hepatocyte vacuolar change

(Brown et al., 1994) (Fig. 9-7A&B). Aspiration of mesenteric fat during the collection process is an artifact that can cause a potential misdiagnosis (Fig. 9-8).

Hepatocellular cytoplasmic rarefaction (lesser cytoplasmic density than normal) that does not form discrete

Text continued on p. 232

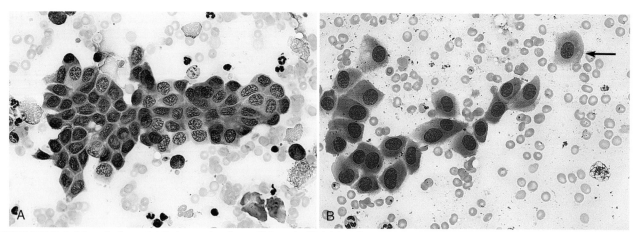

■ **FIGURE 9-4. Mesothelium. A,** Their angular shape (fish scale–like) identifies a sheet of mesothelial cells, probably scraped off during the sampling procedure. They should not be mistaken for a metastatic neoplasm. Note that the cell size approximates that of the hepatocyte. Brownish-stained erythrocytes surround the sheet of cells. (Wright-Giemsa; HP oil.) **B,** A discrete mesothelial cell *(arrow)* has an oval appearance that is punctuated by a pinkish "sunburst" effect at the cytoplasmic border. The cell is reminiscent of plasma cell and, along with the eccentric location of the nuclei of other cell constituents, collectively may be mistaken for a plasma cell tumor. Greenish-stained erythrocytes surround the mesothelial cells. (Wright-Giemsa; HP oil.)

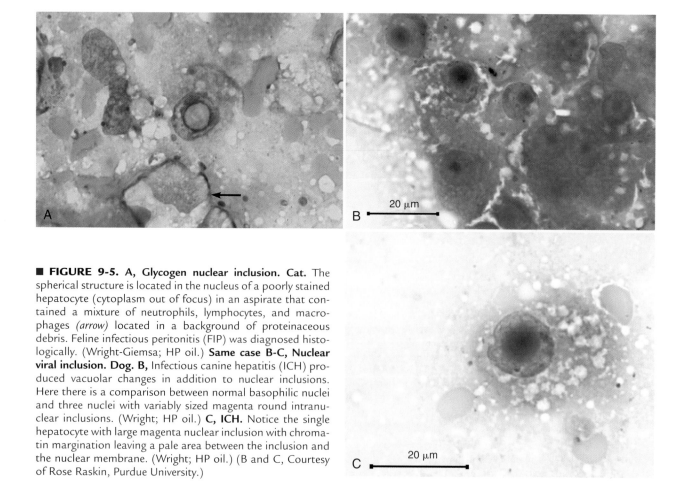

■ **FIGURE 9-5. A, Glycogen nuclear inclusion. Cat.** The spherical structure is located in the nucleus of a poorly stained hepatocyte (cytoplasm out of focus) in an aspirate that contained a mixture of neutrophils, lymphocytes, and macrophages *(arrow)* located in a background of proteinaceous debris. Feline infectious peritonitis (FIP) was diagnosed histologically. (Wright-Giemsa; HP oil.) **Same case B-C, Nuclear viral inclusion. Dog. B,** Infectious canine hepatitis (ICH) produced vacuolar changes in addition to nuclear inclusions. Here there is a comparison between normal basophilic nuclei and three nuclei with variably sized magenta round intranuclear inclusions. (Wright; HP oil.) **C, ICH.** Notice the single hepatocyte with large magenta nuclear inclusion with chromatin margination leaving a pale area between the inclusion and the nuclear membrane. (Wright; HP oil.) (B and C, Courtesy of Rose Raskin, Purdue University.)

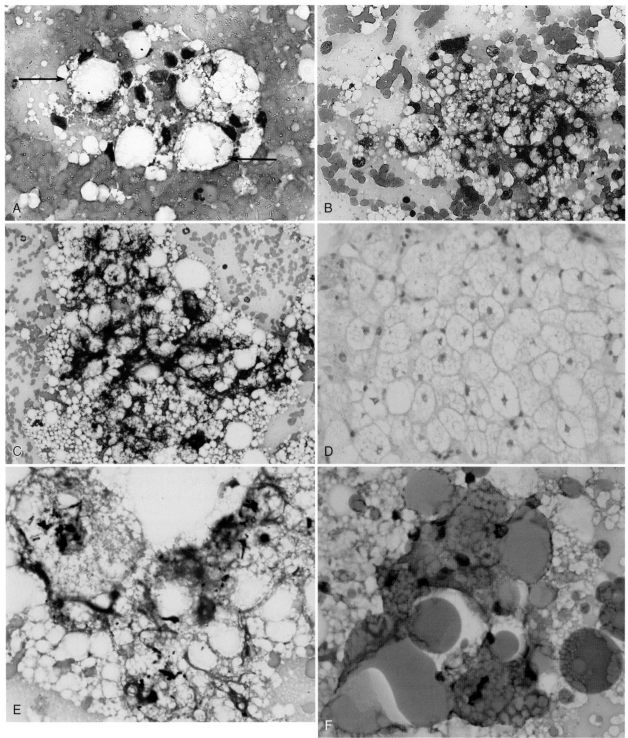

■ **FIGURE 9-6. Lipidosis. Cat. A,** A hepatic aspirate from an icteric 5-year-old cat with a markedly raised serum ALP value and hepatomegaly. The cytoplasm of the hepatocytes is markedly distended by large, clear vacuoles (macrovesicular) that cause nuclear margination or a "signet ring" appearance *(arrows)* and make the hepatocyte difficult to recognize. (Wright-Giemsa; IP.) **B,** Sometimes the hepatocellular cytoplasm is distended by small, variably sized vacuoles (microvesicular). Both cytomorphologic findings of fatty change are consistent with a diagnosis of the feline hepatic lipidosis syndrome. (Wright-Giemsa; IP.) **C,** Another example of feline hepatic lipidosis. Highly vacuolated cells are poorly distinguishable as hepatocytes. (Wright-Giemsa; IP.) **Same case D-F. D,** Tissue section demonstrates the highly vacuolated appearance of hepatocytes in an advanced stage of lipidosis. (H&E; IP.) **E,** Notice the dark pigmented material in the hepatocytes with both microvesicular and macrovesicular vacuolation. (Wright; HP oil.) **F,** The joint application of new methylene blue and oil-red O (ORO) demonstrates stained nuclei and lipoid substances, respectively. Lipids with an affinity for the dye present within microvesicular vacuoles stain dull orange compared with the large free droplets of ORO that stain brightly orange. (NMB/ORO; IP.) (C, Courtesy of Dave Edwards, University of Tennessee. D-F, Courtesy of Rose Raskin, Purdue University.)

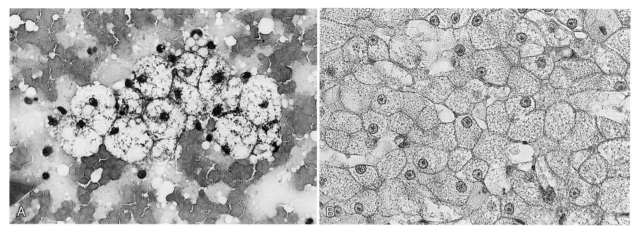

■ **FIGURE 9-7. A, Microvesicular vacuolation. Dog.** Fine-droplet (microvesicular) lipidosis in an aspirate from a puppy with hepatomegaly and ascites is suggestive of a lipid storage disease. (Wright-Giemsa; IP.) **B, Lipid storage disease. Cat.** Note the cytologic features observed in A are similar to a histologic specimen from a kitten with documented lipid storage disease—Niemann-Pick disease type C. (H&E; IP.) (B, Tissue section courtesy of Diane Brown Colorado State University.)

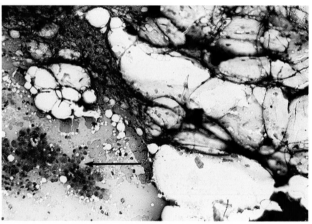

■ **FIGURE 9-8. Mesenteric fat.** Occasionally mesenteric fat is aspirated, which could be confused with hepatic lipidosis. Comparison to a clump of hepatocytes *(arrow)* is helpful in providing a perspective of the much larger size of the mesenteric adipocyte. (Wright-Giemsa; LP.)

vacuoles can be caused by increased glycogen or water content and may occur in both dogs and cats. The latter type of histomorphologic change is also referred to as *hydropic (ballooning) degeneration.* The term *vacuolation* is often used as a nonspecific rubric for cytoplasmic rarefaction. The increased storage of glycogen that occurs in association with either hyperadrenocorticism causing hypercortisolemia or the administration of exogenous corticosteroids is a common cause of hepatocellular cytoplasmic rarefaction in the canine liver (Fig. 9-9A–C) and rarely in cats (Schaer and Ginn, 1999). The unique, robust nature of the canine hepatocyte to store glycogen in response to hypercortisolemia can be sufficiently dramatic to result in generalized hepatomegaly. The volume of the hepatocyte can be increased up to three-fold by excess glycogen accumulation (Kuhlenschmidt et al., 1991). Hepatocytes with excess glycogen are swollen, retain a centrally located nucleus, and lack discrete cytoplasmic vacuoles typically associated with lipid accumulation. A

periodic acid-Schiff (PAS) staining method, with and without amylase (diastase) digestion, is used to distinguish cytoplasmic glycogen from mucin. Glycogen in the hepatocytes is removed by diastase treatment giving a negative reaction to PAS while neutral mucin will be resistant to digestion and thus remain PAS-positive. When hyperadrenocorticism and treatment with glucocorticoid medications have been eliminated as causes of the "vacuolar hepatopathy," a search for an underlying disease is warranted (Sepesy et al., 2006). Various types of hepatocellular injury such as toxic insults and hypoxia will alter the integrity of the cell membrane and cytoplasmic organelles, resulting in increased cellular water content. As a consequence, cytoplasmic rarefaction (hydropic degeneration) is observed morphologically and cannot always be confidently distinguished from the cytoplasmic change associated with increased cytoplasmic glycogen (Fig. 9-10A–C). In aged dogs, hepatic nodular regenerative hyperplasia is common. The number of nodules ranges from a few to many, and they are often composed of hepatocytes with cytoplasmic rarefaction and/or vacuolation (Stalker and Hayes, 2007) (Fig. 9-11A&B).

Pigments

The common types of pigment encountered in hepatocytes are lipofuscin, bile, hemosiderin, and copper. Ceroid pigment is often observed in macrophages. Examples are denoted in Table 9-1. A recent study (Scott and Buriko, 2005) demonstrated through histochemical methods that the green granules found commonly on cytology within canine and feline hepatocytes were not bile pigment as previously suspected but rather lipofuscin.

Lipofuscin is the most common pigment observed in hepatocytes and cytologically appears as small bluish-green to greenish-black granules within the cytoplasm (see Fig 9-2). Histologically, lipofuscin has a yellowish-brown color with H&E and is often located in cytoplasm near bile canaliculi in the centrilobular region. It represents lysosomes filled with indigestible lipid-containing

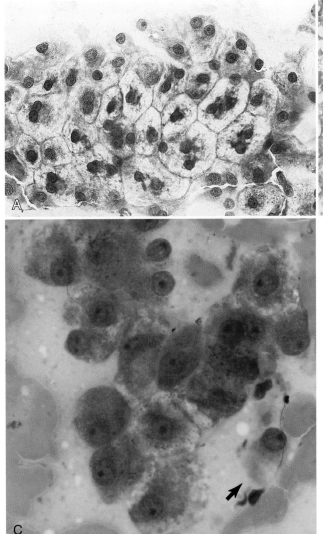

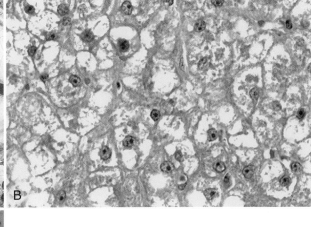

■ **FIGURE 9-9. A-B, Glycogen deposition hepatopathy. Dog.** Uniform sheet of hepatocytes with cytoplasmic rarefaction ("vacuolar change") from a dog with hepatomegaly, markedly raised serum ALP activity, and normal serum bilirubin concentration. The finding is consistent with corticosteroid-induced excess glycogen storage (hepatopathy). (Wright-Giemsa; IP.) **B,** Note the similarities to a histologic specimen from another dog with corticosteroid-induced hepatopathy. (H&E; IP.) **C, Cytoplasmic rarefaction. Imprint. Dog.** Hepatocytes display peripheral cytoplasmic rarefaction in this suspected case of chronic active hepatitis. Note the single columnar biliary cell *(arrow)*. (Wright; HP oil.) (C, Courtesy of Rose Raskin, Purdue University.)

residues. It accumulates as a normal aging product of cell breakdown and is commonly referred to as "wear and tear" pigment. Lipofuscin pigment exhibits autofluorescence when an unfixed specimen is examined under ultraviolet light and stains with the Schmorl ferric-ferricyanide reduction stain and Long Ziehl-Neelsen stain for lipids.

Bile appears as dark greenish-blue to dark bluish-black, variably sized granules. Histologically, the color can range from yellow to yellowish-brown to green with H&E. Bile stains with Hall's stain and van Gieson's method. Retention of bile pigment, referred to as cholestasis, is a consequence of liver pathology resulting in hepatocellular or canalicular accumulation (Fig. 9-12A&B).

Hemosiderin is an insoluble, iron-containing protein produced by the phagocytic digestion of hematin. Hepatic hemosiderin accumulation can be associated with hemolytic disease, prior transfusion, and congenital portosystemic shunts. Cytologically, the color of the variably sized granules or dense clumps of granules ranges from golden brown to bluish-black to black (Fig. 9-13A&B). Histologically, the granules are refractile and have a

golden brown color with H&E. A Prussian blue stain stains the granules dark blue (Fig. 9-13C).

Copper appears cytologically as coarse, variably sized, refractile light bluish-green granules; a crystal-like appearance (Fig. 9-14A). Histologically, copper granules have a bluish-grey to grey appearance with H&E. Rubeanic acid stains the granules bluish-green to greenish-black cytologically (Fig. 9-14B) and a bright reddish-orange color histologically. Copper accumulation may be a cause of liver pathology in certain breeds or may be a consequence of cholestasis.

Ceroid is a pigment that is rich in oxidized lipids and mostly found in macrophages after hepatocellular injury. The granular pigment, which may appear in clumps, has a golden-brown to greenish-yellow color cytologically and golden-brown to brown color with H&E staining. Compared with lipofuscin, which represents a later, more advanced form of oxidized lipid, ceroid appears as an early form of oxidized lipid that stains positive with the Long Ziehl-Neelsen stain method. Although it also exhibits autofluorescence, it does not stain with Schmorl ferric-ferricyanide reduction stain.

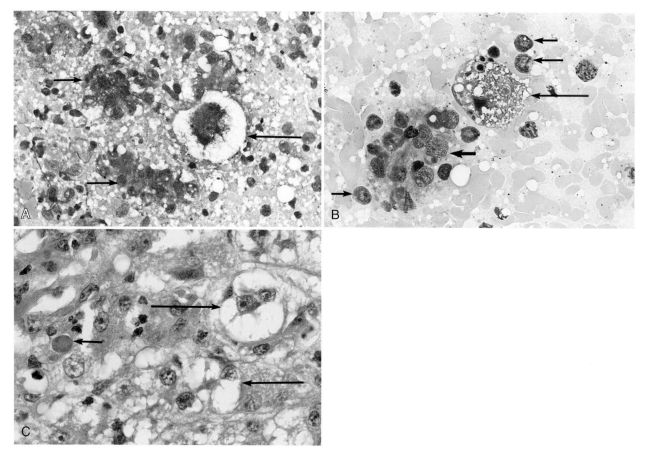

■ **FIGURE 9-10. A-B, Hydropic degeneration. A,** One markedly swollen binucleate hepatocyte demonstrates hydropic (ballooning) degeneration *(long arrow)*. Other hepatocytes *(short arrows)* show less cytoplasmic alteration or appear morphologically normal. Also present are a moderate number of inflammatory cells (difficult to recognize as lymphocytes and neutrophils) surrounded by a bluish-gray background ("dirty appearance"), which is suggestive of necrotic debris. (Wright-Giemsa; IP.) **B,** In another field a hepatocyte is undergoing degeneration, as illustrated by nuclear condensation and fragmentation within a granular, microvacuolated cytoplasm *(long arrow)*. The appearance of its cytoplasm is similar to the "necrotic" background material seen in A. A few inflammatory lymphocytes are in close proximity *(short arrows)*. A small clump of hepatocytes *(thick arrow)* demonstrates regenerative changes consisting of mild anisocytosis and anisokaryosis. The findings along with moderately raised serum ALT and AST activities, mild rise in the serum bilirubin concentration, and only a slight rise in the serum ALP value support a morphologic diagnosis of acute liver injury (hepatitis) (e.g., toxin, drug-induced). (Wright-Giemsa; HP oil.) **C, Ballooning degeneration.** Note histomorphologic similarities to a specimen from a dog with acute liver injury from carprofen administration. Swollen hepatocytes due to ballooning degeneration *(long arrows)* are admixed with lesser affected hepatocytes. A dense-staining eosinophilic structure *(short arrow)* represents a hepatocyte undergoing apoptotic necrosis. (H&E; HP oil.)

Neutrophilic, Lymphocytic, and Mixed Cell Inflammation

The assessment of hepatic inflammation by FNAB often provides an incomplete picture of the pathology because of an inability to evaluate the lobular architecture and assess the magnitude of the inflammatory changes. Confounding factors that are problematic for obtaining diagnostically useful information include the common occurrence of reactive neutrophilic and lymphocytic infiltrates that are associated with the relatively benign condition of nodular regenerative hyperplasia in dogs. Marked blood contamination in a hepatic FNAB from a dog or cat with a high neutrophil count or a cat with a mildly raised lymphocyte count can foster an ambivalent cytologic interpretation.

Neutrophilic or suppurative inflammation is suggested when a high concentration of segmented neutrophils is observed relative to the red blood cell numbers. Finding

neutrophils intimately associated with or within hepatocellular clumps is further supportive evidence. The neutrophils and surrounding tissue should be carefully examined for infectious agents (Fig. 9-15A&B). The anatomic location of the neutrophilic infiltration in the lobule cannot be determined cytologically, precluding differentiation between primarily parenchymal inflammation (hepatitis) versus primarily inflammation of the bile ducts (cholangitis) (Fig. 9-15C&D). Linking the morphologic assessment with the biochemical findings can be of value, especially in the dog. Finding a serum alkaline phosphatase (ALP) value markedly higher than the serum alanine aminotransferase (ALT) value is supportive of cholangitis/cholangiohepatitis, especially if the serum bilirubin concentration is also raised. This generalization of course does not apply to the differential diagnosis of

Text continued on p. 238

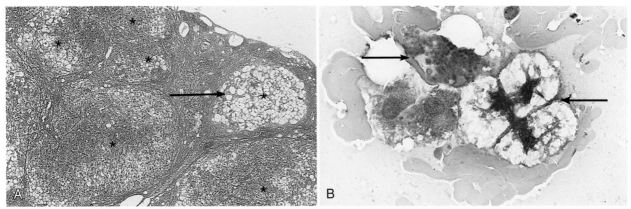

■ **FIGURE 9-11. Nodular regeneration with vacuolar change. Dog. A,** Six nodules of varying size *(asterisks)* can be seen in this wedge biopsy specimen from a clinically healthy 12-year-old mixed-breed dog with mildly raised serum liver enzyme values and numerous hepatic nodules observed at surgery. Note the dramatic variation in hepatocyte morphology among the nodules. If the nodule located to the upper right *(arrow)* was examined cytologically or histologically from a needle biopsy, the findings would be consistent with "vacuolar hepatopathy," suggestive of a metabolic disease. (Gordon & Sweets reticulin; LP.) **B,** Cytologic specimen obtained shows hepatocytes with morphologic characteristics that range from near normal to marked cytoplasmic rarefaction *(long arrow).* A dense clump of platelets *(short arrow)* is a common artifact and should not be confused with a multinucleated cell or infectious agents. (Wright-Giemsa; HP oil.)

TABLE 9-1 Identification of Liver Cell Pigments*

	Lipofuscin	Copper	Hemosiderin	Bile	Ceroid
Cytologic Appearance (Wright)	Bluish-green to greenish-black	Crystal-like, refractile bluish-green to pale blue gray	Golden brown to dark bluish-black	Dark greenish blue Dark bluish-black†	Golden-brown to greenish-yellow
Histologic Appearance (H&E)	Yellowish brown to dark brown	Pale gray to grayish brown	Golden brown	Yellowish-brown Yellow Green	Brown to golden-brown
Cytochemical Stains	Long Ziehl-Neelsen + Schmorl reaction+	Rubeanic acid Orcein method	Prussian blue	Hall van Gieson's method	Long Ziehl-Neelsen + Schmorl reaction −
Interpretation	Normal aging	Abundant amount with chronic hepatitis	Hemolytic anemia Portosystemic shunt Recent transfusion	Cholestasis	Hepatocellular injury
Examples	Fig. 9-2 Fig. 9-19B	Fig. 9-14A Fig. 9-14B	Fig. 9-13A Fig. 9-13B Fig. 9-13C	Fig. 9-12A Fig. 9-12B	Fig. 9-20B

*All pigments are typically located in the cytoplasm of hepatocytes except ceroid, which is mostly located in macrophages. Hemosiderin also may be observed in macrophages (Figure 9-13A).
†Extracellular bile which accumulates in canaliculi appears black (Figure 9-12A&B).

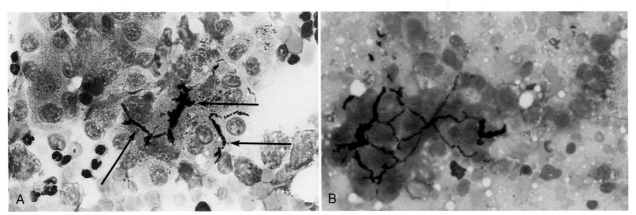

■ **FIGURE 9-12. Bile retention. Dog. A,** In some areas, cholestasis is indicated by black ribbons of inspissated bile that form casts of the biliary canaliculi that course along the surface of hepatocytes *(arrows).* Within some hepatocytes is a fine granular dark material considered to be bile. (Wright-Giemsa; HP oil.) **B,** Marked cholestasis is present in a case of histiocytic sarcoma (formerly termed malignant histiocytosis) (Wright; IP.) (B, Courtesy of Rose Raskin, Purdue University.)

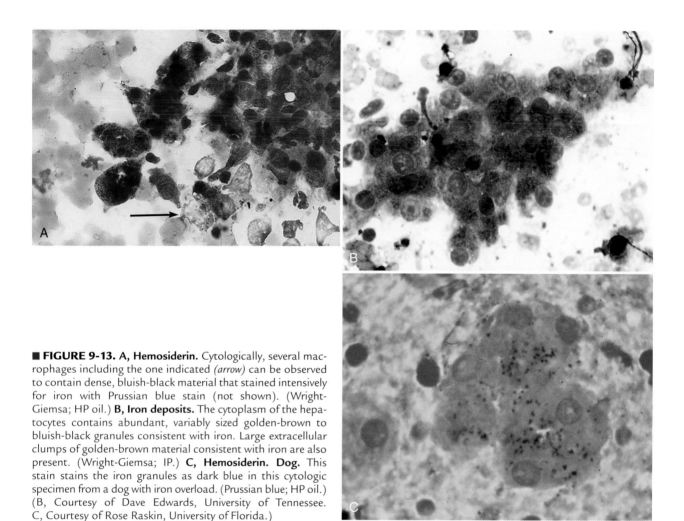

■ **FIGURE 9-13. A, Hemosiderin.** Cytologically, several macrophages including the one indicated *(arrow)* can be observed to contain dense, bluish-black material that stained intensively for iron with Prussian blue stain (not shown). (Wright-Giemsa; HP oil.) **B, Iron deposits.** The cytoplasm of the hepatocytes contains abundant, variably sized golden-brown to bluish-black granules consistent with iron. Large extracellular clumps of golden-brown material consistent with iron are also present. (Wright-Giemsa; IP.) **C, Hemosiderin. Dog.** This stain stains the iron granules as dark blue in this cytologic specimen from a dog with iron overload. (Prussian blue; HP oil.) (B, Courtesy of Dave Edwards, University of Tennessee. C, Courtesy of Rose Raskin, University of Florida.)

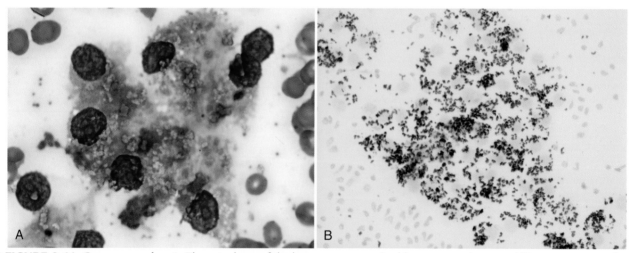

■ **FIGURE 9-14. Copper granules. A,** The cytoplasm of the hepatocytes contains blue-grey angular crystal-like structures consistent with copper granules. (Wright-Giemsa; HP oil.) **B,** Copper granules stain black, indicating a positive reaction with rubeanic acid stain. (Rubeanic acid; IP.) (A and B, Courtesy of Dave Edwards, University of Tennessee.)

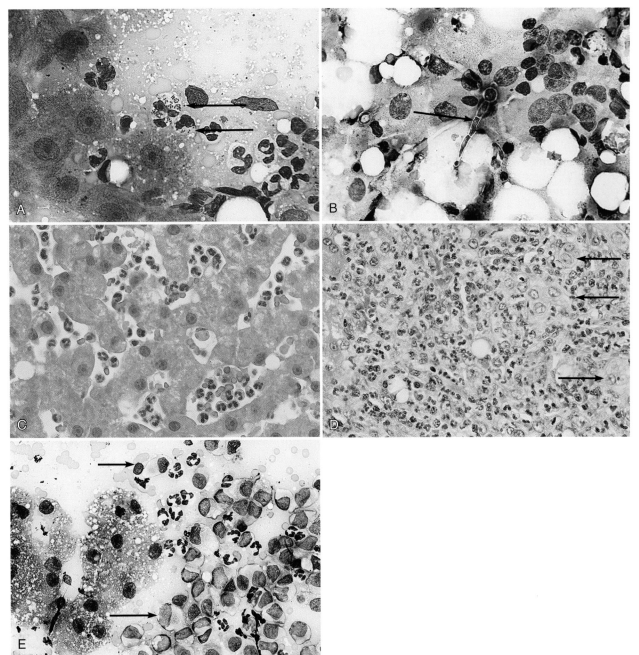

■ **FIGURE 9-15. A, Bacterial suppurative hepatitis. Cat.** The presence of neutrophils intimately associated with hepatocytes is indicative of suppurative hepatitis. Note the paucity of erythrocytes, which indicates that the majority of the neutrophils are not a component of blood contamination. Note two neutrophils packed with bacteria *(arrows)*. This cat also had moderately raised serum ALT and AST values, a slightly raised serum ALP value, a mild rise in the serum bilirubin concentration, and a mild neutrophilia. (Wright-Giemsa; HP oil.) **B, Mycotic hepatitis. Dog.** Neutrophils were prominent in areas (not shown) of this aspirate from a dog with moderately raised liver enzyme tests and hypoechoic foci with ultrasound examination. A mycotic agent *(long arrow)* was discovered after additional searching. A diagnosis of hepatic hyalohyphomycosis, a term applied to opportunistic infections caused by nondematiacious fungi with hyaline hyphal elements as the basic tissue form, was subsequently made based on the culture of *Paecilomyces* species from tissue obtained at surgery. (Wright-Giemsa; HP oil.) **C-D, Suppurative hepatitis. Cat.** Contrast the following histologic findings in two icteric cats with moderately raised serum liver enzyme values. The neutrophilic inflammation **(C)** primarily involves the parenchyma (sinusoidal leukostasis, suppurative hepatitis) versus **(D)** primarily bile duct inflammation (suppurative cholangitis/cholangiohepatitis). The inflammation in **(C)** was secondary to acute pancreatitis that was presumptively diagnosed by ultrasonography, while severe enteritis diagnosed with biopsy was associated with the cholangitis/cholangiohepatitis. Arrows in **(D)** identify bile ductular epithelial cells. (H&E; HP oil, IP, respectively.) **E, Mixed cell inflammation. Cat.** Neutrophils and histiocytes may be a prominent component of the mixed cell inflammation in cats with FIP involving the liver. This touch imprint is from one of several small white foci on the surface of the liver. The histiocytes are the large mononuclear cells (compare to the size of the neutrophils) with oval to reniform nuclei composed of bland homogenous chromatin surrounded by a moderate amount of bluish-gray cytoplasm *(long arrows)*. A lesser number of small mononuclear cells (lymphocytes) are admixed *(short arrows)*. Similar lesions were located on the kidney and in the mesentery in this case of noneffusive feline infectious peritonitis confirmed histologically. (Wright-Giemsa; IP.)

the feline lipidosis syndrome, primarily a hepatocellular disease, in which the serum ALP activity is often dramatically raised in association with hyperbilirubinemia. Neutrophilic inflammation can be a component of either a sterile inflammatory process—e.g., acute pancreatitis (Fig. 9-15C), feline neutrophilic cholangiohepatitis (Fig. 9-15D), feline infectious peritonitis (FIP) (Fig. 9-15E), or septic inflammation (Fig. 9-15A). Sampling a solitary hypoechoic structure in the hepatic parenchyma in association with neutrophilia and/or fever is a relative contraindication and should be approached with caution because of the potential of rupturing an abscess and inducing peritonitis.

The occurrence of a predominantly uniform population of small lymphocytes with or without a few plasma cells in attendance, referred to as *lymphocytic portal hepatitis,* is a common finding in older cats (Fig. 9-16A) (Gagne et al., 1996, 1999; Weiss et al., 1995). The lymphocytic or nonsuppurative inflammation is confined to the portal tract and does not demonstrate piecemeal necrosis (lymphocytic inflammation in the portal tract that streams into surrounding parenchyma and is associated with liver cell necrosis) (Fig. 9-16B). Clinical studies suggest that it may not be associated with any clinical signs, may be associated with a variety of extrahepatic diseases, and may be slowly progressive. The frequency with which the pathology is responsible for illness is not known even when accompanied by raised serum ALT and/or ALP values. The peripheral lymphocyte count is not increased, differentiating it from chronic lymphocytic leukemia with liver involvement. An examination for an extrahepatic disease (e.g., pancreatitis, enteritis, neoplasia) should be thorough before ascribing the illness to primary liver disease. Occasionally the lymphocytic inflammation is dramatic and causes icterus (Fig. 9-16C). This disease usually affects middle-aged dogs and has a breed predilection (Guilford, 1995; Sevelius and Jonsson, 1995). It is not known if the pathology is a more severe form of lymphocytic portal hepatitis or another syndrome. Microscopic examination of a liver biopsy, preferably a wedge biopsy, is the only way to assess the extent of the disease. The cytologic finding of predominantly small lymphocytes is not common in the dog and should be followed by histologic examination for chronic progressive hepatitis (Fig. 9-17A–C). The cytologic evaluation of liver together with Ki-67 immunochemistry can improve the diagnostic accuracy of cytology and rule in or out liver neoplasia (Neumann and Kaup, 2005).

Relatively equal numbers of lymphocytes and neutrophils in a feline liver cytology specimen is suggestive of feline infectious peritonitis or a chronic form of neutrophilic cholangiohepatitis (Fig. 9-18A&B). If the latter is suspected, a search for an extrahepatic disease such as enteritis or pancreatitis is warranted (Weiss et al., 1996). Studies suggest that the syndrome is initially characterized by a prominent neutrophilic inflammation involving bile ducts with periportal necrosis, as shown in Figure 9-15D, followed by the infiltration of a lymphocytic inflammatory component. The etiopathogenesis of the feline neutrophilic cholangiohepatitis syndrome is not known. Clinical

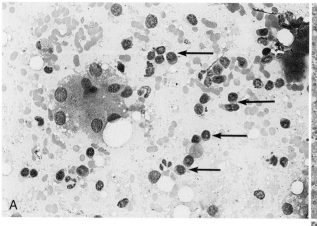

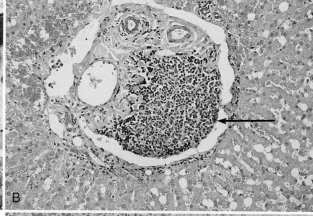

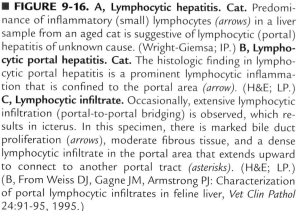

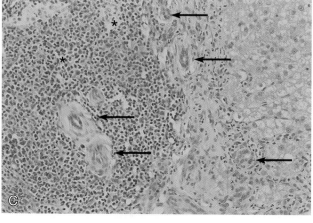

■ **FIGURE 9-16. A, Lymphocytic hepatitis. Cat.** Predominance of inflammatory (small) lymphocytes *(arrows)* in a liver sample from an aged cat is suggestive of lymphocytic (portal) hepatitis of unknown cause. (Wright-Giemsa; IP.) **B, Lymphocytic portal hepatitis. Cat.** The histologic finding in lymphocytic portal hepatitis is a prominent lymphocytic inflammation that is confined to the portal area *(arrow).* (H&E; LP.) **C, Lymphocytic infiltrate.** Occasionally, extensive lymphocytic infiltration (portal-to-portal bridging) is observed, which results in icterus. In this specimen, there is marked bile duct proliferation *(arrows),* moderate fibrous tissue, and a dense lymphocytic infiltrate in the portal area that extends upward to connect to another portal tract *(asterisks).* (H&E; LP.) (B, From Weiss DJ, Gagne JM, Armstrong PJ: Characterization of portal lymphocytic infiltrates in feline liver, *Vet Clin Pathol* 24:91-95, 1995.)

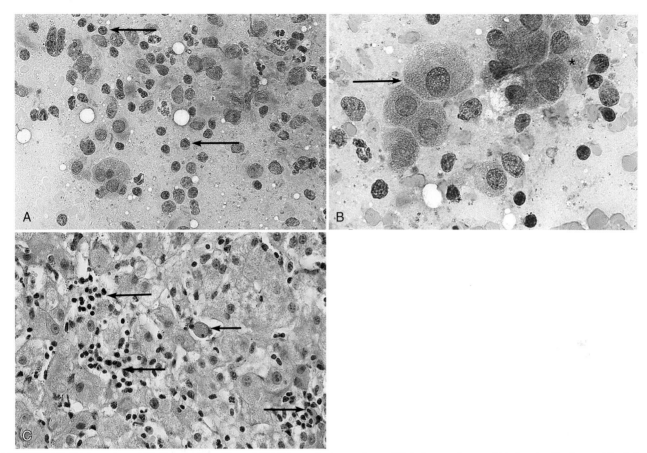

■ **FIGURE 9-17. Lymphocytic inflammation. Dog. A-B,** This cytologic specimen **(A)** is from a 5-year-old Labrador Retriever with clinical lethargy, reduced appetite, and persistent mild to moderate abnormal ALT and AST values documented several times over 6 weeks. Small lymphocytes are the predominant inflammatory cell *(arrows)* and **(B)** are intimately associated with the hepatocytes *(asterisk).* Lesser numbers of neutrophils are also present. The mild to moderate hepatocellular anisocytosis and anisokaryosis *(arrow)* **(B)** are suggestive of a regenerative (or reparative) response. (Wright-Giemsa; IP, HP oil, respectively.) **C,** Microscopic examination of a liver biopsy confirmed the presence of chronic progressive liver disease and defined the extent of the inflammation, bridging necrosis, and fibrotic changes. These are important prognostic criteria that cannot be assessed cytologically. Notable histopathologic findings in this photomicrograph include severe piecemeal necrosis *(long arrows)* (lymphocytes streaming from the portal tracts into the surrounding parenchyma and associated hepatocellular necrosis), increased fibrosis, and apoptotic necrosis *(short arrow).* The dog died of liver failure 7 months later. (H&E; IP.)

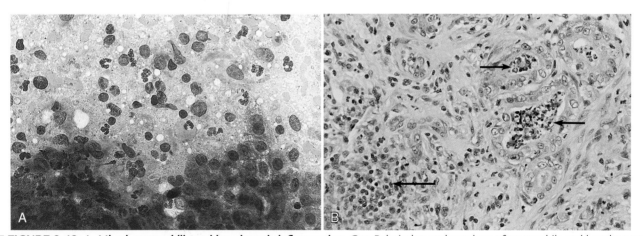

■ **FIGURE 9-18. A, Mixed neutrophilic and lymphocytic inflammation. Cat.** Relatively equal numbers of neutrophils and lymphocytes with occasional histiocytes were observed in this specimen from a cat with moderately raised serum liver enzyme values. Although inflammatory liver disease is identified, the lobular location and the magnitude of the inflammation cannot be determined. (Wright-Giemsa; IP.) **B, Mixed cell inflammation. Cat.** The portal tract is markedly distended by a mixed cell inflammation, bile duct proliferation, and periductal fibrosis. A predominance of lymphocytes is observed in the lower left of center *(long arrow),* while neutrophils invade the bile ducts that contain necrotic debris *(short arrows).* (H&E; IP.) Histology is required to assess the magnitude of the inflammation and degree of fibrosis. The morphologic diagnosis of this specimen is suppurative (neutrophilic) cholangiohepatitis. (B, From Weiss DJ, Gagne JM, Armstrong PJ: Characterization of portal lymphocytic infiltrates in feline liver, *Vet Clin Pathol* 24:91-95, 1995.)

studies suggest that it can be associated with a variety of extrahepatic diseases, notably pancreatitis and inflammatory bowel disease. Mixed cell inflammation (lymphocytes, neutrophils, macrophages) of varying magnitude is a relatively common reaction of the canine liver to both intrahepatic and extrahepatic pathology. In the aged dog, mixed cell inflammation is more likely to be encountered in association with nodular regenerative hyperplasia (see below). If no extrahepatic disease values remain raised on at least three time points over at least 4 weeks, and the patient is clinically ill, histologic examination of preferably a wedge biopsy is required to further characterize the pathology. In both the dog and cat, mixed cell inflammation can be associated with mycotic, protozoal, and mycobacterial infections for which special stains can aid in their recognition. Extra time should be taken to examine the extracellular areas and the cytoplasm of plump macrophages for the presence of these infectious agents. One example is *Cytauxzoon felis* that invades endothelial macrophages which develop into schizonts containing merozoites that infect erythrocytes. Diagnosis in a recently deceased cat is assisted by making imprints of tissues such as the liver, lung, and spleen to identify the presence of the schizont stage (Fig. 9-19). Small numbers of eosinophils may be a constituent of nonspecific mixed inflammatory cell reactions in the dog and cat. A prominent eosinophilic component is observed in cats with the hypereosinophilic syndrome and liver flukes (especially Florida and Hawaii) and in dogs and cats with eosinophilic enteritis (Hendrick, 1981).

Nodular Regenerative Hyperplasia

Nodular regenerative hyperplasia is a common pathology of unknown cause in the older dog, generally older than 8 years of age (Stalker and Hayes, 2007). The number of nodules ranges from a few to too numerous to count and the nodules range in size from microscopic to macroscopic causing distortion of the hepatic surface (see Fig. 9-11A). Their gross color depends on the tissue

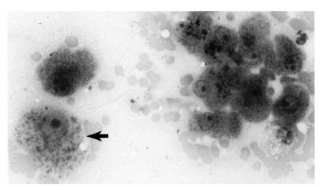

■ **FIGURE 9-19. Cytauxzoonosis schizont. Cat.** This imprint was taken at necropsy of the liver from an infected cat. Several of the hepatocytes contain coarse pigmented granules suggestive of bile or lipofuscin. A single schizont of intermediate stage of maturation is present with developing merozoites (purple granules) within a macrophage *(arrow)*. Note the prominent nucleolus of the infected macrophage. (Wright; IP.) (Courtesy of Rose Raskin, University of Florida.)

constituency—light brown to yellow if the hepatocellular cytoplasm is filled with glycogen or lipid and dark brown if blood is a prominent component. Morphology can vary from nodule to nodule and is probably one of the more common reasons for a histologic diagnosis of "vacuolar hepatopathy" in the aged dog without hyperadrenocorticism or for the administration of corticosteroid medications. In this relatively benign condition, hepatocellular cytoplasmic changes can range from severe rarefaction suggestive of excess glycogen storage or ballooning degeneration to vacuolar change consistent with lipid accumulation foci of lipid-filled and/or pigment-filled macrophages are common (Fig. 9-20A&B; see Fig 9-13A). Inflammatory cells, neutrophils, and lymphocytes of varying magnitude are often attendant to these foci (Fig. 9-20A). Extramedullary hematopoiesis can be found, most often in the compressed portal areas. Granulopoiesis is most common and is composed predominantly of segmented and band neutrophils that could easily be mistaken cytologically for neutrophilic inflammation (Fig. 9-20B). Megakaryocytes are the next most common cell type found in these areas of extramedullary hematopoiesis (Fig. 9-20C). Although hematopoietic precursor cells have been demonstrated in the liver of adult animals (Crosbie et al., 1999), the mechanism responsible for the formation of the extramedullary hematopoietic tissue is not known.

Amyloidosis

Hepatomegaly can be a consequence of the deposition of amyloid A protein (AA amyloid) and is classified as reactive (secondary) amyloidosis. Amyloid A protein is an amino-terminal fragment of an acute-phase reactant protein, serum amyloid A protein (SAA), that is made by hepatocytes in response to macrophage-derived cytokines interleukin-1, interleukin-6, and tumor necrosis factor. This systemic syndrome develops secondary to chronic extrahepatic inflammation (e.g., osteomyelitis), and is a familial disease in the Chinese Shar-Pei dog and Abyssinian cat. The syndrome has also been described in Oriental shorthair and Siamese cats (Loeven, 1994; Zuber, 1993; DiBartola et al., 1986). Cytologically, serpiginous swirls of eosinophilic material are observed in close approximation of hepatocytes (Fig. 9-21A). Histochemical staining with Congo red examined by a polarizing filter to detect birefringence is helpful to diagnose the presence of amyloid (Fig. 9-21B&C).

Extramedullary Hematopoiesis

The adult liver retains its ability to produce hematopoietic cells (Crosbie et al., 1999). The canine liver appears to occasionally develop extramedullary hematopoiesis, notably granulopoiesis, as a nonspecific reaction to chronic hepatic pathology. Late stages of the erythroid series are the predominant cell type in the liver in association with anemia but both granulocytic and megakaryocytic cell types can be observed. As mentioned previously, segmented and band neutrophils along with lesser numbers of megakaryocytes can be observed in the liver of dogs with nodular regenerative hyperplasia

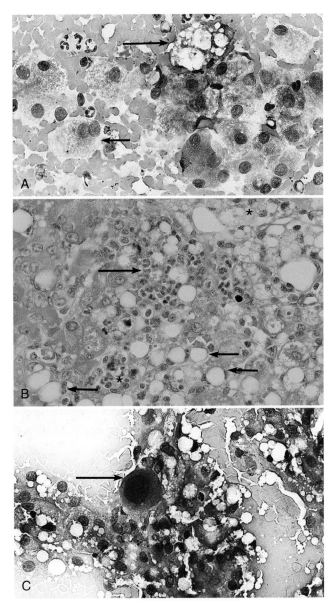

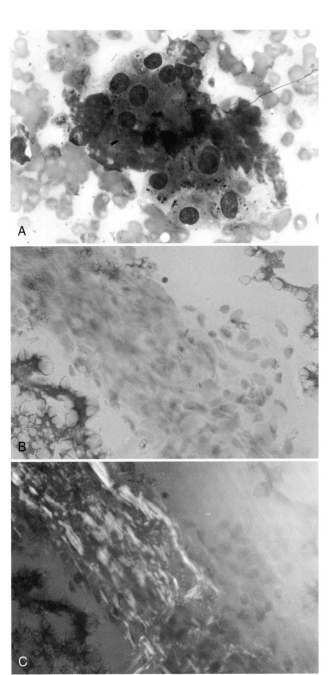

■ **FIGURE 9-20. Nodular regenerative hyperplasia. Dog. A,** This specimen is from an 11-year-old mixed-breed dog with a mildly raised serum ALT value, moderately raised serum ALP value, and variable echogenicity with possible nodules noted by ultrasound. Approximately equal numbers of neutrophils and lymphocytes are scattered amongst the hepatocytes and there is a clump of foamy (vacuolated) macrophages present *(long arrow)*. Hepatocytes show mild cytoplasmic rarefaction and some are binucleated *(short arrow)*. These findings are nonspecific but compatible with nodular regenerative hyperplasia. (Wright-Giemsa; IP.) **B,** Diagnosis was confirmed with a subsequent wedge biopsy. Notable microscopic findings in this specimen include a foci of extramedullary hematopoiesis (granulopoiesis) that is composed of segmented, band, and metamyelocyte neutrophils *(long arrow)*, hypertrophy of hepatic stellate cells (Ito cell, lipocyte, vitamin A-storage cell) *(short arrows)*, and a foci of macrophages filled with golden-brown material consistent with ceroid pigment *(asterisks)*, some of which are vacuolated (upper right) similar to those observed in the cytologic specimen. (H&E; IP.) **C,** Megakaryocyte *(arrow)*, not to be confused with a multinucleated giant cell, is observed in this cytologic specimen from a 10-year-old Labrador Retriever mixed-breed dog with nodular regenerative hyperplasia confirmed histologically. Many of the hepatocytes contain variably sized cytoplasmic vacuoles consistent with lipid. (Wright-Giemsa; IP.)

■ **FIGURE 9-21. A, Hepatic amyloidosis. Dog.** This specimen is from a Chinese Shar Pei dog with hepatomegaly and abnormal liver tests. Amyloid appears as swirls of eosinophilic material which courses between hepatocytes. Hepatocytes have pigmented granules consistent with lipofuscin. (Wright-Giemsa; HP oil.) **B, Amyloidosis.** Amyloid in this cytologic specimen stains an orange-red color. (Congo red; IP.) **C, Amyloidosis.** When a polarizing filter is used with a cytologic specimen stained with Congo red stain, the amyloid material appears birefringent. (Congo red/polarized; IP.) (A-C, Courtesy of Dave Edwards, University of Tennessee.)

(see Fig. 9-20B&C). A predominance of a uniform population of immature hematopoietic precursors is suggestive of neoplastic disease. The cytologic finding of virtually all bone marrow cellular elements along with adipocytes from a nodular hepatic mass is suggestive of a myelolipoma, an uncommon tumor.

NEOPLASIA

Hepatocellular Neoplasia

Hepatocellular-derived neoplasia is more common than neoplasia originating from epithelium of the biliary system in the dog (Straw, 1996; Strombeck and Guilford, 1996). The hepatocellular adenoma (hepatoma) is usually a single mass involving one liver lobe and, because it can be as large as 15 cm, is often first detected as an abdominal mass. It is composed of relatively normal-appearing hepatocytes that can demonstrate mild anisocytosis and anisokaryosis. The differentiation of a hepatic adenoma from nodular regeneration is not possible cytologically and is often problematic histologically. The histologic features of no portal tracts or hepatic venules and relatively sharp demarcation support a histologic diagnosis of hepatic adenoma. It has not been shown to progress to a carcinoma. The hepatocellular carcinoma is also usually a single mass that grossly appears to involve only one liver lobe. It can be composed of relatively normal-appearing hepatocytes or obviously malignant ones (Fig. 9-22A–C). When the cell type is relatively well-differentiated, histologic features of poor demarcation, metastatic islands surrounding the primary, and vascular invasion are required for differentiation from an adenoma and a definitive diagnosis

of malignancy. A paraneoplastic hypoglycemia in association with hepatocellular carcinoma has been attributed to secretion of insulin-like growth factor type II (Zini et al., 2007).

Bile Duct Neoplasia

Cholangiocellular neoplasia, originating from epithelium of the biliary system, is the most common nonhematopoietic hepatic neoplasm in cats (Straw, 1996). It usually does not cause hepatic enlargement. Cytologically, both adenomas and carcinomas are composed of relatively normal-appearing bile duct epithelial cells that exfoliate in small sheets, clusters, or in tubular or acinar formations. In contrast to hepatocytes, these cells tend to be more tightly packed with only a minimal amount of relatively clear cytoplasm. Cholangiocellular adenoma is usually confined to one lobe and is an incidental finding. Cystic formation is common and the size varies from small blister-like accumulations to fluid-filled masses as large as a liver lobe. When aspirated, the fluid can either have a bile-like appearance or a mucinous character. Because the cyst has a thin wall, the large ones are especially prone to rupture. A benign variation, the cystadenoma, is usually multilocular and lined by a mucosa that morphologically resembles

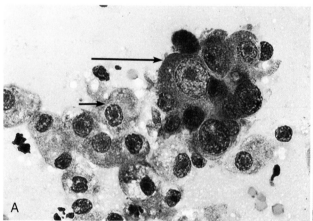
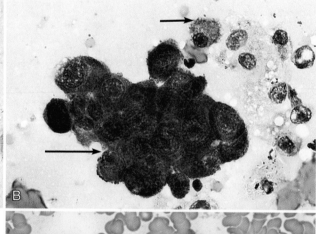
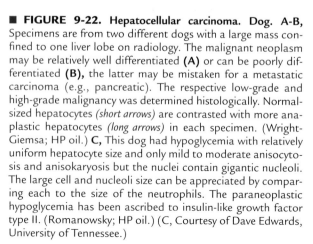
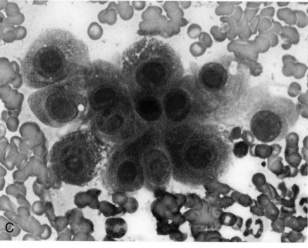

■ **FIGURE 9-22. Hepatocellular carcinoma. Dog. A-B,** Specimens are from two different dogs with a large mass confined to one liver lobe on radiology. The malignant neoplasm may be relatively well differentiated **(A)** or can be poorly differentiated **(B),** the latter may be mistaken for a metastatic carcinoma (e.g., pancreatic). The respective low-grade and high-grade malignancy was determined histologically. Normal-sized hepatocytes *(short arrows)* are contrasted with more anaplastic hepatocytes *(long arrows)* in each specimen. (Wright-Giemsa; HP oil.) **C,** This dog had hypoglycemia with relatively uniform hepatocyte size and only mild to moderate anisocytosis and anisokaryosis but the nuclei contain gigantic nucleoli. The large cell and nucleoli size can be appreciated by comparing each to the size of the neutrophils. The paraneoplastic hypoglycemia has been ascribed to insulin-like growth factor type II. (Romanowsky; HP oil.) (C, Courtesy of Dave Edwards, University of Tennessee.)

biliary epithelium (Fig. 9-23). Histologic examination is required for a definitive diagnosis. Cholangiocellular carcinoma is often multiple to diffuse in appearance, involves all lobes of the liver by the time it is detected, and has an umbilicated appearance at the surface of the liver. Because of its invasiveness, it is most likely to cause clinical disease leading to cytologic examination. The sheets or tubular formations of densely packed epithelial cells usually do not demonstrate dramatic characteristics of malignancy cytologically (Fig. 9-24A&B). Malignancy is implicit when combined with either sonographic or visual evidence of diffuse disease involving all lobes of the liver. Histologic examination is required for a definitive diagnosis.

Hepatic Carcinoid

The hepatic carcinoid is a rare, malignant neuroendocrine tumor in the dog and cat. The solitary tumor arises from enterochromaffin cells located in the biliary system (Fig. 9-25A&B). Note cytological similarity to other neuroendocrine tumors such as carotid body tumor (see Figure 16-9) and pheochromcytoma (see Figure 16-11). A silver stain, e.g., Churukian-Schenck method, is helpful to demonstrate the fine neuroendocrine granules (Fig. 9-25C).

Hepatic Lymphoma and Hematopoietic Neoplasia

Hepatic lymphoma is usually a component of multicentric lymphoma although occasional apparent primary disease has been diagnosed (Twedt and Meyer, personal observation). Uniform hepatomegaly is usually present with all lymphoma types. The diffuse infiltration and noncohesive nature of the cell type affords abundant exfoliation of the immature lymphocyte (Figs. 9-26 and 9-27A&B). Under the recent reclassification

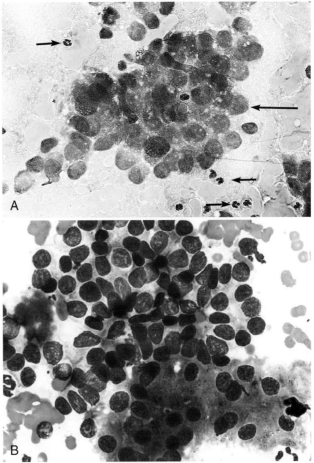

■ **FIGURE 9-24. A, Cholangiocarcinoma. Dog.** This biliary carcinoma appears as a dense aggregate of large epithelial cells with minimal cytoplasm *(long arrow)*. The cells often do not show obvious cytologic criteria of malignancy other than inappropriate large size and overgrowth of neighboring cells. Several neutrophils *(short arrows)* provide a comparative perspective of the abnormally large size of the neoplastic cells and emphasize the importance of defining size relationships with a "cell micrometer" cytologically. Contrast these findings with normal-sized biliary epithelial cells in Figure 9-3A. (Wright-Giemsa; IP.) **B, Biliary carcinoma. Cat.** The neoplastic cells have large nuclei with a scant rim of pale-staining cytoplasm. Despite only demonstrating mild to moderate anisocytosis and anisokaryosis, the abnormally large size is indicative of neoplasia; contrast their inappropriate size to the hepatocytes in the lower part of the specimen. The fine bluish granules in the cytoplasm of the hepatocytes are consistent with lipofuscin pigment. (Romanowsky; HP oil.) (B, Courtesy of Dave Edwards, University of Tennessee.)

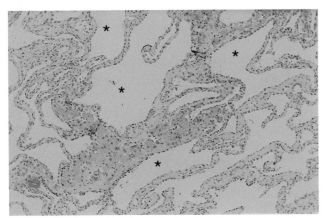

■ **FIGURE 9-23. Cystadenoma. Cat.** This liver biopsy is from a 12-year-old cat with oral disease but otherwise clinically healthy. Mildly raised serum liver enzyme tests were noted on a preanesthetic examination. Multiple fluid-filled lesions were noted on ultrasound examination and clear, acellular fluid was aspirated with ultrasound guidance. A cystadenoma was diagnosed histologically. Note multiple cystic spaces *(asterisks)*. (H&E; IP.)

of human lymphoma is the category of hepatosplenic T-cell lymphoma (Fig. 9-28A&B), a highly aggressive form of disease, for which two similar-appearing cases in dogs have been reported (Cienava et al., 2004; Fry et al., 2003). The use of immunochemistry with multiple antibodies is necessary to define the specific subtypes of lymphoma. For more information about the technique see Chapters 4 and 17. Lymphocytic portal hepatitis is a relatively benign, common finding in older cats and is composed cytologically of mature, small to medium-sized lymphocytes. While cytologic

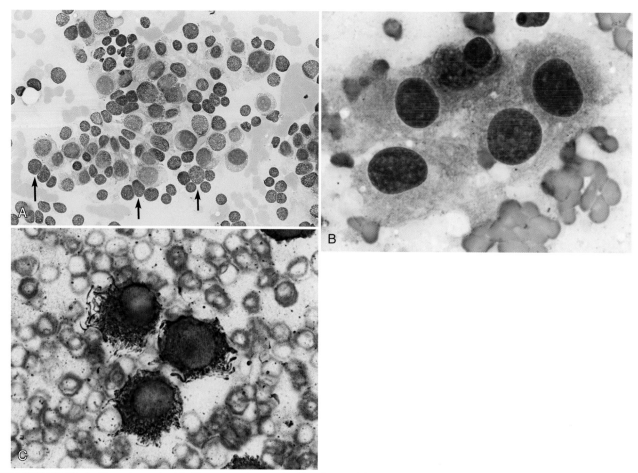

■ **FIGURE 9-25. A, Hepatic carcinoid.** These round to oval cells, obtained from a solitary hepatic mass, have features consistent with a hepatic carcinoid, a neuroendocrine tumor characterized by a naked nuclei cytomorphology. There is moderate to marked anisocytosis, anisokaryosis, and variable nucleus-to-cytoplasm ratio. The nucleus is composed of delicate chromatin surrounded generally by scant amounts of clear to lightly basophilic cytoplasm often with indistinct cytoplasmic borders. Their fragile nature is suggested by frequent free nuclei located at the periphery *(three arrows)* giving them a small lymphocyte-like appearance. (Stain; magnification.) **B, Metastatic carcinoid. Imprint.** These large round cells with round nuclei composed of delicate, open chromatin surrounded by confluent cytoplasm are from a heart base tumor that metastasized to the liver. Noteworthy are the abundant, fine eosinophilic neuroendocrine granules located in the cytoplasm. A hepatocyte at the top center of the cell cluster contrasts with the large size of the neoplastic cells. (Stain; magnification.) **C, Hepatic carcinoid.** Cells react positively to a argyrophilic (silver) stain which demonstrates the neuroendocrine granules. (Stain; magnification.) (B and C, Courtesy of Dave Edwards, University of Tennessee.)

■ **FIGURE 9-26. Lymphoma. Dog. Aspirate.** Sample from a 3-year-old Labrador Retriever with icterus, hepatomegaly, mildly elevated liver enzyme activities, and total bilirubin of 3.1 mg/dl (N <0.6 mg/dl). Lymphoma is indicated by the presence of numerous medium to large lymphocytes *(short arrows)*. A small, dark-staining lymphocyte *(thick arrow)* is a useful "micrometer" for assessing size and immature morphologic features of the neoplastic cells. The binucleated hepatocyte *(long arrow)* contains a small amount of bluish-black granular pigment consistent with bile retained secondary to cholestasis. Small globs of irregularly shaped, metachromatically stained material represent the gel used for the ultrasound examination *(asterisks)*. (Wright-Giemsa; HP oil.)

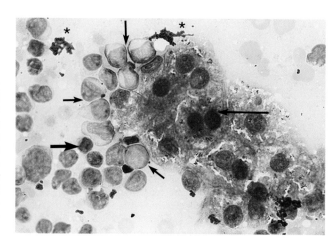

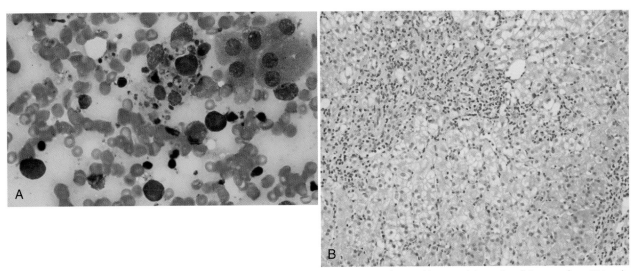

■ **FIGURE 9-27. Lymphoma. Dog. A,** A small cluster of hepatocytes is present along with several large (nuclei more than 3× red cell diameter) and deeply basophilic neoplastic lymphoid cells. The background contains numerous basophilic cytoplasmic fragments. (Wright-Giemsa; HP oil.) **B,** A needle-cut biopsy demonstrates a multifocal to coalescing distribution of basophilic neoplastic lymphoid cells. Notice the focal vacuolar change to the hepatic parenchyma. (H&E; IP.) (A and B, Courtesy of Rose Raskin, Purdue University.)

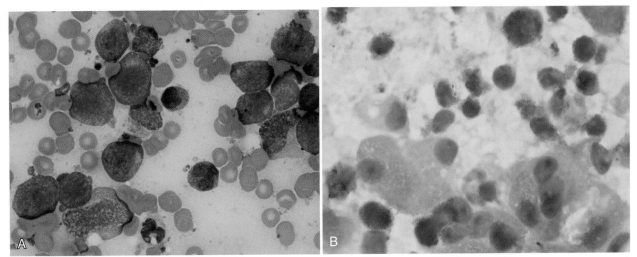

■ **FIGURE 9-28. Hepatosplenic lymphoma. Dog. A,** A monomorphic population of large mononuclear cells that measure more than 3 times the diameter of an erythrocyte. Nuclei are round with occasional indentation and the cytoplasm is generally scant and moderately basophilic. Nucleoli are prominent and frequently multiple. The large size and nuclear irregularly suggest a histiocytic appearance. (Wright; HP oil.) **B,** Notice the positive-stained large and medium sized round cells and negative-stained hepatocytes. (AEC, anti-TCRγδ; HP oil.) (A and B, Courtesy of Rose Raskin, Purdue University.)

confusion should not commonly occur, indecision should be resolved by the histologic examination of a wedge biopsy (see Fig. 9-16B&C). Finding the same cell population in another organ also supports a lymphoid malignancy.

Acute myeloid leukemia can involve the liver, resulting in hepatomegaly. An immature cell type of hematopoietic origin can usually be identified in a cytologic specimen from the liver (Fig. 9-29). Additional examination of the peripheral blood cells and/or bone marrow with special stains may be necessary to differentiate myeloid from lymphoid leukemia. In contrast, the invasion

of the liver by neoplastic mast cells can be readily identified with cytology (Fig. 9-30A&B). Disseminated histiocytic sarcoma is another discrete cell tumor that can involve both the canine and feline liver (Fig. 9-31A&B). When bizarre cell forms are present, neoplasia is readily recognized but the cell type may be problematic. A more uniform population of malignant histiocytes may resemble an acute myeloid or lymphoid leukemia and require special staining procedures for differentiation. Immunocytochemistry can distinguish between dendritic and macrophagic origin of the histiocytic population (Fig. 9-32A&B).

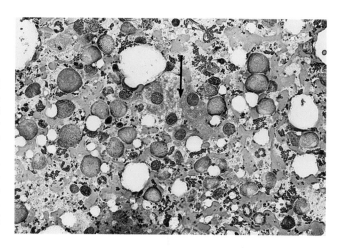

■ **FIGURE 9-29. Acute myelogenous leukemia. Cat.** Large, round to oval, immature discrete cells outnumber hepatocytes *(arrow)* in this liver aspirate from a cat with hepatomegaly, nonregenerative anemia, and neutropenia. The cytologic features are most consistent with an immature cell type of hematopoietic origin. Similar cells were found in the aspirate from the bone marrow and cytochemical stains were used to confirm a diagnosis of acute myelogenous leukemia. A large amount of variably sized, irregular clumps of metachromatic material (ultrasound gel) is located amongst the cells. The large clear spaces are consistent with extracellular lipid that was probably admixed with the specimen from the mesenteric fat during the sampling procedure. (Wright-Giemsa; IP.)

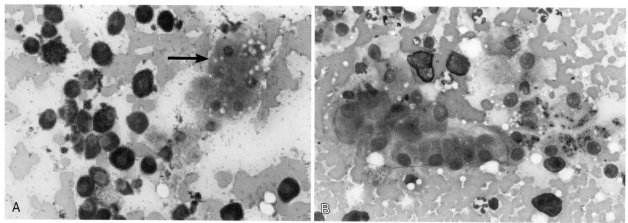

■ **FIGURE 9-30. Mast cell tumor. Cat. A,** Marked numbers of mast cells in this hepatic aspirate causing hepatomegaly is diagnostic of mast cell neoplasia. Hepatocytes *(arrow)* contain a small number of discrete vacuoles compatible with cytoplasmic lipid. (Wright-Giemsa; IP.) **B,** Hepatic mast cell tumor composed of immature, moderately granular mast cells showing anisocytosis and variable cytoplasmic granularity. The hepatocytes to the left of center contain bluish-black cytoplasmic granules consistent with bile or lipofuscin pigment. (Wright-Giemsa; HP oil.) (B, Courtesy of Dave Edwards, University of Tennessee.)

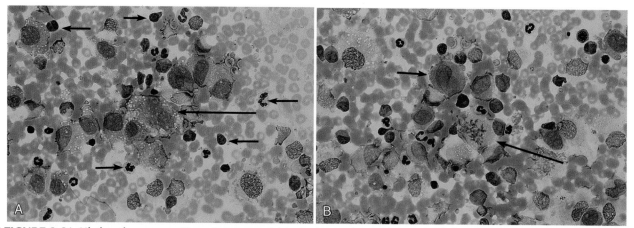

■ **FIGURE 9-31. Histiocytic sarcoma. Dog. A,** Large, variably sized, round to oval, immature discrete cells containing a round to oval to reniform nucleus surrounded by a moderate amount of bluish-gray cytoplasm was the prominent cytologic feature in this liver aspirate from an icteric 5-year-old Rottweiler with hepatomegaly. The cell near the center resembles an immature macrophage *(long arrow)*. Neutrophils and lymphocytes *(short arrows)* indicate concomitant mixed cell inflammation. They are also useful micrometers contrasting the gigantic size of the neoplastic cells. Greenish-colored erythrocytes are prominent in the background. (Wright-Giemsa; IP.) **B,** An atypical mitotic figure *(long arrow)* and another immature gigantic monocytoid cell *(short arrow)* are observed in other areas of the specimen. The findings are indicative of disseminated histiocytic sarcoma (formerly malignant histiocytosis), which was confirmed at necropsy. (Wright-Giemsa; IP.)

Metastatic Epithelial and Mesenchymal Neoplasia

Metastatic lesions to the liver can be either carcinomas or sarcomas. Because of the vascular and lymphatic relationships, metastasis to the liver is most common from primary cancers involving the pancreas and intestinal tract (Fig. 9-33A–C). Often the cell type present cannot definitively identify the primary neoplastic site cytologically. The objective of cytology is to identify a neoplastic lesion as part of a staging process or prompt additional diagnostic efforts if the primary lesion is occult.

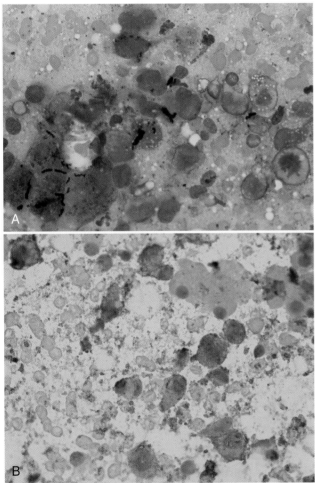

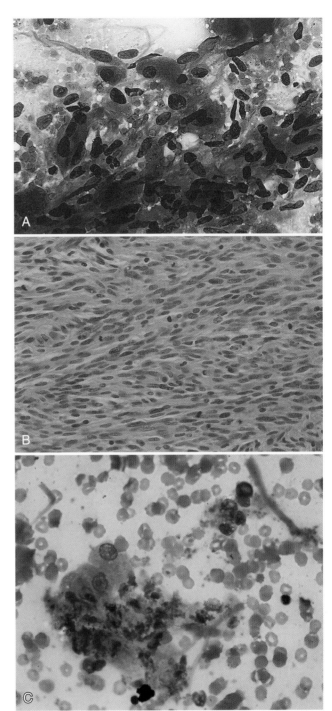

■ **FIGURE 9-32. Histiocytic sarcoma. Dog. A,** A pleomorphic population of irregularly shaped large round cells is present along side of hepatocytes that display marked cholestasis as indicated by the prominent black-green canaliculi. Indented and multilobulated nuclear shapes are common as well as an abnormal mitotic figure on the right lower edge. (Wright; HP oil.) **B,** Notice the positive-stained large pleomorphic round cells and negative-stained hepatocytes. The reaction along with other immunocytochemical stains supports dendritic origin. (AEC, anti-CD1c; HP oil.) (A and B, Courtesy of Rose Raskin, Purdue University.)

■ **FIGURE 9-33. Metastatic leiomyosarcoma. Dog. A,** Spindle-shaped cells were the only cell type present in this liver aspirate from a dog with anorexia, weight loss, microcytic anemia, normal serum liver enzyme values, and variable echogenicity on ultrasound examination. A metastatic spindle cell tumor was diagnosed cytologically. (Wright-Giemsa; IP.) **B,** An ulcerated intestinal mass was biopsied at surgery and determined to be a leiomyosarcoma (H&E; IP.) **C,** A second case shows the basophilic strands of smooth muscle cytoplasm mixed with a cluster of hepatocytes. The site of tumor origin was the jejunum. (Wright; HP oil.) (C, Courtesy of Rose Raskin, Purdue University.)

REFERENCES

Brown DE, Thrall MA, Walkley SU, et al: Feline Niemann-Pick disease type C, *Am J Pathol* 144(6):1412-1415, 1994.

Cienava EA, Barnhart KF, Brown R, et al: Morphologic, immunohistochemical, and molecular characterization of hepatosplenic T-cell lymphoma in a dog, *Vet Clin Pathol* 33:105-110, 2004.

Crosbie OM, Reynolds M, McEntee G, et al: In vitro evidence for the presence of hematopoietic stem cells in the adult human liver, *Hepatology* 29:1193-1198, 1999.

DiBartola SP, Tarr MJ, Benson MD: Tissue distribution of amyloid deposits in Abyssinian cats with familial amyloidosis, *J Comp Pathol* 96:387-398, 1986.

Evans GH, Harries SA, Hobbs KEF: Safety and necessity for needle biopsy of liver tumors, *Lancet* 1:620, 1987.

Ferreri JA, Haardam E, Kimmel SE, et al: Clinical differentiation of acute necrotizing from chronic nonsuppurative pancreatitis in cats: 63 cases (1996-2001), *J Am Vet Med Assoc* 223:469-474, 2003.

Fry MM, Vernau W, Pesavento PA, et al: Hepatosplenic lymphoma in a dog, *Vet Pathol* 40:556-562, 2003.

Gagne JM, Armstrong PJ, Weiss DJ, et al: Clinical features of inflammatory liver disease in cats: 41 cases (1983-1993), *J Am Vet Med Assoc* 214:513-516, 1999.

Gagne JM, Weiss DJ, Armstrong PJ: Histopathologic evaluation of feline inflammatory liver disease, *Vet Pathol* 33:521-526, 1996.

Guilford WG: Breed associated gastrointestinal disease. In Bonagura J, Kirk RW (eds): *Kirk's current veterinary therapy XII*, WB Saunders, Philadelphia, 1995, pp 695-697.

Hendrick M: A spectrum of hypereosinophilic syndromes exemplified by six cats with eosinophilic enteritis, *Vet Pathol* 18:188-200, 1981.

Ishak K: Chronic hepatitis: morphology and nomenclature, *Mod Pathol* 7:690-713, 1994.

Ishii H, Okada S, Okusaka T, et al: Needle tract implantation of hepatocellular carcinoma after percutaneous ethanol injection, *Cancer* 82:1638-1642, 1998.

Kuhlenschmidt MS, Hoffmann WE, Rippy MK: Glucocorticoid hepatopathy: Effect on receptor-mediated endocytosis of asialoglycoproteins, *Biochem Med Metab Biol* 46:152-168, 1991.

Loeven KO: Hepatic amyloidosis in two Chinese shar pei dogs, *J Am Vet Med Assoc* 204:1212-1216, 1994.

Meyer DJ: Hepatic pathology. In Guilford WG, Center SA, Strombeck DR, et al (eds): *Strombeck's small animal gastroenterology*, ed 3, WB Saunders, Philadelphia, 1996, pp 633-653.

Navarro F, Taourel P, Michel J, et al: Diaphragmatic and subcutaneous seeding of hepatocellular carcinoma following fine-needle aspiration biopsy, *Liver* 18:251-254, 1998.

Neumann S, Kaup F: Usefulness of Ki-67 proliferation marker in the cytologic identification of liver tumors in dogs, *Vet Clin Pathol* 34:132-136, 2005.

Owens SD, Gossett R, McElhaney MR, et al: Three cases of canine bile peritonitis with mucinous material in abdominal fluid as the prominent cytologic finding, *Vet Clin Pathol* 32:114-120, 2003.

Roth L: Comparison of liver cytology and biopsy diagnoses in dogs and cats: 56 cases, *Vet Clin Pathol* 30:35-38, 2001.

Rothuizen R, de Vries-Chalmers Hoynck van Papendrecht R, van den Brom WE: Postprandial and cholecystokinin-induced emptying of the gallbladder in dogs, *Vet Rec* 126:505-507, 1990.

Schaer M, Ginn PE: Iatrogenic Cushing's syndrome and steroid hepatopathy in a cat, *J Am Anim Hosp Assoc* 35:48-51, 1999.

Schiff ER, Schiff L: Needle biopsy of the liver. In Schiff L, Schiff ER (eds): *Diseases of the liver*, ed 7, JB Lippincott, Philadelphia, 1993, pp 216-225.

Scott M, Buriko K: Characterization of the pigmented cytoplasmic granules common in canine hepatocytes, *Vet Clin Pathol* 34 Suppl:281-282, 2005 [abstract].

Sepesy LM, Center SA, Randolph JF, et al: Vacuolar hepatopathy in dogs: 336 cases (1993-2005), *J Am Vet Med Assoc* 229:246-252, 2006.

Sevelius E, Jonsson LH: Pathogenic aspects of chronic liver disease in the dog. In Bonagura J, Kirk RW (eds): *Kirk's current veterinary therapy XII*, WB Saunders, Philadelphia, 1995, pp 740-742.

Stalker MJ, Hayes MA: Liver and biliary system. In Maxie MG (ed): *Jubb, Kennedy, Palmer's pathology of domestic animals*, ed 5, vol 2, Elsevier Limited, Philadelphia, 2007, pp 297-388.

Stockhaus C, Teske E, Van Den Ingh T, et al: The influence of age on the cytology of the liver in healthy dogs, *Vet Pathol* 39:154-158, 2002.

Stockhaus C, Van Den Ingh T, Rothuizen J, et al: A multistep approach in the cytologic evaluation of liver biopsy samples of dogs with hepatic disease, *Vet Pathol* 41:461-470, 2004.

Straw RC: Hepatic tumors. In Withrow SJ, MacEwen EG (eds): *Small animal clinical oncology*, ed 2, WB Saunders, Philadelphia, 1996, pp 248-252.

Strombeck DR, Guilford WG: Hepatic neoplasms. In Guilford WG, Center SA, Strombeck DR, Williams DA, Meyer DJ (eds): *Strombeck's small animal gastroenterology*, ed 3, WB Saunders, Philadelphia, 1996, pp 847-859.

Wang KY, Panciera DL, Al-Rukibat RK, et al: Accuracy of ultrasound-guided fine-needle aspiration of the liver and cytologic findings in dogs and cats: 97 cases (1990-2000), *J Am Vet Med Assoc* 224:75-78, 2004.

Weiss DJ, Gagne JM, Armstrong PJ: Characterization of portal lymphocytic infiltrates in feline liver, *Vet Clin Pathol* 24:91-95, 1995.

Weiss DJ, Gagne JM, Armstrong PJ: Relationship between inflammatory hepatic disease and inflammatory bowel disease, pancreatitis, and nephritis in cats, *J Am Vet Med Assoc* 209:1114-1116, 1996.

Zini E, Glaus TM, Minuto F, et al: Paraneoplastic hypoglycemia due to an insulin-like growth factor type-II secreting hepatocellular carcinoma in a dog, *J Vet Intern Med* 21:193-195, 2007.

Zuber RM: Systemic amyloidosis in Oriental and Siamese cats, *Aust Vet Pract* 23:66-70, 1993.

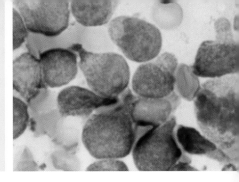

CHAPTER 10

Urinary Tract

Dori L. Borjesson and Keith DeJong

Fine-needle aspiration (FNA) of the kidneys and bladder to obtain cells for cytologic evaluation is a simple, rapid, safe, and relatively inexpensive procedure. The primary indications for cytologic examination of the urinary tract include unilateral or bilateral renomegaly, discrete bladder masses or bladder wall thickening, and urethral masses. Cytologic evaluation of the urinary tract can frequently distinguish between common causes of organ enlargement (inflammation, cyst, and neoplasia), direct further diagnostics (e.g., culture or biopsy), or prevent needless surgical intervention (e.g., in cases of metastatic neoplasia).

NORMAL ANATOMY AND HISTOLOGY

The urinary system is composed of kidneys, ureters, the urinary bladder, and the urethra. The kidney has four basic morphologic components: glomeruli, tubules, interstitium, and blood vessels (Fig. 10-1). The functional unit of the kidney is the nephron. Each nephron is composed of a glomerulus and renal tubule system. The glomerulus is a capillary tuft lined by fenestrated endothelium that is intimately associated with tubule epithelial cells. Components of the glomerulus (Fig. 10-2), including the endothelium, basement membrane, and specialized epithelial cells known as podocytes, make up the filtration barrier of the kidney (Jones et al., 1997).

The renal tubule is divided into distinct functional segments including the proximal convoluted tubule, loop of Henle (ascending and descending limbs), distal convoluted tubule, and the collecting ducts. Reflective of function, the epithelial cells lining the tubules vary from a single layer of cuboidal cells with a brush border in the proximal convoluted tubules to columnar epithelium with no brush border in the distal convoluted segments (Fig. 10-3). Caudate transitional cells line the renal pelvis and calyces. Similarly, the mucosa of the ureters, urinary bladder, and urethra are lined almost exclusively by transitional epithelial cells. Renal interstitial tissue is composed of connective tissue (mesenchymal cells), an extensive capillary network, lymphatic tissue, and smooth muscle cells (Jones et al., 1997; Borjesson, 2003).

SPECIALIZED COLLECTION TECHNIQUES

Sampling method for obtaining cytologic specimens depends on lesion location but may involve either direct mass FNA or traumatic catheterization in the case of a urethral mass or bladder mass in the area of the trigone. Conversely, renal biopsy is frequently indicated in dogs and cats with glomerular disease (and proteinuria) or acute renal failure. Biopsy can be performed with ultrasound guidance or using surgical methods. The increased risks associated with biopsy include the transection of blood vessels or the renal pelvis with resultant hemorrhage, hydronephrosis, or hematuria (Borjesson, 2003). A recent multi-institutional study found complication rates for renal biopsy at 13.4% and 18.5% of dogs and cats, respectively (Vaden et al., 2005). The most common complication was hemorrhage. There have been a number of recent published reviews comparing renal biopsy methods to optimize specimen procurement and minimize biopsy-induced complications (Vaden et al., 2005; Rawlings et al., 2003; Vaden, 2004).

For FNA, manual kidney immobilization and blind percutaneous aspiration can be used to obtain samples for cytologic review, especially in cats. However, this technique is best reserved for diffuse lesions that result in renomegaly as focal lesions may be missed and there is an increased risk of inadvertent puncture or laceration of major blood vessels. Ultrasound-guided FNA is recommended as it is minimally invasive and has a low complication rate. The primary potential complication is hemorrhage; as such, a clotting profile may be indicated.

For ultrasound-guided aspiration, the patient is maintained in dorsal recumbency. If changes are bilateral, aspiration of the caudal pole of left kidney is recommended as it decreases the risk of accidental aspiration of bowel and pancreas. The needle is directed from the cortex of the caudal pole, ventral to dorsal. The needle can be angled from medial to lateral to avoid hitting a large renal vessel. Care should be taken to avoid hitting the renal pelvis. Begin with 25- to 27-gauge, 1.5-inch

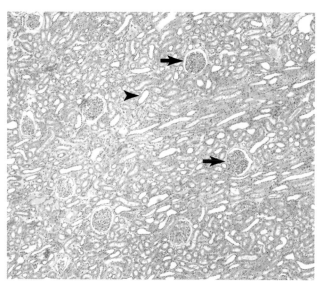

■ **FIGURE 10-1. Tissue section of normal canine kidney.** Numerous glomeruli *(arrows)* are found amidst renal tubules *(arrowhead)* sectioned longitudinally. Tubules are lined mostly by a single layer of cuboidal epithelial cells. (H&E; IP.)

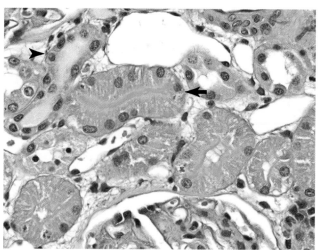

■ **FIGURE 10-3. Tissue section of canine renal tubules.** Note the proximal tubules with the characteristic pink, thick brush border *(arrow)* adjacent to a distal tubule with a single layer of epithelial cells and no brush border *(arrowhead)*. (H&E; HP oil.)

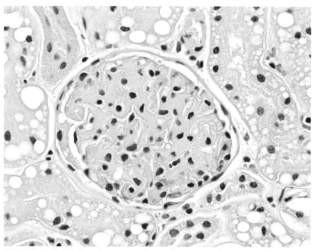

■ **FIGURE 10-2. Tissue section of a normal feline glomerulus.** Higher-power magnification of a glomerulus with a central capillary tuft lined by fenestrated endothelium (not demonstrated). Normal feline renal tubular cells with intracytoplasmic lipid vacuoles surround the glomerulus. (H&E; HP oil.)

needle. If sample of adequate cellularity is not obtained, a larger bore needle can be used. The best results are obtained if multiple preparations are made and one slide is rapidly stained with either a Romanowsky stain or New methylene blue to assess sample adequacy (Borjesson, 2003).

Regardless of the type of mass, aspiration of both the central and peripheral areas is recommended. Frequently the center of a mass may consist solely of necrotic debris or inflammatory cells resulting in a nondiagnostic sample. Although purulent inflammation and necrosis can be associated with malignancy, abundance of either frequently masks the primary disorder. Thus, multiple aspirations in different areas of the mass

are almost always recommended to maximize cellular yield and diagnostic potential as well as to differentiate between primary and secondary inflammation (Borjesson, 2003). If fluid is obtained, a direct smear can be made immediately and the remaining fluid can be placed into EDTA to prevent clotting. Both sediment and cytocentrifuged smears can then be prepared, especially if the sample is of low cellularity. Finally, impression smears can be made from renal biopsy specimens. Cytologic evaluation of impression smears can aid in rapid diagnosis of infectious agents or neoplasia (Borjesson, 2003).

Cells from masses within the bladder can be readily obtained using ultrasound-guided FNA or traumatic urethral catheterization. Occasionally, tumor cells can be noted in urine sediment; however, the submission of urine for cytology rarely results in a definitive diagnosis of neoplasia. Traumatic urethral catheterization can provide adequate and diagnostic samples; however, many of the cells obtained may be superficial and reactive transitional epithelial cells. As such, traumatic catheterization can result in a false negative cytology report due to sample bias with the primary mass not being successfully sampled. Although a few cases of tumor implantation along the ventral abdominal wall following direct FNA of bladder masses have been reported (Nyland et al., 2002), this complication is rare and likely does not affect the clinical outcome. As such, ultrasound-guided FNA may remain the best method for obtaining tissue-associated cells and maximizing cellular yield for cytologic review.

NORMAL RENAL CYTOLOGY

Renal aspirates are typically of low cellularity and usually contain small clusters of renal tubular cells admixed with blood. As the kidneys are highly vascular, blood is generally due to iatrogenic hemorrhage at the time of sampling. Tubular cells generally exfoliate singly or in small clusters of round to oval to columnar epithelial cells. They have abundant basophilic, occasionally vacuolated, cytoplasm that surrounds a uniform, round, often eccentrically placed nucleus (Fig. 10-4). Feline tubular cells are cytologically similar except that cats normally have lipid deposition within their renal tubules. Lipid droplets appear as prominent, variably sized, intracytoplasmic, clear, punctate vacuoles (Figs. 10-5 and 10-6). Fully intact renal tubules arranged in cohesive linear structures may also be present (Fig. 10-7). Tubular cells can also contain dark, intracytoplasmic granules that should not be confused with a well-differentiated melanocyte tumor (Fig. 10-8). Glomeruli may exfoliate singly or in dense, deeply basophilic, rounded clusters, and have very uniform round to oval nuclei (Fig. 10-9).

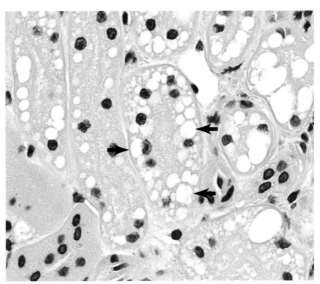

■ **FIGURE 10-6. Tissue section of feline renal tubules.** Note the intracytoplasmic, variably sized lipid droplets that appear as clear, punctate vacuoles within these proximal renal tubule cells from a feline kidney section *(arrows)*. (H&E; HP oil.)

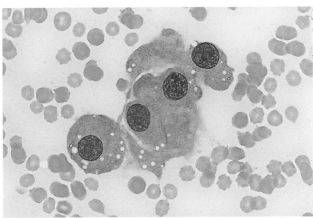

■ **FIGURE 10-4. Canine renal tubular epithelial cells.** Depicted is a small cluster of renal tubular cells that vary from round to columnar in appearance. The background erythrocytes provide a perspective on cell size (Wright-Giemsa; HP oil.)

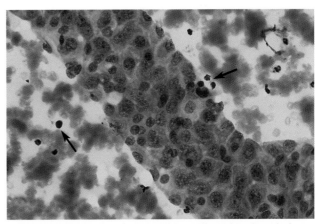

■ **FIGURE 10-7. Intact renal tubule.** Cells within the tubule are minimally pleomorphic. Cell nuclei are round and uniform with small regular nucleoli. The large size is suggestive of a collecting duct or distal tubule. Leukocytes provide a perspective of size *(arrows)*. (Wright-Giemsa; HP oil.)

NON-NEOPLASTIC AND BENIGN LESIONS OF THE URINARY TRACT

Bladder

Polypoid Cystitis, Transitional Cell Polyps, and Papilloma

Hyperplastic and benign mass lesions of the bladder are an uncommon but important subset of bladder diseases that may mimic malignant neoplasia. Polypoid cystitis is characterized by inflammation, epithelial proliferation, and development of a non-neoplastic mass. Similar to most diseases of the urinary bladder, these dogs present with hematuria or recurrent urinary tract infection. However, unlike transitional cell neoplasia, these masses are

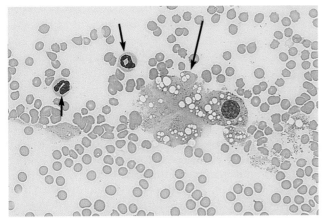

■ **FIGURE 10-5. Feline renal tubular epithelial cells.** Note the intracytoplasmic, variably sized lipid droplets that appear as clear, punctate vacuoles within the renal tubule cells. Free vacuolated cytoplasm from a ruptured cell is also present *(long arrow)*. The size of the tubular cells can be compared to the neutrophils present *(short arrows)*. (Wright-Giemsa; HP oil.)

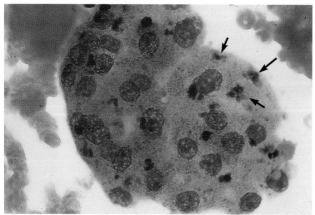

■ **FIGURE 10-8. Intact renal tubule.** The dark, intracytoplasmic granules *(arrows)* of the cells composing this segment of a tubule are indicative of the ascending loop of Henle or distal tubules as the site of origin. The possibility of a well-differentiated melanocyte tumor could be an initial misleading impression. (Wright-Giemsa; HP oil.)

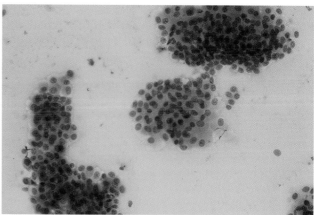

■ **FIGURE 10-10. Transitional cell hyperplasia or benign polyps.** Epithelial hyperplasia or polyp formation is distinguished from malignant epithelial neoplasia by the distinctive, regular clustering pattern and uniform appearance of the epithelial cells. (Wright-Giemsa; IP.)

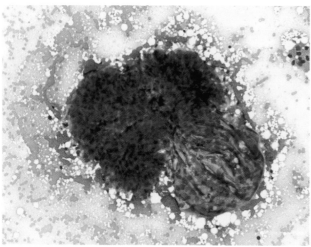

■ **FIGURE 10-9. Intact Glomerulus.** A single intact glomerulus with capillary tuft and associated tubule epithelial cells. (Wright-Giemsa; LP.) (From Friedrichs KR: Laboratory medicine—yesterday today tomorrow: renal resplendence, *Vet Clin Pathol* 36[1]:7, 2007.)

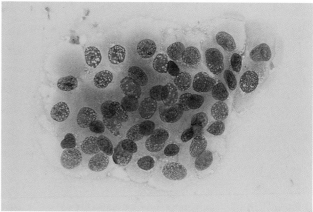

■ **FIGURE 10-11. Transitional cell hyperplasia or benign polyps.** The transitional cells within this epithelial cluster have round to oval uniform nuclei. The chromatin is coarse (a common cytomorphologic feature of the urothelial system) without obvious nucleoli. Cell-cell borders are often readily observed and there is only mild pleomorphism. Contrast the features of this cell cluster to the cells in Figures 10-20 to 10-24. (Wright-Giemsa; HP oil.)

most frequently located cranioventrally in the bladder rather than in the trigone region (Martinez et al., 2003).

Transitional cell hyperplasia and benign transitional cell polyps can exfoliate in large cellular sheets with mild pleomorphism (Fig. 10-10). Nuclei are generally uniform with coarse, ragged chromatin patterns (Fig. 10-11). Transitional cell papillomas may also occur and are characterized by varying size clusters of uniform transitional epithelial cells. These cells are cuboidal to polyhedral and show mild anisokaryosis with an increased nuclear-to-cytoplasmic ratio (Fig. 10-12). Differentiation between the benign processes of hyperplasia, polyps, and papillomas cannot be made cytologically. Often these processes can be difficult to differentiate from neoplastic processes because close proximity to urine causes mild to marked cellular disruption, making definitive identification problematic (Fig. 10-13).

Renal

Cysts

Renal cysts can be acquired or congenital and single or numerous. They are thin walled and contain fluid that is generally viscous or watery and clear or yellow tinged. Although readily evaluated cytologically, clinical history and ultrasound examination may be sufficient for a diagnosis, especially in the case of polycystic disease. Cytologic evaluation of cysts is utilized only when necessary to distinguish between abscesses, neoplasia, or primary cystic disease (Borjesson, 2003).

Cytologically, cysts have low to moderate cellularity with a dense, stippled background consistent with increased protein. Nucleated cells consist primarily of activated macrophages with many large vacuoles that

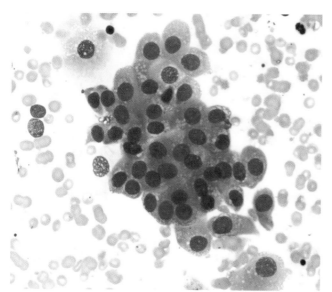

■ FIGURE 10-12. Transitional cell papilloma. Epithelial polyp formation or hyperplasia is distinguished from malignant epithelial neoplasia by the uniform appearance of the epithelial cells. These cells show mild anisokaryosis and anisocytosis with a mildly increased nuclear-to-cytoplasmic ratio. Note the cytoplasmic vacuoles that can be seen in cells from the urothelial system. Contrast the features of this cell cluster to the cells in Figures 10-20 to 10-24. (Wright-Giemsa; HP oil.)

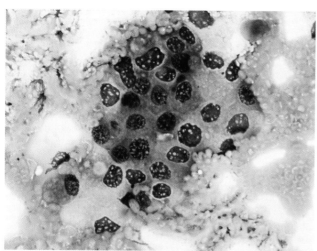

■ FIGURE 10-13. Degenerate transitional cells. Prolonged exposure to urine causes mild to marked cellular disruption, inhibiting definitive cytologic characterization. Common alterations include coarse chromatin, clear vacuoles within the cytoplasm and/or nucleus, and irregular nuclear margins. (Wright-Giemsa; HP oil.)

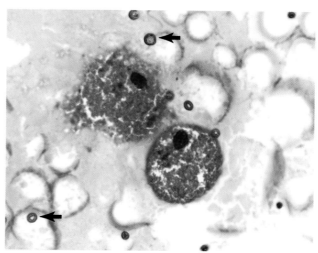

■ FIGURE 10-14. Renal cyst. Cystic fluid is often of low cellularity with a highly proteinaceous background. This cystic fluid is characterized by the presence of large activated and phagocytic macrophages that have abundant cytoplasm containing dark pink material. Note the size of the scattered erythrocytes (*arrows*) in comparison to the macrophages. (Wright-Giemsa; HP oil.)

Crystals

Crystals are rarely noted in cytologic preparations from renal aspirates. However, their presence can be very useful in the diagnosis of nephrotoxicosis. Oxalic acid, a metabolite of ethylene glycol, can precipitate in renal tubules as calcium oxalate crystals (Fig. 10-15A&B). Cytologically, these crystals will appear clear, with barely perceptible, ragged to linear borders (Fig. 10-16A). These crystals are readily visualized under polarized light (Fig. 10-16B).

Acute renal disease and intratubular crystals have also been associated with outbreaks of nephrotoxicosis due to ingestion of contaminated pet food. Pale green to yellow-golden, round to dumbbell-shaped crystals have been identified on renal histology (Fig. 10-17A&B) and in urine sediment cytology. These crystals are suggestive of those formed from the combined precipitation of melamine and cyanuric acid and may be readily misclassified as green-tinged calcium carbonate crystals or smooth ammonium biurate crystals. Earlier reports may also have misclassified these crystals as being associated with a mycotoxin (Jeong et al., 2006).

Inflammation

Pyelonephritis is an infectious tubulointerstitial disease that generally results from an ascending infection of the lower urinary tract. Marked suppurative inflammation is easily diagnosed cytologically and is characterized by increased numbers of neutrophils with scattered activated macrophages (Fig. 10-18). Often, nuclear morphology is degenerate. When the underlying etiology is bacterial infection, intracytoplasmic bacteria can be noted including *Mycobacterium* sp. (Fig. 10-19). Bacterial culture and sensitivity is recommended regardless of the presence of bacteria. Similarly, systemic algal (e.g., *Prototheca zopfii*), fungal (e.g., *Cryptococcus neoformans*

often contain pink secretory material and heme breakdown products, hemosiderin, and hematoidin if hemorrhage is a component of the disease process (Fig. 10-14). Some neoplastic processes have a cystic component; however, the neoplastic cells may or may not exfoliate into the fluid. Therefore, aspiration of the wall or more solid components of a cystic structure should be performed.

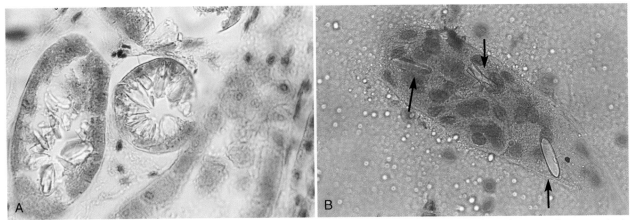

■ **FIGURE 10-15. Ethylene glycol toxicosis. Dog. Same case A-B. A, Tissue section of renal tubule.** Calcium oxalate monohydrate crystals are imbedded in two renal tubules taken at necropsy from the same animal as in Figure 11-16B. (H&E; HP oil.) **B, Touch imprint of renal tubule.** Calcium oxalate monohydrate crystals are imbedded in the renal tubules *(arrows)*. (New methylene blue; HP oil.) (A and B, Courtesy of Denny Meyer.)

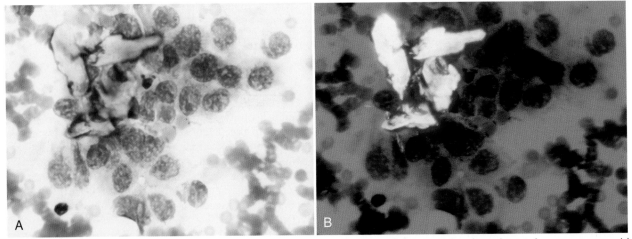

■ **FIGURE 10-16. Ethylene glycol toxicosis. Cat. Same case A-B. A, Tissue aspirate.** Irregular shaped crystals were present within renal tubular epithelium from an animal diagnosed histologically with oxalate crystals at necropsy. (Wright-Giemsa; HP oil.) **B, Tissue aspirate, polarized.** A polarizing filter demonstrates that the irregular-shaped crystals present within renal tubular epithelium were refractive as expected for calcium oxalate. (Wright-Giemsa; HP oil.) (A and B, Courtesy of Rose Raskin, University of Florida.)

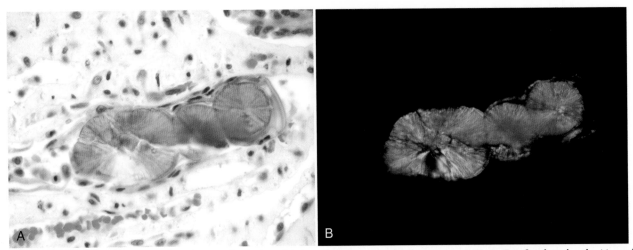

■ **FIGURE 10-17. Tissue section of canine renal tubules with intratubular crystals. Same case A-B. A, Pet food toxicosis.** Note the large, yellow to golden, round to oval, crystals filling this renal tubule and compressing renal tubule epithelial cells. These crystals are presumed to form secondary to melamine and cyanuric acid precipitation associated with consumption of tainted dog food in 2007. Acute tubular necrosis is present but not depicted here. **B, Polarized.** Polarized light demonstrates a colorful refractivity of crystals within the tubules. (A and B, Courtesy of Jessica Hoane, Michigan State University.)

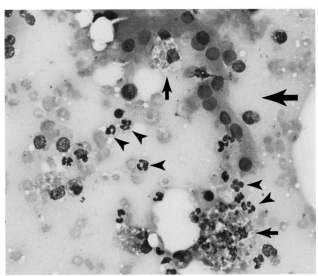

■ **FIGURE 10-18. Pyelonephritis.** Note the small, cohesive cluster of basophilic renal tubular cells *(big arrow)* admixed with a population of nondegenerate neutrophils *(arrow heads)*. Large, foamy macrophages *(small arrows)* containing smooth, blue cellular debris are also present. (Wright-Giemsa; HP oil.)

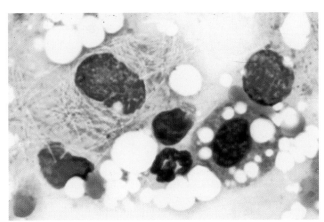

■ **FIGURE 10-19. Mycobacterial nephritis. Aspirate. Cat.** One intact macrophage contains *Mycobacterium* sp. as demonstrated by negative-staining streaks within the cytoplasm. Also present is a renal epithelial cell shown with multiple discrete vacuoles along with a neutrophil and small lymphocyte. This animal had a systemic infection. (Wright-Giemsa; HP oil.) (Courtesy of Rose Raskin, University of Florida.)

and *Aspergillus* spp.), protozoal (e.g, *Leishmania*) (Zatelli et al., 2003), and amebic (e.g., *Balamuthia mandrillaris)* (Foreman et al., 2004) infections can localize in the kidneys and be readily diagnosed cytologically. Cytology is characterized by mixed inflammation, clusters of renal tubular cells, and the presence of organisms. Samples obtained by FNA can also be submitted for fungal culture or other diagnostic techniques (e.g., polymerase chain reaction). Finally, feline infectious peritonitis is uncommonly diagnosed using cytology. Aspirates have a mixed pyogranulomatous inflammation with a basophilic, proteinaceous background. Findings should be interpreted in light of clinical signs and other laboratory tests.

NEOPLASIA

Renal

Primary renal tumors are rare in dogs and cats (Bryan et al., 2006; Henry et al., 1999). Tumors can arise from epithelial, mesenchymal, or embryonal tissue of mixed origin. The vast majority of primary renal tumors in both dogs and cats consist of malignant epithelial tumors (renal cell carcinomas, transitional cell carcinomas, and adenocarcinomas) (Bryan et al., 2006; Henry et al., 1999). Other tumors include fibromas, sarcomas—including hemangiosarcoma (Henry et al., 1999), fibrosarcoma, leiomyosarcoma (Sato et al., 2003), osteosarcoma, and others—and nephroblastoma. Renal lymphoma, a common entity in cats, may represent primary renal disease or be a manifestation of multicentric disease (Henry et al., 1999).

Malignant renal epithelial neoplasms often exfoliate well for cytologic evaluation. In general, renal carcinomas are characterized by high cellularity with many cells observed in variably sized, loose aggregates to poorly cohesive clusters (Figs. 10-20 to 10-22). Due to the number of single, occasionally round cells present in renal cell carcinomas, they can be mistaken for nephroblastomas, round cell tumors, or tumors of neuroendocrine origin. Individual cells are generally cuboidal with mild to occasionally marked anisocytosis and anisokaryosis (see Fig. 10-21). The cells in general have variable nuclear-to-cytoplasmic ratios with a moderate amount of often deep blue cytoplasm and round to polygonal nuclei. A variety of paraneoplastic syndromes have been reported secondary to renal cell carcinomas including hypertrophic osteopathy (Peeters et al., 2001), leukocytosis (Peeters et al., 2001), and polycythemia (Bryan et al., 2006; Henry et al., 1999).

Transitional cell carcinoma (TCC) may exfoliate in small sheets, loose aggregates, or as individual cells. Single

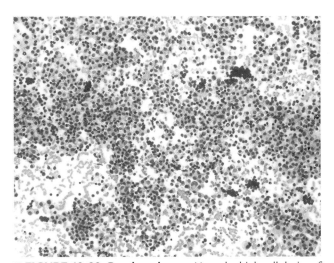

■ **FIGURE 10-20. Renal carcinoma.** Note the high cellularity of the sample. Neoplastic cells are found individually and in loose clusters or sheets. Cells are only minimally pleomorphic. With renal tumors, it can be difficult to differentiate between poorly cohesive carcinomas (depicted here), nephroblastomas, and other round cell tumors. (Wright-Giemsa; IP.)

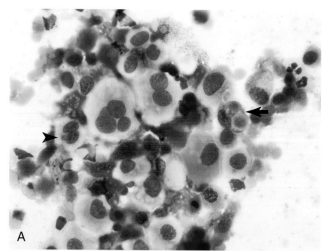

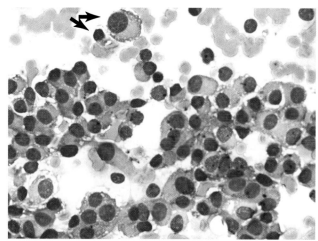

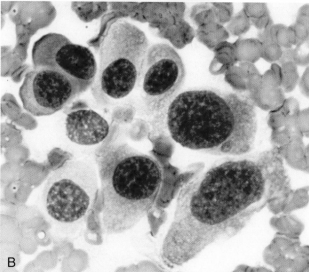

■ FIGURE 10-21. Renal carcinoma. This cluster of poorly cohesive cuboidal cells have moderately increased nuclear-to-cytoplasmic ratios with mild to occasionally marked anisocytosis and anisokaryosis *(arrows)*. Contrast these cellular features of malignancy to the benign characteristics of the cell cluster in Figs. 10-10 to 10-12. (Wright-Giemsa; HP oil.)

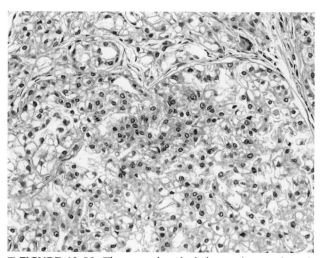

■ FIGURE 10-22. Tissue section depicting canine renal carcinoma. The mass is composed of haphazard tubules and structures lined by polygonal cells supported by a fibrovascular stroma. Individual cells have centrally located round to oval nuclei with dispersed chromatin and occasional prominent nucleoli. Cytoplasm is abundant and varies from clear to eosinophilic and granular. Anisokaryosis is moderate. (H&E; HP oil.)

■ FIGURE 10-23. Transitional cell carcinoma. A, This cluster of transitional cells contains numerous criteria of malignancy including: marked anisocytosis and anisokaryosis, variable nuclear-to-cytoplasmic ratio, pleomorphic and multiple nuclei, and *micronuclei (arrowhead)*. Note the characteristic pink, cytoplasmic inclusions *(arrow)*. Contrast the features of these cells with the features of the cells in Figs. 10-10 to 10-12. (Wright-Giemsa; HP oil.) **B, Urinary bladder. Dog.** This group of transitional epithelial cells appeared individualized with marked anisocytosis and anisokaryosis, variable nuclear-to-cytoplasmic ratio, and pleomorphic nuclei. Contrast the features of these cells with the features of the cells in Figs. 10-10 to 10-12. (Wright-Giemsa; HP oil.) (B, Courtesy of Rick Alleman, University of Florida.)

cells are large and can be cuboidal, polygonal, or even spindle-shaped. Transitional cells have a variable to low nuclear-to-cytoplasm ratio (with abundant cytoplasm) however they are often markedly pleomorphic with numerous and strong criteria of malignancy including marked anisocytosis and anisokaryosis, pleomorphic nuclei and prominent and multiple nucleoli (Fig. 10-23A&B). Characteristic pink homogenous to granular cytoplasmic inclusions are often noted in TCC (see Fig. 10-23A, *arrow*).

Renal nephroblastomas are composed of mixed cell populations including blastemal, epithelial, and mesenchymal elements (Henry et al., 1999). Cytologically,

the predominant cell types are usually the blastemal or epithelial components as cells tend to exfoliate singly or in loose aggregates and sheets. As with renal cell carcinomas, cells from this tumor can mimic round cell neoplasia (e.g., lymphoma or tumors of neuroendocrine origin). Cells are generally polygonal to cuboidal with a high nuclear-to-cytoplasmic ratio, a scant amount of pale blue cytoplasm, and mild anisokaryosis and anisocytosis. Nucleolar criteria of malignancy are generally absent (Fig. 10-24). Histopathology and immunohistochemistry are often necessary for definitive characterization.

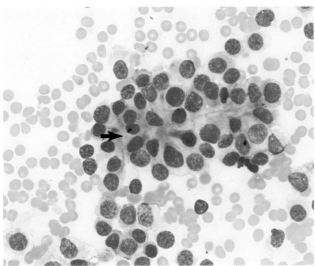

■ **FIGURE 10-24. Nephroblastoma.** This cluster of polygonal to cuboidal cells have high nuclear-to-cytoplasmic ratios with mild anisocytosis and anisokaryosis. Note the pink extracellular matrix material (stroma or basement membrane) coursing through the cluster *(arrow)*. Nuclei are round to polygonal, chromatin is stippled, and nucleoli are not obvious. (Wright-Giemsa; HP oil.)

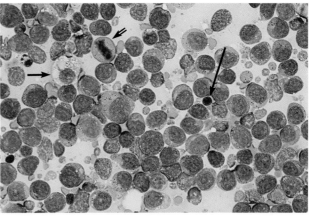

■ **FIGURE 10-25. Renal lymphoma.** This sample contains a dense population of discrete cells with cytomorphologic features consistent with large, immature lymphocytes. Note the marked pleomorphism, smooth, homogeneous nuclear chromatin, and relatively abundant basophilic cytoplasm as compared to a small, mature lymphocyte *(long arrow)*. The presence of pink cytoplasmic granules is a less common feature of lymphoma. These cells are differentiated from renal tubular cells by their abundance and the high nuclear-to-cytoplasmic ratio. An activated macrophage *(short arrow)* and a mitotic figure *(double arrow)* are also seen. (Wright-Giemsa; HP oil.)

Nephroblastomas are characterized by positive vimentin staining of the mesenchymal cells and positive cytokeratin staining of the epithelial cells present within the tumor (Bryan et al., 2006).

Renal lymphoma aspirates generally contain a homogeneous population of discrete cells with cytomorphologic features consistent with large, immature lymphocytes. There can be numerous lysed cells with "smudge cells" in the background. Neoplastic lymphocytes often show moderate to marked pleomorphism, have nuclei composed of homogeneous smooth chromatin, and have a small to moderate amount of basophilic cytoplasm (Fig. 10-25). Occasionally prominent nucleoli can be seen, and rarely the neoplastic lymphocytes may contain bright pink cytoplasmic granules (Fig. 10-26).

Renal sarcomas often exfoliate poorly. They are composed of spindle cells observed individually or in variably sized aggregates. Nuclear-to-cytoplasmic ratios are high with small amounts of moderate to deep blue, often wispy cytoplasm and round to oval to polygonal nuclei with prominent nucleoli. Anisocytosis and anisokaryosis are often marked (Fig. 10-27). Cytology alone cannot distinguish between metastatic sarcomas and sarcomas arising from renal vessels or smooth muscle.

Ureters

Primary ureteral neoplasia is very rare with ureteral invasion by neoplastic processes originating from the bladder (especially transitional cell carcinoma) being far more common (Deschamps et al., 2007). Only 15 documented cases of primary ureter neoplasia in dogs have been reported in the literature, composed mainly of benign neoplasms, primarily fibroepithelial polyps.

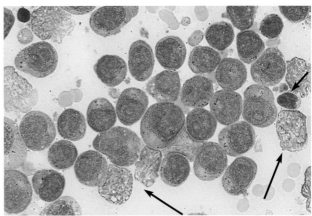

■ **FIGURE 10-26. Renal lymphoma.** A relatively normal, small, mature lymphocyte *(arrow)* accentuates the immature features of the neoplastic lymphocytes. In addition to the features described in Fig. 10-25, prominent nucleoli can be seen in some of the malignant cells, and the pink cytoplasmic granules are more readily observed. Five or six lacy, pink, ovoid formations, sometimes referred to as "basket cells" or "smudge cells," represent free nuclear chromatin from lysed cells *(long arrow)*. It is a frequent finding in aspirates from tissues comprised of fragile cells such as lymphoma. (Wright-Giemsa; HP oil.)

Bladder and Urethra

Tumors of the urinary bladder are infrequent in dogs and cats. However the most common bladder tumor in both dogs and cats is TCC (Mutsaers et al., 2003; Norris et al., 1992; Wilson et al., 2007). Squamous cell carcinomas; malignant tumors of muscle origin (Alleman et al., 1991)— e.g., leiomyosarcoma and rhabdomyosarcoma (Fig. 10-28A&B); lymphoma (Fig. 10-29); and metastatic disease are less frequently encountered. Transitional cell

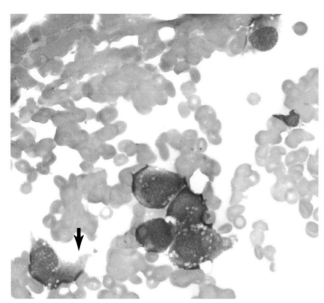

■ **FIGURE 10-27. Renal sarcoma.** Cells of mesenchymal neoplasia tend to exfoliate singly or in small aggregates rather than cohesive clusters. Cell shape may vary from round to oval to spindle-shaped. A cytologic impression of mesenchymal cells is endorsed by finding cells with wispy tails *(arrow).* Cytologically, malignancy is characterized by variable, often high nuclear-to-cytoplasmic ratios, moderate to deep blue, wispy cytoplasm that often contains numerous uniform punctate vacuoles, cellular pleomorphism, and moderate anisokaryosis and anisocytosis, and variable staining intensity. (Wright-Giemsa; HP oil.)

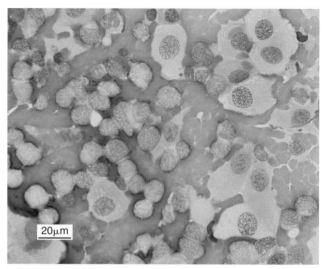

■ **FIGURE 10-29. Urinary bladder. Imprint. B-cell lymphoma. Dog.** Traumatic urinary catheterization resulted in tissue pieces that were imprinted for cytologic examination of a bladder mass. Large numbers of a uniform population of intermediate-sized lymphoid cells are present among the clustered (not shown) and individualized transitional epithelium. Immunocytochemistry demonstrated CD3 negative and CD79a positive lymphoid cells supportive of B-cell origin. Several of the lymphoid cells have a plasmacytoid appearance. (Wright-Giemsa; HP oil.) (Courtesy of Rose Raskin, University of Florida.)

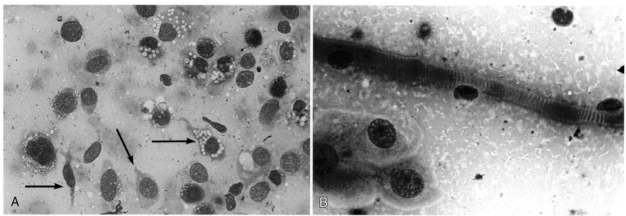

■ **FIGURE 10-28. A, Bladder leiomyosarcoma.** Neoplastic mesenchymal cells tend to exfoliate individually or in small aggregates. Cell shape varies from round to oval to spindle-shaped *(arrows).* Cytologically, malignancy is characterized by moderate anisokaryosis, anisocytosis, cellular and nuclear pleomorphism, and variable nuclear-to-cytoplasm ratios. The pink to blue proteinaceous background that contains pink to basophilic amorphous debris (dirty appearance) is consistent with necrotic debris. Malignant cells from mesenchymal tissue can show uniform punctate cytoplasmic vacuoles, as illustrated by some of these cells. (Wright-Giemsa; HP oil.) **B, Bladder rhabdomyosarcoma. Aspirate. Dog.** A single muscle fiber with striations is present along with three transitional epithelial cells and a lymphocyte. Histopathology confirmed the diagnosis of a skeletal muscle malignant neoplasm for the mass in the urinary bladder. (Wright-Giemsa; HP oil.) (B, Courtesy of Rose Raskin, University of Florida.)

carcinoma in the dog is most commonly associated with the trigone region of the bladder, while the opposite is true in the cat (Mutsaers et al., 2003; Wilson et al., 2007). Transitional cell carcinomas appear cytologically similar (see Fig. 10-23A&B) whether they originate in the kidneys or bladder (see full cytologic description in renal

section above). The diagnosis of canine TCC can frequently be made cytologically as the majority of patients present with high-grade disease and large masses (Mutsaers et al., 2003). However, in addition to cytology, the veterinary bladder tumor antigen test (V-BTA, Alidex Inc, subsidiary of Polymedco, Redmond, WA) can be used to noninvasively detect tumor analytes present in urine. This test is suitable to screen for TCC in dogs in the absence of moderate to marked hematuria, pyuria, glucosuria, or proteinuria (Borjesson et al., 1999). However the specificity of the test declines rapidly if dogs have non-TCC urinary tract disease (Borjesson et al., 1999; Henry et al., 2003). Finally, cyclooxygenase-2 (COX-2), uroplakin III, and cytokeratin 7 show promise as useful immunohistochemical stains to verify tumors of urothelial origin in histology sections if needed (Khan et al., 2000; Knottenbelt et al., 2006; Ramos-Vara et al., 2003).

REFERENCES

Alleman AR, Raskin RE, Uhl, EW, et al: What is your diagnosis? Bladder mass from an 11-month-old dog, *Vet Clin Pathol* 20:44,49-50, 1991.

Borjesson DL: Renal cytology, *Vet Clin North Am Small Anim Pract* 33:119-134, 2003.

Borjesson DL, Christopher MM, Ling GV: Detection of canine transitional cell carcinoma using a bladder tumor antigen urine dipstick test, *Vet Clin Pathol* 28:33-38, 1999.

Bryan JN, Henry CJ, Turnquist SE, et al: Primary renal neoplasia of dogs, *J Vet Intern Med* 20:1155-1160, 2006.

Deschamps JY, Roux FA, Fantinato M, et al: Ureteral sarcoma in a dog, *J Small Anim Pract* 48(12):699-701, 2007.

Foreman O, Sykes J, Ball L, et al: Disseminated infection with Balamuthia mandrillaris in a dog, *Vet Pathol* 41:506-510, 2004.

Henry CJ, Turnquist SE, Smith A, et al: Primary renal tumours in cats: 19 cases (1992-1998), *J Feline Med Surg* 1:165-170, 1999.

Henry CJ, Tyler JW, McEntee MC, et al: Evaluation of a bladder tumor antigen test as a screening test for transitional cell carcinoma of the lower urinary tract in dogs, *Am J Vet Res* 64:1017-1020, 2003.

Jeong WI, Do SH, Jeong da H, et al: Canine renal failure syndrome in three dogs, *J Vet Sci* 7:299-301, 2006, pp 1111-1147.

Jones TC, Hunt RD, King NW: *Veterinary pathology*, ed 6, Baltimore, Williams & Wilkins, 1997.

Khan KN, Knapp DW, Denicola DB, et al: Expression of cyclo-oxygenase-2 in transitional cell carcinoma of the urinary bladder in dogs, *Am J Vet Res* 61:478-481, 2000.

Knottenbelt C, Mellor D, Nixon C, et al: Cohort study of COX-1 and COX-2 expression in canine rectal and bladder tumours, *J Small Anim Pract* 47:196-200, 2006.

Martinez I, Mattoon JS, Eaton KA, et al: Polypoid cystitis in 17 dogs (1978-2001), *J Vet Intern Med* 17:499-509, 2003.

Mutsaers AJ, Widmer WR, Knapp DW: Canine transitional cell carcinoma, *J Vet Intern Med* 17:136-144, 2003.

Norris AM, Laing EJ, Valli VE, et al: Canine bladder and urethral tumors: a retrospective study of 115 cases (1980-1985), *J Vet Intern Med* 6:145-153, 1992.

Nyland TG, Wallack ST, Wisner ER: Needle-tract implantation following US-guided fine-needle aspiration biopsy of transitional cell carcinoma of the bladder, urethra, and prostate, *Vet Radiol Ultrasound* 43:50-53, 2002.

Peeters D, Clercx C, Thiry A, et al: Resolution of paraneoplastic leukocytosis and hypertrophic osteopathy after resection of a renal transitional cell carcinoma producing granulocyte-macrophage colony-stimulating factor in a young Bull Terrier, *J Vet Intern Med* 15:407-411, 2001.

Ramos-Vara JA, Miller MA, Boucher M, et al: Immunohistochemical detection of uroplakin III, cytokeratin 7, and cytokeratin 20 in canine urothelial tumors, *Vet Pathol* 40:55-62, 2003.

Rawlings CA, Diamond H, Howerth EW, et al: Diagnostic quality of percutaneous kidney biopsy specimens obtained with laparoscopy versus ultrasound guidance in dogs, *J Am Vet Med Assoc* 223:317-321, 2003.

Sato T, Aoki K, Shibuya H, et al: Leiomyosarcoma of the kidney in a dog, *J Vet Med A Physiol Pathol Clin Med* 50:366-369, 2003.

Vaden SL: Renal biopsy: methods and interpretation, *Vet Clin North Am Small Anim Pract* 34:887-908, 2004.

Vaden SL, Levine JF, Lees GE, et al: Renal biopsy: a retrospective study of methods and complications in 283 dogs and 65 cats, *J Vet Intern Med* 19:794-801, 2005.

Wilson HM, Chun R, Larson VS, et al: Clinical signs, treatments, and outcome in cats with transitional cell carcinoma of the urinary bladder: 20 cases (1990-2004), *J Am Vet Med Assoc* 231:101-106, 2007.

Zatelli A, Borgarelli M, Santilli R, et al: Glomerular lesions in dogs infected with Leishmania organisms, *Am J Vet Res* 64:558-561, 2003.

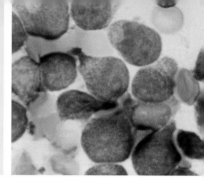

11

Microscopic Examination of the Urinary Sediment

Denny J. Meyer

The urine specimen has been referred to as a liquid tissue biopsy of the urinary tract, painlessly obtained (Haber, 1988). The routine urinalysis is composed of two major components—the macroscopic and the microscopic evaluations. The chapter will focus on findings that can be microscopically observed in the urinary sediment. The evaluation of the physical characteristics and interpretation of alterations detected by reagent test-strip methodologies can be found elsewhere (Meyer and Harvey, 2004). Microscopic examination of urine sediment should be conducted on every urinalysis even if no abnormalities are detected by the reagent test-strip. Studies indicate that up to 16% of urine samples with unremarkable reagent test-strip findings can have positive microscopic findings, notably pyuria and bacteriuria (Barlough et al., 1981; Fettman, 1987). The findings of another study support the recommendation to routinely examine microscopically and culture the urine of dogs with hyperadrenocorticism and diabetes mellitus since clinical signs of bacterial cystitis often are not present (approximately 95% of the cases) and bacteriuria or pyuria may not be observed (approximately 19% of the cases) (Forrester et al., 1999). Bacteria are never considered a normal finding in urine collected by percutaneous cystocentesis even when clinical signs of cystitis are absent (Forrester et al., 1999).

Free catch, catheterization, and percutaneous cystocentesis are the techniques used to obtain urine. The latter method is the surest way to avoid contamination. The specimen should be processed and examined within minutes of collection for the most accurate semiquantitative assessment of the findings. Casts are the most labile constituent and begin to lyse within 2 hours. Cells loose their integrity within 2 to 4 hours depending on the osmolality of the urine. Refrigeration of the urine specimen (for up to 6 hours) is a good way to preserve the physiochemical properties and crystals and delay cellular degeneration. Urine pH will be minimally affected if preserved by refrigeration for up to 24 hours (Raskin et al., 2002).

Lowering the temperature of urine enhances crystal formation, resulting in an inaccurate semiquantitative assessment of their true numbers physiologically. A consistent volume of urine, generally 5 ml, should be routinely assessed so that the findings can be semiquantitated and compared to reference values as well as followed in a patient under treatment (Osborne and Stevens, 1999).

Following centrifugation of the urine specimen in a conical-tipped tube, most of the supernatant is decanted to leave an equal amount of sediment and urine. The sediment is resuspended by flicking the tube several times with the finger. One unstained drop is placed on a clean glass slide with a pipette, a coverslip is applied, and the specimen is examined. Subdued microscopic lighting is required to accentuate the elements in the sediment. The microscope's condenser must be lowered and the iris diaphragm partially closed in order for the constituents to be most conspicuous (Fig. 11-1A). Phase-contrast microscopy accentuates the outline of even the most translucent constituents, simplifying the detection of casts and bacteria. Polarized microscopy is used to enhance the identification of crystals.

A water-based stain (Sedi-Stain, BD Clay Adams, Sparks, MD, or 0.5% new methylene blue) can be used to accentuate cellular detail. One drop of stain is added to the resuspended sediment, mixed by flicking the tube with the finger, allowed to incubate for 2 to 3 minutes, and one drop of the stained sediment placed on a clean glass slide with a pipette. Stain precipitate will develop over time in the bottle and microscopically appear similar to bacteria (Fig. 11-1B). When precipitate is observed, new stain must be employed or the current stain passed through a filter. It is good practice to initially examine an unstained specimen followed by the examination of a stained preparation when there are findings that require additional definition or as a learning tool. A cytology preparation of the sediment is another approach to characterize organisms (Figs 11-2 to 11-3), cells (Fig. 11-4A–D), or the composition

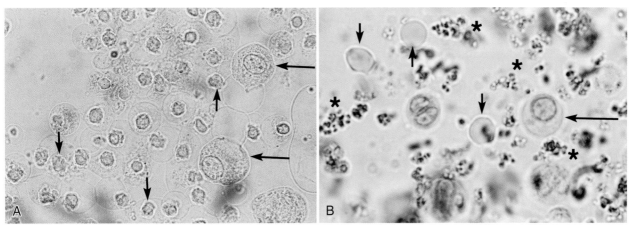

■ **FIGURE 11-1. A, Unstained specimen.** This unstained urine sediment illustrates the enhanced contrast of the cellular constituents when the microscope's condenser is lowered. Crenated erythrocytes are predominant (*short arrows*) and two plump epithelial cells with granular-appearing cytoplasm are present *(long arrows)*. (Unstained; HP oil.) **B, Stained specimen.** Applying stain to the specimen highlights cellular detail. An epithelial cell *(long arrow)* and erythrocytes are present *(short arrows)*. The stain must be kept free of precipitate. As illustrated in this photomicrograph, the stain particles are distracting and give the misleading impression of bacteria *(asterisks)*. (Sedi-Stain; HP oil.)

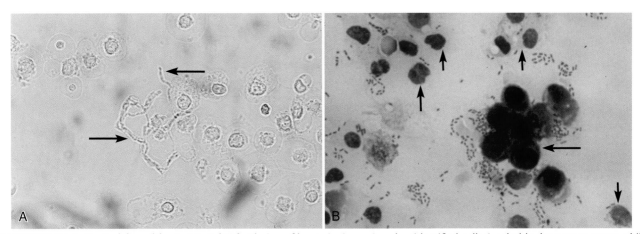

■ **FIGURE 11-2. Bacterial cystitis. A, Unstained.** Chains of bacteria *(arrows)* and unidentified cells (probably degenerate neutrophils with a mononuclear cell appearance and crenated erythrocytes) are observed in this unstained urine sediment obtained by percutaneous cystocentesis. Identification of the cell type is not important in this setting and, in fact, may be impossible owing to changes induced by the physiochemical nature of the urine. (Unstained; HP oil.) **B, Stained.** Romanowsky-stained cytologic preparation of an infected urine specimen highlights the bacteria and a clump of uniform epithelial cells *(long arrow)*. The majority of the cells, presumably neutrophils, have swollen, rounded nuclei or have lysed owing to the hostile environment and cannot be identified *(short arrows)*. In other fields, some of these cells retained slight segmentation and many were observed to contain bacteria supporting their classification as a neutrophil. Again, identification of the cell type is not important in this setting. (Wright; HP oil.)

of casts that are not readily recognized in an unstained preparation. One drop of *unstained,* resuspended sediment is placed near the frosted end of the slide and spread with another slide or a compression (squash) preparation is made, air-dried, and stained (refer to Chapter 1). Often the constituents will wash off during the staining process because of the low-protein nature of the specimen. Serum-coated slides should be used to "glue" the constituents in the sediment to the surface of the slide (refer to Chapter 1, Key Point).

KEY POINT To accentuate the constituents in the unstained urine sediment, the iris diaphragm is partially closed and the substage condenser of the microscope is lowered. This is a dynamic process conducted while viewing the specimen to determine the most advantageous contrast.

Lipid droplets (Fig. 11-5A–C) will resemble cells but are generally more variable in size. Erythrocytes, leukocytes

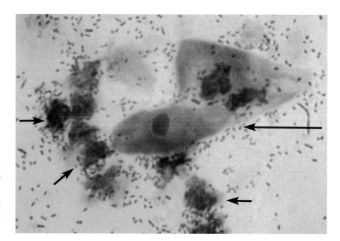

■ **FIGURE 11-3. Contaminated urine specimen, free catch, stained.** The presence of mature squamous epithelial cells *(long arrow)* suggests the probability of bacterial contamination. Six or seven distorted nuclei, presumably neutrophils, are also observed *(short arrows)*. No bacteria or neutrophils were observed in a second specimen obtained via percutaneous cystocentesis. (Wright; HP oil.)

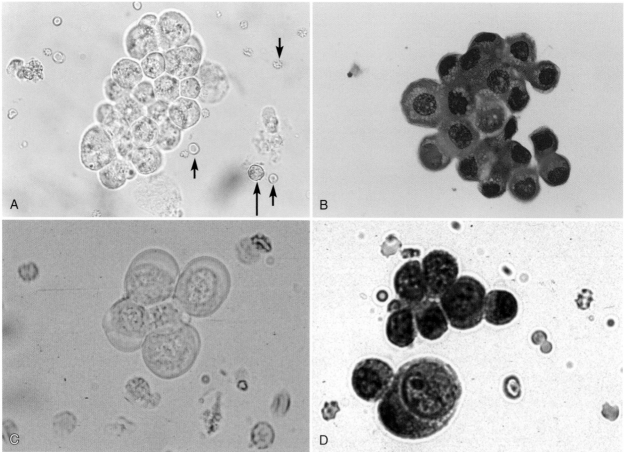

■ **FIGURE 11-4. A, Epithelial cell cluster, unstained.** Epithelial cells demonstrate mild to moderate anisocytosis (20 to 40 μm in diameter). Erythrocytes (approximately 5 to 7 μm in diameter, *short arrows*), some with a smooth surface and some with a crenated appearance and a neutrophil (approximately 10 to 12 μm in diameter, *long arrow*) are observed. The cytoplasmic granules of the neutrophil were in random motion (Brownian movement); sometimes referred to as a "glitter cell." These granules should not be mistaken for bacteria. Note the size relationship of the erythrocyte vs. the neutrophilic leukocyte vs. the epithelial cells. (Unstained; HP oil.) **B, Cytology preparation, hyperplastic epithelial cells, stained.** A drop of the sediment was placed on a glass slide (the surface of which was first coated with a thin layer of serum and air dried), spread, air dried, and stained as a routine cytologic preparation. The stained preparation facilitates the cytologic assessment for criteria of malignancy. The mild to moderate anisocytosis, anisokaryosis, and variable nuclear-to-cytoplasmic ratio were considered to be consistent with hyperplasia of transitional epithelial cells. (Wright; HP oil.) **C, Epithelial cell cluster, unstained.** Epithelial cells demonstrate more variability in cell size and nuclear-to-cytoplasmic ratio. Atypical cell clusters should be investigated further with a cytologic prepreparation of the sediment stained with a Romanowsky stain. (Unstained; HP oil.) **D, Cytology preparation, carcinoma, stained.** Same case as in C. The cytologic criteria for malignancy are more evident in the stained preparation which in this epithelial cell cluster include high and variable nuclear-to-cytoplasmic ratios, prominent nucleoli, and coarse chromatin. Transitional cell carcinoma was suspected cytologically. (Wright-Giemsa; HP oil.) (C and D, Courtesy of Rose Raskin, University of Florida.)

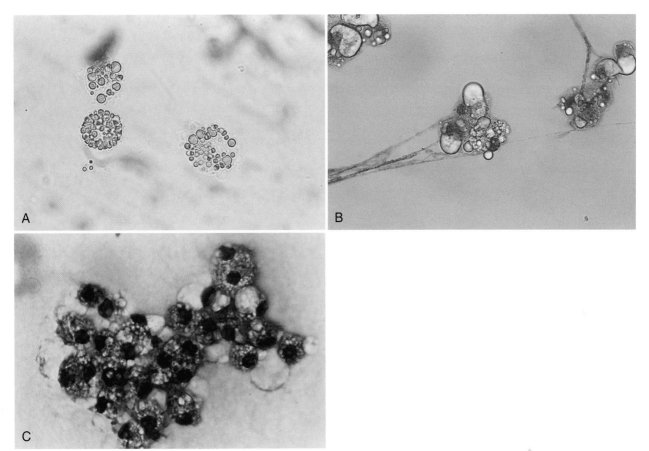

■ **FIGURE 11-5. Lipid droplets.** Lipid vacuoles in epithelial cells may be a prominent cytomorphologic feature in feline urine sediments. They are identified by their size variation and refractile nature when focusing up and down. **A,** Unstained; HP oil. **B,** New methylene blue; HP oil. **C,** Wright (the alcohol-based stain that dissolves the lipid droplets, resulting in punctate holes in the cytoplasm of the cells); HP oil.

(see Fig. 11-2A), and casts (Figs. 11-6 to 11-10) are expressed as the number observed per high-power field (HPF, 40× objective) (Box 11-1). The matrix of all casts is formed by Tamm-Horsfall protein, a glycoprotein secreted by the ascending loop of Henle and possibly the distal tubule. See Meyer and Harvey (2004) for a more detailed discussion of Tamm-Horsfall protein. Crystals are expressed as few (occasional), moderate, or many per low-power field (LPF, 10× objective). The urine pH, temperature, and specific gravity affect the solubility of crystals (Graff, 1983). Struvite (Fig. 11-11) (magnesium ammonium phosphate; triple phosphates is a misnomer), amorphous phosphate (Fig. 11-12A), calcium phosphate (Fig. 11-12B), ammonium urate (Fig. 11-13A–C) (also referred to as *ammonium biurate*), and calcium carbonate (Fig. 11-14) have propensity to form in neutral pH or alkaline urine. Ammonium urate crystals are uncommon in healthy dogs and cats. An exception is ammonium urate crystalluria in apparently healthy Dalmatians and Bulldogs. Dalmatians have an in-born error of uric acid metabolism in which uric acid is not changed to allantoin and results in hyperuricosuria and the predisposition to ammonium urate and uric acid crystalluria. In other breeds, the water-soluble allantoin that is formed is excreted in the urine. Ammonium urate crystalluria is associated with congenital

portosystemic vascular anomalies (shunts) and with liver insufficiency secondary to reduced hepatocellular mass (e.g., cirrhosis). Urine with a neutral or acidic pH tends to favor the formation amorphous urates (Fig. 11-15A), sodium urate (Fig. 11-15B–D), uric acid (Fig. 11-15E), calcium oxalate (Fig. 11-16A–E), bilirubin (Fig. 11-17A&B), cystine (Fig. 11-18), calcium hydrogen phosphate dehydrate (brushite) (Fig. 11-19), sulfa (Fig. 11-20A&B), and tyrosine (Fig. 11-21). A *lignin test* is used as a screening test for sulfonamides. To perform the test, place a few urine drops on a blank strip of newspaper followed by a drop of 25% hydrochloric acid in the center of the moist area. Yellow to orange reaction within 15 minutes indicates a positive reaction (Graff, 1983).

In addition to bacteria in the sediment, other infectious agents include yeast or hyphal forms of fungi. Frequently these may reflect stain contaminants or an overgrowth related to excessive antibiotic usage (Fig. 11-22A). Systemic mycosis can result in the shedding of fungal elements in the urine such as *Aspergillus* sp. (Fig. 11-22B). A urine specimen obtained via percutaneous cystocentesis should be used to confirm the finding and rule out contamination. A positive finding should be related to the clinical presentation

Text continued on p. 266

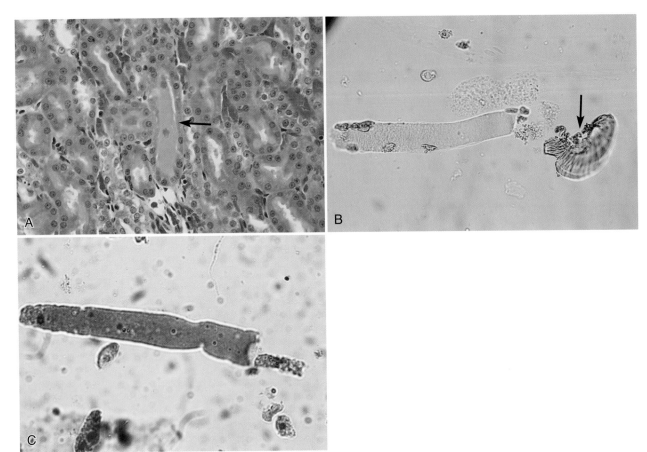

■ **FIGURE 11-6. Hyaline cast. A, Histology.** Casts form in the renal tubules *(arrow)* (ascending limb of the loop of Henle and distal tubule) and reflect their shape. Acidity, solute concentration, and flow rate facilitate the precipitation of protein, resulting in the formation of a cast. (H&E; HP oil.) **B, Unstained with artifact.** Hyaline casts are clear and colorless. They rapidly dissolve, especially in alkaline urine. An occasional cast per 10× field is normal. Cast formation is increased when abnormal amounts of protein enter the tubules, most often excess albumin. Increased numbers are associated with strenuous exercise, fever, congestive heart failure, diuretic treatment, glomerulonephritis, and amyloidosis. A chip of collection container, likely plastic, is present *(arrow)*. (Unstained; HP oil.) **C, Stained.** Note the smooth, homogenous appearance. (Sedi-Stain; HP oil.)

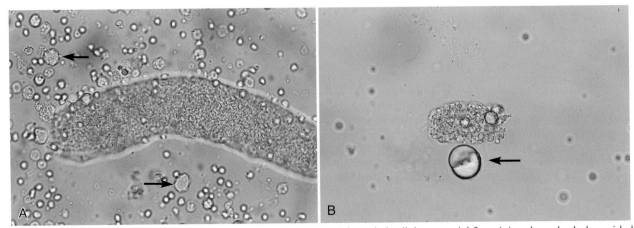

■ **FIGURE 11-7. A, Granular cast, unstained.** Granular casts represent degraded cellular material from injured renal tubular epithelial cells or, less often, inflammatory cells, embedded in a protein matrix. The granularity is sometimes further categorized as fine or coarse but the type of granularity is not of diagnostic importance, but useful rather for prognostic purposes. Nephrotoxins (e.g., gentamicin sulfate, amphotericin B), nephritis, and ischemia are pathologic events that result in their formation. Moderate numbers of epithelial cells *(arrows)*, leukocytes, and erythrocytes (inconspicuous) are present. Marked numbers of brightly refractile lipid droplets are prominent in this specimen. The lipiduria was attributed to the lubricant used to facilitate catheterization. (Unstained; HP oil.) **B, Granular cast with lipid droplets (fatty cast), unstained.** This cast was present in the urine of a dog with the nephrotic syndrome. They can be seen in association with diabetes mellitus and in cats with renal tubular injury. A moderate number of lipid droplets (out of focus) are present. A starch granule (glove powder) is located beneath the cast *(arrow)*. (Unstained; HP oil.)

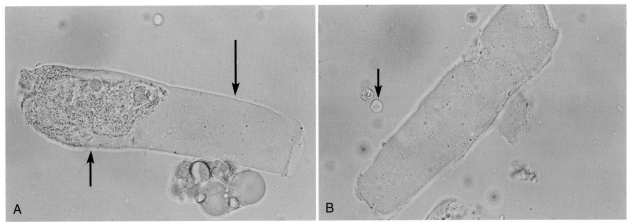

■ **FIGURE 11-8. A, Granular/waxy cast, unstained.** Waxy casts develop from granular casts as illustrated by this cast that has granular cast *(short arrow)* and waxy cast *(long arrow)* characteristics. (Unstained; HP oil.) **B, Waxy cast, unstained.** These casts indicate chronic tubular pathology since additional time is required for their formation. Implicit in the pathogenesis of their formation is localized tubular obstruction. One sequela is dilation of the tubular lumen, resulting in a wide cast. The term "broad" is sometimes added as a descriptive adjective when the width is two to four times that of a hyaline or granular cast. The magnitude of its width is apparent when contrasted to an erythrocyte *(arrow)*. A "fissure" or crack is often observed (top right). (Unstained; HP oil.)

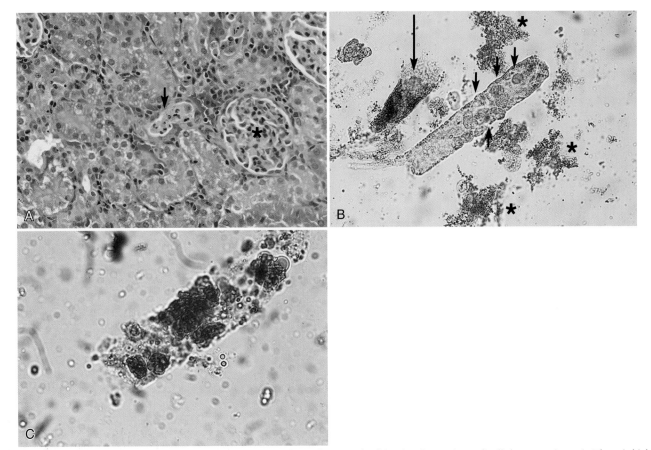

■ **FIGURE 11-9. Cellular cast. A, Histology.** Pyelonephritis has resulted in the formation of cellular cast *(arrow)*. The pinkish protein matrix contains dark-staining neutrophil nuclei and unidentified nuclear debris. A glomerulus is present *(asterisk)*. (H & E; HP oil.) **B, Cytology, unstained.** Cells, most consistent morphologically with epithelial cells, can be seen embedded in the cast matrix *(short arrows)*. The finding is suggestive of acute tubular necrosis. A fragmented granular cast *(long arrow)* and amorphous debris (unrecognizable granular material) *(asterisks)* is observed. (Unstained; HP oil.) **C, Cytology, stained.** A stained specimen further supports the identity of cells in the cast as epithelial cells (when focused up and down). A few lipid droplets are observed. (Sedi-Stain; HP oil.)

(e.g., spondylitis, longterm corticosteroids treatment, diabetes mellitus).

Parasites such as *Pearsonema plica* (formerly *Capillaria*) or *P. feliscati* (Fig. 11-23A&B) produce football-shaped eggs that are occasionally seen. The dog or cat may acquire infection after ingesting infected earthworms or earthworm-associated material. Adult *Pearsonema* spp. develop in the urinary bladder mucosa and may cause minor irritation with subsequent cystitis. Eggs may appear in the urine within two months following infection. This form of urinary nematode appears to be more common in the southeastern U.S. Other parasites such as microfilaria may be incidental from bleeding into the urine (Fig. 11-24).

Other incidental findings in the urine can include dye crystals, starch granules, plant fibers, and pollen (Fig. 11-25A&D).

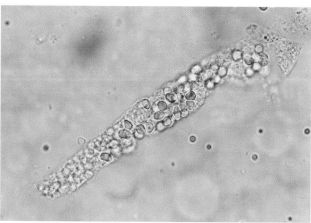

■ **FIGURE 11-10. Red cell cast, unstained.** A fragile and uncommon finding, they indicate acute intrarenal injury. The urine specimen is from a dog that had been traumatized (hit by car). A few lipid droplets are present. Note that they are more refractile than erythrocytes and vary in size. (Unstained; HP oil.)

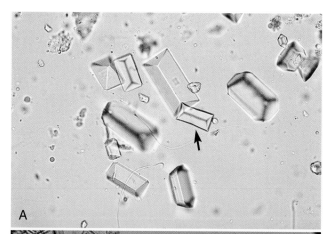

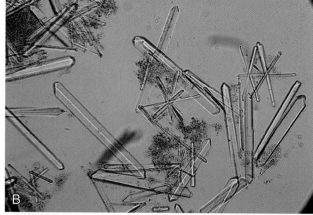

■ **FIGURE 11-11. A, Magnesium ammonium phosphate (struvite) crystalluria.** These crystals have been misnamed as triple phosphates. The small crystal in the center *(arrow)* illustrates the form that has been referred to as a "coffin lid" appearance (closed casket as viewed from the top). They can be a normal finding in dogs and cats or be associated with struvite uroliths (sterile and infected). They tend to be found in urine with a pH >7. (Unstained; HP oil.) **B, Struvite crystals.** Present are a variety of shapes, including rodlike in this specimen and a "fern leaf" appearance (not shown). Small islands of reddish-stained amorphous phosphates are present. (Sedi-Stain; HP oil.)

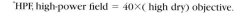

BOX 11-1   Normal Number of Cells per HPF* in a Urine Sediment and the Interpretation of Increased Numbers

Erythrocytes (RBCs)
<5; varying degrees of crenation are often observed due to the physiochemical environment of the urine (see Fig. 11-1A). Increased numbers indicate bleeding associated with (1) renal pathology: glomerular or tubulointerstitial disease, calculus, renal vein thrombosis, vascular dysplasia, trauma—an erythrocyte cast is indicative of intrarenal pathology (see Fig. 11-10); (2) lower urinary tract disease: acute and chronic infection, calculus, neoplasia, hemorrhagic cystitis; or (3) contamination from the genital tract—collect urine via percutaneous cystocentesis.

Leukocytes (WBCs)
<5; the neutrophil is the most common leukocyte. Its nuclear segmentation may be lost as a result of the physiochemical environment of the urine and appear round to oval, resulting in an epithelial cell-like appearance but with less cytoplasm (see Fig. 11-2B). However, it has less cytoplasm compared to an epithelial cell. Increased numbers are associated with (1) renal disease: pyelonephritis—leukocyte cast may be found (see Fig. 11-9A&B)—calculus; (2) lower urinary tract disease: acute and chronic cystitis, calculus, neoplasia; and (3) contamination from the genital tract—collect urine via percutaneous cystocentesis.

Transitional Epithelial Cells
<2; mild size variation is normal, with the larger ones located in the urinary bladder and urethra and the smaller ones located in the renal pelvis and tubules. Epithelial cells with "tails" (cytoplasmic projection) are called *caudate epithelial cells* and have been associated with an origin from the renal pelvis. However, size and shape do not reliably indicate the anatomic site of origin. Transitional cell hyperplasia (see Fig. 11-4B) is readily stimulated by inflammation (e.g., secondary to infection), irritation, and cyclophosphamide.

Squamous Epithelial Cells
0; these large, polygonal, angular cells are often present in free-catch and catheterized specimens and may be prominent during estrus (see Fig. 11-3). Finding bacteria along with squamous epithelial cells is suggestive of contamination, and the examination of a specimen collected via cystocentesis is prudent.

*HPF, high-power field = 40×(high dry) objective.

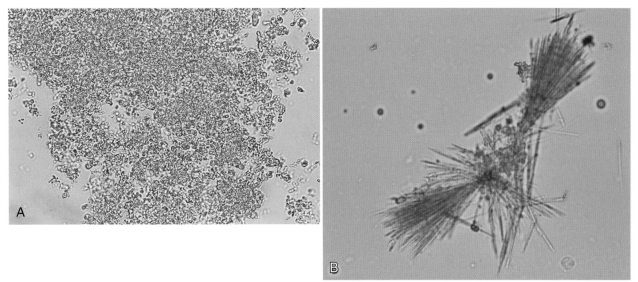

■ **FIGURE 11-12. A, Amorphous phosphate crystals.** They have no known diagnostic importance but should not be mistaken for bacterial colonies. They are distinguished from amorphous urate crystals by their lack of color, formation in alkaline urine, and solubility in acetic acid. (Unstained; ×500.) **B, Calcium phosphate crystals, pH 8.5. Dog.** These clusters of colorless, long, needle-shaped crystals were present in alkaline urine from an Airedale Terrier with elevated liver enzymes and anemia. (Unstained; IP.) (B, Courtesy of Rose Raskin, Purdue University.)

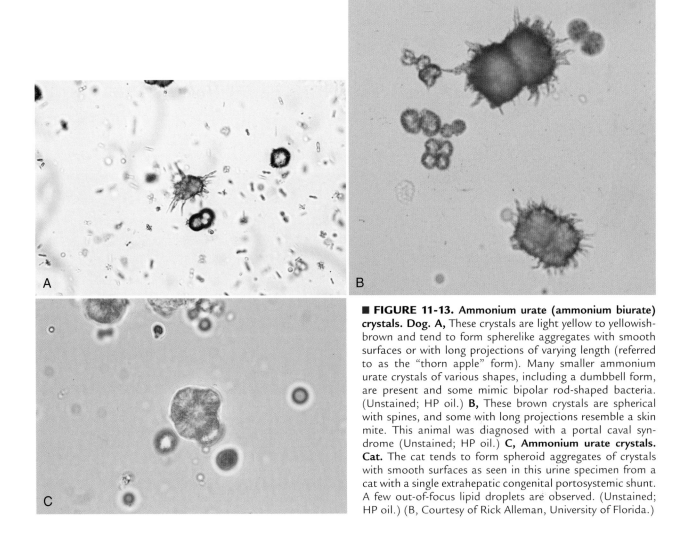

■ **FIGURE 11-13. Ammonium urate (ammonium biurate) crystals. Dog. A,** These crystals are light yellow to yellowish-brown and tend to form spherelike aggregates with smooth surfaces or with long projections of varying length (referred to as the "thorn apple" form). Many smaller ammonium urate crystals of various shapes, including a dumbbell form, are present and some mimic bipolar rod-shaped bacteria. (Unstained; HP oil.) **B,** These brown crystals are spherical with spines, and some with long projections resemble a skin mite. This animal was diagnosed with a portal caval syndrome (Unstained; HP oil.) **C, Ammonium urate crystals. Cat.** The cat tends to form spheroid aggregates of crystals with smooth surfaces as seen in this urine specimen from a cat with a single extrahepatic congenital portosystemic shunt. A few out-of-focus lipid droplets are observed. (Unstained; HP oil.) (B, Courtesy of Rick Alleman, University of Florida.)

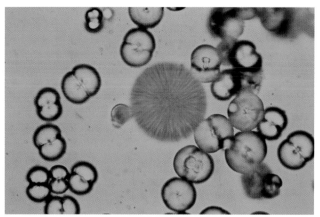

■ FIGURE 11-14. Calcium carbonate crystals. Calcium carbonate crystals are not observed in dog or cat urine but are observed in the urine of horses, rabbits, and guinea pigs. (Unstained; HP oil.)

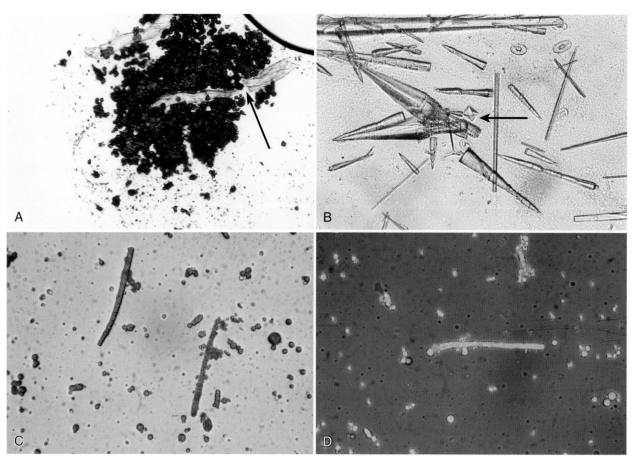

■ FIGURE 11-15. A, Amorphous urate crystals; cotton fiber. Sodium, potassium, magnesium, and calcium urate salts form a granular precipitate that is yellowish to dark brown. They can appear similar to amorphous phosphate crystal precipitates. A congenital portosystemic shunt was diagnosed (markedly abnormal serum bile acids concentration; portogram) in the Yorkshire terrier from which this specimen was obtained. A cotton fiber is trapped within the crystals *(arrow)*. (Unstained; HP oil.) **B, Sodium urate crystals.** These crystals were observed in association with ammonium urate uroliths in a Bulldog. A calcium oxalate dihydrate crystal is also observed *(arrow)*. (Unstained; HP oil.) **Same case C-D. Sodium urate crystals, pH 6.0, unstained. Dog. C, Nonpolarized.** Two forms of sodium urate crystals are shown from the urine of a Dalmatian. The stick shapes and round spheres changed after a short period into rhomboid uric acid forms (not shown). (Unstained; HP oil.) **D, Polarized. Dog.** Under polarized light, these crystals were highly reflective, consistent with urates. (Unstained; HP oil. C and D, Courtesy of Rose Raskin, Purdue University.)

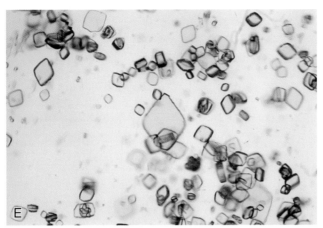

■ **FIGURE 11-15, cont'd. E, Uric acid crystals.** These crystals are uncommonly observed in the dog and cat; however, common in humans owing to the difference in purine metabolism. They have the same associations as listed for ammonium urate crystals. (C and D, Courtesy of Rose Raskin, Purdue University.)

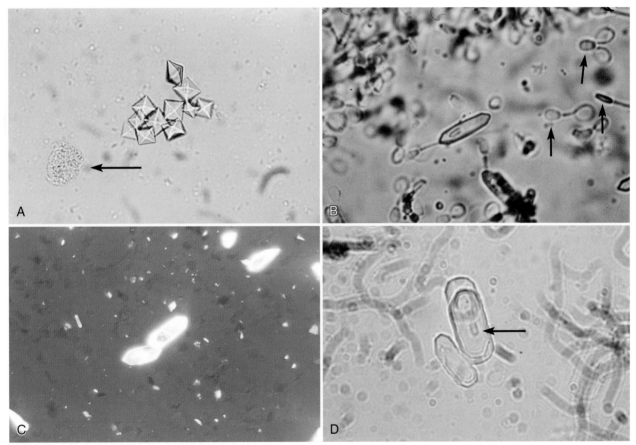

■ **FIGURE 11-16. A, Calcium oxalate dihydrate crystals. Dog.** This photomicrograph illustrates the classical "Maltese cross" form in an apparently healthy animal. They can be found in the urine of apparently healthy dogs and cats, and in association with calcium oxalate urolithiasis and ethylene glycol toxicity. The latter should be promptly considered in a dog or cat with acute renal failure. A fragment of a granular cast is located to the lower left *(arrow)*. (Unstained; HP oil.) **Same case B-C. Calcium oxalate monohydrate crystals. Dog. B, Spermatozoa.** These crystals have been erroneously referred to as hippuric acid. These crystals, alone or in combination with the dihydrate form, are observed in association with ethylene glycol toxicity. They have pointed ends (hippuric acid-like appearance) and often a small projection ("raised lid") is observed on one end. Numerous spermatozoa are observed *(arrows)*. Spermatozoa can be observed in the urine of male dogs collected by cystocentesis. (Unstained; HP oil.) **C, Polarized.** Same specimen as in B. Polarization accentuates the "raised lid"-type projection noted on one end of the crystal. (Polarized; HP oil.) **D, Calcium oxalate monohydrate crystals. Cat.** This crystal is associated with ethylene glycol toxicity. The calcium oxalate monohydrate in the cat is wider than the canine counterpart and has *(arrow)* rounded ends. The "raised lid" effect on one end is apparent on the larger of the two crystals. The out-of-focus elongated material is artifact (dust in the camera optics). (Unstained; HP oil.)

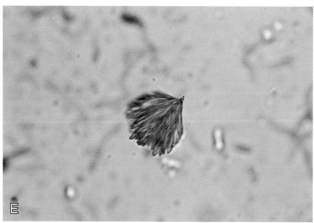

■ **FIGURE 11-16, cont'd. E, Calcium oxalate monohydrate crystals. Dog.** Fan-shaped aggregate of calcium oxalate monohydrate crystals associated with calcium oxalate uroliths. Fan-shaped crystals are also associated with the use of sulfa-containing antibacterials. (Unstained; HP oil.)

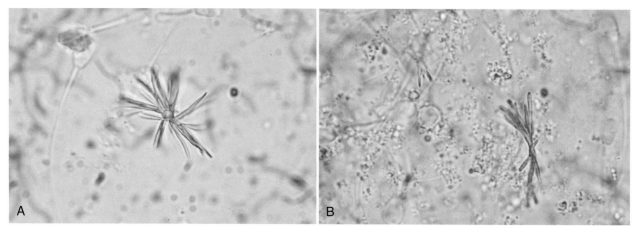

■ **FIGURE 11-17. A-B, Bilirubin crystals.** Bilirubin can crystallize in association with bilirubinuria. The causes of bilirubinuria should be explored. (Unstained; HP oil.)

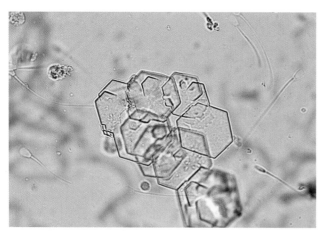

■ **FIGURE 11-18. Cystine crystals.** Cystine crystalluria is always an abnormal finding and indicative of the metabolic disorder of cystinuria. Cystine crystalluria may or may not be associated with cystine uroliths. (Unstained; HP oil.)

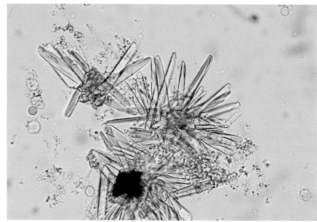

■ **FIGURE 11-19. Calcium hydrogen phosphate dehydrate (brushite) crystals.** This form of calcium phosphate crystals is observed in urine specimens from apparently healthy dogs and in association with calcium phosphate uroliths and calcium phosphate/calcium oxalate uroliths. They tend to form in urine with an acid pH. (Unstained; HP oil.)

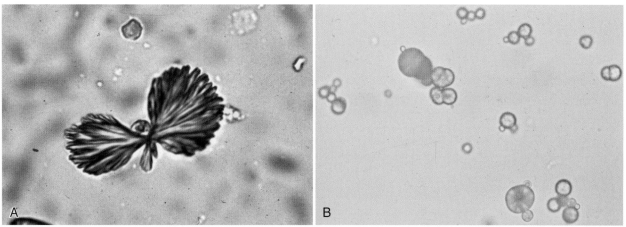

■ **FIGURE 11-20. Sulfa crystals, unstained. A,** One form of sulfa crystals that may result from sulfonamide administration is shown. These yellow crystals resemble bundles or wheat sheaves. A lignin test used as a screening test for sulfonamides was positive in this case. (Unstained; HP oil.) **B,** Another form of sulfa crystals is shown that resembles calcium carbonate crystals; however, they are more yellow in color. Spherical forms with radiating streaks appear singly or attached to each other. A lignin test was positive for this sample. (Unstained; HP oil.) (A and B, Courtesy of Rose Raskin, University of Florida.)

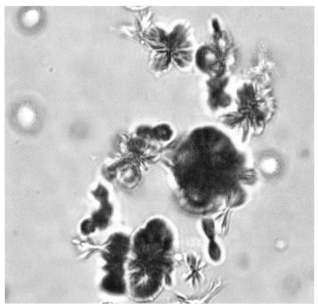

■ **FIGURE 11-21. Tyrosine-like crystals, unstained. pH 6.5. Dog.** This Golden Retriever presented with lymphoma and exhibited elevated liver enzymes and bilirubinuria. The crystals resemble bilirubin crystals with multiple short needles; however, they did not appear golden yellow and were arranged in dense, dark-colored clusters that measured 15 to 30 μm in diameter. The clear, circular shapes in the background are erythrocytes. (Unstained; HP oil.) (Courtesy of Rose Raskin, Purdue University.)

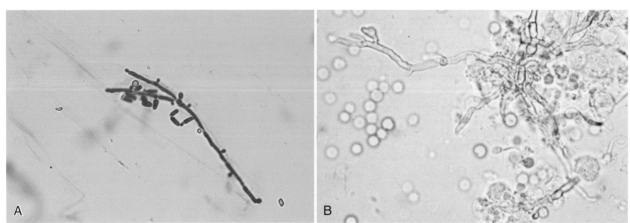

■ **FIGURE 11-22. A, Budding yeast pseudohyphae.** A pseudohyphal form of yeast is suggested by the lack of distinct segmentation. Other forms of yeast can appear morphologically similar to lipid droplets or erythrocytes (not shown). Both yeast and fungi in urine sediments usually represent contaminants. If a stain is used, it should be also examined for fungal growth. (New methylene blue; HP oil.) **B, *Aspergillus* sp., inflammation, unstained. Dog.** Septated hyphal forms are present in the urine of an animal with disseminated *Aspergillus* sp. infection. Diagnosis was confirmed by urine culture. A group of red cells is seen at the left while large, clear, slightly granular leukocytes are closely associated with the infectious agent. (Unstained; HP oil.) (B, Courtesy of Rose Raskin, University of Florida.)

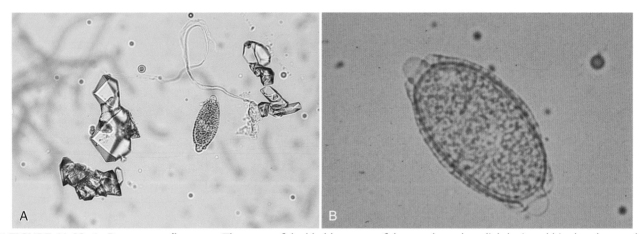

■ **FIGURE 11-23. A, *Pearsonema plica* ovum.** The ovum of the bladder worm of dogs and cats has slightly tipped bipolar plugs and a granular appearance. These features help distinguish it from pollen grain contaminants. Aggregates of magnesium ammonium phosphates crystals are also observed. (Unstained, HP oil.) **B, *Pearsonema feliscati*, unstained. Cat.** Close-up magnification demonstrates the tilted terminal plugs which helps identifies the ovum. No clinical signs were associated with this animals. (Unstained; HP oil.) (B, Courtesy of Rose Raskin, University of Florida.)

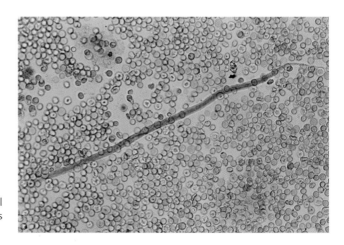

■ **FIGURE 11-24. Microfilaria of *Dirofilaria immitis*.** An incidental finding in this dog with hemorrhagic cystitis. Numerous erythrocytes are observed. (New methylene blue; IP.)

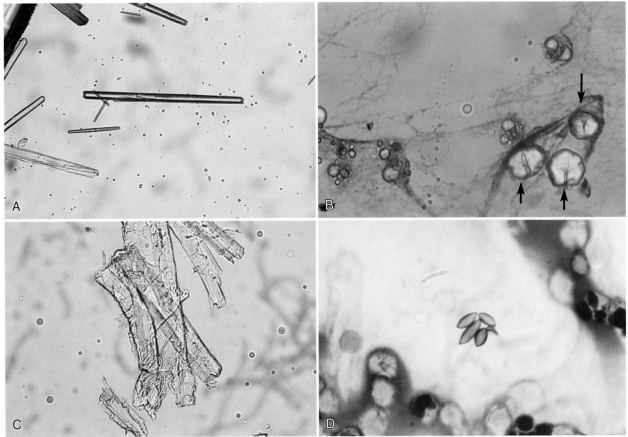

■ **FIGURE 11-25. A, Radiopaque contrast dye crystals.** These needle-shaped crystals were observed in urine in association with the use of an iodinated radiopaque contrast agent used for an excretory urogram. (Unstained; HP oil.) **B, Starch granules** (glove powder) *(arrows)*. These structures are contaminants. An "x" with a central depression can be observed by focusing up and down on the granules. Poorly formed wisps of mucus stain but variably sized refractile lipid droplets do not stain with the water-based stain. (New methylene blue; HP oil.) **C, Cotton fibers.** Cotton fibers from clothing or gauze pads can mimic hyalin/granular casts or crystals. (Unstained; HP oil.) **D, Pollen grains.** Pollen grains of various sizes and morphology can contaminate urine. They are often ovoid or round. (New methylene blue; HP oil.)

REFERENCES

Barlough JE, Osborne CA, Steven JB: Canine and feline urinalysis: value of macroscopic and microscopic examinations, *J Am Vet Med Assoc* 184:61-63, 1981.

Fettman MJ: Evaluation of the usefulness of routine microscopy in canine urinalysis, *J Am Vet Med Assoc* 190:892-896, 1987.

Forrester SD, Troy GC, Dalton MN, et al: Retrospective evaluation of urinary tract infection in 42 dogs with hyperadrenocorticism or diabetes mellitus or both, *J Vet Intern Med* 13:557-560, 1999.

Graff SL: *A handbook of routine urinalysis*, JB Lippincott, Philadelphia, 1983, pp 83-107.

Haber MH: Pisse prophesy: A brief history of urinalysis. In Haber MH, Corwin HL (eds): *Clinics in laboratory medicine*, WB Saunders, Philadelphia, 1988, pp 415-426.

Meyer DJ, Harvey JW: Evaluation of renal function and urine. In Meyer DJ, Harvey JW (eds): *Veterinary laboratory medicine: interpretation and diagnosis*, ed 3, Elsevier, St. Louis, 2004, pp 225-236.

Osborne CA, Stevens JB: *Urinalysis: a clinical guide to compassionate patient care*, Bayer, Shawnee Mission, KS, 1999, pp 125-179.

Raskin RE, Murray KA, Levy JK: Comparison of home monitoring methods for feline urine pH measurement, *Vet Clin Pathol* 31:51-55, 2002.

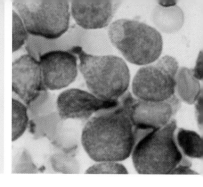

CHAPTER 12

Reproductive System

Laia Solano-Gallego

FEMALE REPRODUCTIVE SYSTEM: MAMMARY GLANDS, OVARIES, UTERUS, AND VAGINA

Mammary Glands

Mammary gland lesions are common in female dogs and cats. Mammary gland enlargement may be related to a wide variety of disease processes, including cysts, inflammation, hyperplasia, and benign or malignant neoplasia. Important information in the investigation of mammary gland disease includes history, breed, and age; whether the gland was intact or older when the dog or cat was neutered; date of last estrus, pregnancy, or hormone therapy; size, number, and consistency of lesion(s); attachment to underlying tissue; rate of growth; presence of ulceration; and evidence of metastasis (Baker and Lumsden, 1999). Ancillary diagnostic tests used to evaluate mammary lesions include a thorough evaluation of health status involving a complete physical examination, complete blood count, serum biochemical profile, urinalysis and/or coagulation profile, imaging, cytology, and histopathology.

While histopathology and, more recently, cytology have been used to accurately classify mammary lesions as cysts, inflammation, or hyperplasia/neoplasia, determination of the malignant potential of mammary neoplasia can be difficult. Histopathology may often show poor correlation between histologic diagnosis of malignant neoplasia and biologic behavior. While a few studies have compared cytologic evaluation of mammary neoplasms with histologic analysis, no reports have related biologic behavior with cytologic diagnosis. However, the ease of obtaining cytologic specimens from mammary lesions, the low invasive nature, and relatively small expense make exfoliative cytology a useful diagnostic tool in the evaluation of mammary disease. When combined with history, signalment, and clinical findings, cytologic examination of mammary aspirates is particularly useful for differentiation between neoplastic disease, cystic lesions, or mastitis. Exfoliative cytology is also useful for evaluation of regional lymph nodes, distant metastatic sites, and

neoplastic effusions associated with mammary malignancies. Unfortunately, use of cytology to evaluate mammary neoplasms can be difficult, and definitive diagnoses may not always be possible. Some of these difficulties are related to sample collection and others are simply inherent in the nature of mammary neoplasia. With an understanding of the potential difficulties of mammary cytology, the cytopathologist can provide useful diagnostic information concerning mammary gland disease.

Cytologic samples from mammary lesions may be obtained by expressing material from the gland, imprints or, more commonly, fine-needle aspiration (FNA) of the affected area. Proper sample collection is important for cytology to be useful in the evaluation of mammary tumors. Because of the considerable tissue heterogeneity that may be present within mammary tumors, sampling of multiple areas within a single tumor and similar samplings of additional tumors are very important. Care should also be taken to aspirate the periphery of a mammary mass as opposed to fluctuant areas within a solid lesion or the center of large tumors. These areas tend to yield fluid of low cellularity or necrosis resulting in a nondiagnostic sample.

Normal Anatomy and Histology

Mammary glands are compound tubuloalveolar glands that are believed to be extensively modified sweat glands (Banks, 1986). In dogs and cats, five pairs of mammary glands are arranged as bilaterally symmetrical rows extending from the ventral thorax to the inguinal region. During pregnancy and lactation, the mammary glands undergo marked hypertrophy and hyperplasia to produce immunoglobulin-containing colostrum followed by milk.

Histologically, mammary glands are composed of a secretory component consisting of alveolar secretory epithelial cells and the initial portion of the intralobular ducts (Banks, 1986) (Figs. 12-1 to 12-3). The secretory portion of the glands is drained by the ductular system, composed of nonsecretory columnar and cuboidal epithelium. Reticular connective tissue supports the alveoli and smaller ducts. Bundles of smooth muscle and elastic

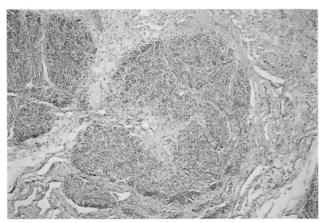

■ **FIGURE 12-1. Normal, inactive mammary gland. Tissue section. Dog.** Lobules of glandular tissue are surrounded by abundant interlobular connective tissue. (H&E; LP.)

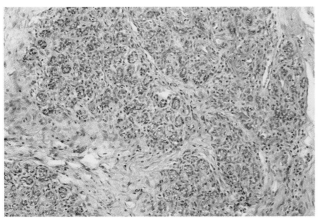

■ **FIGURE 12-2. Normal, inactive mammary gland. Tissue section. Dog.** The glandular portion of mammary tissue is composed of alveoli (acini) and intralobular ducts, which are lined by cuboidal to columnar epithelium. The interlobular ducts, composed of nonsecretory columnar and cuboidal epithelium, drain the alveoli. Reticular connective tissue supports the alveoli and smaller ducts. Bundles of smooth muscle and elastic fibers surround the large ducts. (H&E; IP.)

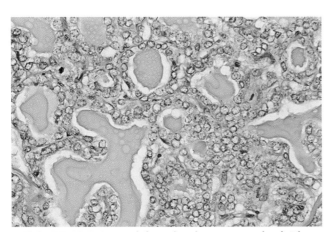

■ **FIGURE 12-3. Normal, lactational mammary gland. Tissue section. Dog.** The secretory portion of the gland is well developed and connective tissue elements are decreased. The alveolar lumens contain bright-pink secretory material. (H&E; HP oil.)

fibers surround the large ducts. Myoepithelial cells can be found between the alveolar epithelial cells and the underlying basement membrane. The normal histology of mammary gland from immature female dogs and sequential microscopic changes that occur during different stages of the estrous cycle are reviewed elsewhere (Rehm et al., 2007).

Normal Cytology

Normal mammary secretions are characterized cytologically by low numbers of sloughed secretory epithelial cells known as foam cells as well as macrophages and occasional neutrophils on an eosinophilic to basophilic proteinaceous background. Foam cells are large, individualized cells characterized by round to oval, eccentrically located nuclei and abundant amounts of vacuolated cytoplasm (Allison and Maddux, 2008). These cells may also contain amorphous, basophilic secretory material (Fig. 12-4). Foam cells resemble and can be difficult to distinguish from reactive macrophages. FNA cytology of normal mammary tissue usually reveals small amounts of blood with no to low numbers of nucleated cells and moderate to large amounts of basophilic, proteinaceous material, clear lipid droplets, and adipocytes (Allen et al., 1986). Small sheets and clusters of mammary secretory epithelial cells that are uniform in size and shape may be seen occasionally in aspirates of normal mammary tissue. Secretory epithelial cells exhibit round, dark nuclei and moderate amounts of basophilic cytoplasm. Acinar formations may be noted. Ductular epithelial cells are characterized by oval, basal nuclei with scant amounts of cytoplasm. Myoepithelial cells may be seen as darkly staining, oval free nuclei or as spindle-shaped cells (Allison and Maddux, 2008).

Mammary Cysts

Mammary cysts or fibrocystic disease (FCD), also known as blue dome cyst or polycystic mastopathy, is a form of mammary dysplasia in which dilated ducts expand to

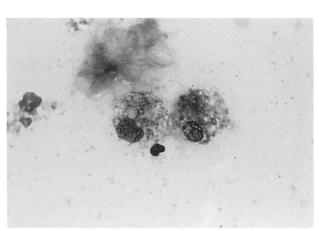

■ **FIGURE 12-4. Mammary gland aspirate. Foam cells. Cat.** The two foam cells have eccentrically located nuclei, low nuclear-to-cytoplasmic ratios, clear cytoplasmic vacuoles, and abundant amounts of basophilic secretory material. The background has a lightly basophilic, proteinaceous appearance consistent with normal mammary aspirates. (Wright-Giemsa; HP oil.)

form cavitary lesions (Brodey et al., 1983). FCD generally occurs in middle-aged to older animals, although the disease has been reported in dogs of 1 year of age. Formation of FCD may have a hormonal component as administration of medroxyprogesterone has been associated with development of FCD in dogs. In dogs, rapid growth during estrus and regression during metestrus has been noted. The rapid growth of cysts during estrus may be associated with rupture of the cysts. Ovariohysterectomy should be considered when mammary cysts grow and regress in association with the estrous cycle, particularly if multiple glands are involved. FCD is considered a benign lesion in dogs; however, the disease has been associated with development of mammary gland carcinoma.

Mammary cysts may present as a well-circumscribed, single cystic nodule or as a flat, rubbery, multinodular mass. The nodule(s) exhibit slow, expansile growth and the overlying skin may develop a blue color, hence the term *blue dome cyst* (Brodey et al., 1983). Mammary cysts may be classified as simple cysts characterized by a single layer of flattened lining epithelium or papillary cysts containing papillary outgrowths of the lining epithelial cells. Aspiration of mammary cysts typically yields a green-brown or blood-tinged fluid containing low numbers of foam cells and pigment-laden macrophages (Allison and Maddux, 2008). Neutrophils may be increased if inflammation is also present. Cholesterol crystals, which appear as large, rectangular crystalline structures often with a notched corner, may be present as a result of breakdown of cellular membranes within the cyst (Fig. 12-5). Epithelial cells derived from the cystic lining may be noted, particularly if the cyst has a papillary component. These cells tend to occur in dense sheets and clusters and may display some mild variation in nuclear size and shape. Mammary cysts may coexist with benign and/or malignant mammary tumors (Brodey et al., 1983). Therefore, aspiration or biopsy of solid areas of a mass associated with a cyst or other mammary masses should be performed to rule out the presence of concurrent mammary neoplasia.

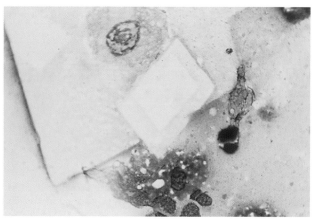

■ **FIGURE 12-5. Mammary cyst aspirate. Cholesterol crystals. Cat.** The clear, rectangular crystals are of varying size. Two foam cells are adjacent to the crystals. (Wright-Giemsa; HP oil.)

Mammary Gland Hyperplasia

Hyperplastic and dysplastic lesions of mammary glands include unilobular and multilobular hyperplasia, adenosis, and epitheliosis (Misdorp et al., 1999). These lesions occur in dogs and less commonly in cats (Yager et al., 1993). Mammary hyperplasia is characterized by proliferations of secretory or ductular epithelium or myoepithelial cells resembling the physiologic hyperplasia of pregnancy with some mild histologic atypia. Cytologically, these lesions may be difficult to distinguish from each other and from benign neoplasms such as adenomas or papillomas. Moderate to large numbers of epithelial cells arranged in sheets and clusters can be aspirated from hyperplastic mammary tissue. These cells, which are similar in appearance to normal mammary epithelial cells, display round nuclei with fine to lightly stippled chromatin of uniform size and shape and scant to moderate amounts of basophilic cytoplasm. Foam cells and macrophages may also be noted.

In cats, a form of mammary hyperplasia occurs that has been variously identified as fibroepithelial hyperplasia, feline mammary hypertrophy, mammary fibroadenomatous hyperplasia, or feline mammary hypertrophy/fibroadenomatous complex. Feline mammary fibroepithelial hyperplasia (MFH) is a clinically benign, fairly common condition affecting estrous-cycling or pregnant female cats usually less than 2 years of age (Mesher, 1997). MFH has also been reported in older intact and neutered cats of either gender receiving progesterone-containing compounds, such as megestrol acetate (Hayden et al., 1989) or depot medroxyprogesterone acetate (Loretti et al., 2005). MFH is considered a form of mammary dysplasia characterized by a rapid, abnormal growth of one or more mammary glands. In contrast to a neoplastic process, paired glands often exhibit a similar degree of enlargement (Lana et al., 2007). MFH is notable for a marked intralobular ductular proliferation identical to the ductular proliferation seen during the progesterone-influenced early stages of pregnancy (Misdorp et al., 1999). This typical histologic appearance, the occurrence in cycling females or cats administered progesterone, and the identification of progesterone receptors in MFH lesions from female and male cats have led to the belief that development of MFH involves endogenous or exogenous progesterone. MFH usually regresses over time without treatment, although secondary infections may require appropriate antibiotic therapy. Ovariohysterectomy, performed via a flank incision if the glands are greatly enlarged, will often result in regression of lesions and will prevent future recurrences (Lana et al., 2007). However, some cats do not respond to withdrawal of progestogens or ovariectomy and can be treated successfully with the progesterone receptor blocker aglépristone (Görlinger et al., 2002).

The cytologic appearance of MFH (Fig. 12-6) has been reported (Mesher, 1997). Aspirated material of a histologically confirmed MFH lesion consisted of a very uniform population of cuboidal epithelial cells arranged in thick clusters. The cuboidal epithelial cells were characterized by dense, round nuclei with small nucleoli and scant amounts of basophilic cytoplasm. A mesenchymal

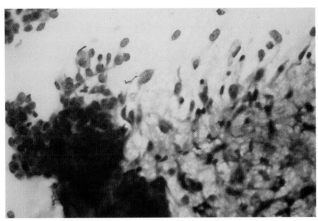

■ **FIGURE 12-6.** **Mammary fibroepithelial hyperplasia. Tissue aspirate. Cat.** Sheet of epithelial cells and spindle cells in pink extracellular material. The epithelial cells are uniform in size and shape and the spindle cells display some mild anisokaryosis. (Wright; HP oil.) (From Mesher CI: What is your diagnosis? A 14-month-old domestic cat, *Vet Clin Pathol* 26:4, 13, 1997.)

population of spindle-shaped cells with narrow oval nuclei, one to two nucleoli, and tapering cytoplasm was also present. The mesenchymal cells displayed moderate variation in nuclear size (anisokaryosis) and cellular size (anisocytosis). Moderate amounts of pink extracellular matrix were associated with the mesenchymal cells. These cytologic findings correlated with the histologic findings of hyperplastic ductular epithelium (cuboidal epithelial population) and proliferation of edematous stroma (mesenchymal cells with extracellular matrix). The presence of abundant stromal elements helps to differentiate MFH from mammary neoplasia, which generally contains scant stromal material. Cytologic recognition of the characteristic cell types from mammary masses in a cat with appropriate signalment and clinical history can be considered highly suggestive of MFH, thus eliminating the need for mammary gland excision and allowing for appropriate medical and/or surgical management.

Mammary Gland Inflammation/Infection

Inflammation of the mammary glands is referred to as *mastitis* and may present as a focal lesion or may involve one or more glands. Mastitis may infrequently occur from hematogenous spread of organisms, nonlactation-associated trauma, fight wounds, or infected neoplasms. *Dirofilaria repens* infection of the mammary gland in the bitch (Manuali et al., 2005) and mastitis due to *Toxoplasma gondii* in a cat (Park et al., 2007) have been recently reported. Mastitis is most often associated with postparturient lactation. It can also occur during pseudopregnancy, as well after early weaning of puppies. It is thought to result from entry of infectious organisms through the teat orifice or damaged overlying skin (Gruffydd-Jones, 1980). Neonatal morbidity or mortality may be the first indication of mastitis. Clinical signs associated with mastitis include swollen, painful glands that result in discomfort while nursing. The glands may become abscessed or gangrenous with necrosis of

overlying skin. The bitch or queen may also present with clinical signs of systemic illness such as anorexia, fever, vomiting, or diarrhea. A complete blood count may reveal an inflammatory leukogram characterized by either an increase in segmented and nonsegmented (band) neutrophils or a degenerative left shift with a predominance of immature neutrophils, especially if gangrenous mastitis is present (Ververidis et al., 2007).

Cytologic examination of secretions from inflamed and/or infected mammary glands is usually diagnostic; however, FNA may be needed for focal lesions. Large numbers of neutrophils are present, which may exhibit degenerative changes of karyolysis and karyorrhexis. Reactive macrophages, small lymphocytes, and plasma cells may also be seen, particularly with more chronic lesions. Infectious organisms may be visualized within neutrophils and, less commonly, macrophages, indicating a septic process. Various bacteria have been incriminated as etiologic agents of disease such as *Staphylococcus* spp., *Streptococcus* spp., and *E. coli*. Other types of bacteria and fungi can be isolated (Allison and Maddux, 2008). *Staphylococcus intermedius* is the most common cause of clinical and subclinical mastitis in the dog (Schafer-Somi et al., 2003). Culture and sensitivity of milk, inflamed mammary secretions, or aspirated material are warranted to determine appropriate antibiotic therapy.

The need for antibiotic therapy to treat bacterial mastitis depends on the severity of the lesions. Systemic antibiotic therapy is based upon culture and sensitivity results. Abscessed glands will need to be surgically débrided or drained. Warm, moist topical packs may be used for gangrenous mastitis, and the necrotic tissue can be excised or allowed to slough. Supportive care, including intravenous fluid therapy, may be necessary for the bitch or queen as well as nursing puppies or kittens. Also, puppies or kittens may require appropriate antibiotic therapy and should be weaned and reared by hand.

Some noninfectious inflammatory conditions of mammary glands have been described. Focal mastitic lesions may leave residual fibrotic nodules consisting of epithelial cell metaplasia, pigment-laden macrophages, nondegenerate neutrophils, small lymphocytes, and plasma cells (Allison and Maddux, 2008). Unlike mammary gland tumors, fibrotic nodules tend to occur in young dogs, do not increase in size, and are usually associated with a previous history of mastitis (Brodey et al., 1983).

Neoplasia

Canine Mammary Gland Tumors

Following skin tumors, mammary neoplasms are the second most common tumor in dogs and the most commonly seen tumor in bitches (Misdorp, 2002). Mammary gland tumors (MGT) rarely occur in male dogs with a reported annual incidence of 4 in 100,000 while the annual incidence is 207 in 100,000 in female dogs (Saba et al., 2007; Lana et al., 2007). Many of the MGT reported in male dogs have been associated with small tumor sizes, benign or well-differentiated malignant epithelial tumors, nondefinitive evidence of metastatic disease at diagnosis, and intense estrogen-receptor positivity. The median age for development of canine mammary gland tumors is 10 to 11 years of age, with rare occurrence in bitches younger than 4 years old. Breed tendencies for MGT have been reported with a predisposition in several spaniels breeds, the Poodle, Dachshund, and other breeds (Sorenmo, 2003) and with a greater prevalence of malignant tumors in large breeds than in small breeds (Itoh et al., 2005). A heritable, familial tendency for development of mammary neoplasms in Beagles has been suggested (Benjamin et al., 1999). Development of MGT appears to have a hormonal component as evidenced by the sparing effect of ovariohysterectomy in first estrus cycles and by the increased length of survival time in dogs spayed less than 2 years before mammary carcinoma surgery when compared with dogs spayed longer than 2 years before tumor surgery or intact dogs (Sorenmo et al., 2000). Estrogen and progesterone receptors have been identified in normal, hyperplastic/dysplastic mammary tissue and a majority of mammary neoplasms (Lana et al., 2007; Millanta et al., 2005; de las Mulas et al., 2005). Interestingly, hormone receptor expression, which is a characteristic feature of mature mammary epithelial cells, tends to be decreased or absent in poorly differentiated tumors and metastatic lesions. It is well known that progesterone or synthetic progestins administration increases the incidence of MGT in dogs (Misdorp, 1991). Mechanisms involved in the progesterone-induced mammary gland tumors include an upregulation of growth hormone production by mammary epithelial cells (van Garderen and Schalken, 2002) and a rise in blood levels of insulin-like growth factor I (IGF-I) and IGF-II (Lana et al., 2007). Growth hormone and IGF may increase proliferation of susceptible or transformed mammary epithelial cells, resulting in neoplasia. Other risk factors to develop MGT are obesity at 1 year of age and low-fat/low-protein diet (Sorenmo, 2003). Other molecule targets have been investigated to elucidate prognosis or the pathways of tumorigenesis such as cyclooxygenase-2 (Millanta et al., 2006a), heat-shock proteins (Romanucci et al., 2006), VEGF (Millanta et al., 2006b), p53, BRCA1, c-erbB-2 , antiapoptotic and proapoptotic proteins (Lana et al., 2007), beta-catenin, E-cadherin and *Adenomatous Polyposis Coli* (APC) (Restucci et al., 2007) and connexin (Torres et al., 2005), as well as several proliferation markers such as proliferating cell nuclear antigen (PCNA) and Ki-67 (Lana et al., 2007). Immunocytochemical Ki-67 marker seems to be useful to identify malignant canine tumors and patient poor outcome (Zuccari et al., 2004).

Mammary tumors can present as single, firm, well-circumscribed masses to multiple, infiltrative nodules involving one or more glands. In animals with benign mammary tumors, the tumor is small, well circumscribed, and firm on palpation. Clinical findings associated with malignant neoplasms include a tumor diameter greater than 5 cm, recent rapid growth, ill-defined boundaries, infiltration of surrounding tissue, erythema, ulceration, inflammation, and edema. However, most benign and malignant canine mammary tumors exhibit none of these signs with the exception of dogs with advanced metastatic disease or inflammatory mammary carcinomas that typically have systemic signs of illness when they are diagnosed (Lana et al., 2007).

The majority of mammary neoplasms occur primarily in the caudal glands, presumably because of the larger amount of glandular tissue present (Sorenmo, 2003). Multiple mammary neoplasms are common, with 50% to 60% of dogs presenting with more than one mammary tumor. Multiple MGT in a dog are often not of the same histologic type and may exhibit differing biologic behaviors (Benjamin et al., 1999). Thus, a thorough search for additional tumors should be undertaken if a mammary mass is found, and separate cytologic and/or histologic analyses should be performed on each mammary tumor.

The ultimate goal of clinical, cytologic, and histologic evaluation of mammary gland neoplasms is to accurately predict the biologic behavior of the tumor. The World Health Organization International Histological Classification of Mammary Tumors of the dog and the cat combines histiogenic and descriptive morphologic classification, incorporating histologic prognostic features that have been associated with increasing malignancy (Misdorp et al., 1999). Most mammary gland tumors are of epithelial origin. Some tumors are composed of both epithelial and myoepithelial tissue, with areas of cartilage and bone, and a few tumors are of purely mesenchymal origin. About 50% of canine MGT have been classified as malignant based on histologic appearance (Brodey et al, 1983). While some classifications of mammary gland tumors, such as carcinosarcomas or sarcomas, have a consistently poor prognosis, histologic evidence of malignancy does not always imply a malignant course (Lana et al., 2007). In fact, only 50% of histologically diagnosed mammary carcinomas result in tumor-associated deaths (Brodey et al., 1983). Morphologic criteria of malignancy, such as cellular pleomorphism, mitotic activity, and individual grades of anaplasia, are not sufficient criteria for diagnosis of carcinomas. Instead, infiltration into skin and soft tissues and invasion of tumor cells into blood or lymphatic vessels have been identified as best histologic evidence of malignancy in mammary tumors (Misdorp, 2002). When stromal invasion is present, 80% of affected dogs will be dead within 2 years while, in the absence of stromal invasion, 80% of affected dogs will be alive after 2 years (Yager et al., 1993). Using stromal invasion as the primary criteria for malignancy, a lifespan study of over a thousand beagles was reported that correlated the various histologic classifications of epithelial mammary tumors with biologic behavior (Benjamin et al., 1999). Specifically, the study showed that ductular carcinomas accounted for 65.8% of all fatalities due to mammary neoplasia, even though these tumors composed only 18.7% of all mammary carcinomas. Of the malignant tumors, squamous cell carcinomas exhibited the lowest metastatic rate (20%), with carcinosarcomas exhibiting the highest rate of metastasis (100%). Ductular carcinomas metastasized more frequently than adenocarcinomas, 45% versus 35%, respectively.

Accurate and diagnostic exfoliative cytology of mammary tumors is associated with difficulties. Mesenchymal tumors or tumors with a fibrous or scirrhous component may not exfoliate well, leading to a poorly cellular sample inadequate for diagnosis. Tissue imprints or smears of tissue scrapings taken from biopsy samples may improve cytologic diagnosis in these cases; however, imprints generally do not yield as good a sample for evaluation as aspirates (Baker and Lumsden, 1999). Also, mammary hyperplasia, dysplasia, benign tumors, and well-differentiated carcinomas tend to form a continuum of morphologic appearance, making cytologic differentiation of these lesions difficult (Benjamin et al., 1999). Lastly, the presence of stromal invasion, one of the most important criteria for determining the malignant potential of a mammary neoplasm, cannot be assessed by the cytologist. All of these factors can result in either false-positive or false-negative diagnosis of malignant mammary tumors using aspiration cytology. A few studies have examined the accuracy of cytology for detecting mammary malignancies as compared to histologic findings. Allen et al (1986) reported cytologic sensitivities for detecting malignancies of 25% and 17% and specificities of 62% and 49% for the two cytopathologists involved in the study. Positive (PPV) and negative (NPV) predictive values were generally similar between the two pathologists, with PPVs of 90% and 100% and NPVs of 75% and 59% (Allen et al., 1986). The diagnostic accuracy was reported as 79% and 66%. In another study, the sensitivity for cytologic detection of mammary malignances was found to be 65% with a specificity of 94% (Hellman and Lindgren, 1989). The PPV was reported as 93% with an NPV of 67% and diagnostic accuracy of 79%. In a recent study, cytologic and histologic diagnostic agreement was 67.5%. However, when suspicious and insufficient/inadequate samples were excluded, a 92.9% agreement rate was obtained (Cassali et al., 2007). The same authors reported a sensitivity and specificity for the diagnosis of malignant tumors of 88.6% and 100%, respectively, and a sensitivity of 100% and specificity of 88.6% for the diagnosis of benign lesions. These studies did not correlate cytologic diagnosis with disease-free intervals or survival times, thus the use of cytologic criteria to accurately predict the biologic behavior of MGT is uncertain. Recent studies demonstrated that cells in malignant epithelial mammary tumors had significantly more irregular nuclear shapes that did control epithelial cells or cells in benign tumors based on differences in fractal dimension and on nuclear diameter and roundness. These morphometric parameters could help in the preoperative cytologic evaluation of canine mammary gland tumors (Simeonov, 2006a, Simeonov, 2006b).

Cytologic examination of most mammary tumors reveals a background containing variable amounts of blood, basophilic proteinaceous material, lipid, and foam cells. Aspirates of benign epithelial tumors (adenomas and papillomas) typically reveal moderate to large numbers of epithelial cells arranged in sheets and clusters (Fig. 12-7). These cells are uniform in appearance with smooth nuclear chromatin and occasionally prominent, single, small, round nucleoli (Allison and Maddux, 2008). Acinar structures may be seen in samples from adenomas and palisade; papillary and trabecular cell arrangement can be observed in other benign epithelial tumors (Masserdotti, 2006). Benign complex adenomas or papillomas, fibroadenomas, and benign mixed tumors may yield sheets and clusters of uniform-appearing epithelial cells and

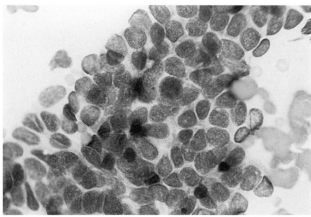

■ **FIGURE 12-7. Mammary adenoma. Tissue aspirate. Cat.** Sheet of epithelial cells with cells that are of uniform size and shape with a high nuclear-to-cytoplasmic ratio and fine nuclear chromatin. The cytoplasm is lightly basophilic and scant in amount. (Wright-Giemsa; HP oil.)

individualized or clumped spindle-shaped cells of myoepithelial (complex tumors) or mesenchymal (mixed tumors) origin. Myoepithelial cells may also appear as oval free nuclei (Allison and Maddux, 2008). Examination of mixed mammary tumors may reveal the presence of cartilage or bone elements such as osteoblasts, osteoclasts, hematopoietic cells, and/or bright-pink extracellular material representative of osteoid (Fernandes et al., 1998) (Figs. 12-8 and 12-9). Mixed mammary tumors can be difficult to diagnose using exfoliative cytology. For instance, the presence of spindle-shaped cells may not be sufficient for diagnosis of mixed or complex tumors. Allen et al. (1986) have noted that spindle cells were identified in the mammary tumors evaluated in their study, yet the presence of these cells did not correlate significantly with histologic classification of complex or mixed tumors. Aspirates of mixed tumors also may not reveal all of the cells composing the tumor. In a case report, aspiration of a mammary mass in a dog revealed the presence of osteoblasts displaying moderate anisokaryosis and

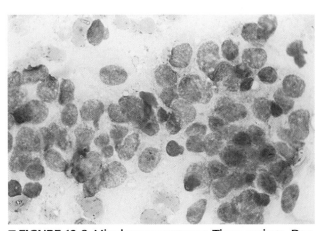

■ **FIGURE 12-8. Mixed mammary tumor. Tissue aspirate. Dog.** Epithelial cells display slightly coarse nuclear chromatin, high nuclear-to-cytoplasmic ratios, and mild to moderate anisokaryosis and anisocytosis. (Wright-Giemsa; HP oil.)

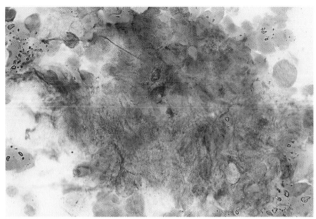

■ **FIGURE 12-9. Mixed mammary tumor. Tissue aspirate. Dog.** Clump of spindle-shaped cells associated with large amounts of extracellular pink material from the same aspirate shown in Figure 12-8. (Wright-Giemsa; HP oil.)

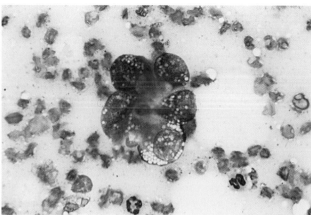

■ **FIGURE 12-11. Mammary adenocarcinoma. Tissue aspirate. Dog.** An acinar structure is shown. Note the presence of punctate cytoplasmic vacuoles as well as prominent nucleoli and moderate anisokaryosis. (Wright-Giemsa; HP oil.)

anisocytosis, osteoclasts, hematopoietic cells, and pink extracellular material (Fernandes et al., 1998). No epithelial cells were noted in the sample. Thus, the multiple differentials included benign or malignant mixed mammary tumor, osseous metaplasia, and osteosarcoma. Histopathology confirmed that the neoplasm was a benign mixed mammary tumor.

Malignant mammary tumors may be diagnosed based on the cytologic appearance of the cell types present and the observation of more than three criteria of malignancy. Adenocarcinomas are characterized by epithelial cells arranged in sheets (Fig. 12-10) and clusters, or sometimes individualized. Acinar arrangements (Fig. 12-11) may be observed (Masserdotti, 2006). The epithelial cells are typically round, with round to oval, eccentrically located nuclei and moderate amounts of basophilic cytoplasm that may contain amorphous basophilic secretory product and/or clear vacuoles (Allison and Maddux, 2008) (Fig. 12-12). Some of these vacuoles may appear as punctate vacuoles of variable number or as a diffuse clearing of the cytoplasm that

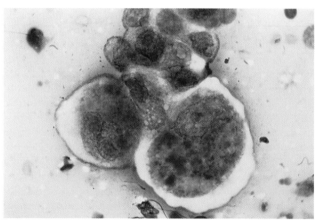

■ **FIGURE 12-12. Mammary adenocarcinoma. Tissue aspirate. Dog.** Marked anisokaryosis and anisocytosis of the epithelial cells are noted. These epithelial cells contain basophilic secretory material as well as diffuse peripheral cytoplasmic vacuolation. (Wright-Giemsa; HP oil.)

distends the cell and displaces the nucleus peripherally. Criteria of malignancy that may be seen in these cells include increased nuclear-to-cytoplasmic ratio; moderate to marked variation in nuclear and cell size; nuclear molding; large, prominent, multiple, and/or abnormally shaped nucleoli; and binucleation and multinucleation. Increased mitotic activity and abnormal mitotic figures may be present (Figs. 12-13 and 12-14). Ductular carcinomas typically present with sheets and clusters of pleomorphic epithelial cells with high nuclear-to-cytoplasmic ratios and round, basal nuclei. These cells usually display more than three malignant criteria. Acinar structures, secretory product, and cytoplasmic vacuoles are not characteristic features of ductular carcinomas. Papillary and trabecular cell arrangements can be observed in malignant epithelial tumors (Masserdotti, 2006).

Anaplastic carcinomas may present with very large, extremely pleomorphic epithelial cells occurring singly and in small clusters (Allison and Maddux, 2008). These cells tend to have bizarre nuclear and nucleolar forms.

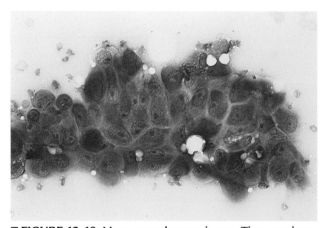

■ **FIGURE 12-10. Mammary adenocarcinoma. Tissue aspirate. Dog.** Sheet of epithelial cells displaying prominent cell-to-cell junctions. These cells also exhibit prominent, large nucleoli, moderate anisokaryosis, and deeply basophilic cytoplasm. (Wright-Giemsa; HP oil.)

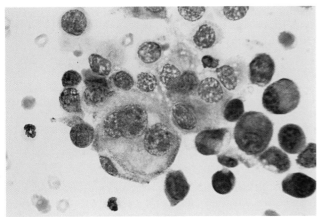

■ FIGURE 12-13. Mammary carcinoma. Tissue aspirate. Dog. Marked anisokaryosis, anisocytosis, prominent nucleoli, coarse nuclear chromatin, and binucleation are present in cells that also display poor cellular adhesion. (Wright-Giemsa; HP oil.)

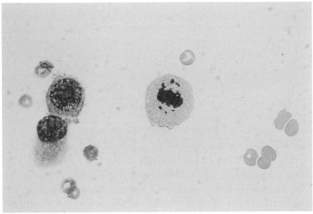

■ FIGURE 12-14. Mammary carcinoma. Tissue aspirate. Dog. Abnormal mitotic figure with lag chromatin from same specimen as shown in Figure 12-13. Lag chromatin results from abnormal formation of the mitotic spindle apparatus. Abnormal mitotic figures are considered one criterion of malignancy. (Wright-Giemsa; HP oil.)

Multinucleation and abnormal mitotic figures are frequently seen. Inflammatory carcinomas, which are a locally aggressive form of mammary carcinoma, also present with large, pleomorphic epithelial cells exhibiting various criteria of malignancy as well as large numbers of nondegenerate neutrophils and macrophages (Lana et al., 2007). The cytologic appearance of inflammatory carcinoma may resemble mastitis. However, history, signalment, and presence of very anaplastic epithelial cells should be helpful for differentiation of these two conditions.

Squamous cell carcinomas of the mammary gland appear cytologically similar to those found in other body sites. The malignant squamous cells tend to occur individually or in small sheets. The nuclei may vary from small and pyknotic to large, round, and immature with prominent nucleoli. The nuclear-to-cytoplasmic ratio is variable and binucleation may be noted. The cytoplasm of the tumor cells is moderately to deeply basophilic

(nonkeratinized) or may have a blue-green color characteristic of keratinization. Mammary squamous cell carcinomas may ulcerate, leading to the presence of inflammatory cells and phagocytized bacteria in the cytologic sample (Allison and Maddux, 2008).

Aspirates of malignant mixed mammary tumors may reveal epithelial cells and spindle-shaped, individualized cells of mesenchymal origin with one of these populations displaying nuclear and cellular criteria of malignancy. However, the presence of either population or predominance of one cell type over the other may depend on the area of tumor aspirated (Allison and Maddux, 2008). In carcinosarcomas, both epithelial and mesenchymal populations should display malignant features. Mammary sarcomas, such as osteosarcoma, fibrosarcoma, and liposarcoma, are of similar cytologic appearance to those found in other body sites. Sarcomas tend to exfoliate poorly, often resulting in samples of low cellularity. Depending on the type of tumor, pink extracellular material or lipid may be present in the background. In general, sarcomas are characterized by spindle-shaped to irregular cells arranged individually and in small clumps. The cytoplasm of these cells is moderately to deeply basophilic and the cytoplasmic borders tend to be indistinct. The cells display cytologic features of malignancy similar to those described for epithelial neoplasms.

Feline Mammary Gland Tumors

Mammary tumors are the third most common tumor in the cat, after hematopoietic neoplasms and skin tumors (Misdorp, 2002; Hayes and Mooney, 1985). The median age for MGT development in the cat is 10 years of age or older. Almost all (99%) of feline MGT occur in intact females (Lana et al., 2007). Domestic short hair and Siamese cats appear to have higher incidence rates (Hayes et al., 1981).

Development of feline MGT is thought to have a hormonal component. Intact females have an almost seven-fold greater risk of developing mammary neoplasms as compared to neutered females, and ovariohysterectomy has been reported to decrease the risk of MGT to 0.6% compared to intact females (Hayes et al., 1981). Regular, but not irregular, administration of exogenous progesterone was associated with a significantly increased risk of benign mammary tumors and mammary carcinomas in cats (Misdorp, 1991). Hormone receptor analysis has shown that normal feline mammary tissue contains estrogen and progesterone receptors in levels similar to those found in the dog (Millanta et al., 2005). However, unlike canine MGT, the majority of feline mammary neoplasms express very low levels of estrogen and progesterone receptors, which may be related to the high rate of malignancy found with mammary neoplasia in the cat. Other molecule targets have been investigated to elucidate prognosis or the pathways of tumorigenesis such as cyclin A, Cox-2 (Millanta et al., 2006b), HER2, VEGF and E-cadherin (Lana et al., 2007).

In contrast to the dog, the majority of feline mammary tumors are malignant with some studies reporting a greater than 80% incidence of malignant neoplasms (Hayes et al., 1981). Adenocarcinomas are the most prevalent malignant mammary tumor followed by carcinomas and sarcomas (MacEwen et al., 1984). Recently, secondary or postsurgical inflammatory carcinomas (Pérez-Alenza et al., 2004) and lipid-rich carcinoma (Kamstock et al., 2005) have been described, for the first time, in cats. Malignant MGT in cats tend to grow rapidly and metastasize to regional lymph nodes, lung, pleura, liver, diaphragm, adrenal glands, and kidneys (Lana et al, 2007). The single most important prognostic indicator for feline MGT is tumor size at time of diagnosis. Median survival times for cats with mammary tumors greater than 3 cm, between 2 and 3 cm, and less than 2 cm is 6 months, 2 years, and greater than 3 years, respectively (MacEwen et al., 1984). Thus, early diagnosis and treatment is very important for feline mammary malignancies.

The cytologic features of benign and malignant mammary neoplasms in the cat are similar to those described in the dog (see Figures 12-10, 12-13, 12-14). The reliability of cytologic criteria to differentiate between hyperplasia, benign tumors, and malignancies in the cat does not appear to have been reported (Baker and Lumsden, 1999). Given the high rate of mammary malignancy in cats, cytologic findings of a benign-appearing population of epithelial cells, particularly in an older cat with no history of progesterone administration, should be treated with some caution. In these cases, samples should be submitted for histopathologic examination to rule out the presence of a malignancy.

Treatment considerations will follow clinical and cytologic and/or histologic identification of a mammary neoplasm in a dog or a cat. If a malignancy is present, staging the extent of the disease should include three-view thoracic radiographs or CT scan of the lungs and any other potential metastatic sites as well as cytologic analysis of regional lymph nodes, metastatic lesions, and/or body cavity effusions. It has been proposed that treatment guidelines for malignant canine mammary gland tumors be based on tumor size, histopathologic type, and differentiation (Sorenmo, 2003). Surgical excision is the treatment of choice for both canine and feline mammary neoplasms. In dogs, it is recommended to perform ovariohysterectomy if intact in all malignant canine mammary gland tumors and to institute chemotherapy in an undifferentiated carcinoma in stage I (Sorenmo, 2003). There is limited information regarding efficacy of adjuvant therapy involving chemotherapeutics, radiation, or immune stimulation in canine and feline mammary malignancies. However, the combination of surgery and adjunctive doxorubicin chemotherapy resulted in improved long-term survival in cats with mammary gland adenocarcinoma (Novosad, 2003; Novosad et al., 2006). In addition, the combination of surgery and adjunctive 5-fluorouracil and cyclophosphamide chemotherapy demonstrated significant survival improvement in dogs with mammary gland carcinomas stage III/IV when compared with surgery alone (Karayannopoulo et al., 2001). In contrast, chemotherapy did not lead to an improved outcome in dogs with invasive malignant mammary gland tumors (Simon et al., 2006). The use of antiestrogens, such as tamoxifen, has been documented in a small number of clinical cases, with somewhat conflicting results in regard to tumor response. These drugs can be associated with undesirable estrogen-related side effects (Novosad, 2003).

Ovaries

Cytology is a valuable tool for diagnosis of ovarian tumors and ovarian cystic disease as recently demonstrated in a study with a diagnostic accuracy of cytology of 94.7% (Bertazzolo et al., 2004).

Special Collection Techniques

There is little information on ovarian cytology collection techniques. Ovarian biopsy is performed and surgical technique is well described elsewhere (Root Kustritz, 2006). Cytologic samples can be made by ultrasound-guided percutaneous fine-needle aspiration or intraoperatively during exploratory laparotomy.

Normal Anatomy and Histology

The ovary is composed of three broad embryologic origins: 1) the epithelium, which includes the outer layer lining (surface) epithelium of the modified mesothelium, the rete ovarii (remnants of the mesonephric tubules), and in the bitch, the subsurface epithelial structures; 2) the germ cells; 3) the ovarian stroma including the sex cords, which together contribute the endocrine apparatus of the ovary (MacLachlan and Kennedy, 2002). Each ovary lies within an ovarian bursa, an extension of the mesosalpinx, which is a fold of the peritoneum. Cuboidal epithelium called germinal epithelium covers the cortex of the ovary, and a layer of dense connective tissue, the tunica albuginea, is present underneath the epithelium. The canine ovary has small ingrowths of the ovarian surface that are called subsurface epithelial structures. The cortex of the ovary contains follicles, stromal connective tissue, and blood vessels. The ova develop in follicles that are of four types: primordial, primary, secondary, and tertiary. Each developing follicle has the oocyte, multiple layers of granulosa cells, and more peripheral thecal connective tissue cells (Fig. 12-15). Ovulation occurs when the follicle ruptures, releasing the ovum and allowing the space to fill with blood and luteal cells to form the corpus hemorrhagicum and the corpus luteum, respectively. In bitches and queens, cords of epithelial cells called interstitial glands, which are cells of an endocrine type, occur throughout the stroma. A medulla consisting of richly vascularized loose connective tissue, lymphatics, and nerves lies internal to the ovarian cortex. Channels lined by cuboidal epithelium called rete ovarii are present in this region (Foster, 2007).

The normal histology of ovaries from immature female dogs and sequential microscopic changes that occur during different stages of the estrous cycle are reviewed elsewhere (Rehm et al., 2007).

Normal Cytology

Cytology of normal ovarian tissue usually reveals small amounts of blood with no to moderate numbers of nucleated cells and moderate to large amounts of basophilic, proteinaceous material and clear lipid droplets. Normal ovaries are characterized cytologically by low to

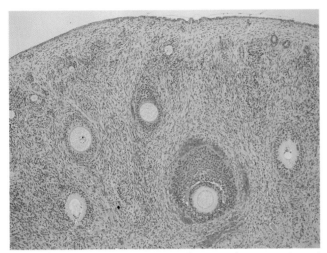

■ **FIGURE 12-15. Normal ovary. Tissue section. Dog.** Several developing follicles, each with an oocyte surrounded by a layer of granulosa cells, are present within the stroma of the ovarian cortex. The cortex is lined by a simple layer of cuboidal epithelium. (H&E; LP.) (Courtesy of Dr. Carlo Masserdotti.)

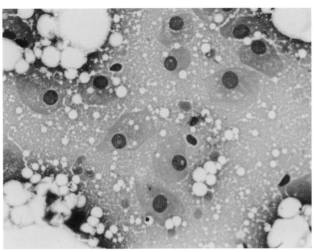

■ **FIGURE 12-17. Normal ovary. Cytologic preparation. Dog.** The basophilic background contains variable sized lipid droplets and red blood cells. Several singly luteal cells characterized by abundant pale basophilic cytoplasm with small clear discrete vacuoles and eccentric round to oval nuclei. (May-Grünwald-Giemsa; IP.)

moderate numbers of one or more of the following cells based on the stage of the estrous cycle: adipocytes, individual fibrocytes/fibroblasts, small monolayered cohesive sheets of nonreactive mesothelial cells, granulosa cells that are uniform in size and shape and are arranged in acinar formations or in small loosely to cohesive aggregates, and singly luteal cells characterized by abundant pale basophilic cytoplasm with small, clear, discrete vacuoles and eccentric round to oval nuclei (Figs. 12-16, 12-17, 12-18, 12-19).

Cysts

Cysts in and around the ovary are a common finding during ovariohysterectomy in dogs and cats. There are two types of cysts: intraovarian and paraovarian. Intraovarian cysts include cystic rete ovarii, subsurface epithelial structure (only dog), vascular hematomas, and

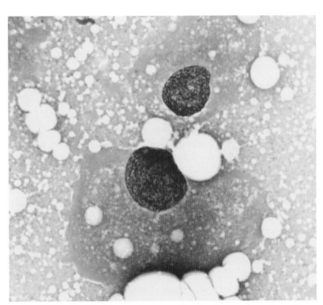

■ **FIGURE 12-18. Normal ovary. Cytologic preparation. Dog.** The basophilic background contains variable sized lipid droplets. Two singly luteal cells characterized by abundant pale basophilic cytoplasm with small, clear, discrete vacuoles and eccentric round to oval nuclei. (May-Grünwald-Giemsa; HP oil.)

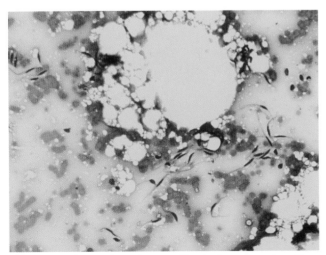

■ **FIGURE 12-16. Normal ovary. Cytologic preparation. Dog.** The basophilic background contains red blood cells, variable sized lipid droplets, and cellular debris. Numerous fibrocytes/fibroblasts are noted. (May-Grünwald-Giemsa; IP.)

adenomatous hyperplasia of the rete ovarii (Foster, 2007; Klein, 2007).

Inflammation

Oophoritis, or inflammation of the ovary, is rare in domestic animals. Bacterial oophoritis occasionally is found in cats and dogs (Foster, 2007). The inflammation is around the ovary and within the uterine tube, suggesting that the causative bacteria ascended from uterus (Van Israel et al., 2002). In cats, feline infectious peritonitis can cause oophoritis.

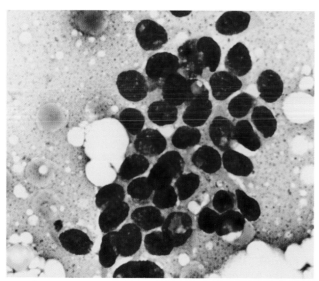

■ **FIGURE 12-19. Normal ovary. Cytologic preparation. Dog.** Cells that are uniform in size and shape and are arranged in small, loose aggregates are consistent with granulosa cells. (May-Grünwald-Giemsa; HP oil.)

Ovarian Neoplasia

Tumors of the ovary are uncommon in dogs and cats accounting for 0.5% to 6.3% of all canine tumors and 0.8% of all feline tumors (McEntee, 2002). The actual frequency of ovarian tumors may be underestimated as ovaries are not routinely sectioned at necropsy and are more commonly examined only if there is a gross lesion. In addition, the low frequency is affected by the fact that many companion animals are neutered at an early age. There are four main categories of ovarian tumors including epithelial, germ cell, sex cord–stromal, and mesenchymal. There are several other miscellaneous neoplastic diseases of the ovaries (mixed tumors and metastatic nonovarian malignant neoplasms). Clinical signs typically occur secondary to a space-occupying mass or to an effusion related to metastasis. Clinical signs in dogs with functional tumors secondary to excessive estrogen and/or progesterone production include signs of persistent estrus, pyometra, and bone marrow toxicity. Ovarian tumors can be an incidental finding at the time of ovariohysterectomy or necropsy (Klein, 2007).

Epithelial Tumors

Epithelial tumors include papillary adenomas/cystadenomas, papillary adenocarcinoma, cystadenocarcinoma, rete adenomas, and undifferentiated carcinomas (MacLachlan and Kennedy, 2002) and account for 40% to 50% of canine ovarian tumors. Fifty percent of malignant epithelial tumors metastasize by implantation or lymphatic or vascular invasion. These tumors occur in older female dogs with a median age of 10 to 12 years (McEntee, 2002). Epithelial tumors are extremely rare in cats (Klein, 2007).

Papillary adenocarcinoma has been recently described cytologically. Cells are arranged in macro- to micropapillary forms (Masserdotti, 2006), acinar or tubular patterns, in cohesive clusters sometimes tridimensional, and

occasionally as single cells (Figs. 12-20, 12-21, 12-22). Cells are round to polyhedral with a single oval nucleus. Nuclear chromatin is reticular to coarse. Nucleoli are indistinct to prominent single or multiple. Mild to marked anisokaryosis and anisocytosis are present. The cytoplasm is scarce to moderate and sometimes with finely discrete, clear vacuoles. Occasionally, large intracytoplasmatic vacuoles or signet ring cells are observed (Bertazzolo et al., 2004; Hori et al., 2006).

Sex-cordal Stromal Tumors

Sex-cordal stromal tumors include granulosa cell tumors, luteomas (also called interstitial gland, lipid, or interstitial cell tumors), and thecomas. In the dog, granulosa cell tumors account 50% of ovarian tumors and occur in elderly bitches with a median age of 10 to 12 years. Seventy-seven percent of granulosa cell tumors produce estrogens and/or progesterone and up to 20% are malignant. Granulosa cell tumor is the most common sex-cordal stromal tumor in older cats and more than 50% are malignant. Reported

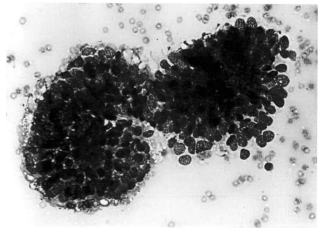

■ **FIGURE 12-20. Ovarian papillary adenocarcinoma. Cytologic preparation. Dog.** A cluster of cohesive neoplastic epithelial cells are arranged in a papillary pattern. (May-Grünwald-Giemsa; IP.) (Courtesy of Dr. Walter Bertazzolo.)

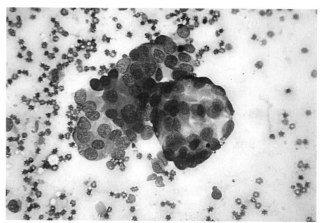

■ **FIGURE 12-21. Ovarian papillary adenocarcinoma. Cytologic preparation. Dog.** Shown is a round papillary cluster of cohesive neoplastic epithelial cells known as a "cell ball." (May-Grünwald-Giemsa; IP.) (Courtesy of Dr. Walter Bertazzolo.)

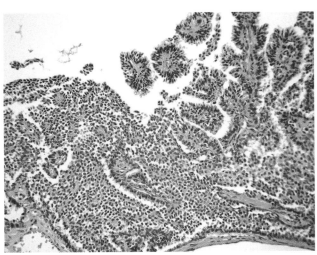

■ FIGURE 12-22. Ovarian papillary adenocarcinoma. Tissue section. Dog. There is dense proliferation of hyperchromic epithelial cells, some of which display acinar formations. (H&E; LP.) (Courtesy of Dr. Walter Bertazzolo.)

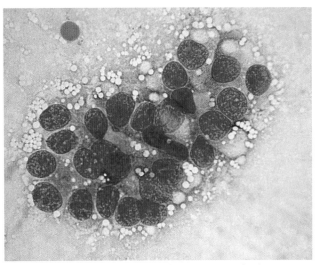

■ FIGURE 12-23. Granulosa cell tumor. Cytologic preparation. Dog. A loosely monolayered aggregate of granulosa cells with a moderate amount of finely vacuolated cytoplasm is present. Cells are arranged in an acinar pattern. (May-Grünwald-Giemsa; HP oil.) (Courtesy of Dr. Walter Bertazzolo.)

metastatic sites include peritoneum, lumbar lymph nodes, omentum, diaphragm, kidney, pancreas, spleen, liver, and lungs (McEntee, 2002). Granulosa cell tumors may be confused sometimes with ovarian epithelial tumors even in histological preparations. Useful immunohistochemical markers to distinguish these two tumors are cytokeratin 7 and inhibin-α. Ovarian epithelial tumors cells are positive to cytokeratin 7 and negative to inhibin-α while granulosa tumor cells and thecomas are negative to cytokeratin 7 and positive to inhibin-α (Riccardi et al., 2007; Klein, 2007).

Cytologically, granulosa tumor cells are usually in monolayered, loosely cohesive clusters and often have acinar to tubular pattern (Fig. 12-23). Cells are arranged sometimes in an acinar pattern surrounding amorphous eosinophilic extracellular material called Call-Exner–like bodies. Capillary-like structures are occasionally evident inside large clusters of cells (Fig. 12-24). Single cells appear from round to polyhedral. Nuclei are round to oval with indistinct nucleoli and mild to moderate cellular atypia. The cytoplasm is scarce to moderate with variable amounts of vacuolated cytoplasm (Bertazzolo et al., 2004).

Feline luteomas have been recently cytologically described. Large round to oval cells arranged individually or in loose clusters are observed. Nuclei are central to eccentric with granular chromatin with prominent, small, central nucleoli. Anisokaryosis is mild to moderate. Cytoplasm is lightly basophilic with many variably sized clear vacuoles and occasionally small purple granules (Choi et al., 2005).

Germ Cell Tumors

Germ cell tumors include dysgerminoma (counterpart of the testicular seminoma), teratoma, and teratocarcinoma. Dysgerminoma represent a less-differentiated tumor than mature teratoma. Germ cell tumors comprise 6% to 20% of canine ovarian neoplasms and 15% to 27% of feline ovarian neoplasms. The median age of dogs with dysgerminoma is 10 to 13 years and with teratomas is 4 years. The age of cats that have been reported to have dysgerminomas

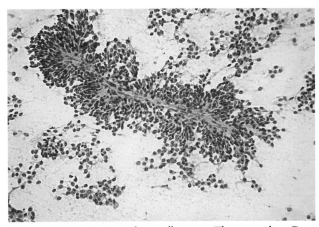

■ FIGURE 12-24. Granulosa cell tumor. Tissue section. Dog. A large cluster of granulosa cells appears with a perivascular pattern. (H&E; LP.) (Courtesy of Dr. Walter Bertazzolo.)

ranges from 1 to 17 years with a median of 5 years. Metastasis is reported to develop in 10% to 20% of canine dysgerminomas with regional lymph nodes, liver, brain, and kidney as the primary sites. Young cats (5 to 8 months) and dogs have teratomas (McEntee, 2002; Klein, 2007).

Dysgerminomas are seen cytologically as a predominant population of markedly pleomorphic, large, round to polygonal cells arranged singly or in loose aggregates. Cells range from 20 to 70 μm of diameter. Nuclei are large and round to oval with chromatin stippled to reticular (Figs. 12-25 and 12-26). Nucleoli are prominent multiple and of variable shape and size. Aberrant mitotic figures and bi- or multinucleated cells are commonly noted. Anisocytosis and anisokaryosis are marked. The cytoplasm is scant clear to blue-gray with variably distinct margins. Occasionally eosinophilic, granular, intracytoplasmic material is

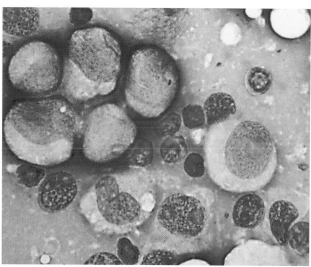

■ **FIGURE 12-25. Ovarian dysgerminoma. Cytologic preparation. Dog.** Large neoplastic cells are round and are arranged singly. Nuclei are pleomorphic in shape and located centrally or eccentrically with a stippled to coarse chromatin pattern and prominent nucleoli. Anisokaryosis and anisocytosis are moderate to marked. The cytoplasm is moderate to abundant and pale basophilic. Lysed cells and small lymphocytes are present. (May-Grünwald-Giemsa; HP oil.) (Courtesy of Dr. Walter Bertazzolo.)

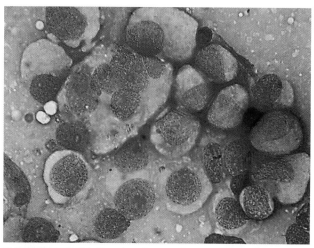

■ **FIGURE 12-26. Ovarian dysgerminoma. Cytologic preparation. Dog.** Note the multinucleated cell with marked anisokaryosis and anisocytosis. (May-Grünwald-Giemsa; HP oil.) (Courtesy of Dr. Walter Bertazzolo.)

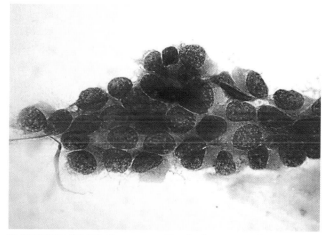

■ **FIGURE 12-27. Teratoma. Cytologic preparation. Dog.** A cluster of cohesive epithelial basal-like cells is shown. (May-Grünwald-Giemsa; HP oil.) (Courtesy of Dr. Walter Bertazzolo.)

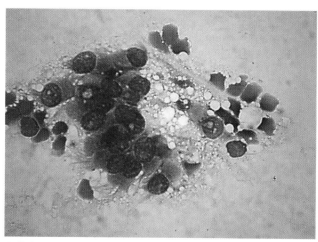

■ **FIGURE 12-28. Teratoma. Cytologic preparation. Dog.** Epithelial cells have a basally polarized round to oval nucleus with an evident eosinophilic brush border suggestive of differentiation towards respiratory epithelium. (May-Grünwald-Giemsa; HP oil.) (Courtesy of Dr. Walter Bertazzolo.)

noted. Small lymphocytes can be observed (Bertazzolo et al., 2004; Brazzell and Borjesson, 2006).

Cytologically, teratomas are seen in a necrotic background, moderate neutrophilic-macrophagic inflammation, clusters of sebocytes or other mature epithelial cells, abundant keratin debris, and mature keratinocytes (Figs. 12-27, 12-28, 12-29, 12-30) (Bertazzolo et al., 2004).

Surgery remains the mainstay of treatment of ovarian tumors. A complete ovariohysterectomy is recommended. Careful examinations of all serosal surfaces and removal or biopsy of any lesions suspected of metastatic disease are recommended for staging purposes. Successful palliation with chemotherapy has been reported but no standard recommendations have been established (Klein, 2007).

Uterus

Indications for uterine cytology/biopsy include evaluation of degree of cystic endometrial hyperplasia, inflammation, neoplasia, and prognostic assessment for fertility (Root Kustritz et al., 2006).

Special Collection Techniques

Cells may be collected at the time of hysterotomy or be retrieved transcervically (Root Kustritz, 2006). This last technique involves visualizing the cervix with a rigid endoscope and passing a catheter through the cervix into the uterus. Samples for microbiology and cytology are

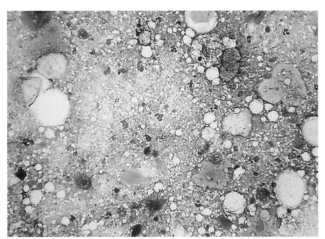

■ **FIGURE 12-29. Teratoma. Cytologic preparation. Dog.** Necrotic background, keratin debris, neutrophils and macrophages are evident. (May-Grünwald-Giemsa; IP.) (Courtesy of Dr. Walter Bertazzolo.)

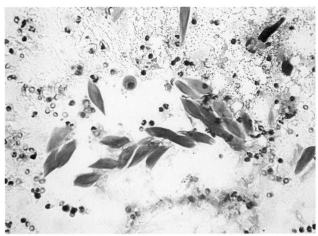

■ **FIGURE 12-30. Teratoma. Cytologic preparation. Dog.** Keratinocytes, keratin debris, neutrophils, and red blood cells are seen. (May-Grünwald-Giemsa; IP.) (Courtesy of Dr. Walter Bertazzolo.)

obtained by the infusion and aspiration of sterile normal saline. This technique allows uterine microbiology and cytology of the normal bitch throughout the reproductive cycle (Watts et al., 1997, 1998). Complications include vaginal inflammation, tearing, and endometritis mainly when samples are taken in anestrus (Watts et al., 1997). Another technique is hysteroscopy, performed in anesthetized bitches with a laparoscope and air insufflation of the uterus. Side effects are petechiae or ecchymosis on endometrium in 50% of bitches (Gerber and Nöthling, 2001).

Normal Anatomy and Histology

Cats and dogs have a bicornuate uterus with uterine horns and a uterine body. The uterine tubes have four regions: the infundibulum, ampulla, isthmus, and uterotubal junction. It is supported by a mesosalpinx. The mesosalpinx of the dog completely surrounds the ovary and has a

large amount of fat; a small hole connects the bursa to the abdominal cavity. The infundibulum surrounds the ovary. The wall of the uterus has three layers: the outer perimetrium (serosa), middle myometrium, and inner endometrium (mucosa). The perimetrium is composed of loose connective tissue and covered by peritoneal mesothelium. The myometrium is divided into a thick, inner circular layer and a thin, outer longitudinal layer (Fig. 12-31). A richly vascularized and well-innervated stratum vasculare usually separates the muscle layers. The epithelium of the endometrium is simple cuboidal or columnar in the bitch and queen depending of the estrus cycle. Simple, branched endometrial glands extend into the lamina propria. The cervix is the structure that separates the external genitalia from uterus and is an effective barrier from the external environment. The cervix does not have transverse folds and tends to open dorsally (Foster, 2007). The normal histology of uterus from immature female dogs and sequential microscopic changes that occur during different stages of the estrous cycle are reviewed elsewhere (Rehm et al., 2007).

Normal Cytology

The normal endometrial epithelial cells vary morphologically throughout the reproductive cycle and have signs of epithelial degeneration defined as nuclear pyknosis, karyorrhexis or karyolysis, and/or cytoplasmic clear vacuoles during late diestrus and during early and mid-anestrus following diestrus and postpartum. The number of degenerating epithelial cells decreases with time until late anestrus, when all endometrial epithelial cells are cuboidal to low columnar and lack signs of degeneration. Endometrial epithelial cells are arranged in monolayered, cohesive clusters and acinar forms are

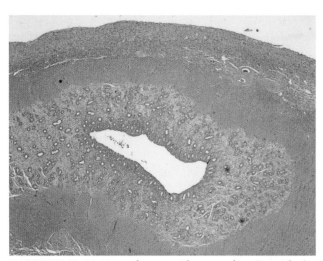

■ **FIGURE 12-31. Normal uterus. Tissue section. Dog.** The inner mucosa or endometrium is lined by cuboidal or columnar epithelium. The uterine glands present in the mucosa extend deep into the lamina propria as tubular formations. The dense area surrounding the endometrial glands is the myometrium, which consists of two encircling layers of smooth muscle. The outermost layer is the perimetrium or mesothelial-lined serosa. (H&E; LP.) (Courtesy of Dr. Carlo Masserdotti.)

commonly seen. Single cells are less frequently observed. The endometrial epithelial cells are low columnar during proestrus and estrus and columnar during early diestrus and pregnancy. During proestrus, estrus, early diestrus, and pregnancy, the cells have intact nuclei and uniformly staining cytoplasm. The nuclei of normal endometrial epithelial cells are usually round or oval with fine, stippled chromatin. The nuclei of degenerated endometrial cells are often of irregular shape and pyknotic. Neutrophils are the most common leucocytes observed during proestrus, estrus, diestrus, and early pregnancy, and lymphocytes and macrophages are frequently seen during anestrus. Erythrocytes are present in variable numbers at all stages of the reproductive cycle. Spermatozoa are observed in samples collected during estrus and early pregnancy in bitches that had their last mating 1 to 3 days previously. Bacteria are commonly observed during proestrus and estrus. Cornified cervical or vaginal cells are present during proestrus and estrus (Watts et al., 1998).

Microorganisms are frequently recovered from the uterus during proestrus and estrus, but rarely at other stages of the reproductive cycle. The uterine microflora often reflects the vaginal microflora during proestrus and estrus (Watts et al., 1997).

Inflammation

Cystic Endometrial Hyperplasia-Pyometra Complex and Metritis

Cytologic examination of vaginal discharges or uterus samples may be useful for diagnosis of inflammatory disease of the uterus in dogs and cats. Cystic endometrial hyperplasia-pyometra complex is a disease that is mainly characterized by progesterone-induced hyperplasia of the endometrium with cystic dilatation of the endometrial glands and inflammation of the uterus with purulent content in the uterine lumen (pyometra) leading to several clinical signs (Agudelo, 2005). The common presentation of pyometra involves older, unbred bitches presenting from 4 weeks to 4 months following estrus with mild to severe evidence of systemic illness (Smith, 2006). Clinical signs may include anorexia, depression, polyuria, and/or polydipsia and abdominal distention with or without vaginal discharge (open and closed-cervix pyometra, respectively). Typically, the bitch is afebrile and will often have leukocytosis, although leukopenia is also less commonly reported. Prerenal azotemia commonly accompanies the dehydration present. This systemic disease may result in death due to toxemia, renal disease, and peritonitis. There is an increased risk of pyometra in some breeds. Cystic endometrial hyperplasia-pyometra complex is considered to be less common in cats, probably because cats are induced ovulators, which limits uterine exposure to progesterone. The disorder is extensively reviewed elsewhere (Agudelo, 2005). *Escherichia coli* is the most frequently isolated microorganism in canine and feline pyometras (Hagman and Kühn, 2002). Anecdotally, *Tritrichomonas foetus* infection and cholesterol granuloma have been reported independently in the uterus of two different cats with pyometra (Dahlgren et al., 2007; Zanghì et al., 1999).

Treatment of choice for pyometra is ovariohysterectomy with supportive therapy including appropriate antibiotic administration. The combination of a prolactin inhibitor, prostaglandin, and an antibiotic treatment in bitches with pyometra appears to have been effective in rapid clinical improvement, terminating the luteal phase and promoting uterine evacuation. This combination may be useful not only in bitches that are required for future breeding, but also in bitches that are a high anesthetic risk (England et al., 2007).

Metritis usually follows parturition and is characterized by a systemically ill animal with a malodorous uterine/vaginal discharge. The treatment of metritis is also ovariohysterectomy if the owner is not interested in further breeding or if severe systemic illness is present. Nursing puppies or kittens should be weaned and hand-raised.

Large numbers of neutrophils, many of which are degenerate (Olson et al., 1984b), characterize smears prepared from vaginal discharges resulting from open-cervix pyometra or metritis. Bacteria may be seen extracellularly and within the neutrophils. Muscle fibers from decomposing fetuses may rarely be visible in samples from metritis (Allison et al., 2008).

Uterine Neoplasia

Uterine tumors occur infrequently in dogs and cats accounting for 0.3% to 0.4% and 0.2% to 1.5% of all canine and feline tumors, respectively. Middle-aged to older animals are most commonly affected (Klein, 2007). In the dog, uterine leiomyomas are reported most common and leiomyosarcomas are comparatively rare. These tumors are of similar cytologic appearance to those found in other body sites. Uterine carcinomas are rare (McEntee, 2002). In cats, both leiomyoma and endometrial adenocarcinoma are reported with similar frequencies (Miller et al, 2003). A complete ovariohysterectomy is recommended, and attempts should be made to remove all tumors and metastatic foci (Klein, 2007).

Vagina

Examination of exfoliated vaginal cells for staging the estrous cycle is one of the most common uses of cytology in veterinary practice. This technique is easy to perform and, with some experience, can be successfully used by the clinician to optimize breeding of client animals. Cytologic examination of vaginal mucosal imprints and discharges is also useful for evaluation of vaginal inflammation and neoplasia of the female reproductive tract (Root Kustritz, 2006).

Special Collection Techniques

Several techniques have been described for obtaining vaginal cells for cytologic examination (Mills et al., 1979). Most commonly, a saline-moistened cotton swab or thin glass rod with a rounded tip is directed craniodorsally into the caudal vagina. The vestibule and clitoral fossa should be avoided since keratinized superficial squamous cells present in these sites may alter cytologic interpretations. Once craniad to the urethral orifice, vaginal cells are obtained by gently passing the swab or glass rod over the epithelial lining (Root Kustritz, 2006). In an alternate method of sample collection, a small glass bulb pipette containing sterile saline is passed into the caudal vagina and cells are obtained by repeatedly flushing and aspirating the saline fluid (Olson et al., 1984a). Once collected, the exfoliated cells are gently transferred onto a clean microscope slide for staining. In addition, endoscopic vaginoscopy is a useful diagnostic procedure for evaluating the nature and the extent of disease in the vestibule and vagina and for obtaining adequate samples for microscopic evaluation. The technique is reviewed in depth elsewhere (Lulich, 2006). Although several types of stains have been used for cytologic evaluation of vaginal cells, Romanowsky-type stains or aqueous-based Romanowsky stains are most commonly used. These stains are easy to use in a clinical setting and provide good morphologic detail for determining the degree of maturation of the epithelial cells. Papanicolaou or trichrome stains have also been used for estrous cycle staging. These stains impart a distinctive orange staining to the keratin precursors abundant in superficial cells. The ratio of orange or eosinophilic cells to noneosinophilic cells, termed the *eosinophilic index,* can be used to assess the degree of maturation of the epithelial cells and subsequently stage the estrous cycle. However, these stains may yield variable staining results and the need for multiple solutions limits their practical use. However, an ultrafast modified Papanicolaou stain seems to be a useful technique in the study of vaginal cytology as a tool for assessing the estrous cycle in the bitch (Perez et al., 2005). Indications for vaginal culture include any disorder of the genitourinary tract associated with vulvar discharge and anterior vaginal culture in proestrus for diagnosis of uterine infection (Root Kustritz, 2006). The vagina is not sterile and larger numbers of normal flora are routinely cultured from the caudal vagina than the cranial vagina and during estrus than diestrus or anestrus. However, a larger number of organisms are retrieved from bitches with reproductive tract disease than from normal bitches. It is important to provide a quantitative culture result due to the fact that reproductive tract infection is caused by overgrowth of normal flora.

Normal Anatomy and Histology

The vagina is a musculomembranous canal extending from the uterus to the vulva. The vaginal wall is composed of an inner mucosal layer, a middle smooth muscle layer, and an external coat of connective tissue and peritoneum (cranially) (Banks, 1986). The mucosal layer consists of stratified squamous epithelium, which undergoes characteristic morphologic changes in association with the estrous cycle. Although the mucosa is typically nonglandular, intraepithelial glands have been observed during estrus in the dog. The vulva is anatomically similar to the caudal vagina. The vulva is composed of the vestibule containing the urethral orifice, the clitoral fossa, and the labia. The mucosa is lined by stratified squamous epithelium; some keratinized epithelial cells may be found in the vestibule and clitoral fossa (Allison et al., 2008)

Vestibular glands within the submucosal layer of the vestibule are responsible for mucus production, which is most notable during estrus and at parturition (Banks, 1986). The normal histology of vagina from immature female dogs and sequential microscopic changes that occur during different stages of the estrous cycle are reviewed elsewhere (Rehm et al., 2007).

Normal Cytology

Four types of vaginal epithelial cells may be identified by exfoliative cytology. In order from the deepest and most immature cells to the most superficial and mature, these cells are basal, parabasal, intermediate, and superficial.

Basal cells are located along the basement membrane and give rise to the other epithelial cell types seen in a vaginal smear (Allison et al., 2008). Round nuclei and scant amounts of basophilic cytoplasm characterize these small cells. Because of their deep location, basal cells are rarely seen in vaginal preparations.

Parabasal cells are the smallest of the epithelial cells seen in routine vaginal cytologic samples. These cells have a high nuclear-to-cytoplasmic ratio, round nuclei of uniform size and shape, and basophilic cytoplasm. Parabasal cells or intermediate cells containing cytoplasmic vacuoles are called *foam cells;* the significance of the vacuoles is unknown (Olson et al., 1984a). These cells may be associated with diestrus and anestrus. Large numbers of parabasal cells may be seen in vaginal smears of prepubertal animals and should not be confused with neoplastic cells (Feldman and Nelson, 2004).

Intermediate cells may vary in size, but are generally twice the size of parabasal cells. The nuclear-to-cytoplasmic ratio is decreased with abundant amounts of blue to blue-green (keratinized) cytoplasm. The cytoplasmic borders are round to irregular and folded (Baker and Lumsden, 1999). Intermediate cells may also be called *superficial intermediate* or *transitional intermediate cells* (Allison et al., 2008).

Superficial cells are characterized by small round to pyknotic nuclei, abundant amounts of light blue to blue-green (keratinized) cytoplasm, and angular to folded cell borders. Some superficial cells contain dark-staining bodies of unknown significance (Olson et al., 1984a). As superficial cells age and become degenerate, the nuclei are lost and the cells become anucleated. Superficial cells with pyknotic nuclei and anucleated superficial cells have the same physiologic significance (Allison et al., 2008). Folded, angular cells with pyknotic or absent nuclei are called anuclear squames or anuclear superficial cells (Feldman and Nelson, 2004).

Metestrum cells are large, intermediate vaginal cells that appear to have one or more neutrophils contained within their cytoplasm. These cells are usually seen in diestrus or vaginitis and such cells are rarely observed in early proestrus (Feldman and Nelson, 2004).

Staging the Canine Estrous Cycle

Duration, cytologic appearance, and hormonal status of the different stages of canine estrous cycle are described in Table 12-1.

TABLE 12-1 Duration, Cytologic Appearance, and Hormonal Status of Stages of Canine Estrous Cycle

Stages and Duration of Estrous Cycle		CYTOLOGIC APPEARANCE					Hormonal Status
		Epithelial Cells	Neutrophils	Red Blood Cells	Bacteria	Background	
Proestrus (9 days; range 3–17 days)	Early	Mixture of parabasal, intermediate and few superficial cells	Present	May be abundant or absent. Usually present	Present	Granular or dirty appearance. Mucus can be present	Rising concentrations of estradiol and low concentrations of progesterone
	Late*	Mixture of superficial (>80%) and intermediate cells	Few or none	May be abundant or absent. Usually present	Present	Clear	
Estrus (9 days; range 3–21 days)		>80% superficial and anuclear squames cells. <5% parabasal or intermediate cells	Absent	Present or absent	Present	Clear	Declining estradiol concentrations and rising progesterone concentrations
Diestrus (2 months)		Abrupt 20% decrease in superficial cells and 15–20% increase in small, intermediate cells	Frequently present (few to many)	May be present but usually none	Present. Ingested bacteria within neutrophils may be seen	May contain large amounts of debris	High to low concentrations of progesterone
Anestrus (4.5 months)		Predominance of parabasal and intermediate cells. Superficial cells absent	Absent or low numbers	Absent	Absent or low numbers	Clear or granular	Low concentrations of progesterone

*It is not possible to distinguish late proestrus from estrus with vaginal cytology.

Proestrus

Proestrus (Figs. 12-32 and 12-33) is characterized by rising concentrations of estradiol and low progesterone concentrations (Freshman, 1991). As the estradiol concentrations increase, the vaginal epithelium proliferates and red blood cells move via diapedesis through uterine capillaries (Baker and Lumsden, 1999). In early to mid proestrus, neutrophils and a mixture of parabasal, intermediate, and superficial epithelial cells (Olson et al., 1984a) characterize the vaginal smear. As proestrus progresses, the neutrophils decrease in number and superficial epithelial cells begin to predominate.

Estrus

For optimal breeding efficiency, sperm should be present in the female reproductive tract as near to ovulation as possible. Although vaginal cytology has been shown to be a more accurate indicator of estrus (Fig. 12-34) and,

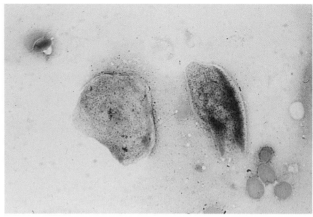

■ **FIGURE 12-34. Estrus. Vaginal smear. Dog.** Shown are anucleated (cornified) superficial epithelial cells along with the presence of red blood cells in the background. (Wright-Giemsa; HP oil.) (Sample provided by Rolf Larsen, University of Florida.)

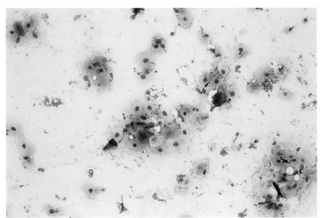

■ **FIGURE 12-32. Proestrus. Vaginal smear. Dog.** There are intermediate epithelial cells with lower numbers of superficial cells. Red blood cells are present. The background has a basophilic appearance due to the presence of mucus. (Wright-Giemsa; HP oil.) (Sample provided by Rolf Larsen, University of Florida.)

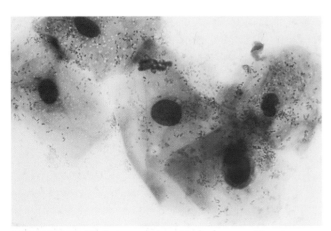

■ **FIGURE 12-33. Late proestrus. Vaginal smear. Dog.** Intermediate and superficial cells appear with round to pyknotic nuclei and moderately basophilic cytoplasm with angular to folded borders. The cells are associated with large numbers of bacteria. (Wright-Giemsa; HP oil.) (Sample provided by Rolf Larsen, University of Florida.)

subsequently, ovulation than behavioral signs, evidence of vaginal maturation or cornification is not closely associated with ovulation. Maximum cornification of vaginal superficial cells ranges from 6 days before the luteinizing hormone (LH) peak to 3 days after the LH peak (Olson et al., 1984a). Since ovulation usually occurs 1 to 2 days after the LH peak, vaginal cytology is not an accurate predictor of ovulation. Ova are viable for up to 2 days postovulation and sperm may remain viable for up to 4 days within the canine reproductive tract during estrus. Therefore, bitches should be bred every 2 to 3 days during cytologic estrus (greater than 90% superficial cells) for optimal breeding (Freshman, 1991). Use of plasma progesterone concentrations in combination with vaginal cytology more accurately indicates the time of ovulation, allowing for even greater breeding efficiency and more accurate estimation of the time of expected parturition (Wright, 1990).

Diestrus

Diestrus (Figs. 12-35 and 12-36) is the luteal phase (Freshman, 1991). The decrease of superficial cells at the beginning of diestrus is usually more rapid than the increase of superficial cells occurring at estrus. Neutrophils frequently reappear during diestrus. Some neutrophils from normal bitches in diestrus contain ingested bacteria. The cytologic appearance of early proestrus and diestrus can be very similar; thus one vaginal smear is not adequate for differentiation of these two stages (Olson et al., 1984a). Once cytologic evidence of diestrus is apparent, breeding is unlikely to be successful.

Anestrus

Anestrus, the period between the end of diestrus and the beginning of the next proestrus, is a time of uterine involution and endometrial repair (Freshman, 1991).

Staging the Feline Estrous Cycle

Cats are seasonally polyestrous. Coitus is necessary for ovulation, with successive estrous cycles occurring until ovulation takes place (Allison et al., 2008). The

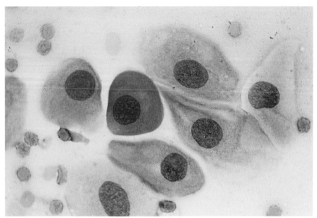

■ **FIGURE 12-35. Diestrus. Vaginal smear. Dog.** Parabasal and intermediate epithelial cells are shown. The parabasal cells have round nuclei, moderate nuclear-to-cytoplasmic ratios, moderately to deeply basophilic cytoplasm, and round cell borders. The intermediate cells are larger with increased amounts of cytoplasm and angular borders. Red blood cells are present in the background. (Wright-Giemsa; HP oil.) (Sample provided by Rolf Larsen, University of Florida.)

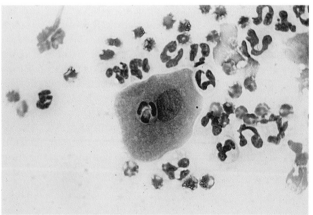

■ **FIGURE 12-36. Diestrus. Vaginal smear. Dog.** Note the large number of neutrophils and red blood cells in the background. An intermediate epithelial cell containing a neutrophil (metestrum cell) is located in the center. These cells are not specific for diestrus and may be found whenever increased numbers of neutrophils are present. (Wright-Giemsa; HP oil.) (Sample provided by Rolf Larsen, University of Florida.)

average duration of estrus is 8 days (range 3 to 16 days) with an intermediate period of 9 days (range 4 to 22 days) if ovulation does not occur. In the presence of ovulation without pregnancy, the return to estrus may be delayed for about 45 days (Olson et al., 1984a). Vaginal cytology has been shown to accurately predict the various stages of the estrous cycle in the cat (Shille et al., 1979; Mills et al., 1979). Collection of smears for cytologic evaluation is similar to those described for the dog; collection of feline vaginal samples may rarely result in ovulation.

Changes in feline vaginal cytology during the estrous cycle are similar to those seen in the dog; however, some differences should be noted. Red blood cells are rarely

seen in smears made at any stage of the cycle. Neutrophils are rare in smears from proestrus and are an inconsistent feature of diestrus. Superficial cells are the predominant cell type seen during estrus. In contrast to dogs, superficial cells comprise only 40% to 88% of the epithelial cells seen during feline estrus (Mills et al., 1979). Anucleated cells increase to about 10% of the epithelial population on the first day of estrus, with a maximum average of 40% anucleated cells by the fourth day of estrus. A prominent clearing of the vaginal smear background in association with estrus has been observed. This clearing occurred in 90% of feline estrus smears and was suggested to be a sensitive indicator of estrus in the cat (Shille et al., 1979).

Inflammation

Vaginitis

Inflammatory disease of the vaginal mucosa is often related to noninfectious factors such as vaginal anomalies, clitoral hypertrophy, foreign bodies, neoplasia, or vaginal immaturity ("puppy vaginitis") (Olson et al., 1984b). Smears for cytologic evaluation of inflammation may be obtained from the vaginal mucosa, vaginal discharges, or FNA of vaginal/vulvar masses. Moderate to large numbers of neutrophils characterize acute vaginitis. In addition to neutrophils, lymphocytes and macrophages may be seen in more chronic inflammatory conditions (Allison et al., 2008). If an infectious component is involved in the inflammatory process, degenerate neutrophils and phagocytized bacteria may be seen (Figs. 12-37 and 12-38). Less commonly, hyphal elements related to fungal infection or pythiosis may be observed. Cytologic specimens may be submitted for silver stains to identify hyphae if fungal infection or pythiosis is suspected (Figs. 12-39 and 12-40).

Treatment of vaginitis should involve identification and correction of any underlying conditions responsible for the inflammation. If sepsis is present, appropriate antibiotic therapy based on culture and sensitivity results should be instituted. Vaginitis can be associated with the

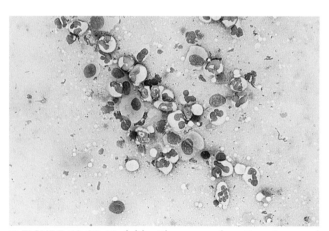

■ **FIGURE 12-37. Vaginitis. Tissue scraping. Dog.** Increased numbers of neutrophils from a vaginal papule. The neutrophils display degenerative nuclear changes of moderate to marked karyolysis. Degenerative changes are typically associated with bacterial infections. A few parabasal and intermediate epithelial cells are also present. (Wright-Giemsa; HP oil.)

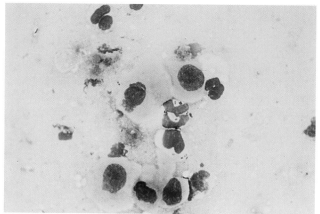

■ **FIGURE 12-38. Septic vaginitis. Tissue scraping. Dog.** Two degenerative neutrophils containing phagocytized bacteria from the vaginal scraping shown in Figure 12-37. (Wright-Giemsa; HP oil.)

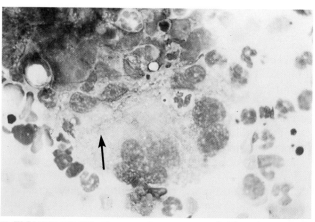

■ **FIGURE 12-39. Pyogranulomatous vaginitis. Tissue aspirate. Dog.** Pyogranulomatous inflammation is present in this specimen from a vulvar mass. Large numbers of neutrophils, lower numbers of eosinophils, and a multinucleated macrophage are present. Pale-staining linear structures suspicious for hyphae are seen associated with the macrophage *(arrow)*. (Wright-Giemsa; HP oil.)

presence of epithelial cells displaying atypical cellular features in response to the inflammatory process. In the absence of a tumor, therapy to alleviate the inflammation should eliminate the atypical cells. However, if an observable mass is present and/or atypical cells remain after appropriate treatment, further tests to rule out the presence of neoplasia should be considered.

Vaginal Neoplasia

Vaginal and vulvar tumors are uncommon and tend to occur in older animals (Olson et al., 1984b; McEntee, 2002). The presenting clinical sign generally is a slow-growing perineal mass. Clinical signs seen less frequently include vulvar bleeding or discharge, an enlarging vulvar mass, dysuria, hematuria, tenesmus, excessive vulvar licking, and dystocia (Klein, 2007). Leiomyomas, fibroleiomyomas, fibromas, and fibropapillomas (polyps) are the most common vaginal neoplasm in dogs and cats (Baker and Lumsden, 1999). These benign mesenchymal tumors are characterized by variable numbers of spindle-shaped cells of uniform size and shape arranged individually and in small clumps (Fig. 12-41). The nuclei are typically oval and scant to moderate amounts of wispy cytoplasm are present. The most common malignant tumor is leiomyosarcoma and distant metastasis has been reported. Other tumors with malignant potential include transmissible venereal tumors (TVT), adenocarcinoma, squamous cell carcinoma, urethral transitional cell carcinoma, osteosarcoma, mast cell tumor, and epidermoid carcinoma (Klein, 2007). The cytologic appearance of these tumors is similar to those found in other body sites. Treatment of vaginal tumors usually involves conservative surgical excision combined with ovariohysterectomy, which is usually is curative for benign tumors (Klein, 2007). In cases of malignant tumors, further evaluation to determine extent of local invasion or metastasis should be performed.

TVT may also be diagnosed using cytologic examination of vaginal smears or fine-needle aspirates. TVT are

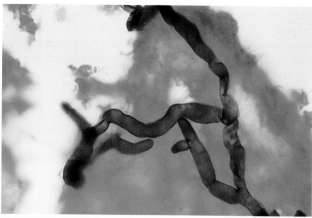

■ **FIGURE 12-40. Fungal vaginitis. Tissue aspirate. Dog.** Special stain of sample shown in Figure 12-39. Positive-staining, poorly septated, linear structures approximately 6 to 8 μm in width are present. Culture confirmed the presence of *Pythium* sp. (Gomori's methenamine silver; HP oil.)

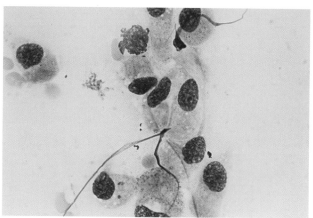

■ **FIGURE 12-41. Vaginal leiomyoma. Tissue imprint. Dog.** The cells are arranged individually or in small clumps and display round to oval nuclei with coarse nuclear chromatin, moderate nuclear-to-cytoplasmic ratios, and inconspicuous nucleoli. The cytoplasm is moderately basophilic and cell borders are indistinct. (Wright-Giemsa; HP oil.)

contagious, sexually transmitted tumors occurring in both genders. The tumors may be located in genital areas and extragenital sites such as the rectum, skin, oral and nasal cavities, and the eyes (Lorimier and Fan, 2007). They appear as firm, friable, tan, ulcerated, and nodular or polypoid masses (Fig. 12-42). In bitches, TVT may spread directly to the cervix, uterus, and oviducts. Although metastasis is uncommon, TVT can spread to regional lymph nodes, skin, and subcutaneous tissue. Other reported metastatic sites include lips, oral mucous membranes, eye, bone, musculature, abdominal viscera, lungs, and the central nervous system. TVT is suspected to be of histiocytic origin based on positive reactions to lysozyme, alpha-1-antitripsin, vimentin, and a macrophage-specific immunostain and negative reaction to immunostains specific for other cell types. Recently described is TVT with intracellular *Leishmania infantum* amastigotes that also suggests a histiocytic origin (Lorimier and Fan, 2007).

Aspirates of TVT generally yield large numbers of individualized, round cells (Figs. 12-43 and 12-44). The nuclei

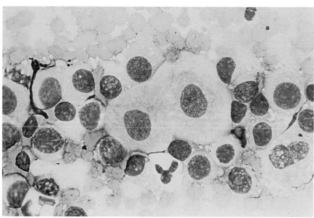

■ FIGURE 12-44. Transmissible venereal tumor. Vaginal mass imprint. Dog. Two intermediate epithelial cells (center) and individualized tumor cells from the same case as shown in Figure 12-43. Note the larger size and increased amounts of cytoplasm in the epithelial cells compared to the tumor cells. (Wright-Giemsa; HP oil.)

are round with clumped nuclear chromatin and single or multiple prominent nucleoli. The nuclei are located eccentrically. Moderate amounts of pale-blue cytoplasm frequently contain multiple punctate vacuoles. Mitotic activity is often high. Inflammation, as indicated by increased numbers of plasma cells, lymphocytes, macrophages, and neutrophils, may be present.

Marginal surgical resection is not considered effective treatment for TVT. The most effective treatments for TVT are chemotherapy and radiation. Single-agent therapy with vincristine has been shown to be very effective for TVT even in cases of metastatic disease. Doxorubicin is the drug of choice for TVT resistant to vincristine (de Lorimier and Fan, 2007).

MALE REPRODUCTIVE SYSTEM: PROSTATE AND TESTES

Prostate Gland

Although the prostate gland is present in cats, the vast majority of prostatic disease is reported in the dog. Therefore, the following discussion of normal and abnormal findings associated with the prostate gland will be limited to the dog. Prostatic disorders are common in middle-aged and older male dogs and have been categorized as hyperplasia, cysts, inflammation, primary and metastatic neoplasia, and squamous metaplasia. More than one prostatic disorder may occur simultaneously (Baker and Lumsden, 1999; Johnston et al., 2000).

The primary presenting clinical findings associated with prostatic disease are signs of systemic febrile illness, lower urinary tract symptoms (hemorrhagic urethral discharge), abnormalities of defecation, and locomotion problems (Dorfman and Barsanti, 1995). Some cases of canine prostatic disease may be present without obvious clinical signs; therefore palpation of the prostate per rectum should be a part of all physical examination in mature intact and neutered male dogs. Normally, the

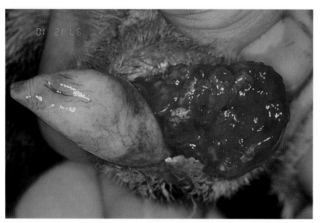

■ FIGURE 12-42. Transmissible venereal tumor. Genital mass. Dog. The mass appears as a soft, friable, hemorrhagic mass on the prepuce.

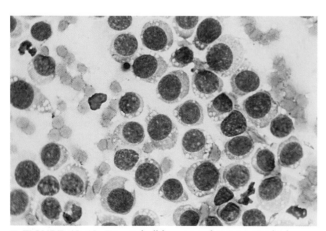

■ FIGURE 12-43. Transmissible venereal tumor. Vaginal mass imprint. Dog. Large numbers of round cells are shown which have round nuclei, coarse nuclear chromatin, variably prominent nucleoli, and scant to moderate amounts of lightly basophilic cytoplasm. Many of the cells contain punctate cytoplasmic vacuoles, which is a characteristic feature of this tumor. (Wright-Giemsa; HP oil.)

prostate should be smooth, symmetrical, and nonpainful. Abdominal palpation can be used to evaluate an enlarged prostate that has moved into the abdominal cavity. Ancillary diagnostic tests that may be used to evaluate suspected cases of prostatic disease include urinalysis, bacterial culture, radiography, and ultrasonography. Complete blood counts and serum biochemical profiles are usually normal in cases of prostatic illness; however, the presence of hemogram and biochemical abnormalities may help in diagnosis (Dorfman and Barsanti, 1995). Cytology, microbiology, and/or histopathology may be necessary for classification of the type of prostatic disease (Baker and Lumsden, 1999). Canine prostatic disease is commonly diagnosed using cytologic techniques, especially now that ultrasound guided FNA is widely available. The diagnostic accuracy of cytology in comparison with histopathologic diagnosis is 80% (Powe et al., 2004). In addition, cytology is a more sensitive method than histology for the detection of bacterial infection.

Special Collection Techniques

Urethral Discharge

Sampling of urethral discharge is a simple method for evaluation of prostatic abnormalities, but is the least effective technique (Baker and Lumsden, 1999). If present, urethral discharge is collected by retracting the prepuce, cleaning the glans, and collecting the discharge into a vial or onto a microscope slide for microscopic evaluation. Some samples may also be collected into sterile containers for bacterial culture and colony counts. Concurrent analysis of urine collected by catheterization or cystocentesis should be performed to differentiate between normal urethral flora and cystitis.

Semen Evaluation

A detailed description of canine and feline semen collection is not fully covered in this text but an in-depth review is available elsewhere (Freshman, 2002; Zambelli and Cunto, 2006). Ejaculate material for evaluation of prostatic disease can be obtained from intact dogs via manual stimulation; however, collection of semen may not be possible if the dog is inexperienced or in pain (Dorfman and Barsanti, 1995). A collection funnel may be used to separate the clear prostatic third fraction of the ejaculate from the sperm-rich first and second fractions (Olson et al., 1987). An aliquot for microbiologic analysis should be placed into a sterile culture tube with the remaining fluid retained for cytologic evaluation. If inflammation is suspected, the cytologic aliquot should be placed into a vial containing EDTA (Baker and Lumsden, 1999). Because of the presence of normal bacterial flora in the lower urethra, a quantitative culture should be performed on the ejaculate fluid. In the presence of inflammatory cells, high numbers (>100,000 cfu/mL) of gram-negative or gram-positive bacteria indicate an infectious process (Root Kustritz, 2006). If cytologic and microbiologic results are equivocal in regards to prostatic infection versus urethral contamination, a quantitative lower urethral culture to compare to the semen culture results may be useful (Dorfman and Barsanti, 1995).

Prostatic Massage

Prostatic massage is used primarily to collect prostatic fluid in dogs unable to ejaculate (Dorfman and Barsanti, 1995). The simplest method for prostatic massage involves passing a urinary catheter, guided by rectal palpation, to the caudal pole of the prostate. A syringe is attached to the catheter and fluid is aspirated as the prostate is gently massaged per rectum (Olson et al., 1987). A few milliliters of sterile saline may be flushed into the catheter and aspirated to facilitate collection of fluid for analysis. Urinary tract infection often accompanies infectious prostatitis, which may confound the results of prostatic massage. For these cases, an alternative massage procedure may be used to determine the source of the infection. The urinary bladder is catheterized, emptied of urine, and flushed with 5 mL of sterile physiologic saline. The fluid from this first flush is collected as the preprostatic massage fraction. The catheter is then retracted to the caudal pole of the prostate. Another 5 mL of sterile physiologic saline is injected through the catheter while the prostate is massaged per rectum. The catheter is then advanced back into the bladder and all the fluid in the bladder is collected. This fluid is the postprostatic massage fraction, which should be relatively free of urinary contamination (Root Kustritz, 2006). Bacterial colony counts and presence or absence of inflammatory cells from the pre- and postprostatic massage fractions can be compared to isolate the source of the infection. Ampicillin, which concentrates in urine but reaches lower concentrations in the prostate owing to its inability to cross the prostatic-lipid barrier, may be administered 1 day prior to prostatic massage to aid in isolation of the source of infection. In general, prostatic massage should be reserved for evaluation of prostatitis in dogs without urinary tract infection or in which the urinary tract infection is controlled. It should be noted that cytologic preparations obtained by catheterization typically yield a mixed population of urothelial cells (Thrall et al., 1985; Powe et al., 2004).

Fine-Needle Aspiration

FNA of the prostate gland has been shown to produce more reliable results and more prostatic cells than prostatic massage (Thrall et al., 1985). If the gland is enlarged, a transabdominal approach may be used. Transperineal and perirectal approaches have also been described (Olson et al., 1987). Ultrasound is particularly useful for guiding the aspiration needle, particularly if focal prostatic disease is present (Zinkl, 2008). The method of aspiration of the prostate gland is similar to that used for other tissues. A 22-gauge needle attached to a 12-mL syringe is directed into the gland and cells and/or fluid are aspirated. A drop of aspirate material or fluid is placed onto a slide. If necessary, any remaining material may then be submitted for culture.

Use of FNA in cases of acute prostatitis or abscessation may be associated with a risk of peritonitis or seeding the infection along the needle tract (Dorfman and Barsanti, 1995). Dogs with suspected prostatic disease presenting with an inflammatory leukogram and fever should not undergo FNA. If purulent fluid is obtained during aspiration of the prostate, aspiration should continue until all pressure is reduced to prevent leakage of the material (Baker and Lumsden, 1999). However, there are numerous reports in the veterinary literature documenting FNA for diagnosis or treatment of prostatic disease with no complications. Ultrasound-guided transabdominal FNA of the prostate is described elsewhere (Root Kustritz, 2006). FNA of the prostate gland has several advantages compared to other collection methods. Identification of squamous epithelial cells from a prostatic aspirate allows diagnosis of squamous metaplasia, whereas the presence of these cells in prostatic massage fluid could be misinterpreted as normal lower urinary tract squamous epithelial cells. Also, the greater cellular detail obtained via FNA increases the confidence of a diagnosis of neoplasia. The primary disadvantage of prostatic FNA is that focal lesions, such as neoplasia, may be missed (Thrall et al., 1985). However, use of ultrasound to guide the aspirate can lessen this possibility.

Normal Anatomy and Histology

The prostate gland secretes a fluid that promotes sperm survival and motility. Normal prostatic fluid is clear and represents the third fraction of the canine ejaculate, although some have suggested that the first fraction also originates from the prostate (Dorfman and Barsanti, 1995). The prostate gland is a glandular, muscular structure completely surrounding the proximal portion of the male urethra (Lowseth et al., 1990). Before 2 months of age, the prostate is located within the abdominal cavity. After breakdown of the urachal ligament until sexual maturity, the prostate lies in the pelvic canal. With increasing age, the prostate enlarges and moves over the pelvic brim into the abdomen. Bladder distension can also pull the prostate cranially into the abdomen.

The prostate gland is composed of compound tubuloalveolar glands radiating from the urethral opening (Figs. 12-45 and 12-46). The secretory alveoli contain primary and secondary enfoldings of epithelium that project into the alveolar lumen. A fibromuscular stroma

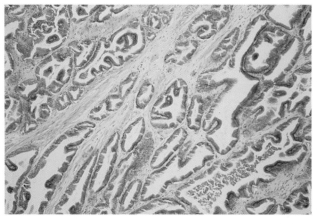

■ FIGURE 12-45. Normal prostate gland. Tissue section. Dog. The tubuloalveolar glands are surrounded by a fibromuscular stroma. Primary and secondary enfoldings of epithelium project into the alveolar lumen. (H&E; LP.) (Case material supplied by Roger Reep and Don Samuelson, University of Florida.)

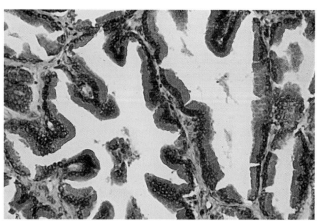

■ FIGURE 12-46. Normal prostate gland. Tissue section. Dog. Higher magnification of specimen in Figure 12-45. Cuboidal and columnar epithelium line the prostatic lumens and ducts. Canine. (H&E; IP.) (Case material supplied by Roger Reep and Don Samuelson, University of Florida.)

surrounds the prostatic ducts, which are lined by cuboidal to columnar epithelium. Transitional epithelium lines the excretory ducts that open onto the urethra (Dorfman and Barsanti, 1995).

Normal Cytology

The number and type of prostatic cells in cytologic samples from the prostate vary depending on the collection technique. Prostatic epithelial cells obtained via aspiration from normal dogs occur in frequent clusters and are cuboidal to columnar. These cells are uniform in size and shape and contain round to oval nuclei, which may be basilar in columnar cells. Nucleoli are usually small and inconspicuous. The cytoplasm is finely granular and basophilic (Thrall et al., 1985). Other cell types that may be seen, particularly from semen samples or prostatic massages, include spermatozoa, squamous epithelial cells, and transitional epithelial cells (urothelial cells) (Zinkl, 2008). Spermatozoa stain blue-green with Romanowsky and modified Romanowsky stains and may adhere to other cells. Squamous cells are large with abundant amounts of blue to blue-green (keratinized) cytoplasm. The nuclei of these cells may be round to pyknotic or absent. Cell borders are typically angular to folded. Transitional cells (urothelial cells) are larger than prostatic epithelial cells and have lighter-staining cytoplasm with a lower nuclear-to-cytoplasmic ratio. Normal ejaculate fluid may contain low numbers of neutrophils and red blood cells. Use of excessive amounts of ultrasound gel during ultrasound-guided FNA can result in large amounts of purple, variably sized, granular background debris that may obscure cellular detail (Zinkl, 2008). To prevent this artifact, excess gel should be removed before inserting the aspiration needle.

Prostatic Cysts

Prostatic cysts may occur as multiple, small cysts associated with benign hyperplasia, large prostatic retention, and periprostatic cysts that can be mineralized or result from osseous metaplasia, and cysts associated with squamous metaplasia. Except for hyperplasia-associated cysts, prostatic cysts account for 2% to 5% of prostatic abnormalities (Dorfman and Barsanti, 1995). Another study reported a prevalence of 14% prostatic cysts in adult, large-breed dogs without genitourinary system problems, and bacterial cultures of prostatic cysts were positive in 42% of cases (Black et al., 1998). Small cysts may be palpated per rectum as small, fluctuant areas in an asymmetrically enlarged prostate. Large, discrete cysts may be palpated in the caudal abdomen or in the perineal area. Unless the cyst(s) become secondarily infected, clinical signs are uncommon (Olson et al., 1987). A bloody urethral discharge, dysuria, and tenesmus may be present owing to increased prostatic size. Recommended treatment is surgical resection, with or without concurrent castration (Johnston et al., 2000). Recently, ultrasound-guided, percutaneous drainage of prostatic cysts appears to be a useful alternative treatment (Boland et al., 2003).

Aspiration of prostatic cysts typically yields variable amounts of serosanguineous to brown fluid (Baker and Lumsden, 1999). Cytologic examination of the fluid usually reveals absent or low numbers of normal-appearing epithelial cells with low to moderate numbers of neutrophils, macrophages, and small lymphocytes and erythrocytes on a red to brown background (Thrall et al., 1985; Boland et al., 2003).

Benign Prostatic Hyperplasia

Benign prostatic hyperplasia (BPH) is a common finding in older intact male dogs. BPH is associated with increases in gland size and weight related to increases in interstitial tissue and gland lumens (Lowseth et al., 1990). Symmetrical cystic dilation of the glands results from increases in the interstitium and gland lumens. The pathogenesis of BPH is not completely understood. However, development of BPH is hormonally dependent and requires the presence of functioning testes (Dorfman and Barsanti, 1995). Dihydrotestosterone is accepted as a key hormone in stimulating enlargement of the canine prostate by enhancing growth in both stromal and glandular components (Johnston et al., 2000). Circulating levels of testosterone are often decreased in older male dogs; however, dihydrotestosterone concentrations are often increased in the hyperplastic tissue (Olson et al., 1987). Nuclear androgen receptor expression is increased in hyperplastic tissue of older Beagles, suggesting increased tissue sensitivity to circulating androgens. Additionally, estrogens appear to act synergistically with androgens in potentiating BPH and may also act directly on the prostate, resulting in stromal hypertrophy and squamous epithelial metaplasia. The treatment of choice for canine BPH is castration or finasteride treatment, as finasteride inhibits conversion of testosterone to dihydrotestosterone, causing prostatic involution via apoptosis (Sirinarumitr et al., 2001).

In men, the prostate is fixed anatomically such that enlargement causes urinary obstruction resulting in the most common presenting sign of dysuria (Lowseth et al., 1990). In dogs, the prostate gland is not fixed so that enlargement occurs in an outward direction resulting in

constipation and tenesmus. Mild hemorrhagic urethral discharge can also be noted (Dorfman and Barsanti, 1995). However, clinical signs are often absent in canine BPH. Palpation of the prostate usually reveals a symmetrically enlarged, nonpainful gland; however, an irregular surface is occasionally felt (Johnston et al., 2000).

Epithelial cells obtained from a hyperplastic prostate gland are generally arranged in variably sized sheets and clusters in a honeycomb pattern (Masserdotti, 2006) (Figs. 12-47 and 12-48). The cells are uniform in appearance with round nuclei and small, round nucleoli. The nuclear-to-cytoplasmic ratio is low to moderate and the cytoplasm is basophilic. Mild increases in cell size and anisokaryosis may be noted (Baker and Lumsden, 1999). Cytologic samples yielding a normal-appearing population of prostatic epithelial cells from an enlarged prostate, particularly if the enlargement is symmetrical,

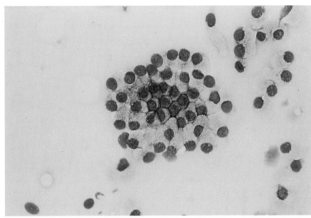

■ **FIGURE 12-47. Benign prostatic hyperplasia. Tissue aspirate. Dog.** Normal-appearing prostatic epithelial cells from an enlarged prostate. The cells are uniform in size and shape and are arranged in clusters and individually. The cluster of cells in the center display a characteristic "honeycomb" appearance. (Wright-Giemsa; HP oil.)

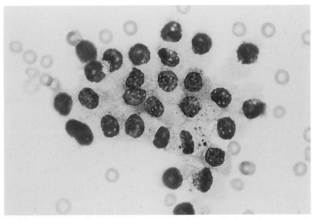

■ **FIGURE 12-48. Benign prostatic hyperplasia. Tissue aspirate. Dog.** Same case as in Figure 12-47. The prostatic epithelial cells display round nuclei, slightly coarse nuclear chromatin, and moderate amounts of lightly basophilic cytoplasm. A few cells contain small amounts of basophilic secretory product. (Wright-Giemsa; HP oil.)

are consistent with a diagnosis of benign hyperplasia (Figs. 12-49 and 12-50).

Squamous Metaplasia

Increased circulating concentrations of estrogen can result in squamous metaplasia of the prostatic epithelium. During this process, the epithelial cells develop staining and morphologic characteristics of squamous epithelial cells. Estrogen receptors, which are present on ductal, stromal, and 10% of the prostatic epithelial cells, may mediate this responsiveness (Baker and Lumsden, 1999).

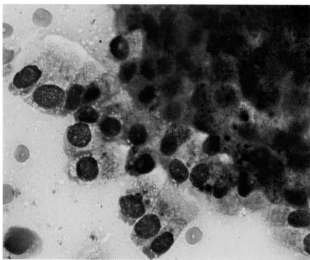

■ **FIGURE 12-49. Benign prostatic hyperplasia. Tissue aspirate. Dog.** Prostatic epithelial cells are columnar and uniform. Note the granulated appearance of the cells and accumulation of secretory pigment in the cell sheets and clusters. (Wright; HP oil.) (Courtesy of Rose Raskin, Purdue University.)

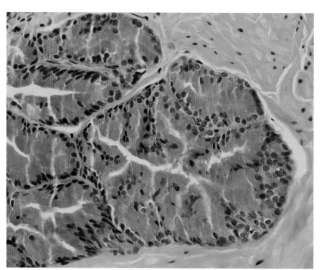

■ **FIGURE 12-50. Benign prostatic hyperplasia, Tissue section. Dog.** Same case as in Figure 12-49. Hyperplastic epithelium is characterized by minimal anaplastic features. Nuclei have less nuclear chromatin density than normal but increased prominence of nucleoli. (H&E; IP.) (Courtesy of Rose Raskin, Purdue University.)

Although chronic irritation and inflammation can result in squamous metaplasia, the most common endogenous source of estrogen is Sertoli cell tumors (Powe et al., 2004). The prostate may be small as a result of decreased concentrations of testosterone or enlarged if cysts or abscessation is present. Clinical signs usually relate to hyperestrogenism. Treatment for squamous metaplasia is removal of the estrogen source.

Prostatic Inflammation

Both acute and chronic infections occur in the canine prostate gland, usually as a result of ascent of normal aerobic urethral bacteria (including *Mycoplasma*) into prostate gland (Johnston et al., 2000). Hematogenous and local spread from other urogenital organs is also possible (Dorfman and Barsanti, 1995). *Escherichia coli* is the most commonly isolated organism from both acute and chronic cases of prostatitis followed by *Staphylococcus aureus, Klebsiella* spp., *Proteus mirabilis, Mycoplasma canis, Pseudomona aeruginosa, Enterobacter* spp., *Streptococcus* spp., *Pasteurella* spp., and *Haemophilus* spp. Anaerobic bacteria or fungal infections also have been observed via hematogenous spread, urethral ascent, or penetration through the scrotum with descending prostate infection from a testicular source. Alteration of normal architecture by diseases such as BPH, squamous metaplasia, and neoplasia can interfere with normal defense mechanisms or provide a medium (i.e., blood in cysts) for bacterial growth (Olson et al., 1987). Coalescing of focal areas of septic prostatitis or infection of prostatic cysts may result in prostatic abscessation (Baker and Lumsden, 1999).

Acute prostatitis is usually associated with systemic signs of illness (fever, anorexia, and lethargy), straining to urinate or defecate, hematuria, edema of scrotum, prepuce, and hind limb or pain on rectal palpation of the prostate gland (Dorfman and Barsanti, 1995). The dog may also experience locomotor problems due to caudal lumbar or abdominal pain. An inflammatory leukogram with or without a left-shift is often present. Clinical signs in dogs with chronic prostatitis may be absent, or there may be recurrent urinary tract infection, poor semen quality with infertility, or sometimes decreased libido (Johnston et al., 2000). Intermittent or constant urethral discharge may also be noted. Prostatic abscesses may present with signs related to enlargement of the prostate (tenesmus, dysuria), constant or intermittent urethral discharge, and evidence of systemic illness related to endotoxemia or peritonitis. Treatment of prostatitis involves appropriate antibiotic therapy as determined by culture and sensitivity. In acute prostatitis, most antibiotics will reach the site of infection since the prostate-lipid barrier is disrupted (Olson et al., 1987). Antibiotics for treatment of chronic prostatitis should be selected for the ability to cross the lipid barrier, which is usually intact, and for the ability to concentrate in the prostate. In addition to appropriate antibiotic therapy, prostatic abscesses can be treated surgically with marsupialization of the gland, placement of a drain, or prostatectomy. All of these surgical procedures are associated with significant complications. Castration should also be performed in dogs with prostatitis (Dorfman and Barsanti, 1995).

Cytologic evaluation of samples from bacterial prostatitis contains large numbers of neutrophils, many of which exhibit degenerative changes of karyolysis and karyorrhexis (Fig. 12-51). Macrophages may also be present, especially in chronic prostatitis (Fig. 12-52). In the absence of previous antibiotic therapy, intracellular and extracellular organisms may be seen (Boland et al., 2003). Epithelial cells that are present may appear normal or hyperplastic as evidenced by increased cytoplasmic basophilia, increased nuclear-to-cytoplasmic ratios, and mild anisokaryosis. Cellular atypia associated with prostatic epithelial cells in the presence of inflammation should be interpreted cautiously to avoid a false-positive diagnosis of neoplasia (Thrall et al., 1985).

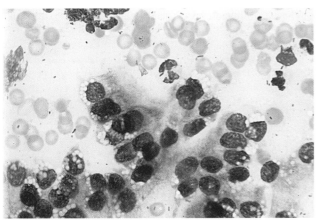

■ **FIGURE 12-51. Septic neutrophilic prostatitis. Tissue aspirate. Dog.** Prostatic epithelial cells and neutrophils are present in this example of acute septic prostatitis. The neutrophils are degenerate as indicated by moderate karyolysis. Bacteria are present in the background and within the neutrophils. (Wright-Giemsa; HP oil.)

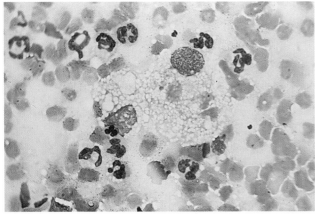

■ **FIGURE 12-52. Mixed cell prostatitis. Tissue aspirate. Dog.** A mixed cell population is present in this case of chronic prostatitis. Increased numbers of neutrophils, the majority of which are nondegenerate, and two reactive macrophages are present. Infectious organisms were not seen in this sample. (Wright-Giemsa; HP oil.)

Prostatic Neoplasia

Prostatic malignant tumors in the dog are rare, with reported prevalences of 0.2% and 0.6% based on necropsy studies (Bell et al., 1991). Adenocarcinoma is the most commonly reported neoplasm of the prostate followed by transitional cell carcinoma arising from the prostatic urethra, but other epithelial neoplasms have been described such as undifferentiated carcinoma and squamous cell carcinoma (Dorfman and Barsanti, 1995; McEntee, 2002). Prostatic intraepithelial neoplasia, a precursor lesion of prostatic carcinoma, has been reported in both normal and neoplastic prostate glands. Other malignant neoplasms have been rarely described such as lymphoma and malignant mesenchymal tumors such as hemangiosarcoma and leiomyosarcoma (Hayden et al., 1999; Teske et al., 2002; Winter et al., 2006; Fan and de Lorimier, 2007).

Prostatic carcinoma most frequently occurs in dogs 8 to 10 years of age (Dorfman and Barsanti, 1995), and neutered dogs are at higher risk (Bryan et al., 2007). Canine prostatic adenocarcinomas arise from ductal epithelium, which is predominantly androgen receptor negative suggesting that androgens may not be required for initiation or progression of this tumor (Fan and de Lorimier, 2007). Most canine prostatic carcinomas are locally invasive and metastatic. Metastases were present at necropsy in 80% to 89% of dogs with prostatic carcinoma and regional lymph nodes and lungs are the most common sites (Cornell et al., 2000). Other sites for metastasis are bone, urinary bladder, and mesentery. Bone metastases are most often located in the pelvis, lumbar vertebrae, and femur and can be lytic or proliferative (Dorfman and Barsanti, 1995). The disease carries a poor prognosis in untreated dogs with survival time of less than 2 months (Bell et al., 1991; Sorenmo et al., 2004).

Canine prostatic carcinoma is an insidious disease, with many dogs showing no evidence of clinical abnormalities until late in the course of the malignancy. The most frequently detected abnormality during physical examination is prostatomegaly, which is identified in 52% of the dogs with carcinoma. The enlargement is primarily asymmetrical (32%); however, sometimes symmetrical enlargement (6%) can be noted (Bell et al., 1991). Other physical abnormalities include depression, painful abdominal palpation, cachexia, pyrexia, dyspnea, dysuria, stranguria, hematuria, tenesmus, weight loss, gait abnormalities, and presence of an abdominal mass (Johnston et al., 2000). Complete obstruction of urinary flow may result in hydroureter, hydronephrosis, and subsequent renal failure (Fan and de Lorimier, 2007).

Therapy for prostatic carcinoma is usually palliative and may include prostatectomy or intraoperative radiation (Dorfman and Barsanti, 1995). However, in humans, epidemiologic and experimental evidence supports the use of nonsteroidal anti-inflammatory drugs (NSAIDs) for the prevention of cancer development. This chemopreventive effect may be partially mediated through the inhibition of cyclooxygenase-2 (COX-2) activity causing the blockade of endogenous prostaglandin E_2 production (Fan and de Lorimier, 2007). Canine normal prostatic tissues have failed to express • COX-2 protein, but it was detected in 75% to 88% of prostatic carcinomas (L'Eplattenier et al., 2007). In addition, a significant increase in survival time in dogs treated with COX-2 inhibitors occurred when compared with untreated dogs (Sorenmo, 2004).

FNA is useful for diagnosis of prostatic neoplasia. Cytologic evaluation of FNA samples from prostatic adenocarcinoma usually reveals large numbers of deeply basophilic epithelial cells arranged in variably sized clusters and sheets (Figs. 12-53 and 12-54). The nuclear-to-cytoplasmic ratio is often high and anisokaryosis and anisocytosis can be moderate to marked. Nuclei are round to pleomorphic and nucleoli are large, prominent, and often multiple. Binucleation may be noted. Adenocarcinoma and transitional cell carcinoma can be difficult to distinguish cytologically, and histopathology may be required for definitive diagnosis (Baker and Lumsden, 1999). Some acinar structures may be noted, which can

help to differentiate the neoplasm from transitional cell carcinoma (Zinkl, 2008). Bell et al. (1991) reported that a diagnosis of neoplasia was established in 15 of 19 (79%) of samples submitted for cytologic analysis from dogs with histologically confirmed prostatic carcinoma. False-negative cytology results could have been related to small sample size, focal distribution of neoplastic lesions, or concurrent prostatitis and/or BPH. Serum and seminal plasma concentrations of acid phosphatase, prostate specific antigen and canine prostate specific esterase have not been shown to be useful in the definitive diagnosis of canine prostatic carcinoma (Gobello et al., 2002).

Testes

Unilateral or bilateral testicular enlargement is the primary indication for FNA and cytologic evaluation of the testes (Zinkl, 2008). Cytology is useful for differentiation between inflammatory or neoplastic conditions that cause testicular enlargement and to classify testicular canine neoplasia (Masserdotti et al., 2005). Testicular FNA has also been shown to be useful for evaluation of male infertility (Dahlbom et al., 1997). Testicular FNA is usually not associated with immediate or long-term adverse effects (Kustritz, 2005).

Special Collection Techniques

Routine FNA with a 20- to 25-gauge needle attached to 5- to 10-mL syringe is used for cytologic sampling of the testes (Kustritz, 2005). Because of the increased fragility of testicular cells, great care should be taken when preparing the slide of aspirated material and some authors recommend avoiding mechanical aspiration to obtain a better cytologic preparation (Masserdotti et al., 2005). The material should be very lightly smeared when preparing the cell monolayer. Alternatively, gentle touch imprints from available tissue may decrease cellular disruption (Baker and Lumsden, 1999). Imprints of testicular biopsies should be made rapidly after removal of the tissue to prevent degeneration of the cells.

Normal Anatomy and Histology

The testes are the site of spermatogenesis in the adult animal and exhibit both exocrine and endocrine function (Banks, 1986). The exocrine portion of the testes is a compound, coiled, tubular gland that produces spermatozoa as its secretory product. The germinal epithelium is actively involved in spermatogenesis. The endocrine portions of the testes are composed of the interstitial (Leydig) cells, which secrete testosterone, and Sertoli (sustentacular) cells, which provide support for the developing sperm (Figs. 12-55 and 12-56).

Normal Cytology

Normal testicular imprints are highly cellular with a predominance of ruptured cells and streaming nuclear material (Baker and Lumsden, 1999). When cells rupture, the nuclear chromatin becomes coarse and nucleoli are prominent. Testicular germinal cells are generally round, with coarse nuclear chromatin, a single large, prominent nucleolus, and moderate amounts of basophilic cytoplasm

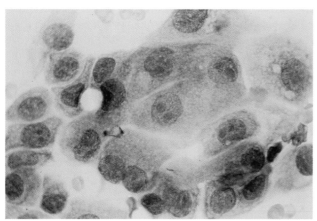

■ **FIGURE 12-53. Prostatic carcinoma. Cytologic preparation. Dog.** Neoplastic epithelial cells display prominent, large, multiple nucleoli, coarse nuclear chromatin, moderate anisokaryosis and anisocytosis, variable nuclear-to-cytoplasmic ratios, and binucleation. (Wright-Giemsa; HP oil.)

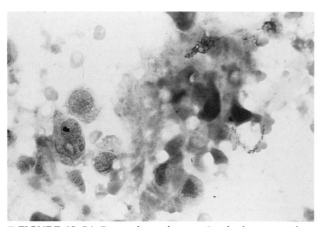

■ **FIGURE 12-54. Prostatic carcinoma. Cytologic preparation. Dog.** Same case as in Figure 12-53. The amorphous basophilic material is compatible with necrosis, which can be found in aspirates of malignant tumors. Cellular features are indistinct. (Wright-Giemsa; HP oil.)

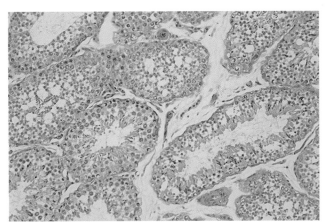

■ **FIGURE 12-55. Normal testes. Tissue section. Dog.** Multiple seminiferous tubules are present, which are surrounded by connective tissue containing low numbers of interstitial cells. (H&E; IP.)

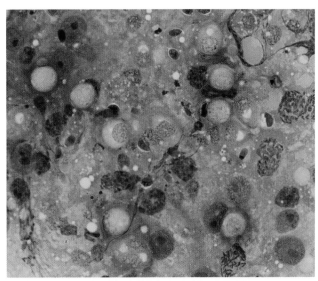

■ **FIGURE 12-57. Normal testes. Tissue imprint. Dog.** Large germinal cells and round spermatocytes are present along with small, densely basophilic spermatids. The background contains few lightly basophilic, detached mature sperm heads. (Wright; HP oil.) (Courtesy of Rose Raskin, Purdue University.)

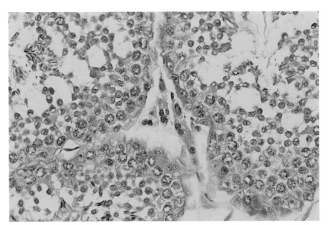

■ **FIGURE 12-56. Normal testes. Tissue section. Dog.** Higher magnification of the seminiferous tubules from the same case as in Figure 12-55. Interstitial cells are seen in the center of the photomicrograph. Spermatocytes as well as early and late spermatids are seen within the tubules. Spermatocytes are characterized by round nuclei and coarse nuclear chromatin. During the maturation process, developing sperm move from the periphery of the tubule to the central lumen. Low numbers of Sertoli cells with smooth nuclear chromatin and single, prominent nucleoli are seen at the periphery of the tubules. (H&E; HP oil.)

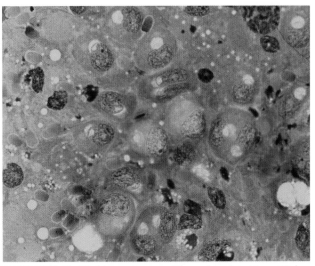

■ **FIGURE 12-58. Normal testes. Tissue imprint. Dog.** Higher magnification of same specimen shown in Figure 12-57. Note large numbers of pale basophilic–staining mature sperm with thin, clear space around the heads. Frequent binucleation is present in the germinal cells that display reticulated chromatin and prominent nucleoli. (Wright; HP oil.) (Courtesy of Rose Raskin, Purdue University.)

(Figs. 12-57 and 12-58). Mitotic activity is often high. More mature stages of developing sperm are characterized by oval, eosinophilic to pale-staining nuclei, and tails may be noted. Small groups of columnar cells, with indistinct cytoplasm and large round nuclei as single nucleoli, recognizable as Sertoli cells, can occasionally be evident. Scattered stellate or caudate Leydig cells, with microvacuolated cytoplasm and round nuclei are sometimes observed (Masserdotti et al., 2005).

Testicular Inflammation

In dogs, inflammatory disease of the testes (orchitis) or epididymis can be due to infection with *Brucella canis* (Wanke, 2004), *Pseudomonas* sp., *E. coli*, or *Proteus* sp. (Ladds, 1993). Orchitis and epididymitis are common in

dogs with clinical patent leishmaniasis (Diniz et al., 2005). Intranuclear or intracytoplasmic inclusions may be seen in cases of distemper-associated orchitis (Ladds, 1993). Orchitis may also be associated with infection by the dimorphic yeast, *Blastomyces dermatitidis*. Orchitis has been recently reported in two dogs with Rocky Mountain spotted fever (Ober et al., 2004). Chronic purulent epididymitis associated with *Mycoplasma canis* infection has been described in one dog (L'Abee-Lund et al., 2003). In cats, orchitis or epididymitis is uncommon and orchitis has been associated with coronavirus infection in one cat (Sigurdardottir et al., 2001) and the isolation of *Sporothrix schenckii* from a testis in another cat (Schubach et al., 2002). Acute orchitis is characterized by a predominance of neutrophils, some of which may exhibit nuclear degenerative changes. Macrophages, including multinucleated giant cells and lymphocytes, may be seen in chronic inflammatory disease or fungal (blastomycosis) or protozoal (such as *Leishmania infantum* [Diniz et al., 2005]) infections. Since the infectious organisms are usually not observed cytologically, culture should be performed to identify the pathogens (Baker and Lumsden, 1999).

Testicular Neoplasia

In the intact male dog, the testis is the second most common anatomic site for cancer development and testicular tumors account for approximately 90% of all cancers of male genitalia (Fan and de Lorimier, 2007). The three most common tumors are Leydig cell tumor/interstitial cell tumor (58%), seminoma (23%), and Sertoli cell tumor (19%) (Masserdotti et al., 2005), although cases of hemangiomas, granulosa cell tumors, teratomas, sarcomas, embryonal carcinomas, gonadoblastomas, lymphomas, and rete testis mucinous carcinomas have been rarely described. More than one type of testicular tumor is common in dogs (McEntee, 2002). Canine testicular tumorigenesis is not well known but it seems that critical cell cycle regulators such as cyclin D1 and E (Murakami et al., 2001) and insulin-like growth factor system (Peters et al., 2003) do not play a role while enhancement of angiogenic processes are observed in some tumors such as seminomas (Restucci et al., 2003). Testicular tumors occur frequently in aged male dogs. Cryptorchid testes have a higher incidence of Sertoli cell tumors and seminomas, with the right testis more frequently being retained and therefore predisposed to tumorigenesis (MacLachlan and Kennedy, 2002). Most primary testicular tumors are locally confined, with fewer than 15% having a metastatic phenotype. In dogs with localized disease, orchiectomy with scrotal ablation remains the treatment of choice and often is curative. Information about appropriate and effective management of metastatic disease is limited, although the use of radiation therapy and chemotherapy has been reported to increase survival time (Fan and de Lorimier, 2007).

Testicular tumors are rare in cats. There are only isolated cases reports of testicular tumors in cats (McEntee, 2002) such as teratoma (Ferreira da Silva, 2002) and interstitial and Sertoli cell tumors (Miller et al., 2007).

High sensitivity (95% for seminoma, 88% for Sertoli cell tumor, and 96% for Leydig cell tumor), and specificity (100%) for the cytologic diagnosis of canine testicular tumors have been reported when compared with histopathologic evaluation. Cytologic evaluation permits accurate diagnosis and is useful in the management of the disease (Masserdotti et al., 2005).

Seminoma

Seminomas arise from neoplastic transformation of the testicular germ cells. The mean age for development of seminoma is 10 years. Other than testicular enlargement, which may not be readily apparent if the tumor involves a cryptorchid testicle, clinical signs related to seminomas are rare. Six to 11% of canine seminomas metastasize, with primary metastatic sites including the inguinal, iliac, and sublumbar lymph nodes and the lungs or abdominal organs (MacLachlan and Kennedy, 2002; McEntee, 2002).

Cytologic differentiation of seminomas from other testicular tumors may be difficult. Cytologic preparations from seminomas often contain large numbers of lysed cells and free nuclei. These cells are large and round and arranged individually or occasionally in small aggregates. The nuclei are large and round, sometimes with irregular outlines. Nuclear chromatin is reticular to coarse and large, prominent nucleoli are commonly present (Fig. 12-59). Moderate anisokaryosis, anisocytosis, and binucleation and multinucleation may be present (Fig. 12-60). The cytoplasm is lightly to moderately basophilic with a moderate to high nuclear-to-cytoplasmic

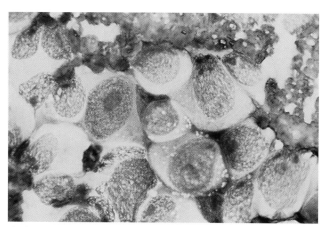

■ **FIGURE 12-59. Seminoma. Tissue aspirate. Dog.** Neoplastic cells appear large with round nuclei, coarse nuclear chromatin, and prominent, large nucleoli. The cytoplasm is lightly basophilic and some cells contain small numbers of punctate cytoplasmic vacuoles. (Wright-Giemsa; HP oil.)

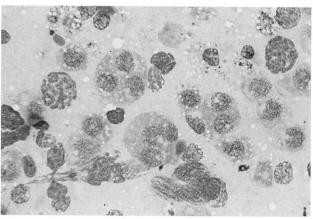

■ **FIGURE 12-60. Seminoma. Tissue aspirate. Dog.** Several multinucleated cells are noted along with the large number of lysed cells and free nuclei in the background. The tendency of testicular cells to rupture can make cytologic evaluation difficult. (Wright-Giemsa; HP oil.)

ratio. The presence of clear macrovacuoles in the cytoplasm is rarely noted. Numerous and aberrant mitoses are often observed. Small lymphocytes are frequently seen in seminomas. Lacy, granular eosinophilic material with the appearance of a tigroid or striped background is occasionally seen (Masserdotti et al., 2005).

Sertoli Cell Tumor

Sertoli cell tumors are fairly common in retained testicles. Most dogs with Sertoli cell tumors are more than 6 years of age with a mean age of 9.5 years, although tumors in dogs as young as 3 years of age have been reported (McEntee, 2002; MacLachlan and Kennedy, 2002). About one third of canine Sertoli cell tumors are associated with excess production of estrogen, although both seminomas and interstitial cell tumors can cause hormonal imbalance. Reductions in the testosterone/estradiol ratio correlate better than absolute increase values of estradiol-17β with clinical signs of feminization including bilaterally symmetric alopecia and hyperpigmentation, a pendulous prepuce, gynecomastia, galactorrhea, atrophic penis, squamous metaplasia of the prostate, and/or bone marrow suppression (Mischke et al., 2002). Metastasis occurs in 10% to 14% of Sertoli cell tumors. Sites of metastasis are iliac lymph nodes primarily, but also other lymph nodes, spleen, liver, and kidney.

Cytologically, variable numbers of round to elongate pleomorphic cells characterize Sertoli cell tumors. These cells may occur individually or in small clusters with palisading formation (Masserdotti, 2006). Nuclei are generally round with fine nuclear chromatin and occasionally one to three prominent, large nucleoli are noted (Fig. 12-61). The lightly basophilic cytoplasm may vary from scant to abundant in amount, sometimes with indistinct margins. The presence of moderate-sized to large cytoplasmic vacuoles (Fig. 12-62) is typical (Masserdotti et al., 2005).

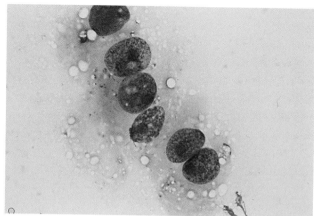

■ **FIGURE 12-62. Sertoli cell tumor. Tissue aspirate. Dog.** A row of tumor cells is shown from the same case as in Figure 12-61. Variably sized cytoplasmic vacuoles are seen in several of the cells. (Wright-Giemsa; HP oil.)

Interstitial Cell Tumors

Interstitial cell tumors are very common in the dog but only 16% of these tumors are associated with testicular enlargement; therefore, they are infrequently aspirated for cytologic analysis (MacLachlan and Kennedy, 2002; Baker and Lumsden, 1999). This tumor has been associated with increased production of testosterone and a high prevalence of prostatic disease and perianal gland neoplasms (McEntee, 2002). Interstitial cell tumors, but not Sertoli cell tumors or seminoma, produce inhibins and 3ß-hydroxsteroid dehydrogenases, which allows discrimination of interstitial cell tumors from other tumors of the canine testes (Taniyama et al., 2001). Cytologic samples from interstitial cell tumors are of variable cellularity. The cells are round or spindle-shaped and usually contain abundant amounts of lightly to moderately basophilic cytoplasm (Fig. 12-63). Perivascular arrangement (Fig. 12-64) is commonly seen

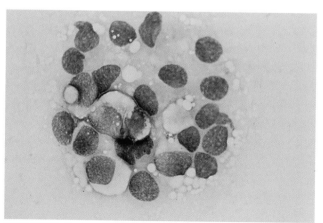

■ **FIGURE 12-61. Sertoli cell tumor. Tissue aspirate. Dog.** This animal presented with infertility, dermatitis with hyperpigmentation, and a testicular mass. The tumor cells have round to oval nuclei, slightly coarse nuclear chromatin, and moderate nuclear-to-cytoplasmic ratios. The nucleoli are small and variably prominent. The cytoplasm is lightly basophilic and cell borders are often indistinct. (Wright-Giemsa; HP oil.)

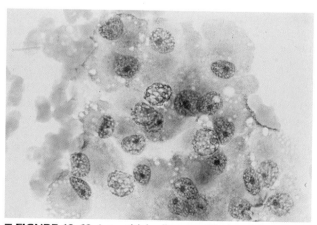

■ **FIGURE 12-63. Interstitial cell tumor. Tissue aspirate. Dog.** A cluster of tumor cells display coarse nuclear chromatin, prominent, single nucleoli, and large amounts of moderately basophilic cytoplasm. The nuclei are often located at the periphery of the cell. Punctate cytoplasmic vacuoles are present in the majority of the cells. (Wright-Giemsa; HP oil.)

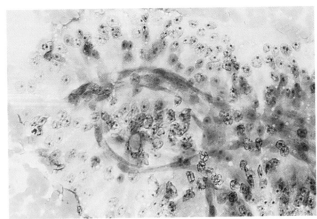

■ **FIGURE 12-64. Interstitial cell tumor. Tissue aspirate. Dog.** Lower magnification of the same case as shown in Figure 12-63. Palisading arrays of interstitial cells surround a central capillary. (Wright-Giemsa; HP oil.)

TABLE 12-2	Canine Spermatozoal Abnormalities	
Location of Abnormality	Primary Abnormalities	Secondary Abnormalities
Head	Pyriform, tapered, narrow, small, giant, round, deformed, double heads	Detached head
Midpiece	Double and swollen midpiece and proximal droplet	Distal droplet
Tail	Tightly coiled and double tails	Bent, reverse, and distal coiled tails
Other		Released acrosome

(Masserdotti, 2006). The nuclei are round to oval with fine, reticular chromatin and small, prominent nucleoli. The presence of nuclear pseudoinclusions is observed in half of the cases. Moderate to marked anisokaryosis and variable nuclear-to-cytoplasmic ratios are seen. Numerous small, uniform cytoplasmic clear vacuoles are common (see Fig. 12-63). Dark, irregularly shaped cytoplasmic granules may be present in some cells (Zinkl, 2008; Masserdotti et al., 2005).

Semen Abnormalities

A detailed description of canine and feline semen collection and evaluation is not offered in this text but in-depth reviews are available elsewhere (Freshman, 2002; Rijsselaere et al., 2005; Zambelli and Cunto, 2006; Axner and Linde Forsberg, 2007; Root Kustritz, 2007). However, the cytologist is occasionally presented with seminal material from dogs or cats with infertility or suspected testicular or prostatic disease; thus the ability to recognize certain abnormalities is useful. Gross evaluation, pH, and light microscopy such as concentration, motility, and morphology are routinely used to evaluate the principal parameters of dog and cat semen. Concentration is usually determined using a counting chamber. Aqueous-based Wright stain or Romanowsky-type stain is often used to assess sperm morphology. In high-quality semen, nearly all of the sperm should be of similar morphology. Spermatozoal abnormalities are considered as primary or secondary and described in Table 12-2. Primary abnormalities occur mostly during defective spermatogenesis and are therefore more serious. Secondary abnormalities may occur during passage through the epididymis (defective maturation) or during collection and preparation of the slide (see Table 12-2). Severe abnormalities include abnormal size or shape of the sperm head or acrosomal cap, proximal or midpiece protoplasmic droplets, and coiled tails (Figs. 12-65 to 12-67). Less severe abnormalities include detached, normal-appearing heads and bent tails (Figs. 12-67 and 12-68). Normal semen samples should have less than 10% and 20% of primary and secondary abnormalities, respectively. Total canine and

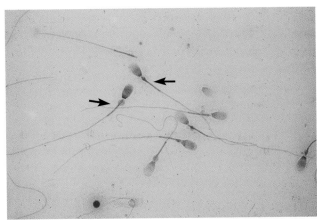

■ **FIGURE 12-65. Primary abnormalities. Semen smear. Dog.** Noninflammatory semen sample from a case of infertility. Sperm have prominent proximal protoplasmic droplets *(arrows)*. (Wright; HP oil.) (Courtesy of Rose Raskin, Purdue University.)

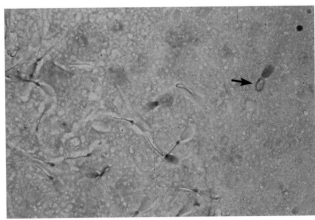

■ **FIGURE 12-66. Primary abnormalities. Semen smear. Dog.** Noninflammatory semen sample from a case of infertility. Against a heavy proteinaceous background, several sperm display tightly coiled tails *(arrow)* and proximal protoplasmic droplets. (Wright; HP oil.) (Courtesy of Rose Raskin, Purdue University.)

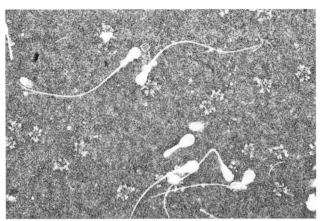

■ **FIGURE 12-67. Primary and secondary abnormalities. Semen smear. Dog.** Noninflammatory semen sample from a case of infertility. Sperm abnormalities include proximal protoplasmic droplets, coiled tails, and bent tails. (India ink; ×250.) (Courtesy of Rose Raskin, Purdue University.)

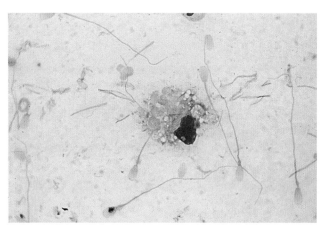

■ **FIGURE 12-69. Inflammation. Semen sample. Dog.** A reactive macrophage and several relatively normal–appearing sperm from the same ejaculate demonstrated in Figure 12-68. (Wright-Giemsa; HP oil.)

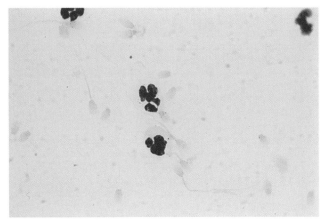

■ **FIGURE 12-68. Inflammation and abnormal sperm. Semen sample. Dog.** An ejaculate sample from an animal with intermittent preputial bleeding. Mildly degenerate neutrophils are present. Several morphologic secondary abnormalities of the sperm (detached heads, bent tails, and coiled tails) are present. (Wright-Giemsa; HP oil.)

feline spermatozoal abnormalities should be less than 20% to 30% (Freshman, 2002).

Cytology of the sperm-rich and prostatic fractions should be evaluated separately by centrifuge or whole sample (less cellularity). Normal cytology of the sperm-rich fraction contains spermatozoa, white blood cells (WBC) (2/hpf to 4/hpf), epithelial cells, bacteria, and red blood cells. Increased or degenerate neutrophils or macrophages or intracellular bacteria indicate inflammation and/or infection (Figs. 12-68 and 12-69). If neutrophils exhibit degenerative changes, a search for infectious organisms should be performed. However, culture of the

fluid may be necessary for identification of pathogens due to the fact that 55% of clinically meaningful aerobic, anaerobic, or myoplasmic bacterial growth has noninflammatory seminal fluid cytology (Root Kustritz et al, 2005). Normal cytology of prostatic fluid is characterized by small amounts of epithelial cells, bacteria, and WBC (2/hpf to 4/hpf) (Freshman, 2002). Lower urinary tract inflammation and/or prostatitis should also be considered when inflammatory cells are present in semen. The presence of abnormal prostatic epithelium in the semen sample warrants further evaluation of the prostate gland (Zinkl, 2008).

Other miscellaneous tests exist to evaluate semen such as live-dead staining with eosin-nigrosin stains, hyposmotic swelling test, and measurement of components of seminal fluid (Root Kustritz, 2007). The most often used seminal markers are alkaline phosphatase (ALP) and carnitine. Both components originate from the epididymis in the dog and have the same application as markers of patency of ductal azoospermia. In an azoospermic semen sample, measurement of ALP or carnitine activity is essential in determining if the azoospermia is due to problems with libido, testicular failure, or ductal blockage. A low ALP or carnitine activity indicates ductal blockage whereas a normal ALP or carnitine activity indicates testicular failure (Gobello et al., 2002; Freshman, 2002).

There are numerous limitations of light microscopical methods such as subjectivity and variability. Recently, several techniques have been described related to the capacity to reach, bind, penetrate, and fertilize an oocyte that may enable more accurate prediction of the fertilizing capacity of semen sample. Conventional light microscopic semen assessment is being replaced by fluorescent staining techniques, computer-assisted sperm analysis systems, and flow cytometry (Rijsselaere et al., 2005).

REFERENCES

Agudelo CF: Cystic endometrial hyperplasia-pyometra complex in cats: a review, *Vet Q* 27:173-182, 2005.

Allen SW, Prasse KW, et al: Cytologic differentiation of benign from malignant canine mammary tumors, *Vet Pathol* 23: 649-655, 1986.

Allison RW, Maddux JM: Subcutaneous glandular tissue: mammary, salivary, thyroid, and parathyroid. In Cowell RL, Tyler RD, Meinkoth JM, DeNicola DB (eds): *Diagnostic cytology and hematology of the dog and cat*, ed 3, St. Louis, 2008, Mosby, pp 112-117.

Allison RW, Thrall MA, Olson, PN: Vaginal cytology. In Cowell RL, Tyler RD, Meinkoth JM, DeNicola DB (eds): *Diagnostic cytology and hematology of the dog and cat*, ed 3, St. Louis, 2008, Mosby, pp 378-389.

Axner E, Linde Forsberg C: Sperm morphology in the domestic cat, and its relation with fertility: a retrospective study, *Reprod Domest Anim* 42:282-291, 2007.

Baker RH, Lumsden JH (eds): *Color atlas of cytology of the dog and cat*, St. Louis, 1999, Mosby, pp 235-251, 253-62.

Banks, WJ (ed): *Applied veterinary histology*, Williams & Wilkins, Baltimore, 1986, pp 348-378, 489-504, 506-23.

Bell FW, Klausner JS, Hayden DW, et al: Clinical and pathologic features of prostatic adenocarcinoma in sexually intact and castrated dogs: 31 cases (1970-1987), *J Am Vet Med Assoc* 199:1623-1630, 1991.

Benjamin SA, Lee AC, Saunders WJ: Classification and behavior of canine mammary epithelial neoplasms based on life-span observations in beagles, *Vet Pathol* 36:423-436, 1999.

Bertazzolo W, Dell'Orco M, Bonfanti U, et al: Cytological features of canine ovarian tumours: a retrospective study of 19 cases, *J Small Anim Pract* 45:539-545, 2004.

Black GM, Ling GV, Nyland TG, et al: Prevalence of prostatic cysts in adult, large-breed dogs, *J Am Anim Hosp Assoc* 34:177-180, 1998.

Boland LE, Hardie RJ, Gregory SP, et al: Ultrasound-guided percutaneous drainage as the primary treatment for prostatic abscesses and cysts in dogs, *J Am Anim Hosp Assoc* 39: 151-159, 2003.

Brazzell JL, Borjesson DL: Intra-abdominal mass aspirate from an alopecic dog, *Vet Clin Pathol* 35:259-262, 2006.

Brodey RS, Goldschmidt MH, Roszel JR: Canine mammary gland neoplasms, *J Am Anim Hosp Assoc* 19:61-90, 1983.

Bryan JN, Keeler MR, Henry CJ, et al: A population study of neutering status as a risk factor for canine prostate cancer, *Prostate* 67:1174-1181, 2007.

Cassali GD, Gobbi H, Malm C, et al: Evaluation of accuracy of fine needle aspiration cytology for mammary tumours: comparative features with human tumours, *Cytopathology* 18:191-196, 2007.

Choi US, Seo KW, Oh SY, et al: Intra-abdominal mass aspirate from a cat in heat, *Vet Clin Pathol* 34:275-277, 2005.

Cornell KK, Bostwick DG, Cooley DM: Clinical and pathological aspects of spontaneous canine prostatic carcinoma: a retrospective analysis of 76 cases, *Prostate* 45:173-183, 2000.

Dahlbom M, Makinen A, Suominen J: Testicular fine needle aspiration cytology as a diagnostic tool on dog infertility, *J Small Anim Pract* 38:506-512, 1997.

Dahlgren SS, Gjerde B, Pettersen HY: First record of natural *Tritrichomonas foetus* infection of the feline uterus, *J Small Anim Pract* 48:654-657, 2007.

de las Mulas JM, Millán Y, Dios R: A prospective analysis of immunohistochemically determined estrogen receptor alpha and progesterone receptor expression and host and tumor factors as predictors of disease-free period in mammary tumors of the dog, *Vet Pathol* 42:200-212, 2005.

de Lorimier LP, Fan TM: Canine transmissible venereal tumor. In Withrow SJ, Vail DM (eds): *Withrow & MacEwen's small animal clinical oncology*, St. Louis, 2007, Saunders, pp 799-804.

Diniz SA, Melo MS, Borges AM, et al: Genital lesions associated with visceral leishmaniasis and shedding of *Leishmania* sp. in the semen of naturally infected dogs, *Vet Pathol* 42: 650-658, 2005.

Dorfman M, Barsanti J: Diseases of the canine prostate gland, *Comp Cont Ed Pract* 17:791-810, 1995.

England GC, Freeman SL, Russo M: Treatment of spontaneous pyometra in 22 bitches with a combination of cabergoline and cloprostenol, *Vet Rec* 160:293-296, 2007.

Fan TM, de Lorimier LP: Tumors of the male reproductive system. In Withrow SJ, Vail DM (eds): *Withrow & MacEwen's small animal clinical oncology*, St. Louis, 2007, Saunders, pp 637-648.

Feldman EC, Nelson RW: Ovarian cycle and vaginal cytology. In Feldman EC, Nelson RW (eds): *Canine andfeline endocrinology and reproduction*, St. Louis, 2004, Saunders, pp 752-775.

Fernandes PJ, Guyer C, Modiano JF: What is your diagnosis? Mammary mass aspirate from a Yorkshire terrier, *Vet Clin Pathol* 27:79, 91, 1998.

Ferreira da Silva J: Teratoma in a feline unilateral cryptochid testis, *Vet Pathol* 39:516, 2002.

Freshman JL: Clinical approach to infertility in the cycling bitch, *Vet Clin North Am Small Anim Pract* 21:427-435, 1991.

Freshman JL: Semen collection and evaluation, *Clin Tech Small Anim Pract* 17:104-107, 2002.

Foster RA: Female reproductive system. In McGavin MD, Zachary JF (eds): *Pathologic basis of veterinary disease*, St Louis, 2007, Mosby, pp 1263-1315.

Gerber D, Nöthling JO: Hysteroscopy in bitches, *J Reprod Fertil* 57:415-417, Suppl, 2001.

Gobello C, Castex G, Corrada Y: Serum and seminal markers in the diagnosis of disorders of the genital tract of the dog: a mini-review, *Theriogenology* 57:1285-1291, 2002.

Görlinger S, Kooistra HS, van den Broek, et al: Treatment of fibroadenomatous hyperplasia in cats with aglépristone, *J Vet Intern Med* 16:710-713, 2002.

Gruffydd-Jones TJ: Acute mastitis in a cat, *Feline Pract* 10:41-42, 1980.

Hagman R, Kühn I: *Escherichia coli* strains isolated from the uterus and urinary bladder of bitches suffering from pyometra: comparison by restriction enzyme digestion and pulsed-field gel electrophoresis, *Vet Microbiol* 84:143-153, 2002.

Hayden DW, Barnes DM, Johnson KH: Morphologic changes in the mammary gland of megestrol acetate-treated and untreated cats: a retrospective study, *Vet Pathol* 26:104-113, 1989.

Hayden DW, Klausner JS, Waters DJ: Prostatic leiomyosarcoma in a dog, *J Vet Diagn Invest* 11:283-286, 1999.

Hayes AA, Mooney S: Feline mammary tumors, *Vet Clin North Am Small Anim Pract* 15:513-520, 1985.

Hayes HM, Milne KL, Mandell CP: Epidemiological features of feline mammary carcinoma, *Vet Rec* 108:476-479, 1981.

Hellman E, Lindgren A: The accuracy of cytology in diagnosis and DNA analysis of canine mammary tumors, *J Comp Pathol* 101:443-450, 1989.

Hori Y, Uechi M, Kanakubo K, et al: Canine ovarian serous papillary adenocarcinoma with neoplastic hypercalcemia, *J Vet Med Sci* 68:979-982, 2006.

Itoh T, Uchida K, Ishikawa K, et al: Clinicopathological survey of 101 canine mammary gland tumors: differences between small-breed dogs and others, *J Vet Med Sci* 67:345-347, 2005.

Johnston SD, Kamolpatana K, Root Kustritz MV, et al: Prostatic disorders in the dog, *Anim Reprod Sci* 60-61:405-415, 2000.

Kamstock DA, Fredrickson R, Ehrhart EJ: Lipid-rich carcinoma of the mammary gland in a cat, *Vet Pathol* 42:360-362, 2005.

Karayannopoulo M, Kaldrymidou E, Constantinidis TC: Adjuvant post-operative chemotherapy in bitches with mammary cancer, *J Vet Med* 48:85-96, Series A 2001.

Klein MK: Tumors of the female reproductive system. In Withrow SJ, Vail DM (eds): *Withrow & MacEwen's small animal clinical oncology*, St. Louis, 2007, Saunders, pp 610-618.

Kustritz MV, Johnston SD, Olson PN, et al: Relationship between inflammatory cytology of canine seminal fluid and significant aerobic bacterial, anaerobic bacterial or mycoplasma cultures of canine seminal fluid: 95 cases (1987-2000), *Theriogenology* 64:1333-1339, 2005.

L'Abee-Lund TM, Heiene R, Friis NF, et al: *Mycoplasma canis* and urogenital disease in dogs in Norway, *Vet Rec* 153:231-235, 2003.

Ladds PW: The male genital system: the testes. In Jubb KVF, Kennedy PC, Palmer N (eds): *Pathology of domestic animals*, ed 4, San Diego, 1993, Academic Press, pp 485-512.

Lana SE, Rutteman GR, Withrow SJ: Tumors of the mammary gland. In Withrow SJ, Vail DM (eds): *Withrow & MacEwen's small animal clinical oncology*, St. Louis, 2007, Saunders, pp 619-636.

L'Eplattenier HF, Lai CL, van den Ham R, et al: Regulation of COX-2 expression in canine prostate carcinoma: increased COX-2 expression is not related to inflammation, *J Vet Intern Med* 21:776-782, 2007.

Loretti AP, Ilha MR, Ordas J, et al: Clinical, pathological and immunohistochemical study of feline mammary fibroepithelial hyperplasia following a single injection of depot medroxyprogesterone acetate, *J Feline Med Surg* 7:43-52, 2005.

Lowseth LA, Gerlach RF, Gillett NA, et al: Age-related changes in the prostate and testes of the beagle dog, *Vet Pathol* 27:347-353, 1990.

Lulich JP: Endoscopic vaginoscopy in the dog, *Theriogenology* 66:588-591, 2006.

MacEwen EG, Hayes AA, Harvey J, et al: Prognostic factors for feline mammary tumors, *J Am Vet Med Assoc* 185:201-204, 1984.

MacLachlan NJ, Kennedy PC: Tumors of the genital systems. In Meuten DJ (ed): *Tumors in domestic animals*, ed 4, Ames, 2002, Iowa State Press, pp 547-573.

Manuali E, Eleni C, Giovannini P, et al: Unusual finding in a nipple discharge of a female dog: dirofilariasis of the breast, *Diagn Cytopathol* 32:108-109, 2005.

Masserdotti C: Architectural patterns in cytology: correlation with histology, *Vet Clin Pathol* 35:388-396, 2006.

Masserdotti C, Bonfanti U, De Lorenzi D, et al: Cytologic features of testicular tumours in dog, *J Vet Med A Physiol Pathol Clin Med* 52:339-346, 2005.

McEntee MC: Reproductive oncology, *Clin Tech Small Anim Pract* 17:133-149, 2002.

Mesher CI: What is your diagnosis? A 14-month old domestic cat, *Vet Clin Pathol* 26:4, 1997.

Millanta F, Calandrella M, Bari G, et al: Comparison of steroid receptor expression in normal, dysplastic, and neoplastic canine and feline mammary tissues, *Res Vet Sci* 79:225-232, 2005.

Millanta F, Citi S, Della Santa D, et al: COX-2 expression in canine and feline invasive mammary carcinomas: correlation with clinicopathological features and prognostic molecular markers, *Breast Cancer Res Treat* 98:115-120, 2006a.

Millanta F, Silvestri G, Vaselli C, et al: The role of vascular endothelial growth factor and its receptor Flk-1/KDR in promoting tumour angiogenesis in feline and canine mammary carcinomas: a preliminary study of autocrine and paracrine loops, *Res Vet Sci* 81:350-357, 2006b.

Miller MA, Hartnett SE, Ramos-Vara JA: Interstitial cell tumor and Sertoli cell tumor in the testis of a cat, *Vet Pathol* 44:394-397, 2007.

Miller MA, Ramos-Vara JA, Dickerson MF, et al: Uterine neoplasia in 13 cats, *J Vet Diagn Invest* 15:515-522, 2003.

Mills JM, Valli VE, Lumsden JH: Cyclical changes of vaginal cytology in the cat, *Can Vet J* 20:95-101, 1979.

Mischke R, Meurer D, Hoppen HO: Blood plasma concentrations of oestradiol-17beta, testosterone and testosterone/oestradiol ratio in dogs with neoplastic and degenerative testicular diseases, *Res Vet Sci* 73:267-272, 2002.

Misdorp W: Progestagens and mammary tumours in dogs and cats, *Acta Endocrinol* (Copenh) 125:27-31, 1991.

Misdorp W: Tumors of the mammary gland. In Meuten DJ (ed): *Tumors in domestic animals*, ed 4, Iowa State Press, 2002, Ames, pp 577-606.

Misdorp W, Else RW, Hellmén E, et al: Histological classification of mammary tumors of the dog and the cat. In *World Health Organization international histological classification of tumors of domestic animals*, Second Series, Vol VII, Armed Forces Institute of Pathology, American Registry of Pathology, Washington DC, 1999.

Murakami Y, Tateyama S, Uchida K: Immunohistochemical analysis of cyclins in canine normal testes and testicular tumors, *J Vet Med Sci* 63:909-912, 2001.

Novosad CA: Principles of treatment for mammary gland tumors, *Clin Tech Small Anim Prac* 18:107-109, 2003.

Novosad CA, Bergman PJ, O'Brien MG: Retrospective evaluation of adjunctive doxorubicin for the treatment of feline mammary gland adenocarcinoma: 67 cases, *J Am Anim Hosp Assoc* 42:110-120, 2006.

Ober CP, Spaulding K, Breitschwerdt EB, et al: Orchitis in two dogs with Rocky Mountain spotted fever, *Vet Radiol Ultrasound* 45:458-465, 2004.

Olson PN, Thrall MA, Wykes PM, et al: Vaginal cytology: Part I, A useful tool for staging the canine estrous cycle, *Compend Contin Educ Pract* 6:288-297, 1984a.

Olson PN, Thrall MA, Wykes PM, et al: Vaginal cytology: Part II, Its use in diagnosing canine reproductive disorders, *Compend Contin Educ Pract* 6:385-390, 1984b.

Olson PN, Wrigley RH, Thrall MA, et al: Disorders of the canine prostate gland: pathogenesis, diagnosis, and medical therapy, *Compend Contin Educ Pract* 9:613-623, 1987.

Park CH, Ikadai H, Yoshida E, et al: Cutaneous toxoplasmosis in a female Japanese cat, *Vet Pathol* 44:683-687, 2007.

Perez CC, Rodriguez I, Dorado J, et al: Use of ultrafast Papanicolaou stain for exfoliative vaginal cytology in bitches, *Vet Rec* 156:648-650, 2005.

Pérez-Alenza MD, Jiménez A, Nieto AI, et al: First description of feline inflammatory mammary carcinoma: clinicopathological and immunohistochemical characteristics of three cases, *Breast Cancer Res* 6:300-307, 2004.

Peters MA, Mol JA, van Wolferen ME: Expression of the insulin-like growth factor (IGF) system and steroidogenic enzymes in canine testis tumors, *Reprod Biol Endocrinol* 1:22-29, 2003.

Powe JR, Canfield PJ, Martin PA: Evaluation of the cytologic diagnosis of canine prostatic disorders, *Vet Clin Pathol* 33:150-154, 2004.

Rehm S, Stanislaus DJ, Williams AM: Estrous cycle-dependent histology and review of sex steroid receptor expression in dog reproductive tissues and mammary gland and associated hormone levels, *Birth Defects Res B Dev Reprod Toxicol* 80:233-245, 2007.

Restucci B, Maiolino P, Martano M, et al: Expression of beta-catenin, E-cadherin and APC in canine mammary tumors, *Anticancer Res* 27:3083-3089, 2007.

Restucci B, Maiolino P, Paciello O: Evaluation of angiogenesis in canine seminomas by quantitative immunohistochemistry, *J Comp Pathol* 128:252-259, 2003.

Riccardi E, Greco V, Verganti S, et al: Immunohistochemical diagnosis of canine ovarian epithelial and granulosa cell tumors, *J Vet Diagn Invest* 19:431-435, 2007.

Rijsselaere T, Van Soom A, Tanghe S, et al: New techniques for the assessment of canine semen quality: a review, *Theriogenology* 64:706-719, 2005.

Romanucci M, Marinelli A, Sarli G et al: Heat shock protein expression in canine malignant mammary tumours, *BMC Cancer* 6:171, 2006.

Root Kustritz MV: Collection of tissue and culture samples from the canine reproductive tract, *Theriogenology* 66:567-574, 2006.

Root Kustritz MV: The value of canine semen evaluation for practitioners, *Theriogenology* 68:329-337, 2007.

Saba CF, Rogers KS, Newman SJ, et al: Mammary gland tumors in male dogs, *J Vet Intern Med* 21:1056-1059, 2007.

Schafer-Somi S, Spergser J, Breitenfellner J, et al: Bacteriological status of canine milk and septicaemia in neonatal puppies—a retrospective study, *J Vet Med B Infect Dis Vet Public Health* 50:343-346, 2003.

Schubach TM, de Oliveira Schubach A, dos Reis RS, et al: *Sporothrix schenckii* isolated from domestic cats with and without sporotrichosis in Rio de Janeiro, Brazil, *Mycopathologia* 153:83-86, 2002.

Shille VM, Lundstrom KE, Stabenfeldt GH: Follicular function in the domestic cat as determined by estradiol-17ß concentrations in plasma: relation to estrous behavior and cornification of exfoliated vaginal epithelium, *Biol Reprod* 21:953-963, 1979.

Sigurdardottir OG, Kolbjornsen O, Lutz H: Orchitis in a cat associated with coronavirus infection, *J Comp Pathol* 124:219-222, 2001.

Simeonov R, Simeonova G: Computerized morphometry of mean nuclear diameter and nuclear roundness in canine mammary gland tumors on cytologic smears, *Vet Clin Path* 35:88-90, 2006a.

Simeonov R, Simeonova G: Fractal dimension of canine mammary gland epithelial tumors on cytologic smears, *Vet Clin Path* 35:446-448, 2006b.

Simon D, Schoenrock D, Baumgartner W, et al: Postoperative adjuvant treatment of invasive malignant mammary gland tumors in dogs with doxorubicin and docetaxel, *J Vet Intern Med* 20:1184-1190, 2006.

Sirinarumitr K, Johnston SD, Kustritz MV, et al: Effects of finasteride on size of the prostate gland and semen quality in dogs with benign prostatic hypertrophy, *J Am Vet Med Assoc* 218:1275-1280, 2001.

Smith FO: Canine pyometra, *Theriogenology* 66:610-612, 2006.

Sorenmo K: Canine mammary gland tumors, *Vet Clin Small Anim* 33:573-596, 2003.

Sorenmo KU, Goldschmidt MH, Shofer SF: Evaluation of cyclooxygenase-1 and cyclooxygenase-2 expression and the effect of cyclooxygenase inhibitors in canine prostatic carcinoma, *Vet Comp Oncol* 2:13-23, 2004.

Sorenmo KU, Shofer FS, Goldschmidt MH: Effect of spaying and timing of spaying on survival of dogs with mammary carcinoma, *J Vet Intern Med* 14:266-270, 2000.

Taniyama H, Hirayama K, Nakada K: Immunohistochemical detection of inhibin-a, -ßB, and -ßA chains and 3ß-hydroxysteroid dehydrogenase in canine testicular tumors and normal testes, *Vet Pathol* 38:661-666, 2001.

Teske E, Naan EC, van Dijk EM, et al: Canine prostate carcinoma: epidemiological evidence of an increased risk in castrated dogs, *Mol Cell Endocrinol* 197:251-255, 2002.

Thrall MA, Olson PN: The vagina. In Cowell RL, Tyler RD, Meinkoth JM (eds): *Diagnostic cytology and hematology of the dog and cat*, ed 2, St. Louis, 1998, Mosby, pp 240-248.

Thrall MA, Olson PN, Freemyer EG: Cytologic diagnosis of canine prostatic disease, *J Am Anim Hosp Assoc* 21:95-102, 1985.

Torres LN, Matera JM, Vasconcellos CH, et al: Expression of connexins 26 and 43 in canine hyperplastic and neoplastic mammary glands, *Vet Pathol* 42:633-641, 2005.

van Garderen E, Schalken JA: Morphogenic and tumorigenic potentials of the mammary growth hormone/growth hormone receptor system, *Mol Cell Endocrinol* 29; 197:153-165, 2002.

Van Israel N, Kirby BM, Munro EA: Septic peritonitis secondary to unilateral pyometra and ovarian bursal abscessation in a dog, *J Small Anim Pract* 43:452-455, 2002.

Ververidis HN, Mavrogianni VS, Fragkou IA, et al: Experimental staphylococcal mastitis in bitches: Clinical, bacteriological, cytological, haematological and pathological features, *Vet Microbiol* 124:95-106, 2007.

Wanke MM: Canine brucellosis, *Anim Reprod Sci* 82-83:195-207, 2004.

Watts JR, Wright PJ, Lee CS: Endometrial cytology of the normal bitch throughout the reproductive cycle, *J Small Anim Pract* 39:2-9, 1998.

Watts JR, Wright PJ, Lee CS, et al: New techniques using transcervical uterine cannulation for the diagnosis of uterine disorders in bitches, *J Reprod Fertil* 51:283-293, Suppl 1997.

Winter MD, Locke JE, Penninck DG: Imaging diagnosis-urinary obstruction secondary to prostatic lymphoma in a young dog, *Vet Radiol Ultrasound* 47:597-601, 2006.

Wright PJ: Application of vaginal cytology and plasma progesterone determinations to the management of reproduction in the bitch, *J Small Anim Pract* 31:335-340, 1990.

Yager JA, Scott DW, Wilcock BP: The skin and appendages: neoplastic disease of skin and mammary gland. In Jubb KVF, Kennedy PC, Palmer N (eds): *Pathology of domestic animals*, ed 4, San Diego, 1993, Academic Press, pp 706-737.

Zambelli D, Cunto M: Semen collection in cats: techniques and analysis, *Theriogenology* 66:159-165, 2006.

Zanghì A, Nicòtina PA, Catone G: Cholesterol granuloma (Xanthomatous metritis) in the uterus of a cat, *J Comp Pathol* 121:307-310, 1999.

Zinkl JG: The male reproductive tract: prostate, testes, and semen. In Cowell RL, Tyler RD, Meinkoth JM, DeNicola DB (eds): *Diagnostic cytology and hematology of the dog and cat*, ed 3, St. Louis, 2008, Mosby, pp 369-377.

Zuccari DA, Santana AE, Cury PM, et al: Immunocytochemical study of Ki-67 as a prognostic marker in canine mammary neoplasia, *Vet Clin Pathol* 33:23-28, 2004.

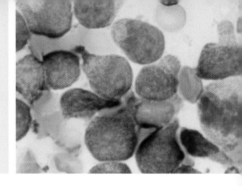

CHAPTER 13

Musculoskeletal System

Anne M. Barger

Lameness is the cardinal clinical sign associated with disease of the musculoskeletal system. Other signs include stiffness, ataxia, weakness, pain, fever, limb and joint swelling, and deformity. Depending on the type of disorder, other organ systems may also be involved, including neurologic, endocrine, urologic, hemolymphatic, digestive, respiratory, and cardiovascular systems. Because of this, an animal with musculoskeletal disease may present with a variety of problems and signs.

Cytology may be a component of the workup in an animal with a suspected musculoskeletal disorder. Material that may be sampled include synovial fluid as well as fine-needle aspirates of soft tissue masses involving muscle or proliferative/lytic lesions of the bone. Cytologic evaluation alone is rarely the sole diagnostic test necessary to completely define a musculoskeletal problem. Other important information includes signalment, history, physical examination, radiographs, complete blood count, and biochemistry. In addition, many lesions will require histopathology for definitive characterization. Some types of muscle, bone, and joint disease cause changes that cannot be detected by cytologic methods.

SYNOVIAL FLUID EVALUATION

Synovial fluid analysis is part of the minimum database when assessing an animal for joint disease. It is important to recognize that evaluation of the synovial fluid is only a component of the workup of an animal with suspected joint disease. The data obtained from joint fluid analysis must be integrated with other clinical and laboratory findings, including appropriate ancillary diagnostic tests (e.g., culture, serology, antinuclear antibody [ANA] titer, rheumatoid factor [RF] titer). Nevertheless, when an animal has suspected joint disease, fluid evaluation is a critical component in determining the cause of disease.

As with other body cavity effusions, a complete fluid analysis is helpful when evaluating a synovial effusion. Routine synovial fluid analysis should include evaluation of color, transparency, protein concentration, viscosity, mucin clot test, nucleated cell count, differential, and cytologic evaluation. These tests are discussed in further detail below. If the sample is limited, the most important component of analysis is the cytology. Typical results for different kinds of joint disease are shown in Table 13-1.

Sample Collection and Handling

Collection of synovial fluid varies to some degree depending on the joint sampled. Descriptions of approaches to various joints have been described. In general, collection of synovial fluid requires the following materials: 3- to 6-mL syringe, 18- to 22-gauge 1-inch needles, and red-top and/or lavender-top tubes. The amount of restraint and necessary levels of sedation and anesthesia will vary from animal to animal. Enough restraint should be used to minimize struggling during collection. In general, many animals will require at least some degree of sedation or anesthesia. Sterile technique is critical when preparing the site and during aspiration. The fur should be clipped and the area of aspiration scrubbed. Care should be taken not to scratch the articular surface during needle insertion. Palpation and slight flexion or hyperextension of the joint will help to identify insertion points of the needle. Aspiration sites for specific joints are described below. The location of aspiration varies with the joint aspirated. The coxofemoral joint can be aspirated cranioproximal to the trochanter major and slightly ventral and caudal. The stifle should be flexed when aspirated. Aspiration can occur medial or lateral to the patellar ligament, midway between the tibia and femur. The tarsocrural joint can be aspirated by hyperextending the joint and inserting the needle lateral or medial to the fibular tarsal bone. To aspirate the shoulder, insert the needle 1 cm distal and slightly caudal to the acromion process. The elbow should be hyperextended and the needle inserted lateral and along side the olecranon. The carpal joints can be simply aspirated by flexing the joint and palpating the joint space. The needle should be advanced slowly through the joint capsule into the joint cavity. The amount of fluid withdrawn depends on the size of animal and joint as well as the amount of

TABLE 13-1   Classification of Synovial Fluid

	Normal	Hemarthrosis	Degenerative Arthropathy	Inflammatory Arthropathy
Appearance	Clear to straw colored	Red, cloudy, or xanthochromic	Clear	Cloudy
Protein	<2.5 g/dl	Increased	Normal to decreased	Normal to increased
Viscosity	High	Decreased	Normal to decreased	Normal to decreased
Mucin clot	Good	Normal to poor	Normal to poor	Fair to poor
Cell count (/μl)	<3000 (dogs) <1000 (cats)	Increased RBCs	1000 to 10,000	5000 to >100,000
Neutrophils	<5%	Relative to blood	<10%	>10 to 100%
Mononuclear cells	>95%	Relative to blood	>90%	10 to <90%
Comments	Only a small amount should be present (<0.5 mL in most joints).	Erythrophagia helps confirm previous hemorrhage.	Synoviocytes are typically macrophages or synovial lining cells found in thick sheets.	Septic and nonseptic etiologies. Bacteria are rarely observed in infected joints.

effusion present. Synovial fluid will be aspirated easily if there is a significant effusion but a few drops may be obtained from joints without an increase in synovial fluid volume. Before removing the needle from the synovial cavity, the plunger of the syringe should be released to remove any negative pressure. Normal synovial fluid has a gel-like consistency that should not be mistaken for a clot. The gel-like consistency will become less viscous when shaken and return to the original viscosity upon standing; this property is referred to as *thixotropy.* Clotting is likely to occur if there is significant blood contamination and inflamed joints may form fibrin precipitates or clots. For these reasons, some joint fluid should be put into an EDTA tube (lavender-top tube). The EDTA will interfere with tests such as the mucin clot test and culturing. The synovial fluid should be refrigerated if not immediately evaluated. For samples that may be cultured dependent on the cytologic findings, the fluid should be put into a red-top tube, left in the sterile syringe, and/or placed in an aerobic culturette. There are advocates of putting fluid in blood culture media to improve the chances for bacterial growth. The laboratory should be contacted for their recommendations. In many smaller animals, only one or two drops of joint fluid can be obtained. In these cases, immediate preparation of direct smears is the critical component of sample management (refer to Chapter 1). Regardless of the amount of fluid collected, it usually is advantageous to make direct smears immediately to best preserve cell morphology. These slides should not be refrigerated before staining.

Appearance and Viscosity

Normal joint fluid is typically present in small amounts (<0.5 mL) and is clear to straw-colored (Fig. 13-1A). Red-tinged fluid indicates hemorrhage or peripheral blood contamination. True hemorrhage will be uniformly discolored throughout aspiration, whereas peripheral blood contamination often occurs at the end of aspiration. This may appear as a red tail or wisp in the fluid. The fluid should be viscous as evident by stringiness when

suspended between fingertips, touched by an applicator stick, or expelled from the syringe (see Fig. 13-1A). The fluid viscosity is related to the concentration and quality of hyaluronic acid. Normal synovial fluid has good viscosity and demonstrates thixotropy (see above).

Healthy synovial fluid should be viscous due to production of mucin. The mucin clot test is done to semi-quantitatively assess the amount and/or degree of polymerization of hyaluronic acid in the joint fluid. Since EDTA interferes with this test, heparin can be used if an anticoagulant is required before performing this test. One to two drops of undiluted joint fluid are added to four to eight drops of 2% acetic acid. In a sample with normal hyaluronic acid concentration and quality, a thick, ropy clot will form (Fig. 13-1B). As the amount and/or quality of hyaluronic acid decreases in various forms of joint disease, the mucin clot is less well formed. This test is typically interpreted as good, fair, or poor. Normal joints have good mucin clot results.

The direct smear of the synovial fluid should also be evaluated for presence of windrowing. In a viscous sample, the cells will often line up in rows or windrow (Fig. 13-2A). Mucinous material can be identified in the background of the direct smears as eosinophilic granular material (Fig. 13-2B&C) or sometimes as proteinaceous crescents.

Cell Counts and Differential

Cell counts and the differential count are done by routine methods. If enough fluid is present, cell counts can be made using a hemocytometer. Some reference laboratories use automated cell counters for cell enumeration. Automated cell counters tend to give a higher cell count than the hemocytometer; however, the difference is not usually great enough to affect the clinical interpretation. The cells may occur in clumps and accurate assessment of cell numbers may be difficult. In an effort to minimize cell clumping, hyaluronidase can be added to the synovial fluid. Various methods have been described. The easiest procedure is to add a small amount of hyaluronidase

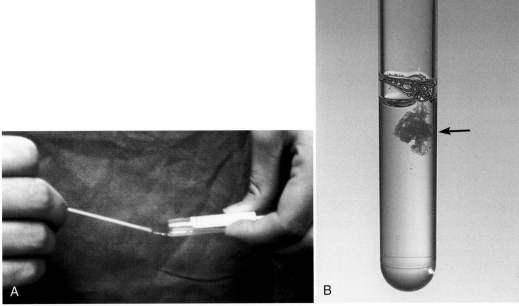

■ **FIGURE 13-1. A, Viscosity test.** A string of viscous material from normal synovial fluid should measure about 2 cm in length when touched with an applicator stick before it snaps apart. **B, Mucin clot test.** This sample is from a normal joint. The mucin clot is thick and ropy indicative of good mucin content and quality *(arrow)*. (A, Courtesy of Rose Raskin, Purdue University. B, Courtesy of Dr. Sonjia Shelly.)

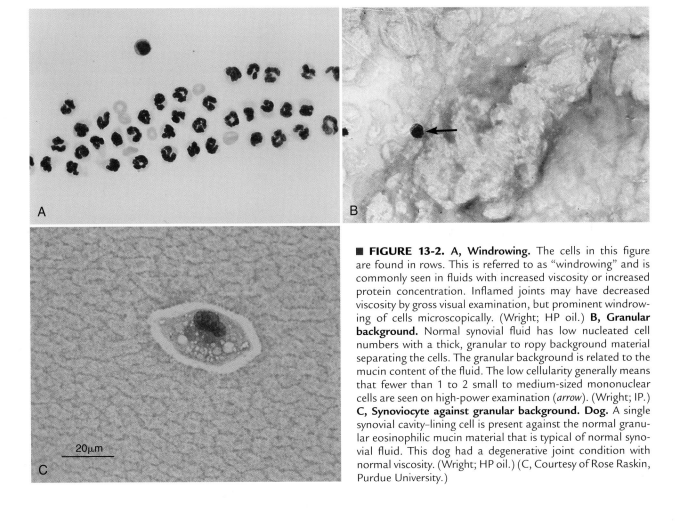

■ **FIGURE 13-2. A, Windrowing.** The cells in this figure are found in rows. This is referred to as "windrowing" and is commonly seen in fluids with increased viscosity or increased protein concentration. Inflamed joints may have decreased viscosity by gross visual examination, but prominent windrowing of cells microscopically. (Wright; HP oil.) **B, Granular background.** Normal synovial fluid has low nucleated cell numbers with a thick, granular to ropy background material separating the cells. The granular background is related to the mucin content of the fluid. The low cellularity generally means that fewer than 1 to 2 small to medium-sized mononuclear cells are seen on high-power examination *(arrow)*. (Wright; IP.) **C, Synoviocyte against granular background. Dog.** A single synovial cavity–lining cell is present against the normal granular eosinophilic mucin material that is typical of normal synovial fluid. This dog had a degenerative joint condition with normal viscosity. (Wright; HP oil.) (C, Courtesy of Rose Raskin, Purdue University.)

powder (amount adherent to an applicator stick) directly into the sample tube, which may result in more accurate cell counts. If only slides are prepared, cell numbers can be roughly estimated by counting the number of cells per low-power field (10×) and multiplying the count by 100 to give an approximate number per µl. However estimates from smears are less accurate and tend to be higher than counts from automated counters. Normal joints will have low nucleated cell numbers, usually fewer than 3000 cells/µl in the dog and 1000 cells/µl in the cat (Pacchiana et al., 2004), although more typically the count is fewer than 500 cells/µl in both species. These counts may vary slightly based on breed, age, body weight, and joint sampled. Consequently, only 1 to 2 cells per high-power field (40×) will be observed depending on the thickness of the direct smear (see Fig. 13-2B). Gibson et al. (1999) demonstrated the variability in performing these estimates by a group of clinicians on synovial fluid. Cells commonly observed in synovial fluid include lymphocytes, macrophages (clasmatocytes), neutrophils, and, occasionally, synovial lining cells that produce glycosaminoglycans. Neutrophils typically account for less than 5% to 10% of nucleated cells in normal joints. If fluid is obtained, both direct smears and concentrated preparations can be evaluated. If available, a cytocentrifuge is useful in preparing concentrated preparations. Concentrated preparations can also be prepared by centrifuging the fluid, pouring of the supernatant, and resuspending the fluid in one or two drops of supernatant. Smears can then be prepared from this concentrated preparation. Concentrated preparations are useful in synovial fluid particularly if the cell count is low (<500 cells/µl).

Protein Concentration

Protein concentration is often measured by refractometry, which usually provides a value that is useful for routine clinical classification and interpretation of the synovial fluid. The most accurate measurement of protein requires chemical methods. Normal synovial fluid generally has a low protein concentration (<2.5 g/dl) or commonly between 1.5 to 3.0 g/dl (MacWilliams and Friedrichs, 2003). Protein concentration will increase with inflammatory disease. False increases in protein can occur with EDTA, especially if a short sample is submitted or if the patient has received an intra-articular injection.

Classification of Joint Disease

The primary goal in synovial fluid evaluation is to distinguish inflammatory joint disease from degenerative joint disease (see Table 13-1). Other types of joint disease that may be distinguished include hemarthrosis and neoplastic disease. Further defining the disease process, as noted above, requires integrating the synovial fluid findings with other historical, physical, and laboratory findings including imaging techniques. It is important to note that synovial fluid analysis alone rarely differentiates or identifies the specific cause from among the multiple etiologic factors involved in inflammatory and noninflammatory joint diseases.

Inflammatory Joint Disease

Inflammatory joint disease is characterized by finding increased numbers of white blood cells, particularly neutrophils (Fig. 13-3), in the joint fluid. Absolute numbers of segmented neutrophils are often moderately to markedly increased. However, the inflammatory process appears to cytologically wax and wane with time and, if polyarticular, involve other joints with varying intensity. Consequently, repeating joint sampling and, more importantly, sampling multiple joints, even if not clinically affected, has diagnostic value. A key point is that inflammatory joint disease has both infectious and noninfectious causes.

Infectious Arthritis

Some cases of joint disease are caused by bacterial (Fig. 13-4) or fungal infection (Fig. 13-5). In general, septic joints have very high cell counts. In most cases, the cells are primarily segmented neutrophils. It is important to evaluate the condition of the neutrophils. Degenerative or karyolytic neutrophils are more commonly observed with septic joints. Degenerate neutrophils have a pale, swollen nucleus with some loss of nuclear segmentation. However, often the majority of the neutrophils will appear nondegenerative in septic arthritis. In one study, *Staphylococcus* sp. was the most common bacterial agent isolated in septic joints (Marchevsky and Read, 1999). Organisms may gain access to joints either hematogenously or via direct inoculation. In addition, there may be infection elsewhere in the body (e.g., endocarditis) with immune complex deposition in the synovial tissue and resultant nonseptic inflammation in the fluid. Bacterial and fungal arthritis most commonly present with solitary joint involvement but on occasion may have multiple joint involvement, especially in young animals. Because infectious and noninfectious arthritis can have a similar presentation, it may be advisable to

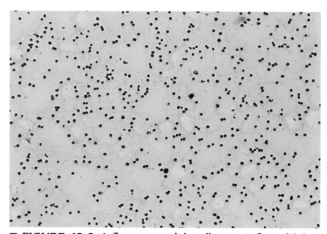

■ **FIGURE 13-3. Inflammatory joint disease.** Inflamed joints have an absolute increase in the numbers of neutrophils and often exceed 50,000/µl, as in this specimen. The total cell number occasionally may be within normal limits (i.e., <3000/µl dogs) in a septic joint but the neutrophil number will represent more than 70% of the total cell number emphasizing the need for microscopic examination. (Wright; IP.)

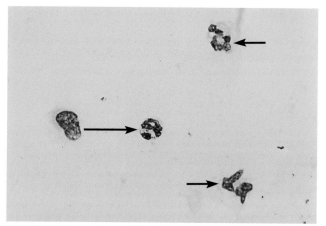

■ FIGURE 13-4. Bacterial arthritis. Bacterial arthritis may be caused by direct inoculation or hematogenous spread. Infected joints typically have high neutrophil counts (>50,000/μl). In this example, the neutrophils display degenerative changes, including nuclear swelling *(short arrows),* and cytoplasmic vacuolization. The presence of degenerative changes strongly supports infection; however, the lack of degenerative changes or observable microorganisms does not rule out the possibility of infection. The bacteria may be located in the joint tissue and not present in the synovial fluid. Rare bacteria were observed after prolonged searching *(long arrow).* (Wright; HP oil.).

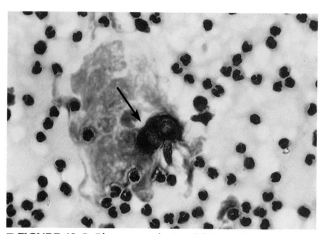

■ FIGURE 13-5. Blastomycosis. In addition to bacteria, other types of infectious agents may also involve the joint. This photomicrograph contains numerous neutrophils that are "rounded up" and almost appear like mononuclear cells owing to the thickness of the smear. In the center of the photo, broad-based budding yeast are found that are consistent with *Blastomyces dermatitidis (arrow).* Fungal organisms may be present infrequently and are best found on low-power examination. As with bacteria, the lack of observable organisms does not rule out infection. Fungal culture is advisable in suspected cases. (Wright; HP oil.).

culture inflamed joints, keeping in mind that a negative culture does not rule out infection as the microorganisms are sometimes limited to the synovial lining tissue. Other types of organisms that have been implicated as causative agents of joint disease include mycoplasma, bacterial L-forms, spirochetes *(Borrelia burgdorferi),* protozoa *(Leishmania donovani),* viruses (calicivirus,

coronavirus), and rickettsia/anaplasma such as *Erlichia canis, Erlichia ewingii* (Fig. 13-6A&B), *Anaplasma phagocytophilum,* formerly *Erlichia equi,* and *Rickettsia rickettsi* (Santos et al., 2006; Harvey and Raskin, 2004). In one study of *E. ewingii* joint infection cases in which the diagnosis was confirmed by polymerase chain reaction testing of peripheral blood, nucleated cell counts ranged from 16,000 to 125,000/μl with 63% to 95% neutrophils (Goodman et al., 2003).

Noninfectious Arthritis

Many animals with inflamed joints have nonerosive disease (Michels and Carr, 1997). Causes of nonerosive polyarthritis include inflammation secondary to infection or neoplasia elsewhere, breed-specific polyarthritis

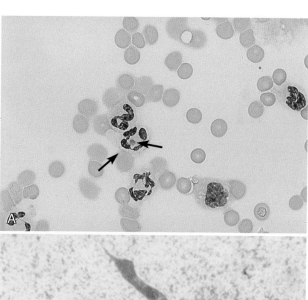

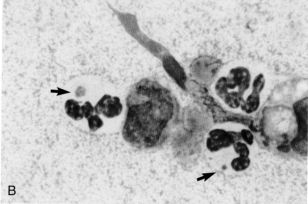

■ FIGURE 13-6. A, Granulocytic ehrlichiosis. Dog. The neutrophil in the center *(arrows)* contains an ehrlichial morula in the cytoplasm. Granulocytic ehrlichiosis may be caused by *A. phagocytophilum* or *E. ewingii.* These organisms may cause joint inflammation as well as a variety of other clinical signs and laboratory problems. It is unusual to find the organisms in clinical samples except for acute infections. Diagnosis is usually based on recognition of clinical signs with appropriate serologic testing. (Wright; HP oil.) **B, *Ehrlichia ewingii* joint infection. Dog.** Pictured are three neutrophils with intracytoplasmic morulae *(arrows).* This stifle synovial fluid had an estimated white cell count of >50,000/μl and a predominance mildly karyolytic neutrophils against an eosinophilic granular background. Diagnosis was confirmed by PCR testing to amplify genus-and species-specific products. (Wright; HP oil.) (B, Courtesy of Rose Raskin, Purdue University.)

(e.g., Beagle, Chinese Shar Pei), drug-induced disease, immune-mediated polyarthritis, and systemic lupus erythematosus. Although crystal-induced arthritis (e.g., gout or pseudogout) has been described in animals, it is infrequent in dogs and cats (deHaan and Andreasen, 1992; Forsyth et al., 2007) (Fig. 13-7A&B). As the name implies, polyarthritis typically affects multiple joints, but on occasion may present with only a solitary affected joint.

Joints affected by immune-mediated disease have increased numbers of nondegenerate neutrophils. In rare cases, increased numbers of lymphocytes and plasma cells may be found. Smaller distal joints are most commonly affected. Diagnosis of immune-mediated disease depends not only on demonstrating joint inflammation, but also on ruling out infection via culture, serology, and/or empiric therapy. Some cases of immune-mediated disease will have ragocytes (Fig. 13-8A–C) or (lupus erythematosus) LE cells (Fig. 13-8D). These are infrequent findings and should not be relied on to make a diagnosis of immune-mediated disease.

Erosive arthritis is suggested when there are lucent cystlike areas in the subchondral bone with narrowing or widening of the joint spaces found on joint radiographs. Types of erosive arthritis described in animals include rheumatoid arthritis, polyarthritis of Greyhounds, and feline chronic progressive polyarthritis (Carr and Michels, 1997). The classic finding is progressive loss of subchondral bone with deformation and destruction of affected joints. Infection or neoplasia may also cause erosive joint disease. Erosive arthritis, as with other types of inflammatory joint disease, is characterized by increased numbers of neutrophils in the synovial fluid. Synovial fluid analysis alone cannot distinguish erosive disease from nonerosive disease and, for this reason, radiographs should be done on animals with inflammatory

joint disease. Other clinical features of noninfectious erosive arthritis include morning stiffness, swelling of same or multiple joints within a 3-month period, symmetric swelling of joints, mononuclear infiltrates observed microscopically in a synovial membrane biopsy, and positive RF titer.

Degenerative Joint Disease

Degenerative joint disease (osteoarthritis, osteoarthropathy) is characterized by degeneration of articular cartilage with secondary changes in associated joint structures. The disorder usually occurs secondary to conditions such as osteochondrosis, hip dysplasia, joint instability, chronic bicipital tenosynovitis, and trauma. Changes in the synovial fluid are not as remarkable as seen with inflammatory disease (Fig. 13-9A&B). A mild increase in the number of mononuclear cells is the predominant finding (Stobie et al., 1995). These cells are likely a mixture of macrophages, lymphocytes, and synovial lining cells (Fig. 13-9C–E). Occasionally osteoclasts can be observed which may suggest erosion of cartilage and exposure of underlying subchondral bone (Fig. 13-10A&B).

Hemarthrosis

If recent trauma has occurred, joint hemorrhage may be appreciated (Fig. 13-11A&B). True hemorrhage must be distinguished from the much more common artifact of blood contamination. This is best done at the time of sample collection. If previous hemorrhage has occurred, the withdrawn fluid will appear xanthochromic (yellowish color due to old hemorrhage) to homogeneously red and cloudy. Besides trauma, other causes of hemorrhagic joint fluid include coagulation defects and neoplasia. A congenital coagulation factor deficiency should be considered in a puppy or kitten that presents with

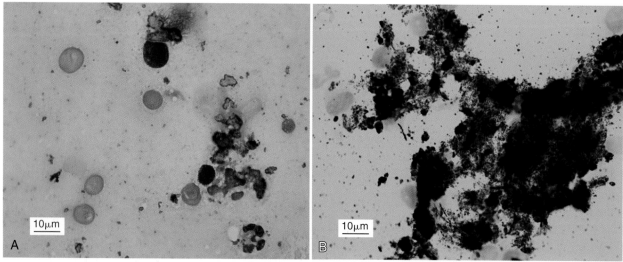

■ **FIGURE 13-7. Same case A-B. A, Mixed inflammation with mineral deposition. Dog.** Neutrophils, mononuclear cells, and several erythrocytes are present within a background containing coarse and fine irregular refractile yellow-green crystalline material. This animal had a history of histoplasmosis and current therapy for lymphoma. (Wright; HP oil.) **B, Calcium deposition. Dog.** Large collections are present of brown, positive-stained granules confirming calcium composition. Also noted are several inflammatory cells indicated by a nuclear counterstain that is associated with the mineral (Von Kossa; HP oil.) (A and B, Courtesy of Rose Raskin, Purdue University.)

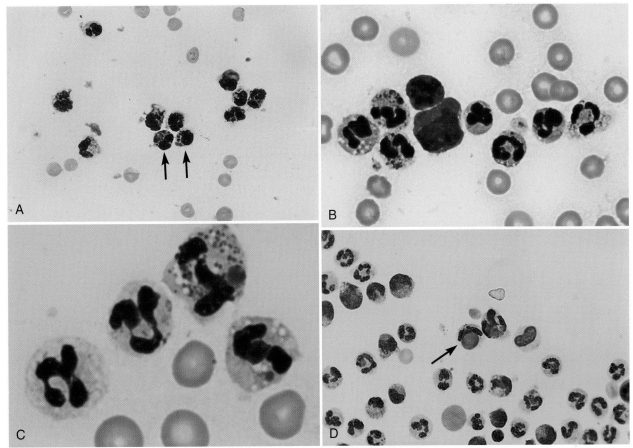

■ **FIGURE 13-8. Same case A-C, Ragocytes. Dog. A,** Ragocytes are neutrophils with multiple small, variably sized, purple cytoplasmic inclusions *(arrows)*. They are thought to represent nuclear remnants or phagocytosed immune complexes. They should be distinguished from bacteria. Observations suggest that these cells are seen more commonly in association with immune-mediated polyarthropathies but are not considered diagnostic. Serologic evaluation for immune-mediated disease and extra-articular nonbacterial infections such as ehrlichiosis and borreliosis is recommended when polyarthritis is identified. (Wright; HP oil) **B,** Neutrophils frequently contain several variably sized, dark, cytoplasmic granules in a case of immune-mediated polyarthropathy. Stifle fluid had WBC 7,400/µl, protein 3.6 g/dl, good mucin clot, 21% nondegenerate neutrophils, 45% small lymphocytes, 34% large mononuclear cells, positive ANA titer, and negative rickettsial titers. (Wright; HP oil.) **C,** Close-up of affected neutrophils containing fragments of nuclear material. (Wright; HP oil.) **D, Lupus erythematosus cell. Dog.** Synovial fluid from a dog with shifting leg lameness. The total cell number is moderately increased and composed of predominantly nondegenerate neutrophils with lesser numbers of lymphocytes and monocytes. The neutrophil in the center contains a large, round, homogeneous eosinophilic inclusion in the cytoplasm that displaces the nucleus to the periphery of the cell membrane *(arrow)*. This is an LE cell. The phagocytized material is thought to be nuclear material that has been structurally altered by antinuclear antibody. The homogeneous, light-staining appearance of the material distinguishes it from normal nuclear material. LE cells are rare, but when found, support the diagnosis of systemic lupus erythematosus. (Wright; HP oil.) (B and C, Courtesy of Rose Raskin, Purdue University. D, Courtesy of Linda L. Werner.)

repeated episodes of hemarthrosis or with hemarthrosis and a history of minimal trauma. Low numbers of red blood cells can be observed in normal synovial fluid but should not be present in high enough numbers to discolor the fluid. Cytologically, hemorrhage can be distinguished from peripheral blood contamination by identification of erythrophagia, hemosiderin-laden macrophages, and other red blood cell pigments such as hematoidin. Occasionally platelets will be observed in samples with severe peripheral blood contamination. Care must be taken not to overinterpret erythrophagia because this can occur *ex vivo* if the sample is not evaluated quickly.

Neoplasia

Normal synovium consists loose connective tissue containing blood vessels, fibroblasts, adipocytes, and histiocytes lined by a layer of synoviocytes. The synoviocytes involves three cell populations: macrophages, antigen-presenting dendritic cells, and glycosaminoglycans-producing cells. In a study of 35 dogs, the most common neoplasm of canine synovium (51%) was of histiocytic origin (Craig et al., 2002). Other neoplasms in this study were (17%) synovial myxomas, (14%) synovial sarcomas, and the remaining 17% were mixed sarcomas including malignant fibrous histiocytoma, fibrosarcoma, chondrosarcoma, and undifferentiated. Immunohistochemical

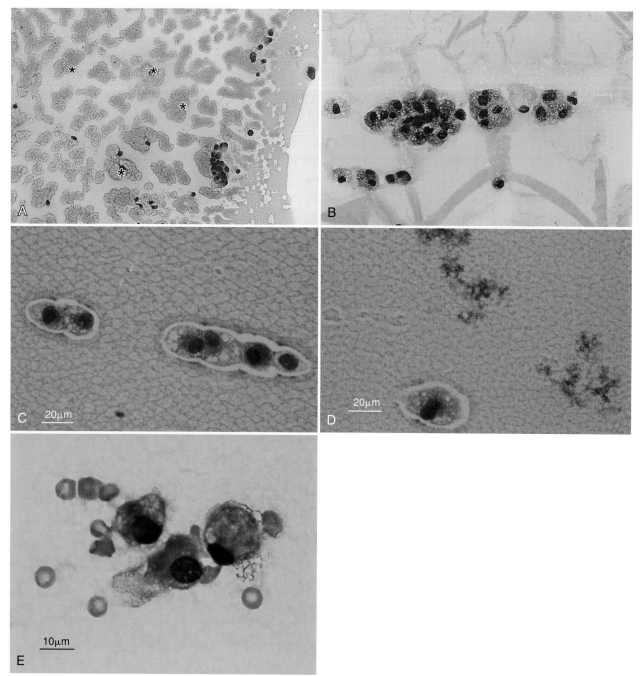

■ **FIGURE 13-9. A-B, Degenerative joint disease. A, Dog.** This sample is from the stifle joint of a large dog with chronic hind limb lameness. Cell numbers appear to be slightly increased although difficult to estimate because of clumping and thickness of the smear. The granular background that includes clumps of mucin *(asterisks)* is suggestive of good mucin content. The majority of the cells are mononuclear with some having a macrophage appearance consistent with a cytologic interpretation of degenerative joint disease. Further evaluation for underlying disease such as osteochondrosis or meniscal disease is warranted. (Wright; IP.) **B,** Joints with degenerative disease typically have increased numbers of macrophages (clasmatocytes) or secreting synoviocytes. The cells are usually large and vacuolated, and contain numerous pink-staining, cytoplasmic granules. Mucin content may remain good as is evident in this figure by the thick, pink background. (Wright; HP oil.) **Same case C-D. Chronic bicipital tenosynovitis. Dog. C,** Windrowing of large mononuclear cells is noted in this shoulder joint fluid specimen with chronic degenerative disease involving the biceps brachii tendon and synovial sheath. It is a common cause for forelimb lameness in adult dogs. (Wright; HP oil.) **D,** A single synoviocyte is shown against the granular background, which contains eosinophilic aggregates of mucin materials likely released from damaged articular surfaces. (Wright, HP oil) **E, Osteoarthritis. Dog.** Three individual large, mononuclear cells are shown from a direct smear of synovial fluid from a joint with a noninflammatory degenerative disease. These are consistent with synoviocytes with phagocytic function. (Wright; HP oil.) (C-E, Courtesy of Rose Raskin, Purdue University.)

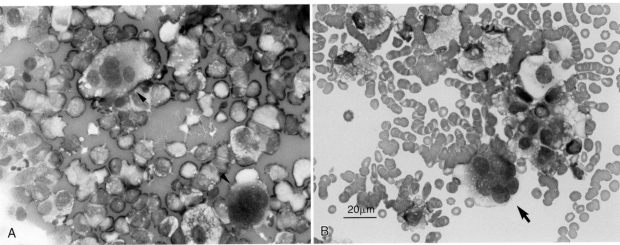

■ **FIGURE 13-10. Osteoclast. A,** In patients with degenerative joint disease or erosion of cartilage, osteoclasts can be observed *(arrows)*. (Wright; HP oil.) **B, Dog.** Same case as in Fig. 13-9E. The arrow indicates a multinucleated osteoclast among the numerous mononuclear cells and erythrocytes. (Wright; HP oil.) (B, Courtesy of Rose Raskin, Purdue University.)

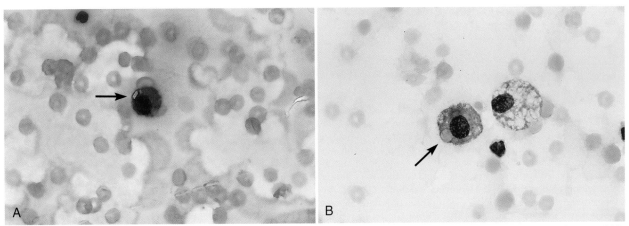

■ **FIGURE 13-11. Hemarthrosis.** Because of the small size of canine and feline joints, it is common to get some degree of blood contamination in most joint aspirates. To help distinguish true hemorrhage from blood contamination, the smears should be routinely examined for erythrophagia, hematoidin crystals, hemosiderin, and platelet clumps. In **(A)**, the macrophage contains a small, golden hematoidin crystal *(arrow)*, while the smaller of two macrophages in **(B)** contains a phagocytosed erythrocyte in the lower left area of its cytoplasm *(arrow)*. These findings indicate that there has been previous hemorrhage in the joint. Potential causes of hemarthrosis include trauma, coagulopathy, and neoplasia. Coagulopathies may have evidence of multiple joint involvement and bleeding elsewhere. Abnormal hemostasis is documented by coagulation testing. (Wright; HP oil.)

staining was necessary to distinguish between the histologic types of synovial tumors as prognosis varied greatly between them. A recommended panel of antibodies is suggested to include cytokeratin (AE1/AE3) for synovial cell sarcoma, CD18 for histiocytic sarcoma, and smooth muscle actin for malignant fibrous histiocytoma. Synovial cell sarcomas may appear most commonly as the spindle cell form (Fig. 13-12A) or alternatively as a mixed spindle and epithelioid variant. Histiocytic sarcomas arise from the antigen-presenting dendritic cells of the synovium layer. These neoplasms are frequently associated with Rottweilers, Bernese Mountain Dogs, and retrievers (Affolter and Moore, 2002). Cytologically, histiocytic sarcoma displays a round cell appearance with anaplastic characteristics including cellular pleomorphism, multinucleation, anisokaryosis, coarse chromatin, and prominent nucleoli with abundant basophilic cytoplasm (Fig. 13-12B&C). Another neoplasm occasionally encountered in the joint is a metastatic form of carcinoma. Cases with metastatic neoplastic cells in synovial fluid have been documented arising from the lung and mammary gland (Meinkoth et al., 1997).

MUSCULOSKELETAL DISORDERS

Aspiration of muscle, connective tissue, or bone lesions is much the same as aspiration of other lesions. Generally there is a mass, evidence of lysis, or swelling that warrants

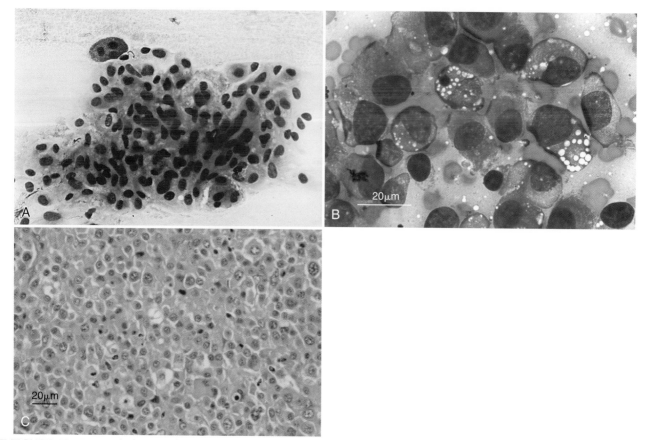

■ **FIGURE 13-12. Neoplasia. A, Synovial sarcoma.** Synovial fluid aspirated from a dog with lameness localized to a solitary joint. The sample is predominated by large sheets of pleomorphic spindle cells that are sometimes separated by a fine, pink, streaming stroma. The cells display moderate pleomorphism. This joint had an associated soft tissue mass that was ultimately diagnosed as synovial sarcoma. The cells in this photograph display some cytologic features of malignancy and may be neoplastic, but could potentially be reactive synovial cells. As with many mesenchymal tumors, it is difficult to definitely diagnose malignancy based solely on cytologic detail. (Wright; HP oil.) **Same case B-C. Histiocytic sarcoma. Dog. B,** An aspirate from a localized soft tissue mass that arose around the joint and infiltrated the muscle revealed a pleomorphic population of round cells. These cells display malignant features of anisokaryosis, variable nuclear-to-cytoplasmic ratio, coarse chromatin, and prominent nucleoli. The abundant basophilic cytoplasm suggests histiocytic origin, which was confirmed by immunohistochemistry. (Wright; HP oil.) **C,** Pleomorphic round cell neoplasm that was negative for CD3, CD79, and MUM1 (lymphoid) antigens and positive for CD45, CD18, E-cadherin (leukocyte, histiocytic, and dendritic cell antigens, respectively). (H&E; IP.) (B and C, Courtesy of Dr. Rose Raskin, Purdue University.)

aspiration. Fine-needle aspiration, fenestration, or impression smears of tissue taken for biopsy are common methods of obtaining a sample. Components of the musculoskeletal system that will be reviewed in this section of the chapter include skeletal muscle and bone.

Skeletal Muscle

Normal cytology of skeletal muscle has a characteristic appearance. Usually a tissue fragment is aspirated and the cytoplasm of the cells stains deeply basophilic (see Figure 2-1). Often, striations can be visualized by focusing up and down on the cell aggregate. The nuclei are round with a condensed chromatin pattern. Myositis is difficult to diagnose with cytology because it is difficult to associate the inflammatory cells with the myocytes (Fig. 13-13). Therefore, cytology is of limited use in

diagnosing myositis. Diagnosis of myositis typically requires consideration of history, signalment, and chemistry findings (increased creatine kinase and aspartate transaminase), as well as electromyographic (EMG), immunologic, and serologic tests. Histopathology is necessary as well for definitive characterization of inflammatory and degenerative muscle lesions.

Tumors arising from skeletal muscle include rhabdomyoma and rhabdomyosarcoma. These neoplasms are uncommon. Cytologically these tumors may appear similar to other mesenchymal tumors. Rhabdomyomas in particular often exfoliate poorly; however, rhabdomyosarcomas can be cellular enough to diagnose as a sarcoma. Usually these cells are round to spindle-shaped with abundant amounts of basophilic cytoplasm and oval nuclei. Occasionally, multinucleated cells are observed, with the nuclei arranged in a row consistent with a straplike

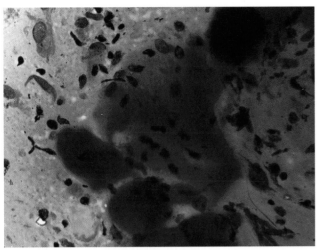

■ **FIGURE 13-13. Suppurative myositis.** Aspirate from a sub-mandibular mass. The background consists of blood and bare nuclei from ruptured cells. Several large blue structures are present, consistent with skeletal muscle fragments. Striations are present and occasionally a basophilic nucleus is present. Additionally, scattered inflammatory cells and few other spindle-shaped cells are identified. This patient had suppurative myositis with secondary fibrosis. (Wright; HP oil.)

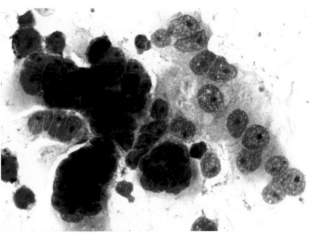

■ **FIGURE 13-14. Rhabdomyosarcoma.** Cytologic preparation of a fine-needle aspirate of a submandibular mass from a 12-month-old dog with multiple oral and facial masses. Large, multinucleated cells and arrangement of nuclei in rows can be seen. (Wright-Giemsa; HP oil.) (From Fallin CW, et al. What is your diagnosis? A 12-month-old dog with multiple soft tissue masses, *Vet Clin Pathol* 24:80, 100-01, 1995.)

cell (Fig. 13-14). This feature has been reported in cytology of rhabdomyosarcomas (Fallin et al., 1995). Rarely, striations are visible within the cytoplasm. Specific diagnosis of a rhabdomyoma or rhabdomyosarcoma on cytology is difficult; however, presence of striations and strap cells can assist with the diagnosis. Histopathology with immunohistochemistry is often necessary for a definitive diagnosis (refer to Chapter 17).

Bone

Fine-needle aspiration of bone is becoming a more commonly used technique (Britt et al., 2007). Aspiration of bone is indicated if an osteolytic or osteoproliferative lesion is observed, which may involve cortical lysis or periosteal bone proliferation. Healthy bone does not exfoliate well; however, inflamed or neoplastic bone exfoliates much more readily. Bone aspiration can be performed with an 18-gauge needle, or if there is considerable lysis a smaller gauge needle may be used. Both aspiration and fenestration techniques can be used to obtain a specimen for cytology. Additionally, imprints of tissue obtained for a biopsy can be used for cytology. Care must be taken to blot as much blood off the biopsy specimen as possible before making the imprints. The bone should be sampled in the center of the lesion rather than on the periphery of the lesion, where there may be a transition between normal and abnormal bone.

Histology of normal bone consists of osteocytes housed in lacunae with low numbers of osteoblasts and osteoclasts. Osteoblasts make osteoid, which appears on cytology and histology as a pink, amorphous, proteinaceous material. On the outer surface of the bone is the periosteum, which consists of fibrous connective tissue. Cytology of normal bone is usually of very low

cellularity and may consist of 1 to 2 cells per slide or less. Usually only the spindle-shaped mesenchymal cells of the periosteum will exfoliate. However, when bone remodeling occurs secondary to trauma, inflammation, or neoplasia, reactive osteoblasts can be observed on cytology. These cells are round with an eccentrically placed nucleus with prominent nucleoli and occasionally prominent Golgi apparatus (Fig. 13-15). It is important not to mistake reactive osteoblasts for neoplastic osteoblasts and sometimes this is quite difficult. The presence of osteoblasts in the absence of inflammation

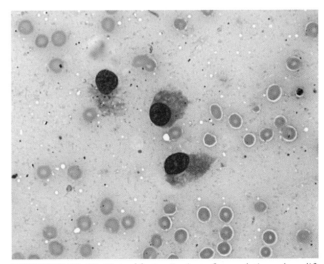

■ **FIGURE 13-15. Osteoblasts.** Aspirate from a lytic and proliferative lesion in the distal radius of a dog. The sample overall is of low cellularity. Pictured are three reactive osteoblasts. These cells commonly have an eccentrically placed nucleus with prominent Golgi apparatus and prominent nucleoli. Care must be taken not to overinterpret reactive osteoblasts for neoplastic cells. (Wright; HP oil.)

and minimal criteria of malignancy should be interpreted with caution.

Cytology of lytic bone exfoliates more readily. Processes associated with bone lysis include inflammation, neoplasia, hypertrophic osteopathy, and aneurismal bone cyst. Osteomyelitis usually consists of suppurative to pyogranulomatous inflammation with varying numbers of neutrophils, macrophages, and multinucleated giant cells depending on the cause of inflammation. Reactive osteoblasts and other mesenchymal cells may also be observed. Osteomyelitis can be caused by bacteria or fungus. Bacterial osteomyelitis can occur uncommonly via hematogenous spread but more commonly secondary to bite wounds, trauma, postsurgical infections, or foreign body. There are many causes of bacterial osteomyelitis; however, organisms commonly associated with osteomyelitis include *Actinomyces* and *Nocardia*. The inflammatory process associated with bacterial osteomyelitis is suppurative rather that pyogranulomatous. It is important to remember when aspirating bone that there is often peripheral blood contamination, and some white blood cells will be observed secondary to the hemodilution. It may be necessary to evaluate a CBC or peripheral blood smear on the patient to determine if there are truly increased numbers of neutrophils within the sample. Observation of intracellular bacteria is diagnostic for bacterial osteomyelitis; however, culture is recommended for all inflammatory bone aspirates.

Fungal osteomyelitis consists of a pyogranulomatous to suppurative inflammatory process and often consists of neutrophils, macrophages, and multinucleated giant cells. Organisms are not always observed in the aspirate so it is important to aspirate more than once and examine all of the slides. Fungal organisms known to cause osteomyelitis include *Blastomyces dermatitidis* (Fig. 13-16A&B), *Cryptococcus* spp., *Coccidioides immitis* (Fig. 13-17A&B), *Histoplasma capsulatum*, and, less commonly, *Candida* spp., *Aspergillus* spp., *Geomyces* spp. (Erne et al., 2007), and *Sporothrix* spp. *Blastomyces* is a round yeast organism with a double-contoured wall and broad-based bud. *Coccidioides* organisms are large (10 to 100μm) blue or clear spheres with finely granular protoplasm. *Histoplasma* organisms by comparison are quite small (2 to 4 μm) and are easily phagocytized by macrophages and can be observed within the cytoplasm of macrophages. The organisms are round with a thin capsule and crescent-shaped, eccentrically placed, eosinophilic nuclei. Cryptococcal organisms are round with a narrow-based bud and thick, nonstaining with Wright stain, mucoid capsule.

Bone tumors often cause boney lysis or proliferation. They can be categorized as primary bone tumors, tumors of bone marrow, tumors that invade bone, or tumors that are metastatic to bone (Rosol et al., 2003). Primary bone tumors include osteosarcoma, chondrosarcoma, fibrosarcoma, hemangiosarcoma, and synovial cell sarcoma (Chun, 2005). Cytologically these tumors can be difficult to differentiate from one another.

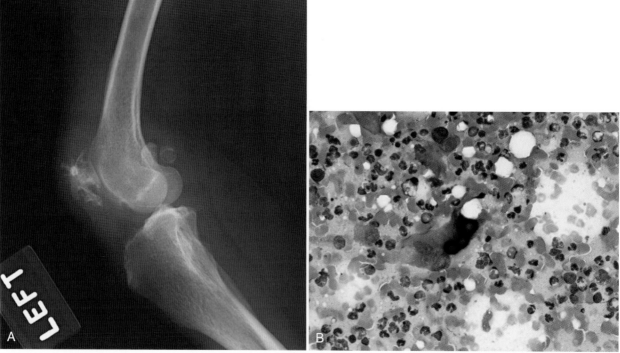

■ **FIGURE 13-16. Blastomycosis. A,** Radiograph from a three-year-old dog with a history of left hind leg lameness. A lytic lesion is noted in the patella. **B,** Fine-needle aspirate of the lytic lesion from A. The sample is cellular and consists of a mixed inflammatory population predominated by neutrophils. Several fungal yeast organisms, consistent with *Blastomyces dermatitidis,* are observed. (Wright; HP oil.) (A, Courtesy of Kristen Odell-Anderson.)

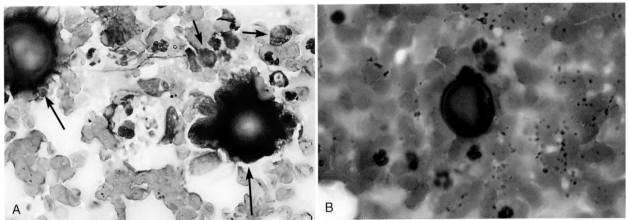

■ **FIGURE 13-17. Coccidioidomycosis. Dog. A,** Aspirate from a lytic lesion in the scapula of a middle-aged dog with pain and lameness of the foreleg. This aspirate contains blood with a mixture of inflammatory cells and smudged nuclei *(short arrow)*. There are two large, blue, spherical structures in this field *(long arrow)* that are *Coccidioides immitis* spherules. The size of the spherules prevents sharp focusing on both the spherules and the background cells. When focusing up and down on these spherules, variable numbers of endospores may be seen within. Aspiration of fungal myelitis lesions does not always yield observable organisms (particularly *Coccidioides*) and if infection is suspected, culture and appropriate serology is indicated. Because of the zoonotic potential of some fungal organisms, extreme care should be taken when culturing these lesions. (Wright; HP oil.) **B,** Aspirate from a lytic lesion in the proximal humerus of a 4-year-old dog with a history of lameness of the left front leg. The cellularity is low and is markedly hemodiluted with many red blood cells observed in the background. Few inflammatory cells and one *Coccidioides immitis* spherule are observed. The spherule is filled with many endospores and occasionally a spherule will rupture, allowing the much smaller endospores to be visualized. It is not uncommon to find low numbers of spherules in a bone aspirate. (Wright; HP oil.)

General cytologic features include round to spindle-shaped cells with basophilic cytoplasm and an eccentrically placed nucleus, with prominent nucleoli (Fig. 13-18A) (Reinhardt et al., 2005). Fibrosarcoma and hemangiosarcoma are less likely to have round cells and the majority of the cells are spindle-shaped. Within the background, osteosarcoma, chondrosarcoma, fibrosarcoma, and synovial cell sarcomas can have varying amounts of eosinophilic proteinaceous material (Fig. 13-18B). This material can also be observed within the cytoplasm of the cells. Chondrosarcomas can have a large amount of matrix in the background, which results in understaining of the cells (Fig. 13-19A–D). In spite of these subtle differences, these tumors can be

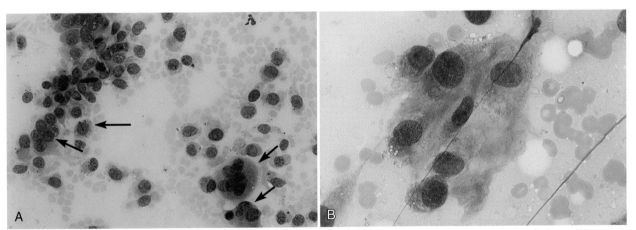

■ **FIGURE 13-18. Same case A-B. A, Bone tumor aspirate cellularity.** Aspirate from a lytic and proliferative lesion of the proximal tibia. The specimen is bloody with high cellularity with a mixture of ellipsoid and multinucleated cells *(short arrows)*. In some areas, there are thick accumulations of cells *(long arrow)*. (Wright; HP oil.) **B, Eosinophilic background matrix.** Shown is a closer view of the background demonstrating a group of individualized cells that are presumptively osteoblasts with swirls of a fine, pink extracellular material around them. Note the large cell size by contrasting them to the greenish-stained erythrocytes. This appearance is most consistent with a sarcoma. It is difficult to cytologically distinguish different types of sarcoma, and additional tests such as radiography and biopsy are necessary for definitive morphologic diagnosis. Histopathology of this lesion indicated osteosarcoma. (Wright; HP oil.)

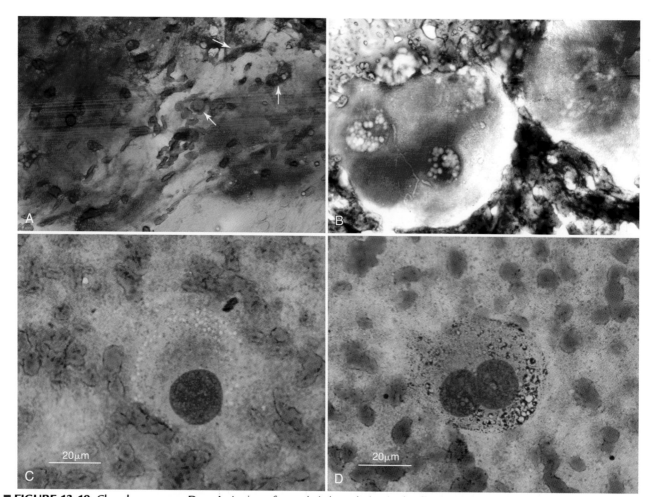

■ **FIGURE 13-19. Chondrosarcoma. Dog. A,** Aspirate from a lytic bone lesion in the distal radius of a 10-year-old Labrador Retriever. The sample is highly cellular. Neoplastic cells *(arrows)* are not stained well because of the abundant amounts of deeply eosinophilic matrix filling the background. The presence of this material is common in bone tumors, particularly chondroma and chondrosarcoma. The cytologic diagnosis of this sample is sarcoma, likely chondrosarcoma. A biopsy with histopathology confirmed the diagnosis of chondrosarcoma. (Wright; HP oil.) **B, Tissue aspirate.** The foamy cytoplasm of the chondrocytes gives the appearance of lacunae within dense, eosinophilic, mucinous material. (Wright; HP oil.) **C, Tissue aspirate.** A composite of two neoplastic chondrocytes is shown. Note the prominent multiple nucleoli, coarse chromatin clumping, and fine eosinophilic-cytoplasmic granularity in the mononuclear cell. (Wright; HP oil.). **D, Tissue aspirate.** The binucleated cell cytoplasm contains dark purple cytoplasmic granularity and the two nuclei have slightly different sizes. (Wright; HP oil.) (B, Courtesy of Rick Alleman, University of Florida. C, Courtesy of Rose Raskin, Purdue University.)

difficult to differentiate cytologically and biopsy with histopathology is an important diagnostic tool. Additional cytochemical testing can be done to improve the sensitivity of cytologic diagnosis of osteosarcoma. Staining of the neoplastic cells for alkaline phosphatase activity with nitroblue tetrazolium chloride/5-bromo-4-chloro-3-indolyl phosphate toluidine salt (NBT/BCIP) increases the sensitivity and specificity of differentiating osteosarcoma from other mesenchymal tumors (Barger et al., 2005). One limitation of this staining technique is that reactive osteoblasts will stain positive as well, so obvious criteria of malignancy must be observed before this test is performed (Fig. 13-20A). Positive staining is indicated by grayish-black staining of the cytoplasm (Fig. 13-20B). Previously unstained

slides must be used. After staining for alkaline phosphatase activity, cells can be lightly counterstained with a Romanowsky stain to examine the positive cells for the appropriate criteria of malignancy.

Lymphoma and plasma cell tumors are considered tumors of bone marrow that can result in bone lysis. The morphology of these cells appears similar to that in other tissues (Fig. 13-21). Plasma cell tumors produce a characteristic punched-out radiographic appearance. A combination of diagnostic tests is necessary to diagnose the plasma cell tumor as multiple myeloma. In addition to radiographs and cytology, protein electrophoresis of serum and urine are recommended.

Squamous cell carcinoma is the most common tumor that can invade bone. Usually the cytology reveals

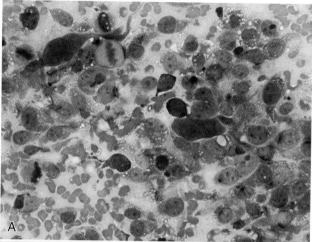

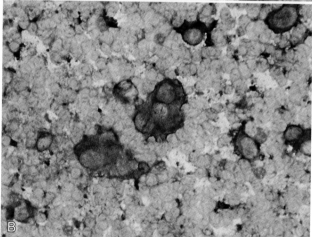

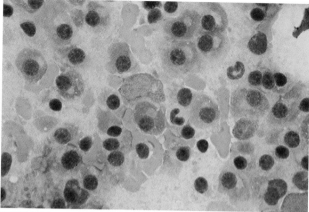

■ **FIGURE 13-21. Multiple myeloma. Dog.** Aspirate from a lytic, "punched-out" lesion in a vertebral spinous process of an 8-year-old dog. The aspirate is predominated by mildly pleomorphic plasma cells. This finding in combination with the presence of lytic bony lesions is diagnostic for multiple myeloma (Wright; HP oil.)

■ **FIGURE 13-20. Osteosarcoma. Dog. Same case A-B. A,** This sample is from a proliferative and lytic lesion in the proximal humerus of a mixed breed dog. The sample is cellular and consists of a population of round and spindle-shaped neoplastic cells. Multiple criteria of malignancy are observed, including prominent and multiple nucleoli, anisocytosis and anisokaryosis, and marked variability in the nuclear-to-cytoplasmic ratio. Small pools of eosinophilic proteinaceous matrix are identified. Cytologic diagnosis is sarcoma. (Wright; HP oil.) **B,** Alkaline phosphatase staining of a previously unstained slide demonstrates a strong positive reaction for alkaline phosphatase activity as indicated by the black staining of the cytoplasm. Combination of Figs 12-16A&B is consistent with osteosarcoma. This diagnosis was confirmed with histopathology. (Alkaline phosphatase; HP oil.)

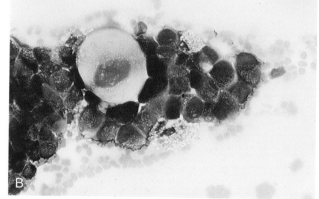

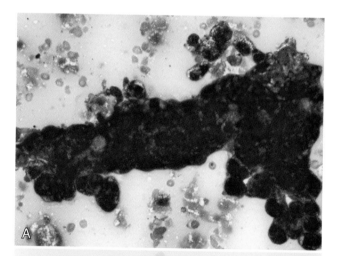

■ **FIGURE 13-22. Metastatic carcinoma. Dog. A,** Aspirate from a lytic lesion in a vertebral body from a dog with a history of prostatic carcinoma. The cohesive nature of these cells is consistent with carcinoma and in this case the most likely diagnosis is metastatic prostatic carcinoma. (Wright; HP oil.) **B,** This sample is from the stifle joint of a 12-year-old Golden Retriever. The joint was swollen and painful with evidence of bony lysis. Numerous clusters of pleomorphic cells are present. These cells display marked anisocytosis and anisokaryosis with prominent, irregularly shaped nucleoli. The atypia of the cells is consistent with the diagnosis of metastatic carcinoma (Wright; HP oil.)

neoplastic squamous cells with rare or no osteoblasts. Cytologic features of this tumor are similar to those in other locations. Many tumors can metastasize to bone but the common tumors that metastasize to bone include prostatic, lung, and mammary carcinomas. Identification of metastatic neoplasms can be difficult because cytology is often accompanied by reactive osteoblasts and osteoclasts. However, a second population of cells can often be differentiated from the reactive population. Epithelial neoplasms are usually clustered, but when they metastasize they may appear more poorly differentiated (Fig. 13-22A&B). Additional stains are very helpful for diagnosis.

REFERENCES

Affolter VK, Moore PF: Localized and disseminated histiocytic sarcoma of dendritic cell origin in dogs, *Vet Pathol* 39:74-83, 2002.

Barger A, Graca R, Bailey K, et al: Utilization of alkaline phosphatase staining to differentiate osteosarcoma from other vimentin positive tumors, *Vet Pathol* 42:161-165, 2005.

Britt T, Clifford C, Barger A, et al: Diagnosing appendicular osteosarcoma with ultrasound-guided fine-needle aspiration: 36 cases, *J Small An Pract* 48:145-150, 2007.

Carr AP, Michels G: Identifying noninfectious erosive arthritis in dogs and cats, *Vet Med* 92:804-810, 1997.

Chun R: Common malignant musculoskeletal neoplasms of dogs and cats, *Vet Clin Sm Anim* 35:1155-1167, 2005.

Craig LE, Julian ME, Ferracone JD: The diagnosis and prognosis of synovial tumors in dogs: 35 cases, *Vet Pathol* 39:66-73, 2002.

deHaan JJ, Andreasen CB: Calcium crystal-associated arthropathy (pseudogout) in a dog, *J Am An Hosp Assoc* 200:943-946, 1992.

Erne JB, Walker MC, Strik N, et al: Systemic infection with *Geomyces* organisms in a dog with lytic bone lesions, *J Am Vet Med Assoc* 230:537-540, 2007.

Fallin CW, Fox LE, Papendick RE, et al: What is your diagnosis? A 12-month-old dog with multiple soft tissue masses, *Vet Clin Pathol* 24:80, 100-101, 1995.

Forsyth SF, Thompson KG, Donald JJ: Possible pseudogout in two dogs, *J Sm An Pract* 48:174-176, 2007.

Gibson NR, Carmichael S, Li A, et al: Value of direct smears of synovial fluid in the diagnosis of canine joint disease, *Vet Rec* 144:463-465, 1999.

Goodman RA, Hawkins EC, Olby NJ, et al: Molecular identification of *Ehrlichia ewingii* infection in dogs: 15 cases (1997-2001), *J Am Vet Med Assoc* 222:1102-1107, 2003.

Harvey JW, Raskin RE: Polyarthritis in a dog, *NAVC Clinician's Brief* 2:37-38, 2004.

MacWilliams PS, Friedrichs KR: Laboratory evaluation and interpretation of synovial fluid, *Vet Clin North Am Small Anim* 33:153-178, 2003.

Marchevsky AM, Read RA: Bacterial septic arthritis in 19 dogs, *Aust Vet J* 77:233-237, 1999.

Meinkoth JH, Rochat MC, Cowell RL: Metastatic carcinoma presenting as hind-limb lameness: diagnosis by synovial fluid cytology, *J Am An Hosp Assoc* 33:325-328, 1997.

Michels GM, Carr AP: Noninfectious nonerosive arthritis in dogs, *Vet Med* 92:798-803, 1997.

Pacchiana PD, Gilley RS, Wallace LJ, et al: Absolute and relative cell counts for synovial fluid from clinically normal shoulder and stifle joints in cats, *J Am Vet Med Assoc* 225:1866-1870, 2004.

Reinhardt S, Stockhaus C, Teske E, et al: Assessment of cytological criteria for diagnosing osteosarcoma in dogs, *J Small An Pract* 46:65-70, 2005.

Rosol TJ, Tannehill-Gregg, LeRoy BE, et al: Animal models of bone metastasis, *Cancer* 97(3 suppl):748-757, 2003.

Santos M, Marcos R, Assuncao M, et al: Polyarthritis associated with visceral leishmaniasis in a juvenile dog, *Vet Parasit* 141:340-344, 2006.

Stobie D, Wallace LJ, Lipowitz AJ, et al: Chronic bicipital tenosynovitis in dogs: 29 cases (1985-1992), *J Am Vet Med Assoc* 207:201-207, 1995.

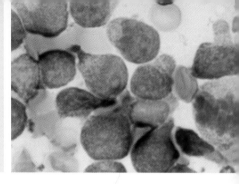

14

The Central Nervous System

Davide De Lorenzi and Maria T. Mandara

CEREBROSPINAL FLUID

Cerebrospinal fluid (CSF) evaluation is a mainstay in the diagnosis of central nervous system (CNS) disease because it is relatively simple to collect and has the potential to provide valuable information. Lesions of the CNS do not consistently cause CSF abnormalities related to the location and extent of the lesion. Although CSF evaluation infrequently provides a definitive diagnosis, it may be of benefit in documenting normal or abnormal features and, in combination with other tests, determining a diagnosis or differential diagnoses (Bohn et al., 2006; Bush et al., 2002; Chrisman, 1992; Cook and DeNicola, 1988; Fenner, 2000; Rand, 1995). CSF collection is recommended as a part of virtually any diagnostic investigation of CNS disease of unknown cause when contraindications to its collection are not present.

The submission of a properly collected specimen is necessary to obtain reliable and accurate information. Proper interpretation of the sample requires knowledge of the clinical presentation, collection site, and specimen-handling considerations. The presence of artifacts or contaminants may interfere with an appropriate interpretation unless the conditions surrounding the collection are known. Experience in interpretation of cytologic specimens from the species of interest and knowledge of the limitations of cytology or types of pathologic processes likely to be reflected in CSF are also important and can only be gained by diligent study of the literature and specimens over time.

Cerebrospinal fluid is formed primarily by the ultrafiltration and secretion through the choroid plexuses of the lateral, third, and fourth ventricles. Other sites that secrete CSF include the ependymal linings of the ventricles and blood vessels of the subarachnoid spaces and pia mater. Fluid then escapes from the fourth ventricle into the subarachnoid spaces and central canal of the spinal cord. It is then absorbed predominantly from the subarachnoid spaces via veins in the arachnoid and subarachnoid villi that project into subdural venous sinuses.

Collection of Cerebrospinal Fluid

Contraindications to CSF Collection

Cerebrospinal fluid collection is not indicated in cases in which a cause is obvious, such as known trauma or intoxication (Parent and Rand, 1994). Because anesthesia is required for collection of CSF in small animals, CSF collection is contraindicated in cases in which anesthesia is contraindicated (Carmichael, 1998; Cook and DeNicola, 1988).

Cerebrospinal fluid collection is contraindicated in cases with increased intracranial pressure. Increased intracranial pressure should be suspected with acute head trauma, active or decompensated hydrocephalus, anisocoria, papilledema, or cerebral edema. Expansile mass lesions and unstable CNS or systemic conditions may result in increased intracranial pressure or decreased pressure in the spinal compartment relative to the intracranial compartment. In these situations herniation of the brain may result in severe compromise of brain function, tetraplegia, stupor/coma, and/or death (Parent and Rand, 1994). Physical and neurologic examination, history, presentation, and results of imaging studies are of benefit in determining if these conditions are likely before the decision to collect CSF.

Even in cases with potential for brain herniation, the risks associated with CSF collection may be acceptable if the cause of patient deterioration is not apparent. Risk of herniation may be reduced by administration of dexamethasone (0.25 mg/kg IV) just before induction of anesthesia and by hyperventilation of the patient with oxygen during the procedure (Fenner, 2000). Except in cases in which dexamethasone is administered prophylactically because of suspected increased intracranial pressure, CSF collection should predate corticosteroid administration because of potential alteration of CSF composition (Rand, 1995).

Complications of CSF Collection

As with any medical procedure, the risks and benefits of CSF collection should be considered for individual cases. The potential exists for iatrogenic trauma to the spinal cord and/or brainstem from the collection needle, but is minimized by attention to anatomic landmarks and careful collection procedures (Carmichael, 1998; Parent and Rand, 1994). Risk of introduction of infectious agents into the CNS is minimized by adherence to the basic principles of aseptic technique and correct preparation of the site of collection (Cook and DeNicola, 1988).

Slight to moderate blood contamination is a common complication of collection associated with penetration of the dorsal vertebral sinuses or small vessels within the meninges; this may complicate interpretation of the fluid analyses and cytology, but has not been found to be harmful to the patient (Carmichael, 1998; Fenner, 2000).

Ketamine should not be used to anesthetize cats for CSF collection because it increases intracranial pressure and may induce seizures; gas anesthesia should be used (Parent and Rand, 1994).

If three unsuccessful attempts at CSF collection occur, abandonment of the procedure is recommended to decrease the probability of repeated penetration of the spinal cord, which may result in serious complications or death. Practice on cadavers before performing collection in live clinical cases has been recommended.

Equipment for CSF Collection

Clippers, scrub, and alcohol to surgically prepare the site of collection are needed. Sterile gloves should be worn during the procedure. A sterile disposable or resterilizable spinal needle with stylet is used. A 20- to 22-gauge, 1.5-inch needle with a polypropylene hub is recommended for most cases, although smaller needles may be needed in very small dogs and cats and longer needles may be needed in large dogs (Carmichael, 1998; Cook and DeNicola, 1988; Parent and Rand, 1994; Rand, 1995). Several needles should be available since replacement may be needed if the needle is inserted off the midline and enters a venous sinus (Cook and DeNicola, 1988).

Sterile plain tubes for collection of CSF are recommended. Some authors indicate that EDTA is not used because clotting is rare and EDTA may falsely elevate the protein concentration of CSF (Parent and Rand, 1994). However, others recommend addition of samples to EDTA if blood contamination is present or if elevated nucleated cell count, bacteria, elevated protein concentration, and/or the presence of fibrinogen are suspected because these may lead to clotting (Carmichael, 1998). If glucose determination is desired, it is recommended to collect CSF into fluoride/oxalate; this may not be necessary if CSF contains few erythrocytes and is analyzed rapidly.

Plastic containers are recommended because leukocytes may adhere to glass. Use of only a few plain, sterile containers makes collection easier and simpler and increases the probability of maximum yield of CSF.

Collection Volume

Carmichael (1998) indicates that approximately 1 mL of CSF per 5 kg of body weight can be collected safely. It may be dangerous to remove more than 1 mL of CSF per 30 seconds, more than 4 to 5 mL of CSF from the dog, more than 0.5 to 1 mL of CSF from the adult cat or more than 10 to 20 drops of CSF from the kitten. Rand (1990) indicates that 1.0 to 1.5 mL of CSF can usually be collected from the cat. The cat may be susceptible to meningeal hemorrhage if too much fluid is withdrawn.

Cerebellomedullary Cistern Collection

Collection at this site is indicated to classify lesions affecting the meninges of the head and neck when the clinical signs involve seizures, generalized incoordination, head tilt, or circling.

Preparation of the site should include clipping of the hair from the head and neck, from the anterior margin of the pinna to the level of the third cervical vertebra and laterally to the level of the lateral margins of the pinnae. This area should be scrubbed for a sterile procedure (Cellio, 2001).

The animal is positioned in lateral recumbency with the head and vertebral column positioned at an angle of approximately 90 degrees. Excessive flexion of the neck may result in elevation of intracranial pressure and increase the potential for brain herniation (Fenner, 2000) or may result in occlusion of the endotracheal tube (Carmichael, 1998). The nose should be held or propped so that its long axis is parallel to the table and it should not be allowed to rotate in either direction. The point of insertion is located on the midline approximately half way between the external occipital protuberance and the craniodorsal tip of the dorsal spine of C2 (axis) and just rostral to the anterior margins of the wings of C1 (atlas). The needle is inserted at the intersection of a line connecting the anterior borders of the wings of the atlas and a line drawn from the occipital crest to the dorsal border of the axis along the midline. Puncture of the skin first with an 18-gauge needle or a scalpel blade is helpful in overcoming skin resistance in thick-skinned animals. Alternatively, the skin can be pinched and lifted so that the needle can be safely pushed through the skin with a twisting motion.

The needle should be inserted with the bevel oriented cranially. It should be held perpendicular to the skin surface and gradually advanced with the stylet in place. Periodically the needle should be stabilized and the stylet withdrawn to determine if CSF is present. Occasionally, a sudden loss of resistance may be felt as the subarachnoid space is entered, but this may not be recognized in all cases. If the collector suspects that the needle has been inserted too deeply, the stylet may be removed and the needle slowly withdrawn a few millimeters at a time, watching for the appearance of fluid in the hub. If the needle hits bone during insertion, slight redirection of the needle cranially or caudally should be attempted to enter the atlanto-occipital space.

If opening pressure readings are taken, CSF fluid sample is taken by directing the flow of CSF through the manometer by way of a three-way stopcock. If pressure readings are not obtained, CSF may be collected directly from the spinal needle hub by dripping into a test tube or gentle aspiration of drops as they collect at the hub using a syringe. Attachment of a syringe to the needle with aspiration of CSF is not recommended because suction may result in contamination with blood or meningeal cells or obstruction of CSF flow by aspirated meningeal trabeculae. Careful aspiration is acknowledged to be necessary for collections in some cases. Passage of the needle through the spinal cord to underlying bone should be avoided at the cerebellomedullary cistern because it may cause damage to the cord and/or cause blood contamination of the CSF sample. On completion of collection of CSF, the needle is smoothly withdrawn. Replacement of the stylet is not necessary.

If the fluid appears bloody at the onset of collection, replacement of the stylet for 30 to 60 seconds may result in clearing of the blood. If the first few drops of CSF are still slightly bloody, they can be collected separately from the following drops that are often clear. If rate of flow of CSF is slow, the needle should be rotated slightly to make sure that it is clear at the luminal tip. If this not effective, rate of flow may be increased by compression of the jugular veins, resulting in expansion of the venous sinuses and increased CSF pressure.

Appearance of abundant fresh blood from the collection needle indicates that the point of the needle is most likely off the midline and in a lateral venous sinus. A new approach with a fresh, clean needle is recommended if the first attempt results in frank blood consistent with puncture of the venous sinus.

Lumbar Cistern Collection

Both cerebellomedullary and lumbar cistern specimens may be collected. Collection of a cerebellomedullary specimen is recommended prior to thoracolumbar myelography to ensure that a diagnostic CSF sample will be obtained because lumbar puncture alone may not be sufficient. The collection of CSF from the lumbar cistern is more difficult and more likely to be contaminated with blood than that from the cerebellomedullary cistern (Chrisman, 1992). Sometimes no fluid or only a very small amount of fluid can be obtained owing to the small size of the lumbar subarachnoid space. Lumbar puncture may be preferred in cases with localized spinal disease because it may be more likely to confirm abnormality than cerebellomedullary cistern collections (Thomson et al., 1990).

The dorsal midline is clipped and prepared between the midsacrum and L3, extending laterally to the wings of the ilium. The animal is placed in lateral recumbency and the back is flexed slightly to open the spaces between the dorsal laminae of the vertebrae. The L5-6 or L6-7 spaces are most commonly used in dogs because the subarachnoid space rarely extends to the lumbosacral junction. In cats collection can frequently be made from the lumbosacral space.

The dorsal spinous process of L7 lies between the wings of the ilia and is usually smaller than that of L6. To collect from the L5-6 intervertebral space, the needle is inserted just off the midline at the caudal aspect of the L6 dorsal spinous process and advanced at an angle cranioventrally and slightly medially to enter the spinal canal between the dorsal laminae of L5 and L6. Misdirection laterally into the paralumbar muscles or underestimation of the length of needle required might result in advancement of the needle to the hub without encountering bone.

Cerebrospinal fluid may be collected from the dorsal subarachnoid space, or the needle may be passed through the nervous structures to the floor of the spinal canal and CSF collected from the ventral subarachnoid space. The stylet is removed and the needle may be carefully withdrawn a few millimeters to allow for fluid flow. The rate of flow is usually slower than from the cerebellomedullary cistern. Rate of flow may be increased by jugular compression.

Cerebrospinal Fluid Opening Pressure

CSF pressure is measured with a standard spinal fluid manometer as the fluid is collected (Simpson and Reed, 1987). CSF opening pressure should be measured to confirm a supposed increase in intracranial pressure due to a space-occupying mass or cerebral edema. Its normal range is less than 170 mmH$_2$O (Lipsitz et al., 1999) and 100 mmH$_2$O, for the dog and cat, respectively (Chrisman, 1991).

Handling of Cerebrospinal Fluid Specimens

Cells lyse rapidly in the low-protein milieu of CSF, so cell counts and cytologic preparations of unfixed fluid should be done within 30 to 60 minutes of collection (Fry et al., 2006). The likelihood of misinterpretation due to sample deterioration depends on the initial protein concentration of the sample and how long analysis is delayed. For example, if the CSF protein concentration is >50 mg/dl, a delay in analysis of <12 hours is unlikely to alter final interpretation. Addition of an equal volume of 4% to 10% neutral buffered formalin or 50% to 90% alcohol is recommended for fixation of specimens that cannot be immediately delivered to a laboratory and processed immediately (Carmichael, 1998). Alternatively, the addition of one drop of 10% formalin to 1 to 2 mL of CSF may be used to preserve cells for cell counts and morphologic examination when submitted to a referral laboratory, keeping in mind that cell counts will be affected but may not be clinically significant. Refrigeration will help retard cellular degeneration. Cellular stability can be increased by addition of fresh, frozen, or thawed serum or plasma (Bienzle et al., 2000) or by addition of 20% albumin (Fenner, 2000). If a CSF sample is not analyzed within 1 hour from collection, Fry and co-workers (2006) recommend to divide the fluid into 2 aliquots, an unadulterated aliquot for total nucleated cell count and protein measurement and an aliquot added with 20% of fetal calf serum (or 10% autologous serum) for differential cell count and morphologic evaluation. For those samples of insufficient volume (<0.5 mL total), hetastarch (1:1) can be added to CSF for all routine assays. In the last situation, the dilutional effect of adding a stabilizing agent must be taken into account when calculating results. Protein and enzyme concentrations in CSF are relatively stable, and submission to the laboratory by routine delivery, postal delivery, or courier is usually sufficient for accurate determinations (Carmichael, 1998).

Laboratory Analysis of CSF

Usually at least 1 to 2 mL of CSF is available from dogs or cats. The analysis for cell counts requires approximately 0.5 mL (500 µl total or 250 µl for duplicate erythrocyte count and nucleated cell count, respectively). The volume required for chemical protein determination will vary, depending on the equipment and method used, but can be expected to be on the order of 200 to 250 µl for large, automated pieces of equipment. Taking these figures into account, approximately 0.25 to 1.25 mL of CSF should be available for cytologic evaluation and/or other tests.

Routine analysis of CSF is recommended in all cases in which it is collected; specialized analyses may be needed in selected cases. Routine analyses of CSF includes the following: macroscopic evaluation, quantitative analysis (erythrocyte count, nucleated cell count, and total protein), and microscopic evaluation as summarized in Table 14-1. If the volume of CSF is small and all tests are not likely to be obtained, the clinician should rank the tests in order of preference when the specimen is submitted to the laboratory. Rand (1995) indicates that the most useful diagnostic tests, in decreasing order, are nucleated and erythrocyte counts, sedimentation cytology, protein concentration, and cytocentrifuge cytology.

Effect of Blood Contamination

Various formulas have been used to predict the effect of blood contamination on protein concentration and nucleated cell count in CSF (Parent and Rand, 1994; Rand et al, 1990). Rand (1995) indicates that red blood cell (RBC) counts greater than 30 cells/µl in CSF will have a profound effect on the total and differential cell counts. However, in a study (Hurtt and Smith, 1997) of iatrogenic blood contamination effects of total protein and nucleated cell counts in CSF, the RBC count was not significantly correlated with nucleated cell count or protein concentration in CSF from clinically normal dogs or those with neurologic disease. The study concluded that high CSF nucleated cell counts and protein concentrations are indicative of neurologic disease, even if samples contain up to 13,200 RBC/µl. Although blood contamination may make interpretation of CSF more difficult, red or pink CSF or CSF with a high RBC count should not be discarded as a useless specimen because cytologic evaluation may detect abnormalities (Chrisman, 1992).

Macroscopic Evaluation

Normal CSF is clear, colorless, and transparent and does not coagulate Deviations from normal should be recorded as part of the macroscopic evaluation and are often graded 1 to 4 + or as slight, moderate, or marked. Turbidity (Fig. 14-1A) is reported to be detectable if greater than 500 cells/µl are present (Fenner, 2000) or if at least 200 leukocytes/µl or 700 erythrocytes/µl are present (Parent and Rand, 1994).

Red to pink discoloration may be associated with iatrogenic contamination with blood or pathologic hemorrhage. Erythrophages or siderophages in a rapidly processed CSF specimen with fixative added immediately following collection support pathologic hemorrhage as an underlying cause. Xanthochromia is the yellow to yellow-orange discoloration (Fig. 14-1B) associated with pathologic hemorrhage due to trauma, vasculitis, severe inflammation, disc extrusion, or necrotic or erosive neoplasia. Occasionally xanthochromia will be seen with leptospirosis, cryptococcosis, toxoplasmosis, ischemic myelopathy, coagulopathy, or hyperbilirubinemia.

Quantitative Analysis

Cell Counts

Erythrocyte and nucleated cell counts are often done using standard hemocytometer techniques. In general, collections from normal animals from the cerebellomedullary cistern have slightly higher numbers of cells and slightly lower protein levels than those from the lumbar cistern.

To count nucleated cells, charge both chambers of the hemocytometer with undiluted CSF and place the unit in a humidified Petri dish for 15 minutes to allow cells to adhere to the glass. All nucleated cells are counted in the 10 large squares (four corner squares and one center square on each side) for a total nucleated cell count per microliter. Cell counts for erythrocytes are performed similarly. A study conducted to evaluate the usefulness of an automated cell counter in counting and differentiating cell types from canine CSF (Ruotsala et al., 2008) determined moderate correlation between this method and a hemocytometer for leukocyte values and excellent correlation for erythrocytes; however, cell differentials were much more variable. Results from this study also suggested that lymphocytes may be underestimated by manual microscopy in favor of large mononuclears.

Reference intervals for feline CSF erythrocyte counts are reported to range from 0 to 30 red blood cells per microliter (Parent and Rand, 1994). Reference intervals for feline CSF nucleated cell counts are reported to be less than 5 cells/µl, 0 to 2 cells/µl (Parent and Rand, 1994), less than 3 cells/µl (Chrisman, 1992), and less than 8 cells/µl (Cook and DeNicola, 1988).

Reference intervals for canine CSF erythrocyte counts are reported to be zero (Chrisman, 1992). Reference intervals for canine CSF nucleated cell counts are reported to be less than 5 cells/µl (Cook and DeNicola, 1988), and less than 6 cells/µl for cerebellomedullary cistern collections or less than 5 cells/µl for lumbar cistern collections (Chrisman, 1992).

Absence of elevation of nucleated cell counts in CSF does not preclude the need for cytomorphologic evaluation with a differential cell count or estimate because abnormalities in cell type or morphology may be present even when CSF nucleated cell counts are within normal limits.

Protein

Reference intervals for CSF total protein values may vary slightly with the laboratory and testing method used, but cerebellomedullary CSF protein is usually less than 25 to 30 mg/dl and lumbar cistern collections less than 45 mg/dl

TABLE 14-1 Routine Evaluation of CSF

Component of CSF Evaluation	Normal CSF	Abnormal CSF	Comments/Notes
Macroscopic Evaluation			
Color	Colorless	Pink, red xanthochromic (yellow to yellow-orange). Occasional gray to green color may be seen.	Compare with tube containing water. Red or pink suggests blood; if due to intact erythrocytes, it will clear with centrifugation. Xanthochromia is an indication of previous hemorrhage with accumulation of oxyhemoglobin or methemoglobin from erythrocyte degradation; may occur with hyperbilirubinemia. May be graded as slight, moderate, or marked.
Turbidity	Clear, turbidity absent	Turbid or cloudy—slight, moderate, or marked	Evaluate ability to read printed words through the tube. Detectable turbidity corresponds to nucleated cell count > 500 cells/µl
Erythrocyte (RBC) count	Zero RBC considered normal, but frequently present in small numbers	Variable	Standard hemocytometer
Nucleated cell count	Most commonly cited reference intervals: 0-5 cells/µl (dog) 0-8 cells/µl (cat)	Variable	Standard hemocytometer
Specific gravity	1.004-1.006	Most within reference interval for normal CSF	Of questionable value because only relatively marked increases in total protein result in changes that are detectable by specific gravity measurement
Total Protein (Microprotein)			
Quantitation	Most commonly cited reference intervals indicate usually <30 mg/dl (cerebellomedullary) or <45 mg/dl (lumbar cistern)	Increased total protein seen in a variety of conditions	Microprotein method and reference values may vary with laboratory; use laboratory-established reference values.

Estimation

Ames Multistix*	Microprotein Concentration		Ames Multistix	Microprotein Concentration	
Trace	<30 mg/dl		2+	100 mg/dl	
1+	30 mg/dl		3+	300 mg/dl	
Trace to 1 + protein on urine dipstick is within normal limits			4+	>2000 mg/dl	

Comments/Notes (Ames Multistix): Most sensitive to albumin; detects ranges of protein that are useful for evaluation of most canine and feline CSF specimens; good correlation with standard dye-binding microprotein determinations.

Component of CSF Evaluation	Normal CSF	Abnormal CSF	Comments/Notes
Microscopic Evaluation			
Cell population	Lymphocytes and monocytoid cells predominate; very few mature, nondegenerated neutrophils may be present. A few erythrocytes may be seen.	Variable	See other sections for more details of cytologic features and specific conditions. Preparatory techniques for concentrating cells: Cytospin preparation; Membrane filter; Sedimentation chamber

* N-Multistix SG, Bayer, Miles, Diagnostic Division, Elkhart, IN.

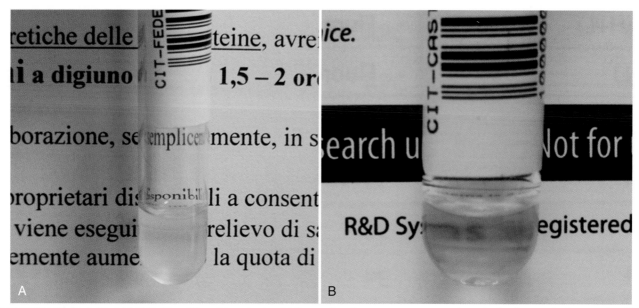

■ FIGURE 14-1. A, Turbid CSF. Dog. There is marked turbidity or cloudiness as apparent against the background of newsprint. This animal had a steroid-responsive meningitis with a count of 760 nucleated cells/μl. Turbidity is reported to be detectable if greater than 200 leukocytes/μl are present. **B, Xanthochromic CSF. Dog.** The fluid has a yellow-orange discoloration and moderate turbidity from a dog with subarachnoidal hemorrhage of inflammatory origin.

in dogs and cats (Chrisman, 1992; Fenner, 2000). Refractometer total protein evaluation is not accurate for assessment of CSF since the concentration of protein is quite low compared to serum or plasma and clinically significant changes may not be easily detectable on the refractometer scale. Special analytic techniques most often available at commercial or reference laboratories and not available in practice are needed owing to the minute protein concentration in CSF. Due to the minute amounts present, CSF protein analysis may be referred to as "microprotein." An estimate of CSF protein content can be obtained using urine dipsticks. A membrane microconcentrator technique followed by agarose gel electrophoresis was recently described for measurement of cerebrospinal fluid proteins in dogs (Gama et al., 2007).

Increased CSF protein concentration may be caused by an alteration in the blood-brain barrier and leakage from plasma or increased local synthesis. Quantitative tests for detection of the components of CSF protein are covered under the heading of Other Tests. Differential diagnoses and examples of processes causing elevated CSF protein are covered under the heading of Protein Abnormalities in CSF.

Albumin accounts for 80% to 95% of the total protein in normal CSF. Qualitative tests to detect increased globulins in CSF are the Pandy and Nonne-Apelt tests. Use of these tests is limited because of the qualitative nature and absence of specificity regarding underlying cause. Normal CSF contains little if any globulin that can be detected by these methods.

Other Tests

Other tests that have been recommended by various authors or used in specific situations include electrophoretic determination of albumin and determination of total immunoglobulin levels. In combination with the serum albumin level and serum immunoglobulin, these can be used to calculate the albumin quotient (AQ) and immunoglobulin G (IgG) index. The AQ is equal to the CSF albumin divided by serum albumin times 100. AQ greater than 2.35 suggests an altered blood-brain barrier with increased protein in CSF associated with leakage from plasma. The IgG index is equal to the (CSF IgG/serum IgG) divided by (CSF albumin/serum albumin). An IgG index greater than 0.272 with a normal AQ suggests intrathecal production of IgG. An increased IgG index and increased AQ are suggestive of an altered blood-brain barrier as the source of IgG (Chrisman, 1992).

Alterations in electrophoretic protein fractions have been reported to be useful in identifying inflammatory, degenerative, and neoplastic disease in combination with clinical signs. In general, dogs with canine distemper often have elevated CSF gamma globulins, most likely related to intrathecal production, while dogs with granulomatous meningoencephalitis (GME) may have elevated CSF beta and gamma globulins (Chrisman, 1992).

In a more recent work, Behr and co-workers (2006) found, using high-resolution protein electrophoresis, a strong linear correlation between CSF total protein concentration and AQ suggesting that an increased CSF total protein concentration is an indicator of blood-brain barrier dysfunction; moreover, although unexpected, the same authors found that electrophoretic profiles in a series of 94 dogs with different neurologic diseases were not characteristic of any particular disease concluding that high-resolution electrophoresis of paired CSF and serum samples cannot be considered a valuable ancillary diagnostic tool for canine neurologic diseases.

Detection of specific antibodies within the CSF and comparison with serum levels may be useful in diagnosis of infectious meningoencephalitides, including infectious canine hepatitis, canine herpesvirus, canine parvovirus, canine parainfluenza virus, canine distemper virus, ehrlichiosis, Rocky Mountain spotted fever, Lyme disease (borreliosis), *Toxoplasma gondii, Neospora caninum, Encephalitozoon cuniculi* infection, *Babesia* spp. infection, cryptococcosis (Berthelin et al., 1994), and blastomycosis. On the contrary, measurement of anticoronavirus IgG in CSF of cats with confirmed feline infectious peritonitis involving the central nervous system is considered of equivocal clinical use (Boettcher et al., 2007). Serial titers for serum IgG to show rising titer are helpful to demonstrate active disease. The presence of IgM in serum or CSF is considered more specific than IgG or total immunoglobulin levels for detection of active disease (Chrisman, 1992).

Glucose measurement in CSF and comparison with serum or plasma glucose levels are frequently cited. Normal CSF glucose is approximately 60% to 80% of the serum or plasma concentration (Fenner, 2000). However, changes in CSF glucose concentration in serum or plasma are not immediately reflected in CSF and may take 1 to 3 hours before they are apparent in CSF (Cook and DeNicola, 1988). The ratio between blood glucose and CSF glucose is frequently reduced in bacterial infections of the CNS in humans and has been reported to occur in some cases of pyogenic infections of the CNS, CSF hemorrhage, or blood contamination that may result in increased utilization of glucose by cells. However, the relationship between bacterial encephalitis and decreased CSF glucose compared with serum or plasma glucose may depend on multiple factors, including the blood glucose level, degree of permeability of the blood-brain barrier, and presence or absence of glycolytic cells or microorganisms. Fenner (2000) states that the reduction in glucose does not occur in dogs. Significant reductions in CSF glucose concentrations have been reported in human malignant disorders involving the leptomeninges and it is considered a relatively specific finding for this condition (Chamberlain, 1995).

Measurement of various electrolytes and enzymes in CSF has been reported. Their interpretation may be limited because of increases associated with altered blood-brain barrier permeability, concurrent evaluation of serum values, low benefit for cost, and poor correlation or specificity for particular pathologic processes or conditions (Chrisman, 1992; Cook and DeNicola, 1988; Parent and Rand, 1994).

Aerobic and anaerobic bacterial cultures are recommended for all CSF samples with degenerated neutrophils or when bacteria are identified cytologically.

Nevertheless, the CSF culture rarely assist in the identification of microorganisms: in a series of 8 confirmed cases of canine bacterial meningoencephalomyelitis, the CSF culture was positive in only 1 sample and the cultured bacteria was *Corynebacterium* spp. (Radaelli and Platt, 2002). Several factors likely contribute to poor culture performance in veterinary medicine —e.g., small volumes of CSF are collected for culture, the organisms are mostly confined to the brain parenchyma, some organisms are slow growing or require nonstandard culture techniques, and animal has received antibiotic therapy before sampling (Fenner, 1998).

Staphylococcus, Streptococcus, Klebsiella, Escherichia coli and *Pasteurella* are aerobic bacteria that may cause CNS infection; *Fusobacterium, Bacteroides, Peptostreptococcus, Clostridium,* and *Eubacterium* are anaerobic species that have been reported.

The immunophenotype of cerebrospinal fluid mononuclear cells in the dog has been examined (Duque et al., 2002). According to authors, the main advantage of standardized immunophenotyping is having a more objective classification of mononuclear cells compared with the relative inconsistency of this classification when based solely on microscopic appearance.

Cytologic Evaluation of CSF

Cytologic evaluation of CSF is recommended for all collections as a valuable part of CSF evaluation. When necessary, clinicians are asked to rank tests in order of preference if less than 1-mL total volume is submitted. Usually, cell counts and total protein concentration are requested, followed by cytology. If additional CSF is available, other tests may be requested, depending on the differential diagnoses suggested by clinical signs, presentation, history, imaging studies, and results of cell counts, protein, and cytologic evaluation. Rand (1995) indicates that the most useful diagnostic tests in decreasing order are nucleated cell and erythrocyte counts, sedimentation cytology, protein concentration, and cytocentrifuge cytology.

Methods of Cytologic Preparation

Standardization of the volume used for cytologic evaluation may be of benefit in minimizing analytic variation and aid in interpretation, although evaluation of multiple preparations or preparations from larger volumes of CSF may increase the likelihood of detection of minor abnormalities. Because CSF is normally of low cellularity and increases in cellularity may not result in large numbers of cells, concentration of the cells is required. Cytocentrifugation, sedimentation, or membrane filtration techniques may be used for concentration of cells.

Cytocentrifugation is most commonly available in reference or commercial laboratories in which the volume of submissions justifies purchase of specialized equipment. The membrane filtration technique requires special staining that is not commonly available in practice, but which may be available at some reference or commercial laboratories. Several sedimentation techniques have been described and are suitable for use in practice or commercial or reference laboratories to which rapid submission of CSF specimens is possible (Cook and DeNicola, 1988; Parent and Rand, 1994). Readers are referred to these sources for more detail on construction of a sedimentation apparatus and preparation of sedimentation specimens. A sample device is demonstrated in Fig. 14-2A&B.

Sedimentation preparations should be made if a specimen cannot be delivered immediately to the laboratory for cytologic processing. Prepared slides can then be sent to a commercial or reference laboratory for interpretation or stained and evaluated by clinicians at the practice.

Cytocentrifuge or sedimentation preparations are most commonly air-dried and stained with Romanowsky stains that are commonly available in commercial or reference laboratories and clinical practice laboratories. Membrane-filtration specimens require wet-fixation and stains appropriate for this method, commonly Papanicolaou, Trichrome, or H & E. Wet-fixation and these staining methods may also be used on cytocentrifuge or

sedimentation preparations and are appropriate for formalin- or alcohol-fixed specimens. Cytocentrifuge or membrane-filtration preparatory and staining techniques may vary with laboratory, technical training, and pathologist preference. Summaries of cytopreparatory and staining techniques for cytospin and membrane filtration specimens and specimens fixed in formalin or alcohol are available from a variety of sources. Interested readers are referred to Keebler and Facik (2008) as a recent comprehensive review.

Special stains may be indicated in some cases. Gram stain may be useful for confirmation and identification of categories of bacteria. India ink or new methylene blue preparations have been reported to be helpful in identification of fungal infections, especially cryptococcosis. Periodic acid-Schiff stain may be used to demonstrate positive intracellular material in dogs with globoid cell leukodystrophy. Luxol fast blue can be used to demonstrate myelin in CSF specimens (Mesher et al., 1996).

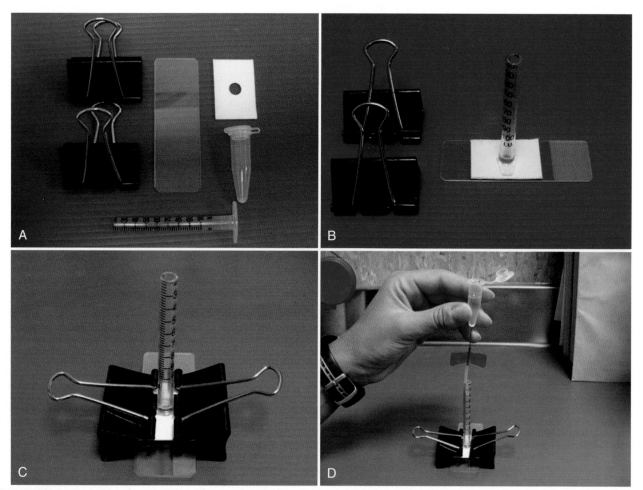

■ **FIGURE 14-2. A-D, In-house CSF sedimentation device. A,** Unassembled sedimentation device with materials needed including 1 mL modified insulin syringe barrel, filter paper with hole punched, glass slide, two binder clips, and Eppendorf tube for CSF collection. **B,** Partially assembled sedimentation device. **C,** Assembled sedimentation device demonstrating the attachment of the binder clips to the barrel flanged portions. **D,** The tube made from the syringe barrel is filled with as little as 100 µl CSF by transfer pipette or as the figure demonstrates using a Butterfly needle. The added fluid is allowed to sit undisturbed for 1 hour. Cells concentrate and settle on to the exposed area of the glass slide.

Cytologic Features of CSF

Several reviews of differential diagnoses and features of normal and abnormal cytology of canine and feline CSF with photomicrographs are available (Baker and Lumsden, 2000; Desnoyers et al., 2008). Cytologic features that may be found in canine and feline CSF are summarized in Table 14-2. Differential diagnoses associated with abnormal CSF findings are summarized in Table 14-3.

Cytologic Features of Normal CSF

Normal CSF from healthy dogs and cats contains primarily mononuclear cells (Fig. 14-3) and is indicated to be a mixture of lymphocytes and large mononuclear (monocytoid) cells. The percentages of lymphocytes and monocytoid cells may vary with the method used for cytologic preparations, but lymphocytes are reported to be the predominant nucleated cell type in normal canine and feline CSF. However, Parent and Rand (1994) report monocytoid cells as the predominant type in normal CSF from healthy cats. They indicate monocytoid cells compose 69% to 100% of the nucleated cells, lymphocytes 0% to 27%, neutrophils 0% to 9% macrophages 0% to 3%, and eosinophils 0% to less than 1% of nucleated cells. Occasional neutrophils or eosinophils as within normal limits may be present as long as these cell types do not represent more than 10% or 1% of the nucleated cells, respectively. Low numbers of mature, nondegenerate neutrophils are occasionally seen in normal CSF from healthy dogs and cats and that rare eosinophils may be present. Occasional choroid plexus cells, ependymal cells, meningeal lining cells, or mitotic figures may be seen in normal CSF from dogs or cats (Chrisman, 1992; Rand, 1995).

Accidental Puncture Contaminants

Christopher (1992) described bone marrow elements as contaminants in canine CSF associated with bone marrow aspiration during lumbar cistern collections of CSF. These may not have been from bone marrow aspiration but possibly from a site of extramedullary hematopoiesis as was discovered in five dogs with hematopoietic elements within the interstitium of the choroid plexus at the level of the 4th ventricle (Bienzle et al., 1995). Myelin-like material, neurons (Fig. 14-4A), and neuropil (Fig. 14-4B) have been reported as contaminants of canine CSF associated with accidental puncture of the spinal cord during cerebellomedullary cistern collection (Fallin et al., 1996) because of the absence of significant neurologic deficits in the patient.

CSF Presentation and Interpretation

Normal CSF Findings in the Presence of Disease

No abnormalities may be detected in CSF in many cases of neurologic disease, although some animals with the same conditions may have abnormalities detected in CSF. CSF abnormality is not detected in the majority of cases of idiopathic epilepsy, congenital hydrocephalus, intoxication, metabolic or functional disorders, vertebral disease, or myelomalacia. A significant proportion of cases with neurologic disease due to feline infectious peritonitis, distemper encephalitis, neoplasia, or GME may have CSF that is within normal limits. In a series of 17 dogs with neurologic symptoms due to spinal arachnoid cysts, CSF analysis was unremarkable (Skeen et al., 2003). Absence of cytologic abnormality does not rule out the possibility of neurologic disease not reflected in the CSF.

Protein Abnormalities in CSF

Elevated total protein may occur in the absence of cytologic abnormalities and may be referred to as "albuminocytologic dissociation." Elevated total protein as the sole abnormality or in combination with increases in nucleated cell count and/or cytologic abnormality in CSF may occur with inflammatory, degenerative, compressive, or neoplastic disease (Carmichael, 1998). Elevated protein may occur in association with increased permeability of the blood-brain barrier, local necrosis, interruption of normal CSF flow and absorption, or intrathecal globulin production (Chrisman, 1992). Elevated CSF protein without increases in CSF nucleated cell count has been reported with viral nonsuppurative encephalomyelitis, or with neoplasia, acute spinal cord injury, and compressive spinal cord lesions. In the cat, CSF protein concentration may provide some help in categorizing disease groups as markedly elevated protein concentrations should increase the index of suspicion only for feline infectious peritonitis (Singh et al., 2005). In a series of 56 cases of canine intracranial meningiomas, increased total protein concentration, in the presence of a normal total nucleated cell count, was detected in 16 (30%) dogs (Dickinson et al., 2006). Elevated total protein without pleocytosis may occur with neoplasia, ischemic myelopathy, postseizure activity, fever, disc extrusion, degenerative myelopathy (Clemmons, 1991), myelomalacia, or GME.

Increased Cell Type Percentages without Increased Total Nucleated Cell Counts

Increased percentages of either neutrophils or eosinophils may occur without an increase in the total white cell count in a variety of neurologic disorders. If blood contamination is ruled out, increased neutrophil percentages greater than 10% to 20% and eosinophil percentages greater than 1% should be considered unusual. Increased neutrophils may indicate mild or early inflammation, a lesion that does not contact the meninges or ependymal cells, or previous use of drugs such as glucocorticoids and antibiotics, which reduce the inflammatory response. Conditions to consider include degenerative intervertebral disc disease, spinal fractures, or cerebrovascular disorders such as infarcts. Increased eosinophils without increased total white blood cell (WBC) count may occur with parasite migration or protozoal disease (Desnoyers et al., 2008).

Pleocytosis

Increases in the total nucleated cell count of the CSF is termed *pleocytosis,* which is further defined by the predominant cell type, that is, neutrophilic, eosinophilic,

Text continued on p. 336

TABLE 14-2   Cytologic Features of Cerebrospinal Fluid in Dogs and Cats

Cell or Feature	Description	Significance
Lymphocytes	Morphologically similar to those in peripheral blood; 9-15 μm in diameter, scant to moderate, pale basophilic cytoplasm with round to ovoid, slightly indented nucleus	Predominant cell type in normal CSF from healthy dogs; present in normal CSF from healthy cats
Reactive lymphocytes	Morphologically similar to those in peripheral blood; greater amount of cytoplasm and more deeply basophilic cytoplasm than normal lymphocytes; may see prominent perinuclear clear zones and coarse chromatin patterns	Not present in normal CSF from healthy animals, but not specific for underlying condition
Monocytoid cells	Large mononuclear cell; 12-15 μm diameter; moderate amount, pale basophilic, often finely foamy cytoplasm; nuclear shape variable to amoeboid; chromatin pattern open to lacy	Present in CSF from healthy animals in low numbers
Activated monocytoid cells	Morphologically resemble macrophages in many sites; larger than "normal" monocytoid cells (>12-15 μm diameter); increased amount of cytoplasm that is often paler than normal and possibly vacuolated; nuclei become round to oval and eccentric; chromatin with increased coarseness	Activation associated with irritation, inflammation, or degenerative processes; often phagocytic; reported in cats to be commonly associated with extensive necrosis
Neutrophils	Morphologically similar to those in peripheral blood; polymorphonuclear leukocytes	May be present in low numbers (up to 25% of total nucleated cells) in normal CSF from healthy animals
Ependymal lining cells	Uniform, round to cuboidal mononuclear cells; individual cells or in cohesive clusters; eccentric, round nuclei; uniformly granular to coarse chromatin; moderate amount of finely granular cytoplasm	May be present in normal CSF from healthy animals in low numbers; not consistently present in normal or abnormal conditions
Choroid plexus cells	Indistinguishable from ependymal lining cells (see above description)	May be present in normal CSF from healthy animals in low numbers; not consistently present in normal or abnormal conditions
Subarachnoid lining cells/ leptomeningeal cells	Mononuclear cells with moderate to abundant pale basophilic cytoplasm; round to oval eccentric nuclei; uniform, delicate chromatin pattern; indistinct cytoplasm margins; single or in small clusters	May be present in normal CSF from healthy animals in low numbers; not consistently present in normal or abnormal conditions
Hematopoietic cells	Morphologically similar to those in bone marrow or other locations	Myeloid and erythroid precursors and erythroblastic island reported as contaminants of canine CSF with lumbar collections
Eosinophils	Morphologically similar to those in peripheral blood; polymorphonuclear leukocytes with eosinophilic granules with shape characteristic for species	Occasionally cells seen in normal CSF from healthy dogs or cats; may be seen as a nonspecific part of an active inflammatory response; also consider parasitic, hypersensitivity, or neoplastic processes (primary or metastatic)
Plasma cells	Morphologically similar to those in other locations; eccentric nuclei with prominent chromatin ("clockface" pattern); moderately abundant cytoplasm, moderately to deeply basophilic with perinuclear clear zone (Golgi apparatus)	Not present in normal CSF from healthy dogs or cats; may be part of nonspecific reactive or inflammatory process with response to antigenic stimulation
Bacteria	Morphology varies with type, may include cocci, rods of various sizes, coccobacilli, or filamentous forms	Not present in normal CSF from healthy dogs or cats; may be contaminants if collection process or tube are not sterile or if CSF collected close to death; pathologic role likely if suppurative meningitis is present and supported by intracellular location
Neural tissue	Nerve cells morphologically similar to those in nervous tissue; very large cell with prominent nucleolus, abundant cytoplasm, and three to four tentacle-like cytoplasmic processes; neuropil/myelin represented by amorphous, acellular background material	Reported as contaminant in canine CSF associated with accidental puncture of spinal cord; myelin fragments may be associated with demyelination
Paracellular coiled "ribbons"	Coiled, homogeneous, basophilic material within phagocytic vacuoles	Reported in CSF obtained at postmortem; hypothesized to represent denatured myelin, myelin figures, or myelin fragments
Neoplastic cells	Abnormal cell type or number for location (benign tumors) or atypical features fulfilling criteria for malignancy (malignant tumors); morphology may vary with cell type of origin and degree of differentiation	May be primary or metastatic; presence requires communication with subarachnoid space or ventricles; absence of tumor does not rule out its presence without contribution of cells to the CSF

TABLE 14-2 Cytologic Features of Cerebrospinal Fluid in Dogs and Cats—cont'd

Cell or Feature	Description	Significance
Fungi/Yeast/Protozoa	Appearance varies with type; may be primary or opportunistic infections	Characteristic morphology associated with various common pathologic organisms; demonstration of organisms in conjunction with clinical signs and results of other testing increases confidence in diagnosis of fungal or protozoal disease
Mitotic Figures	Recognized by characteristic nuclear configurations of cells undergoing mitosis; cell type of origin not identifiable during the mitotic cycle	Rare mitotic figures reported in normal CSF from healthy animals; presence indicates proliferative process, often neoplasia

TABLE 14-3 Differential Diagnoses Associated with Cytologic Features of Inflammation in the CSF

Cytologic Features	Special Considerations or Differential Diagnoses	Comments
Slight to moderate neutrophilic inflammation 25% to 50% neutrophils, with or without elevated CSF protein, with or without pleocytosis	Bacterial, fungal, protozoal, parasitic, rickettsial, or viral infection Neoplasia Other noninfectious conditions	Depends on species, type of infection, focal or diffuse involvement, presence of concurrent necrosis; presence of protozoa or fungi/yeast organisms or intracellular bacteria confirms diagnosis Depends on type of neoplasm, location, presence of concurrent necrosis Neoplastic cells rarely seen in CSF Consider traumatic, degenerative, immune-mediated, associated with metabolic conditions, ischemia
Marked neutrophilic inflammation (suppurative meningitis) Predominance of neutrophils (>50%), often with increased CSF protein	Bacterial infection Severe viral encephalitis Necrotizing vasculitis Steroid-responsive meningitis-arteritis Postmyelography reaction (usually within 24-48 hrs) Neoplasms Trauma Hemorrhage Acquired hydrocephalus	May be focal (abscess) or diffuse (meningoencephalomyelitis); intracellular bacterial confirms diagnosis Especially feline infectious peritonitis (FIP) in cats May have immune-mediated or infectious basis; Bernese Mountain Dogs and Beagles Responsive to glucocorticoids but must rule out infectious causes History of recent, previous myelography Especially meningiomas, but may occur with any neoplasm, especially if associated with necrosis History may be supportive, if trauma was observed History may be supportive; may have traumatic, degenerative, metabolic infectious, neoplastic, or other underlying cause May depend on underlying cause of acquired condition
Mixed cell inflammation with a variety of cell types (no single cell type predominant) Mixture of macrophages, lymphocytes, neutrophils, and sometimes plasma cells, with or without elevated CSF protein, with or without pleocytosis	Often interpreted to represent granulomatous inflammation—consider fungal, protozoal, parasitic, or rickettsial infection Some idiopathic inflammatory or degenerative diseases Inadequately treated chronic bacterial infections or early response to antibacterial treatment	Presence of fungal or protozoal organisms is confirmatory Especially granulomatous meningoencephalomyelitis (GME) History and previous diagnosis helpful
Nonsuppurative inflammation (mononuclear pleocytosis) Pleocytosis with predominance of mononuclear cells, especially lymphocytes	Viral, bacterial, fungal, protozoal, parasitic, or rickettsial infection Necrotizing encephalitis of small-breed dogs Neoplasia Noninfectious or degenerative conditions	Especially non-FIP viral meningoencephalomyelitis in cats and canine distemper infection in dogs Signalment and lymphocytic predominance helpful in diagnosis but definitive diagnosis requires histopathology; not responsive to glucocorticoids Neoplastic cells may rarely be seen in CSF Consider GME; may require elimination of other possible causes and consideration of multiple factors to arrive at a clinical diagnosis
Eosinophilic inflammation Pleocytosis with predominance of eosinophils	Parasitic, protozoal, bacterial, viral, or rickettsial infections Neoplasia Hypersensitivity reaction Inflammatory process	Uncommon manifestation reported with a variety of types of disease Occasionally seen with neoplasia Consider vaccine reactions or other hypersensitivity components associated with infectious or noninfectious origin May be seen as part of a nonspecific inflammatory process

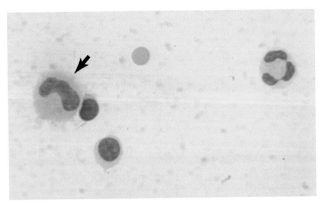

■ FIGURE 14-3. Cell types found in CSF. Dog. Two small mononuclear cells (lymphocytes), one large mononuclear (monocytoid) at *(arrow)*, one nondegenerate neutrophil, and one erythrocyte are present. (Wright-Giemsa; HP oil.)

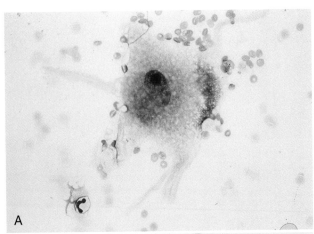

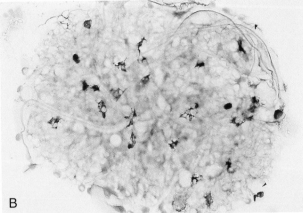

■ FIGURE 14-4. A, Neuron. CSF. Dog. Accidental puncture of nervous tissue during collection at the cerebellomedullary cistern demonstrating the large size of the neuron compared with a neutrophil and erythrocytes. Basophilic granular material within the neuronal cell cytoplasm is presumed to be Nissl bodies. (Wright-Giemsa; HP oil.) **B, Nervous tissue with microglial cells. Dog.** CSF from the same case of a dog with cervical pain as in A. (Wright-Giemsa; HP oil.) (A, From Fallin CW, Raskin RE, Harvey JW: Cytologic identification of neural tissue in the cerebrospinal fluid of two dogs, *Vet Clin Pathol* 25:127-29, 1996.)

mononuclear, or mixed cell pleocytosis. Pleocytosis is graded as mild (6 to 50 cells/µl in dogs and cats), moderate (51 to 200 cells/µl and 51 to 1000 cells/µl, in dogs and cats, respectively), or marked (>200 cells/µl and >1000 cells/µl, in dogs and cats, respectively) (Chrisman, 1992; Singh, 2005).

Neutrophilic Pleocytosis

Neutrophilic pleocytosis has been associated with a wide variety of active inflammatory disorders, including trauma, postmyelographic aseptic meningitis, fibrocartilagineus embolic myelopathy, myelomalacia, hemorrhage, neoplasia, and mycotic and bacterial meningitis (Mariani et al., 2002; Mikszewski et al., 2006). It may be seen with abscesses communicating with the ventricles or subarachnoid space, early viral infections, feline infectious peritonitis, Rocky Mountain spotted fever, discospondylitis, acquired hydrocephalus, necrosis, or GME. Marked neutrophilic pleocytosis is most often found with bacterial or fungal meningoencephalitis, neoplasia (Fig. 14-5), steroid-responsive meningitis, or necrotizing vasculitis (Chrisman, 1992). Demonstration of bacteria, fungi, yeast, or protozoa in CSF can confirm the presence of these infections. A variety of bacterial types—*Cryptococcus, Blastomyces, Histoplasma, Neospora caninum,* and ehrlichial organisms—have been demonstrated in CSF (Gaitero et al., 2006; Singh et al., 2005). Parasites such as *Toxocara canis, Dirofilaria immitis, Cuterebra* larva, or *Cysticercus* that may cause neurologic disease have not been reported to be seen in CSF cytology preparations. The presence of marked neutrophilic pleocytosis or increasing numbers of neutrophils in sequential CSF collections has been reported to be an unfavorable prognostic finding. Neoplasia should be considered as the most likely diagnosis in a cat more than 7 years of age with progressive clinical neurologic signs of greater than 4 weeks' duration (Rand et al., 1994).

Feline infectious peritonitis (FIP), a coronavirus infection, is a common cause of neutrophilic pleocytosis in the cat (Fig. 14-6A&B). The main neurologic signs are

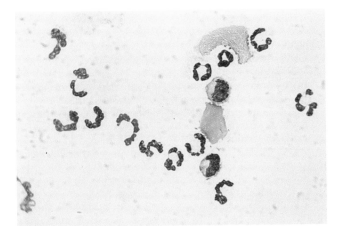

■ FIGURE 14-5. Neutrophilic pleocytosis. CSF. Dog. Nucleated cell count was 1018/µl and 240 mg/dl protein with a history of head tilt and hemiplegia related to a cranial meningioma. Nondegenerate neutrophils composed 83% of the cell population. (Wright-Giemsa; HP oil.)

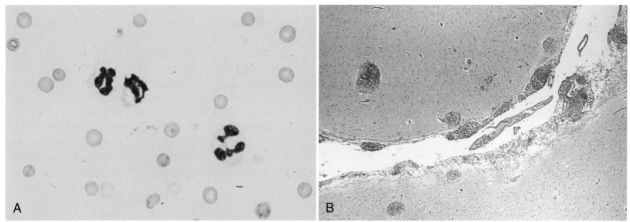

■ **FIGURE 14-6. Neutrophilic pleocytosis. CSF. Cat. Same case A-B. A,** This direct smear is made from fluid from a kitten with 5-day duration of ataxia. A high nucleated cell count supported use of a direct smear to evaluate leukocytes. The case was diagnosed as FIP by positive titer and histologic examination. Numerous erythrocytes and several nondegenerate neutrophils characterize the cells present. Acute hemorrhage was evident but is not demonstrated in this field. (Wright, HP oil) **B,** Section of midbrain and third ventricle demonstrating multifocal perivascular infiltrates in a cat with FIP. The proximity of the infiltrates to the ventricle contributed to the neutrophilic pleocytosis. (H & E; LP.)

depression, tetraparesis, head tilt, nystagmus, and intention tremor (Baroni and Heinold, 1995). It accounted for 44% of 61 feline cases of inflammatory CNS disease (Rand et al., 1994). Parent and Rand (1994) indicate that marked neutrophilic pleocytosis with a nucleated count of more than 100 cells/µl and neutrophils greater than 50% is commonly seen with FIP, along with increased CSF protein (usually greater than 200 mg/dl). They indicate a high probability of FIP if a cat is less than 4 years of age and shows multifocal neurologic signs referable to the cerebellum and/or brainstem, protracted course of illness, and CSF protein greater than 200 mg/dl. Later

in the course of the disease, a mixed cellular population may be found with large mononuclear cells and lymphocytes present to a significant degree (Fig. 14-7A&B). Similar results were found by Singh and others (2005) in a series of 11 cats with FIP. CSF analysis in that study was characterized as suppurative in seven cats, mixed in one, and mononuclear in three. Five cats had marked elevations in the CSF white cells count (>1000 cells/µl), three cats had moderate elevations (51 to 1000 calls/µl), two cats had mild elevations (6 to 50 cells/µl), and one cat had insufficient sample for a white cells count.

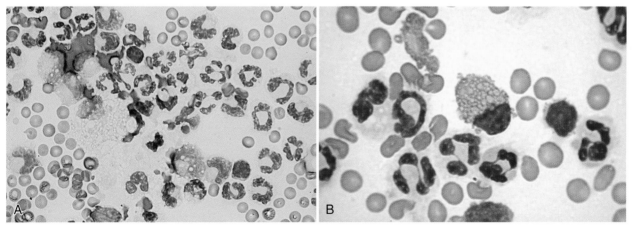

■ **FIGURE 14-7. Mixed cell pleocytosis with neutrophilic predominance. CSF. Cat. A,** Increased numbers of large mononuclear cells consistent with macrophages were present in a cat with fever, high titers for FIP, and histopathologic support of FIP at necropsy. Duration of disease was several months, accounting for the more mononuclear response than the case in Fig. 14-6. (Wright-Giemsa; HP oil.) **B,** Chronicity of infection with FIP is suggested by the presence of plasma cells indicated by the Mott cell (center). Nondegenerate cells and erythrocytes are also seen. Plasma cells are not seen in the CSF of healthy animals but rather in viral infections and tumors. (MGG; HP oil.) (A, Courtesy of Rick Alleman, University of Florida.)

Only 11 of 19 cats in one study (Baroni and Heinold, 1995) demonstrated high serum antibody titers, indicating that CSF analysis was essential for a correct diagnosis. Non-FIP viral meningoencephalitis that involved 37% of the inflammatory cases reported by Rand et al. (1994) was considered most likely with cats less than 3 years of age having progressive neurologic disease and focal neurologic signs referable to the thalamocortex. In these cases, the nucleated cell count was less than 50 cells/μl and CSF protein was less than 100 mg/dl. Non-FIP viral meningoencephalitis usually carries a favorable prognosis for recovery.

Steroid-responsive suppurative meningitis-arteritis (Fig. 14-8) has been recognized in young to middle-aged dogs that present with signs of fever, cervical pain, hyperesthesia, and paresis. CSF pleocytosis is often greater than 500 cells/μl with greater than 75% nondegenerate neutrophils if glucocorticoids have not been recently administered (Chrisman, 1992). Bacteria are not observed or cultured and improvement is often seen within 72 hours following glucocorticoid administration; long-term prognosis is good. One report investigated the immunologic response in these cases finding IgG and IgA synthesis intrathecally and suggested the humoral response is primary, rather than the result of a generalized immune complex disease (Tipold et al., 1995). In another more recent paper Behr and Cauzinille (2006) evaluated clinical findings and prognosis in a series of 12 cases of aseptic suppurative meningitis in juvenile Boxers of which 10 of the dogs exhibited the acute form of the disease and had more than 100 nucleated cells/μl with neutrophils ranging from 72% to 100%. The two other dogs presented with a more chronic form that produced a mixed pleocytosis, with neutrophils about 60% of total nucleated cells. An abnormal cell count of mixed cell population or mononuclear cells in the CSF are seen in

the protracted form, and monitoring of CSF cell count in dogs with this condition seems to be a sensitive indicator of success of treatment (Cizinauskas et al., 2000).

Necrotizing vasculitis, a syndrome of aseptic suppurative meningitis in young Bernese Mountain Dogs involving the leptomeningeal arteries, has been described. Animals presented with severe cervical pain and neurologic deficits. Total WBC counts are generally greater than 1000 cells/μl, with nondegenerate neutrophils predominating. A similar condition has been reported in Beagles and sporadic cases have been described in a variety of other breeds (Caswell and Nykamp, 2003). Clinical improvement occurred with corticosteroid administration.

Bacterial meningoencephalitis (Fig. 14-9A&B) is suspected if greater than 75% neutrophils are present in

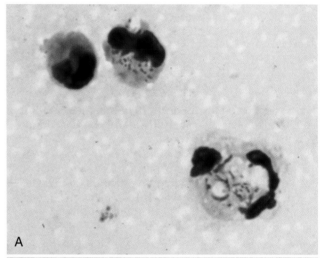

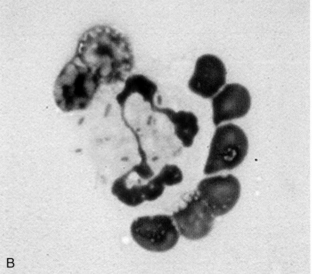

■ **FIGURE 14-9.** A, Neutrophilic pleocytosis. CSF. Cat. Direct smear of cloudy CSF indicated increased cellularity with many degenerate neutrophils present. Associated with the karyolytic neutrophils shown are intracellular, small rod-shaped bacteria that were cultured as *Enterobacter* sp. (Wright; HP oil.) **B, Septic meningoencephalitis. CSF. Bacterial infection. Cat.** Several rod bacteria are present with the cytoplasm of the neutrophil. Several erythrocytes surround the inflammatory cell. (MGG; HP oil.)

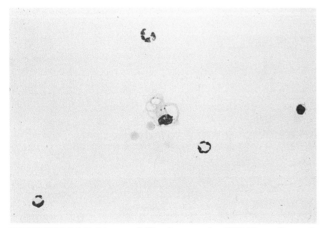

■ **FIGURE 14-8.** Neutrophilic pleocytosis. CSF. Dog. Generalized nonseptic inflammatory response in a 1-year-old dog exhibiting fever and cervical, thoracic, and lumbar pain. Nucleated cell count was 106/μl with 41 mg/dl protein and 3700 RBC/μl. Three nondegenerate neutrophils, one large mononuclear cell, and one lymphocyte are present. Multiple joints were similarly affected in this case. An immune-mediated corticosteroid-responsive meningitis was suspected. (Wright-Giemsa; HP oil.)

the CSF regardless of the total cell count. Bacteremia is usually the cause with septic emboli to the brain as a result. Untreated cases often produce marked pleocytosis with greater than 1000 cells/μl. Intracellular location of bacteria and accompanying inflammation are particularly important in eliminating the possibility of bacterial contamination associated with nonsterile collection technique or nonsterile collection tubes. Neutrophils affected may display mild to severe karyolysis.

Identification of bacteria on CSF cytology is even rarer than positive bacterial culture. Bacteria were identified by using CSF cytology in 62 of 109 (57%) adult humans, 0 of 14 (0%) dogs, and 2 of 5 (40%) cats with confirmed bacterial CNS infection (Messer et al., 2006). The difficulty of identifying bacteria in CSF often forces the clinician to rely on inflammatory changes in the CSF to make a presumptive diagnosis of bacterial CSF infection.

Eosinophilic Pleocytosis

Cerebrospinal fluid pleocytosis that is predominantly eosinophilic is rare. Increased eosinophils in CSF may be present in association with a nonspecific acute inflammatory response, but also can be seen with parasitic, hypersensitivity, neoplastic processes, protozoal infection including toxoplasmosis (Fig. 14-10A&B) and neosporosis, or *Cryptococcus* infection. Steroid-responsive meningoencephalitis with a predominance of eosinophils (Fig. 14-10C) has been described in dogs and cats (Chrisman, 1992). Sometimes migrating internal parasites, *Prototheca* infection, canine distemper virus infection, or rabies may cause eosinophilic pleocytosis (Chrisman, 1992).

Steroid-responsive eosinophilic meningitis has been reported in dogs and cats. Finding greater than 80% eosinophils with mild to marked pleocytosis present and finding no evidence of protozoal, parasitic, or fungal infection usually supports the diagnosis. In the canine study, Golden Retrievers were overrepresented, which may suggest a breed predisposition to this condition (Fig. 14-11). Animals usually respond to glucocorticoid therapy with dramatic decreases in cell numbers and changes in differential percentages. An allergic or type I hypersensitivity reaction is suspected in some cases.

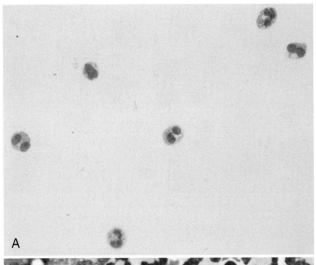

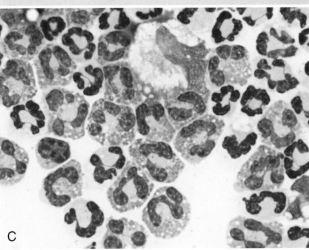

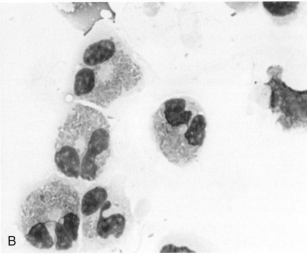

■ **FIGURE 14-10.** Eosinophilic pleocytosis. **A, Cisternal CSF. Dog.** This acutely paraparetic animal with upper motor neuron dysfunction to the rear legs was diagnosed as having toxoplasmosis by serum titer. Total WBC count was 124/μl with high normal protein. Eosinophils accounted for 98% of the cell population. Peripheral eosinophilia was not evident. (Wright-Giemsa; HP oil.) **B, Cisternal CSF. Cat.** Note the predominance of typical bi-lobate eosinophils in the cerebrospinal fluid from this case of toxoplasmosis confirmed by PCR of CSF. (MGG; HP oil.) **C, CSF. Dog.** The nucleated cell count was 125/μl and eosinophils represented 85% of the nucleated cells. Several nondegenerate neutrophils and a large, foamy macrophage are also present. The final diagnosis was eosinophilic steroid-responsive meningoencephalitis. (MGG; HP oil.)

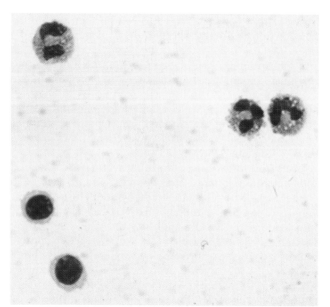

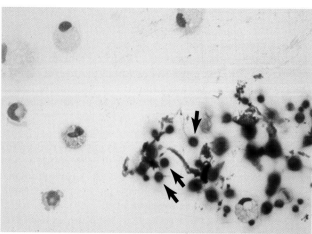

■ **FIGURE 14-12. Cryptococcosis with mononuclear pleocytosis. CSF. Dog.** Clusters of basophilic-staining extracellular yeast forms measuring approximately 10 to 20 μm in diameter are present. Three yeast forms are indicated by arrows. The fluid contained a total nucleated cell count of 60/μl of which 85% were mononuclear phagocytes. Several mononuclear cells are pictured that have abundant foamy to vacuolated pale cytoplasm indicating reactivity. (Wright-Giemsa; HP oil.)

■ **FIGURE 14-11. Eosinophilic pleocytosis. CSF. Dog.** This sample is from a Golden Retriever whose CSF cell count was 43/μl and whose protein was 77 mg/dl. The cell differential indicated 43% eosinophils, 50% lymphocytes, and 7% large mononuclear phagocytes. Three eosinophils and two small lymphocytes are shown. An idiopathic eosinophilic meningoencephalitis associated with this breed was suspected. (Wright-Giemsa; HP oil.)

Mononuclear Pleocytosis

Mononuclear pleocytosis of CSF usually presents with increased lymphocytes in viral, protozoal, or fungal infection, uremia, intoxication, vaccine reaction, GME, and discospondylitis. It may be seen with necrotizing encephalitis, steroid-responsive meningoencephalomyelitis, ehrlichiosis, or treated bacterial meningoencephalitis. However, monocytoid/macrophage cells may also predominate in these conditions and most commonly with cryptococcosis (Figs. 14-12 and 14-13). Mononuclear pleocytosis was noted in two cats with cuterebriasis (Glass et al., 1998) and in another cat with cerebral cholesterol granuloma (Fluhemann et al., 2006). The appearance of CSF macrophages containing vacuoles and pink-purple amorphous granular material in a young cat with mononuclear pleocytosis, elevated protein content, seizures, incoordination, and tremors indicated the presence of a lysosomal storage disease (GM_2-gangliosidosis) (Johnsrude et al., 1996). A recent report of necrotizing meningoencephalitis in a young miniature Poodle demonstrated the predominance and pleocytosis of large granular lymphocytes (Garma-Aviña and Tyler, 1999). The most frequent noninflammatory neurologic diseases of the CNS in the cat are neoplasia and ischemic encephalopathy, which usually present with an elevated CSF protein and slight lymphocytic pleocytosis or normal nucleated cell counts (Rand et al., 1994). Hemorrhagic conditions may be accompanied by a mononuclear pleocytosis composed of foamy macrophages (Fig. 14-14A&B). Mononuclear cells may take on changes that are nonspecific

Necrotizing encephalitis in small breed dogs (Figs. 14-17 and 14-18A–D)—Pugs, Maltese, Shih Tzus, French

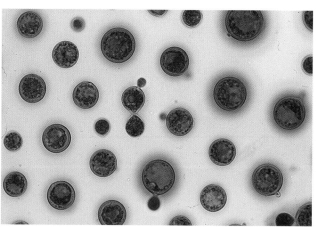

■ **FIGURE 14-13. Cryptococcosis. CSF. Dog.** These spherical organisms display frequent budding. (New methylene blue; HP oil.) (Courtesy of Rick Alleman, University of Florida.)

Bulldogs, and Yorkshire Terriers—is reported to demonstrate multifocal to massive necrosis and nonsuppurative inflammation of the cerebrum and meninges that is fatal or leads to euthanasia (Uchida et al., 1999; Stalis et al., 1995; Timmann et al., 2007; Tipold et al., 1993). These dogs are usually less than 4 years of age and present frequently with seizures, depression, and ataxia; they do not respond significantly to glucocorticoids. The CSF presents with mild to moderate pleocytosis, generally greater than 200 cells/μl, and these are predominantly lymphocytes, generally greater than 70%. CSF protein concentration is often greater than 50 mg/dl. The cause is considered unknown but some Pugs appear to exhibit an autoantibody against astrocytes that has been detected in the CSF by indirect immunofluorescence assay, confirming an immune-mediated syndrome. A similar

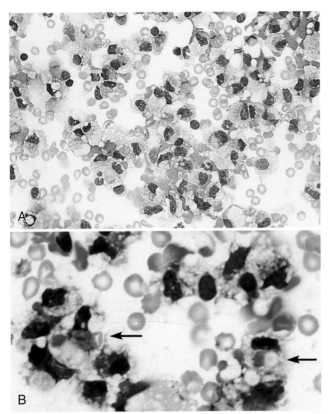

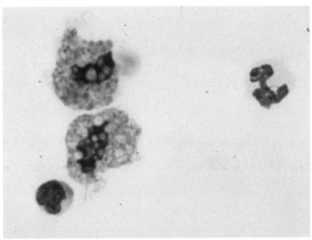

■ **FIGURE 14-16. Granular large mononuclear phagocytes. CSF. Dog.** Highly granulated and phagocytic-appearing cells in a case of suspected granulomatous meningoencephalomyelitis. (Wright-Giemsa; HP oil.) (Courtesy of Rick Alleman, University of Florida.)

■ **FIGURE 14-14. Acute hemorrhage with mononuclear pleocytosis. CSF. Dog. A,** This animal had a history of seizures and dementia. Nucleated cell count was 190/μl and protein 72 mg/dl. Mononuclear phagocytes accounted for 91% of the cell population. (Wright-Giemsa, HP oil) **B,** Same case as A. Several vacuolated, phagocytic macrophages with engulfed erythrocytes (*arrows*) are shown. (Wright-Giemsa; HP oil.)

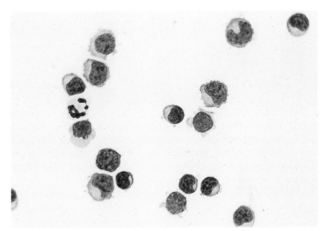

■ **FIGURE 14-17. Lymphocytic pleocytosis. CSF. Dog.** This example of Pug encephalitis is characterized by pleocytosis (265 cells/μl) with lymphocytic predominance (87%). Lymphocytes shown are small to medium size with normal morphology. (Wright-Giemsa; HP oil.)

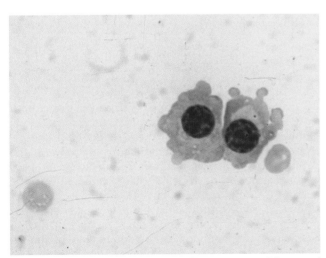

■ **FIGURE 14-15. Flaming plasma cells. CSF. Dog.** High-normal nucleated cell count and increased protein (361 mg/dl) were present in a suspected case of granulomatous meningoencephalomyelitis. The term "flaming" is used to describe the red-pink periphery of the cytoplasm. (Wright-Giemsa; HP oil.)

population of cells may be found in the CSF in GME necessitating a histologic examination of the brain to detect the necrotizing lesions.

Granulomatous meningoencephalomyelitis (GME) (Fig. 14-19) is an idiopathic inflammatory disease of the CNS in primarily young to middle-aged female dogs (Sorjonen, 1990). A study of 42 dogs found a high percentage of affected animals were toy or terrier breeds (Munana and Luttgen, 1998). Clinical signs of fever, ataxia, tetraparesis, cervical hyperesthesia, and seizures have been reported. Designation of the clinical signs into focal or multifocal was helpful in determining prognosis, with dogs having focal clinical signs surviving longer. Lesions are histologically found in both white and gray matter of the brain and predominantly the white matter of the caudal brainstem and spinal cord. The CSF may have a mild to moderate lymphocytic,

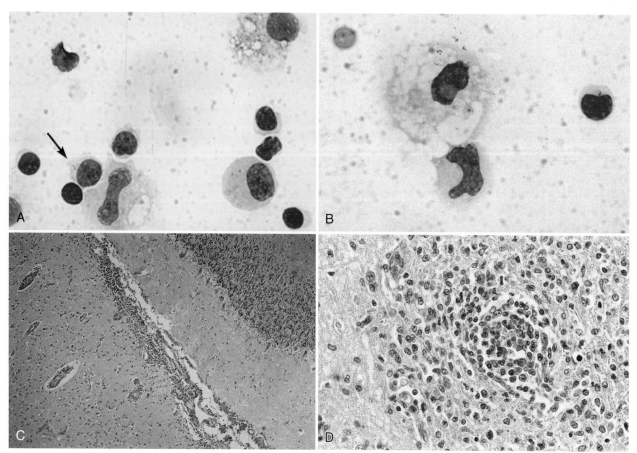

■ **FIGURE 14-18. Lymphocytic pleocytosis. CSF. Dog. Same case A-D. A,** This 6-year-old Maltese presented with acute seizures that were unresponsive to glucocorticoids and anticonvulsants. Fluid indicated total nucleated cell count of 430/µl and 3+ protein on chemistry dipstick. Lymphocytes accounted for 82%, large mononuclear cells 11%, and nondegenerate neutrophils 7% of the cell population. Shown are many lymphocytes, one of which is a granular lymphocyte *(arrow)* and three large mononuclear cells demonstrating various nuclear shapes and cytoplasmic features. (Wright-Giemsa; HP oil.) **B,** Mononuclear pleocytosis is evident in this field with two large mononuclear cells, one of which displays marked cytoplasmic vacuolization consistent with demyelination. One granular lymphocyte and one erythrocyte are also present. (Wright-Giemsa; HP oil.) **C,** Maltese with nonsuppurative necrotizing meningoencephalitis. Dense accumulations of mononuclear cells along the meninges extend into the parenchyma. There is gliosis and neuronal necrosis evident in the parenchyma. (H&E; LP.) **D,** Severe, focally extensive, perivascular meningoencephalitis. Cells present consist mostly of lymphocytes and plasma cells, with smaller numbers of large mononuclear phagocytes. (H&E; HP oil.)

mixed cell pleocytosis, or occasionally neutrophilic predominance (Chrisman, 1992). Nucleated cell counts had a median of 250 cells/µl (range 0 to 11,840) with the majority having counts greater than 100 cells/µl (Munana and Luttgen, 1998). In this same study, dogs with multifocal signs all had pleocytosis, whereas some of the dogs with focal signs had normal cell counts. The predominant cell type was lymphocytic (52%), monocytic (21%), neutrophilic (10%), and mixed cell (17%). CSF protein is variably elevated, with a mean value of 256 mg/dl (range 13 to 1119) as reported by Bailey and Higgins (1986). Differentiation must be made from infectious diseases and idiopathic necrotizing encephalitis, all of which may appear similar cytologically. Electrophoretic separation of CSF proteins in GME has shown increases in the alpha and beta globulin fractions (Sorjonen, 1990); however, these fractions are generally

decreased in canine distemper (Chrisman, 1992). Both GME and canine distemper may have increased gamma globulins. GME lesions involve widely disseminated perivascular, lymphocytic-granulomatous meningeal, and parenchymal infiltrates. Necrosis and demyelination are major features in necrotizing encephalitis and may be present to a minor extent in GME. GME cases with lesions that involve the caudal brainstem or spinal cord progress slowly, permitting longer survival. Radiation has been recommended as an adjunct to treatment, especially in dogs with focal clinical signs. The disease is poorly responsive to glucocorticoids, although an immune-mediated etiology has been suggested (Kipar et al., 1998). In this study, it was determined that the GME inflammatory lesions are composed of predominantly CD3 antigen–positive T-lymphocytes and a heterogeneous population of activated macrophages with

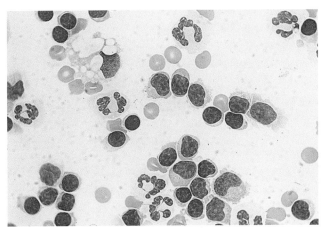

■ **FIGURE 14-19. Mixed cell pleocytosis. CSF. Dog.** This young dog presented with neck pain. Shown are numerous small and medium-sized lymphocytes (70%), several nondegenerate neutrophils (18%), and fewer numbers of large mononuclear cells (12%), one of which demonstrates large cytoplasmic vacuoles. Total WBC count was 208/μl and protein increased to 256 mg/dl. The dog died 5 days later and histopathology indicated an idiopathic condition with moderate to marked, multifocal, nonsuppurative meningoencephalitis and mild, multifocal vacuolization and neuronal necrosis. (Wright-Giemsa; HP oil.)

MHC class II expression suggesting a T-cell–mediated delayed-type hypersensitivity of an organ-specific autoimmune disease.

Canine viral infections such as *canine distemper infection* (Fig. 14-20A&B) and *rabies infection* (Fig. 14-21) each present with CSF that exhibits a lymphocytic pleocytosis. Cell counts may be variable, ranging from normal to greater than 50 cells/μl, and lymphocytes represent the predominant cell population, accounting for greater than

60% of the cells present. One report (Abate et al, 1998) indicated that the CSF in distemper cases had an increase in macrophages, an increase in total protein concentration, an increase of the gamma-globulin fraction by electrophoretic separation, and the presence of cellular inclusions. Another report from Amude et al (2006) describes a marked CSF pleocytosis (554 cells/μl) with protein content within normal limits in a 7-month-old dog with PCR-confirmed viral distemper. In this case, the nucleated cell differential count was 70% lymphocytes, 25% neutrophils, and 5% monocytes. Diagnosis of canine distemper often involves suggestive history, clinical signs, and evidence of serum or CSF IgM in response to active infection by canine distemper virus. In addition, RT-PCR on CSF is considered a useful, fast, and specific method to diagnose canine distemper virus infection (Amude et al., 2006).

Mixed Cell Pleocytosis

Pleocytosis with a mixture of cell types may be seen with a variety of underlying causes including GME, FIP, canine distemper, steroid-responsive meningoencephalomyelitis (Fig. 14-22), toxoplasmosis, neosporosis, Sarcocystosis (Fig. 14-23A–C), encephalitozoonosis, cryptococcosis, blastomycosis, aspergillosis, histoplasmosis, degenerative disc disease, ischemia, and neoplasia (Chrisman, 1992).

Neural Tissue Injury Findings

In addition to blood contamination encountered during collection, the presence of erythrocytes in a cytologic preparation may result from cranial or spinal hemorrhage. Macrophages with engulfed erythrocytes (Fig. 14-24A&B) may be seen in cases of acute spinal cord injury such as intervertebral disc herniation, neoplasia, inflammation, or degenerative conditions. Chronic hemorrhage will be indicated by the presence of hemosiderin-laden macrophages.

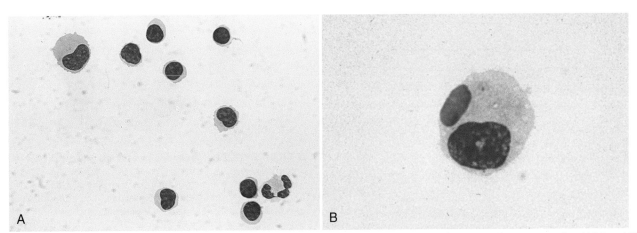

■ **FIGURE 14-20. CSF. Dog. A, Lymphocytic pleocytosis.** Pleocytosis (292 cells/μl), elevated CSF protein concentration (126 mg/dl), and lymphocyte predominance (72%) were detected in a cerebellomedullary cistern sample from a dog with acute ataxia and head tilt. Canine distemper titer levels were present in the CSF suggesting a viral-induced encephalopathy, which responded completely by 6 months with glucocorticoid therapy. Shown are numerous small lymphocytes, one neutrophil, and one large mononuclear cell. (Wright-Giemsa; HP oil.) **B, Distemper inclusion.** Eosinophilic inclusion, the homogenous oval structure above the nucleus within a large mononuclear cell, represents viral proteins from a dog diagnosed with canine distemper. (Wright-Giemsa; HP oil.) (B, From Alleman AR, Christopher MM, Steiner DA, et al: Identification of intracytoplasmic inclusion bodies in mononuclear cells from the cerebrospinal fluid of a dog with canine distemper, *Vet Pathol* 29:84-85, 1992.)

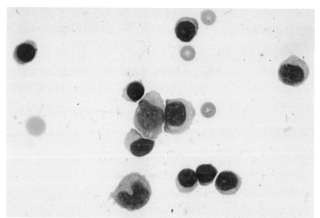

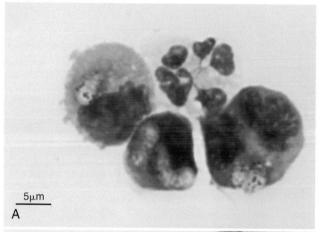

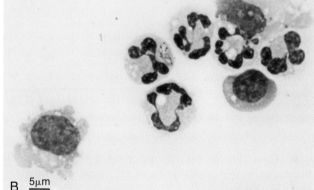

■ **FIGURE 14-21. Lymphocytic pleocytosis. Rabies infection. CSF. Dog.** Six-month-old stray presented with weakness on one hind leg that progressed over the course of a week to bilateral forelimb paresis and later seizures. The clinical presentation of a leg bite wound with cytologic appearance of CSF warranted euthanasia and subsequent diagnosis of rabies. If infectious agents are suspected, gloves and facial mask must be worn when handling diagnostic specimens and cytocentrifugation must be covered to prevent aerosolization. Note the predominance of small lymphocytes in addition to two large mononuclear cells. The nucleated cell count was 1140 cells/μl and protein 366 mg/dl in this fluid. (Wright-Giemsa; HP oil.) (Courtesy of Rose Raskin, University of Florida.)

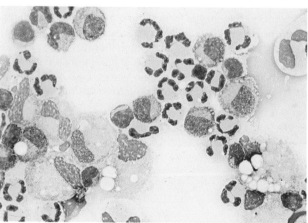

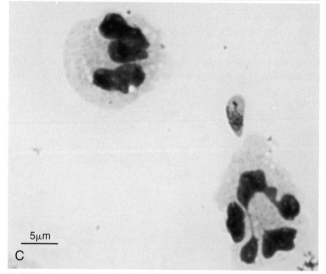

■ **FIGURE 14-22. Mixed cell pleocytosis. CSF. Dog.** This sample is from an adult female Cairn Terrier with 4-month history of neck pain and muscle spasms that were responsive to glucocorticoids. Mononuclear phagocytes (52%) were mostly reactive as indicated by a foamy or vacuolated cytoplasm and evidence of phagocytized debris. Neutrophils composed 35% and lymphocytes 13% of the total cell population. (Wright-Giemsa; HP oil.)

Homogeneous "ribbons" of basophilic material hypothesized to represent degenerated myelin, as myelin figures or myelin fragments (Figs. 14-25A&B and 14-26), have been reported in a postmortem collection of CSF from a dog (Fallin et al., 1996). Spinal cord infarction with diffuse myelomalacia in a dog resulted in the presence of foamy macrophages in the CSF (Mesher et al., 1996). Luxol fast blue staining of the amorphous eosinophilic material found within the macrophages was positive in this case,

■ **FIGURE 14-23. Mixed cell pleocytosis. Cisternal CSF. Cat. Same case A-C. A,** This shows several *Sarcocystis* sp. merozoites within the cytoplasm of three large mononuclear cells. This 5-month-old cat presented with paraparesis and pain upon palpation of the spine. PCR and gene sequencing established the specific diagnosis. (Wright; HP oil.) **B,** This shows rare containment of the *Sarcocystis* merozoite within a neutrophil. Neutrophils appear mostly nondegenerate and account for 80% of the nucleated cell population along with 11% lymphocytes and 9% large mononuclear cells. The cytocentrifuge preparation was highly cellular but insufficient fluid did not allow an accurate cell count. (Wright; HP oil.) **C,** This shows an extracellular, pear-shaped merozoite that measures approximately 2 to 3 × 5 μm (Wright; HP oil.) (A-C, Courtesy of Rose Raskin, Purdue University.)

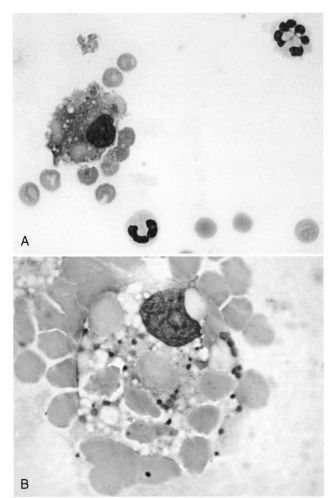

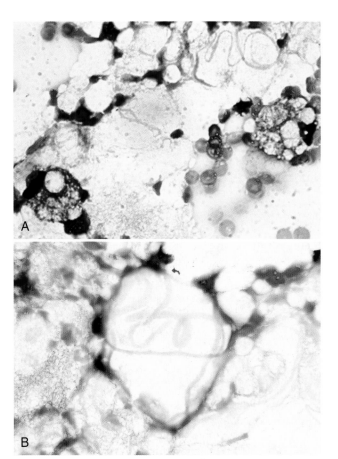

■ FIGURE 14-25. Same case A-B. A, Myelomalacia. CSF. Dog. Patient presented with acute paraplegic and absent deep pain related to a disc protrusion at LI-2. A myelogram confirmed dorsal spinal compression from T11 to L1. A cerebellomedullary cistern sample was taken 4 days postsurgery at the time of euthanasia. Pictured are two macrophages with large lipid-filled cytoplasmic vacuoles and basophilic ribbon material extracellularly. Necropsy confirmed a necrotic spinal cord in the areas shown compressed on the presurgery myelogram. (Wright-Giemsa; HP oil.) **B, Myelin figures. CSF. Dog.** Pictured are basophilic ribbon structures that likely represent phospholipids, derived from damaged cytomembranes. (Wright-Giemsa; HP oil.)

■ FIGURE 14-24. Erythrophagocytosis. CSF. Dog. A, This lumbar site collection was bloody with nucleated cells 84/µl, RBC 7000/µl, and protein 104 mg/dl. A car-related injury caused a thoracic spinal fracture that contributed to the acute hemorrhage exhibited in this example. A macrophage with engulfed red cells is present along with a hypersegmented neutrophil. (Wright-Giemsa; HP oil.) **B,** A macrophage with engulfed red cells is present and surrounded by erythrocytes. (MGG; HP oil.) (A, Courtesy of Rick Alleman, University of Florida.)

suggestive of myelin. Similar myelin-like extracellular material was found in a dog with spinal subdural hemorrhage secondary to an intervertebral disk protrusion (Bauer et al., 2006). Other demyelinating conditions such as degenerative myelopathy may present with free myelin (Fig. 14-27A&B).

Mikszewski et al. (2006) described diagnostic evaluations of five cats with myelomalacia due to fibrocartilagineus embolism. In those animals results of CSF were abnormal in four cats with neutrophilic pleocytosis detected in three cases.

Neural Cystic and Neoplastic Lesion Findings in CSF

Rare developmental defects have been demonstrated within the brain and in one case the CSF contained numerous mature squamous epithelium, consistent with an epidermoid cyst (Fig. 14-28A&B). Spinal arachnoid cysts,

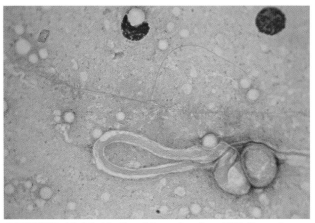

■ FIGURE 14-26. Myelin ribbon. Lumbar CSF. Dog. An eosinophilic ribbon structure is present along with two mononuclear cells. It is likely this represents phospholipids, derived from damaged membranes. (MGG; HP oil.)

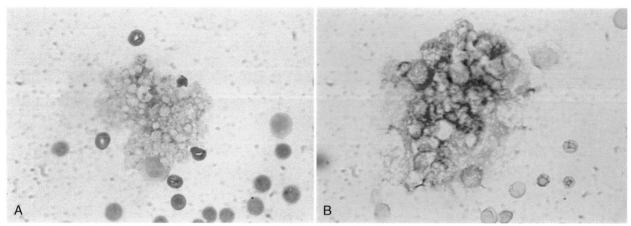

■ **FIGURE 14-27. Myelin. CSF. Dog. Same case A-B. A,** Mixed-breed dog with a history of degenerative myelopathy with normal nucleated cell count and increased protein (62 mg/dl). Foamy, phagocytic macrophages were present (not shown). Collections of eosinophilic foamy material are shown extracellularly. (Wright-Giemsa; HP oil.) **B,** Extracellular material stained positive for myelin. Demyelination was suspected in this dog. (Luxol fast blue; HP oil.)

also referred to as meningeal cysts and leptomeningeal cysts, have been reported as an uncommon cause of neurologic deficits in the dog and cat generally related to a normal CSF analysis (Galloway, 1999).

With neoplasia, more often the protein concentration is elevated, with only occasional neoplastic cells present in the CSF. This will depend on the location of the mass with its proximity to the ventricle, its involvement with the meninges, or its communication with the subarachnoid space in order to have access to the CSF. CSF was collected in 51 dogs with primary intracranial neoplasia in which the fluid was normal in 10% of cases,

characterized by an elevated cell count in 58% of cases, and characterized as albuminocytologic dissociation in 30% of cases. A mixed cell pleocytosis was the most common cytologic abnormality in the 51 samples while cellular atypia or neoplastic cells were detected in only two dogs with CNS lymphoma (Snyder et al., 2006). The authors concluded that in the case of CNS lymphoma, CSF analysis may be helpful in achieving a diagnosis. However, because of the inflammatory nature of CSF seen with primary intracranial neoplasia, this test may not be helpful in differentiating between neoplastic and other inflammatory diseases.

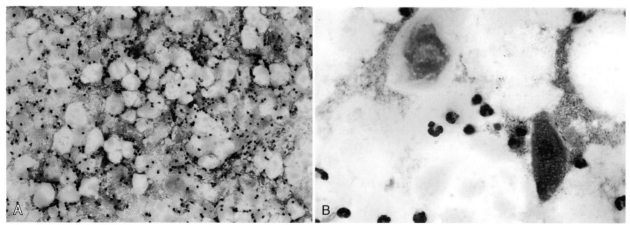

■ **FIGURE 14-28. Epidermoid cyst. CSF. Dog. Same case A-B. A,** Direct smear of creamy, opaque fluid with a nucleated cell count of 80,000/μl taken from the cerebellomedullary cistern of a dog with a 3-month duration of seizures. Numerous large, blue-green cells are evident at low magnification. (Romanowsky-type stain; IP.) **B,** Squamous epithelium is present as keratinized (upper left) and intermediate (lower right) squamous epithelium along with numerous nondegenerate neutrophils. (Romanowsky-type stain; HP oil.) (A-B, From a glass slide submitted by Joseph Spano to the 1988 ASVCP case review.)

Similar results were found in a series of CSF analyses from 28 cats with intracranial neoplasia (Troxel et al., 2003) in that albuminocytologic dissociation was noted in 8 (28.6%) cats. The remaining 20 (71.4%) cats had varied increases in nucleated cell counts while a definitive diagnosis of lymphoma was made in only one cat in which lymphoid blast cells were detected in the CSF.

Dickinson et al. (2006) tested the hypothesis that predominantly neutrophilic pleocytosis is a typical finding in dogs with intracranial meningioma by evaluating the characteristic of cisternal CSF in a series of 56 dogs with confirmed disease. Results were significantly different from those routinely reported in veterinary literature. Pleocytosis was detected in only 27% of dogs, and pleocytosis with a predominance of neutrophils was detected only in 19% of dogs. They concluded in particular that neutrophilic pleocytosis may not be detected in CSF samples from dogs with meningiomas located within the middle or rostral portion of the cranial fossae.

The presence of mitotic cells in the CSF is unusual and often indicates a proliferative population such as a neoplasm. The presence of immature lymphocytes is highly diagnostic for the presence of CNS lymphoma (Figs. 14-29 to 14-31). Well-differentiated lymphoid malignancies may not be readily distinguished from a lymphocytic pleocytosis involving granular lymphocytes (Fig. 14-32A&B). Other round cell tumors (Sheppard et al., 1997; Greenberg et al., 2004) are less common and include encephalic and spinal plasma cell tumors (Fig. 14-33A–C), histiocytic-appearing neoplasms (Fig. 14-33D) that are difficult to distinguish from GME (Zimmerman et al., 2006). Medulloblastoma should be considered as another differential diagnosis for atypical round cells in the CSF of young dogs (Thompson et al., 2003). Rarely, individualized cells from choroid plexus papillomas may be found in the CSF as large round cells (see discussion later under "Neoplasms of Neuroepithelial Cells").

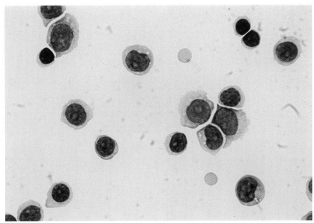

■ **FIGURE 14-30. Lymphoma. CSF. Dog.** Clinical signs involved a head tilt with ataxia of 3 months' duration. Increased protein (170 mg/dl) and pleocytosis (1417 cells/μl) were present in the clear fluid from the cerebellomedullary site. A mixed population of small, well-differentiated lymphocytes and large lymphoid blast cells (greater than 50%) together accounted for 99% of the cell population. Blast cells often contain a single prominent nucleolus. (Wright-Giemsa; HP oil.)

Finding metastatic carcinoma cells in the CSF is confirmed to be the gold standard for the diagnosis of leptomeningeal carcinomatosis in humans. Patients with extensive meningeal involvement are more likely to have a positive CSF cytology (66%) than those with only focal involvement of the leptomeninges (38%). In two cases of canine leptomeningeal carcinomatosis CSF, cytology demonstrated atypical cells with high or normal cell counts (Pumarola and Balash, 1996; Stampley et al., 1986).

CYTOLOGY OF NERVOUS SYSTEM TISSUE

Collection and Cytologic Preparation of Nervous System Tissues

When an intracranial or spinal mass is suspected, the veterinary neurologist often relies on sophisticated imaging such as computed tomography (CT) and magnetic resonance to identify the lesion. Even if imaging can give some information about the location, the size, and the relationship to other surrounding structures, very often the differential diagnosis for the mass found on imaging includes inflammatory (sterile or septic) lesion or benign and malignant tumor.

Since each disease has a different prognosis and requires different therapies, a definitive diagnosis needs to be sought but this can be achieved only by histologic examination. Intraoperative cytology has been applied worldwide in human neuropathology as a method for obtaining a rapid and accurate diagnosis even on very small specimens collected from stereotactic needle biopsy or intracranial and spinal surgery (Di Stefano et al., 1998, Tilgner et al., 2005). In human neurosurgery, where stereotactic biopsies are a routine way of obtaining samples of brain tissue in the least invasive manner possible with the fewest complications, cytology has emerged as the preferred diagnostic

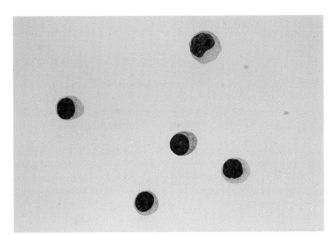

■ **FIGURE 14-29. Lymphocytic pleocytosis. CSF. Cat.** Cerebellomedullary collection contained 60 nucleated cells/μl, protein 140 mg/dl, and 80% lymphocytes in a cat with hind-limb paresis, urinary and fecal incontinence, and flaccid anal tone and tail. Intermediate-sized lymphocytes predominate in the field shown. Myelogram revealed a lumbar spinal cord mass that was cytologically diagnosed as large cell lymphoma. (Wright-Giemsa; HP oil.) (Courtesy of Rick Alleman, University of Florida.)

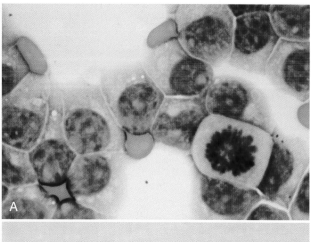

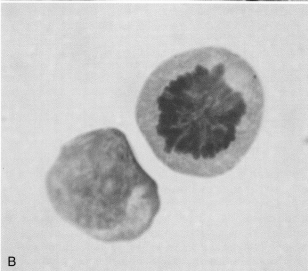

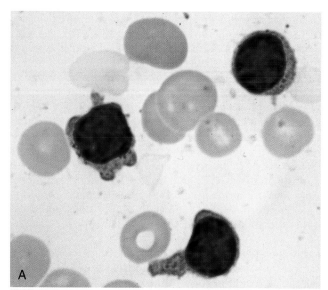

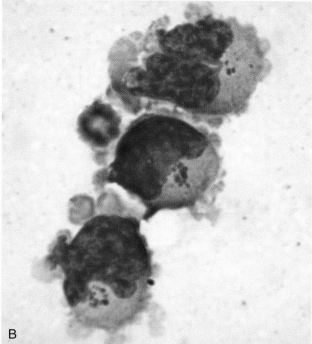

■ **FIGURE 14-31. Lymphoma. Dog. A, CSF.** Cream-colored CSF from the cerebellomedullary cistern of a dog with vestibular deficits. The fluid had marked pleocytosis of 109,400 nucleated cells/μl and increased protein of 220 mg/dl. A monomorphic population composing 92% of the cells involved large lymphoid blast cells with a prominent single nucleolus. Pictured are the blast cells along with a normal-appearing mitotic figure. (Wright; HP oil.) **B, Cisternal CSF.** This dog presented with dementia and circling. Of the two cells shown, the left cell is a blast cell with a single prominent nucleolus. The cell on the right is a normal-appearing mitotic figure, common in neoplastic CSF. (MGG; HP oil.)

■ **FIGURE 14-32. Granular cell lymphoma. CSF. Dog. A,** Shown are three granular cell lymphocytes found in fluid collected from the cerebellomedullary cistern from a dog with granular cell lymphocyte leukemia that originated within the spleen. Two months later the dog presented with dementia and cerebellar signs. The fluid had moderate pleocytosis (32 cells/μl), increased protein (69 mg/dl), few erythrocytes (520/μl) with 91% lymphocytes. The granules are very fine and lightly eosinophilic (most prominent in the uropod or cytoplasmic projection of the lower center cell). (Wright-Giemsa; HP oil.) **B,** Shown are three granular cell lymphocytes with prominent paranuclear eosinophilic granules from a dog with intestinal and splenic granular cell lymphoma. Note the red cell for size comparison. Some artifact is apparent from cytocentrifugation as indicated by the surface blebbing and nuclear incontinence. (MGG; HP oil.)

tool over the traditional frozen section technique (Shah et al., 1998).

Elective employment of smear cytology in neuropathology is based on several considerations: it is very simple and quick to perform, it requires few materials and equipment, and the specimens can be prepared directly in the operating or adjacent room. Small pieces of tissue can be examined and smears can be repeated several times with different portions of the same specimens. Various fast-staining techniques can be used. A recent study confirmed the adequacy of smear preparation for intracranial lesions in dogs and cats. Smear preparations appeared to be of greater diagnostic value, with fewer nondiagnostic specimens, when compared with touch preparations (Long et al., 2002). Moissonnier et al. (2002)

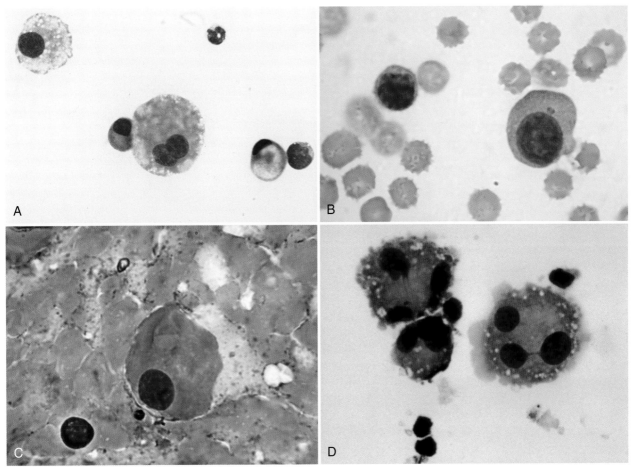

■ **FIGURE 14-33. A, Plasma cell tumor. CSF. Dog.** Two large mononuclear cells and two plasmacytoid cells are shown from the spinal fluid with marked mononuclear pleocytosis (27,600 nucleated cells/µl) and increased protein (greater than 2000 mg/dl). A primary encephalic plasma cell tumor involving the brainstem was diagnosed at necropsy with diagnostic support by electron microscopy and immunocytochemistry. (Wright-Giemsa; HP oil.) **B, Plasma cell. CSF. Dog.** Two lymphoid cells are shown, one of which displays a plasmacytoid appearance with an irregular nuclear outline. (MGG; HP oil.) **C, Spinal plasmacytoma. Lumbar CSF. Dog.** A large atypical plasma cell with pink and blue cytoplasm is shown against a proteinaceous background with numerous erythrocytes. Compare the size of this neoplastic cell with the small lymphocyte on the lower left. (MGG; HP oil.) **D, Multinucleated cells. CSF. Dog.** A tumor of unknown origin in the area of the thalamus produced clinical signs of pain initially and later tetraparesis. The fluid had mild pleocytosis (21 nucleated cells/µl) and elevated protein (70 mg/dl). Large mononuclear cells (59%) predominated followed by lymphocytes (37%). The pleomorphism of the large mononuclear cells along with many giant, multinucleated forms as shown supported a neoplastic process rather than an inflammatory disease. (Wright; HP oil.)

demonstrated that stereotactic CT-guided brain biopsy can be considered as a valued technique in the neurologic workup of patients with brain diseases and an early cytologic assessment is considered important even during conventional intracranial and spinal surgery.

The interpretation of smear samples from nervous system lesions requires considerable experience, not only in general cytology, but also in normal and abnormal cytology of the specific features of nervous system tissue.

Cytology of Normal Nervous System Tissues

Very little information is available on normal nervous tissue cytology in dogs and cats. Cytology of normal cerebral, cerebellar, and spinal cord tissue of these animals

shows a close resemblance to their human counterparts (Herzberg, 1999).

In one study (De Lorenzi et al., 2004) authors collected several samples by core needle biopsy from different areas of brain and cerebellum of dogs and cats without neurologic disorders in five dogs and five cats. From the two edges of the biopsy sample, a small fragment was removed with a scalpel blade and smeared on a glass slide a "squash" or "crush" technique (Fig. 14-34). The small portion (approx. 1 mm³) of the biopsy material was placed between two slides and squashed firmly until it becomes a thin film. Then, with a firm, even motion the slides were quickly pulled apart horizontally. All the cytologic samples were air dried, then placed in an automatic slide stainer with May-Grünwald Giemsa

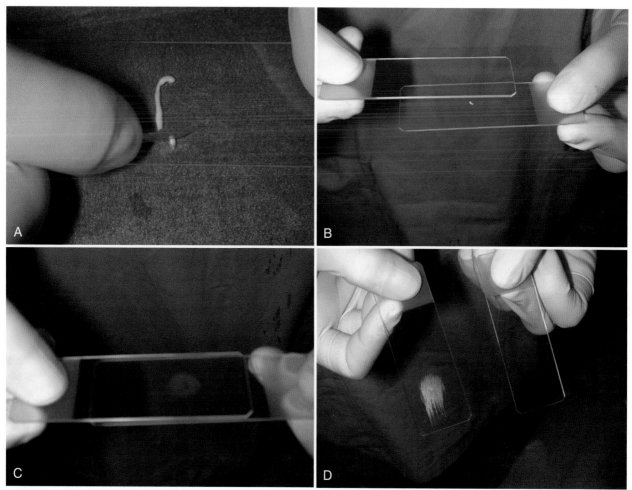

■ **FIGURE 14-34. Squash prep technique. Brain. A,** Cut a tiny portion of the brain tissue biopsy for the smear. **B,** Place the small fragment near the frosted end of a standard glass slide. **C,** Apply pressure using a second slide, maintain compression, then slide the top slide over the held bottom slide. **D,** The tissue is smeared out, resulting in an oval cytologic preparation.

(MGG) stain. The rest of the biopsy was fixed in 10% neutral-buffered formalin, and processed routinely as 5-μm sections stained with H&E, then examined by a neuropathologist to confirm the absence of pathologic changes.

Central Nervous System Cells

Central nervous system cells have two main origins, the neuroectoderm and mesenchyme. Neurons and glial cells (astrocytes, oligodendrocytes, Schwann cells, ependymal cells, and choroid plexus cells) are considered of neuroectodermal origin; meningeal cells and microglia are of mesenchymal origin.

In normal CNS tissue smears it is usually possible to recognize many of cellular and noncellular elements, while it is often difficult to identify the exact nature of every cell. A short description of the normal cytologic features found in this study is provided in the following paragraphs.

Normal cerebral tissue is an easy-to-smear tissue of low cellular density. In general, the grey matter contains neurons and a few nonmyelinated fibers, while the white matter displays myelinated axonal fibers.

Neuropil

Neuropil is the term used to define the dense network of fine glial processes, neuronal processes (axons and dendrites), and fibrils in the gray matter of the CNS (Fig. 14-35A&B). The neuropil is particularly prominent with MGG staining, in which it appears blue-purple. The characteristic and almost distinctive blue staining and foaminess shown by normal neuropil is particularly important to recognize since it is rarely, if ever, present in tumors and in most pathologic lesions.

Neurons

Neurons are the principal components of the CNS. More than any other cell, neurons vary in size from location to location. Most neurons are very large cells (Figs. 14-4A and 14-36), measuring up to 40 μm in diameter, but their size can vary from 5 μm (granular layer of the cerebellum) to 100 μm (motor cortex). Despite this variation in size, neurons share a common morphologic feature in both dogs and cats, which is an angulated shape with multiple and branching cytoplasmic processes composed of dendrites and a single axon. The real number of extensions of these specialized

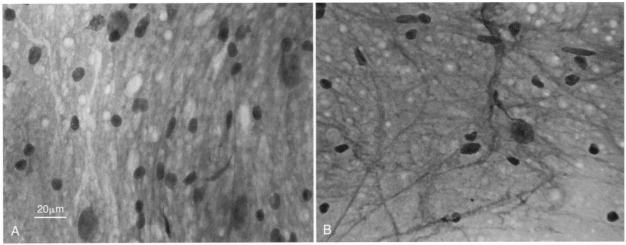

■ **FIGURE 14-35. Neuropil. A, Brain cortex aspirate. Dog.** Accidental puncture of cerebral cortex during aspiration of sinus cavity. Demonstrates the vacuolated foamy and amorphous basophilic appearance of neuronal and glial processes of the gray matter. (Wright; HP oil.) **B, Normal brain cortex. Squash preparation. Cat.** Present is a neuron (large nucleus with prominent nucleolus) and several hyperchromatic glial cell nuclei within a meshwork of fibrillary processes known as neuropil. Blood vessels are present within the neuropil. (MGG; HP oil.) (A, Courtesy of Rose Raskin, Purdue University.)

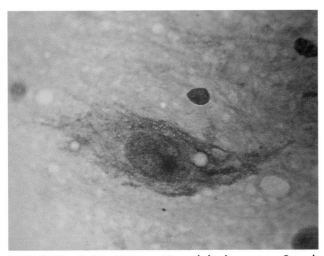

■ **FIGURE 14-36. Neuron. Normal brain cortex. Squash preparation. Cat.** A neuron with a prominent nucleolus is shown. Neurons vary in size and shape depending on location. Common morphologic features shared by most neurons include single, centrally placed nucleus with prominent nucleolus, and angulated cytoplasm. Note the basophilic, granular cytoplasm that is rough endoplasmic reticulum (Nissl substance). Small hyperchromatic glial cell nuclei are noted in the background. (MGG; HP oil.)

structures cannot be evaluated by MGG stain, as special stains are needed for this purpose. All neurons have a very large, centrally placed nucleus and frequently a single, prominent nucleolus. The cytoplasm is usually abundant and granular, due to the presence of Nissl substance, the rough endoplasmic reticulum often so abundant as to obscure the nucleus. In some areas of the brain, the cytoplasm may contain melanin pigments (neuromelanin) and microvacuoles (neuromediators).

Smears from the cerebellar cortex have a highly characteristic appearance as the cellularity is usually higher than in the brain cortex with sheets of small, hyperchromatic granular cells (Fig. 14-37A) from the inner, granular layer that are occasionally intermixed with large Purkinje cells (Fig. 14-37B).

Astrocytes

Astrocytes have a supportive function to neurons and are distributed throughout the nervous system. The characteristic star-shaped appearance cannot be evaluated with MGG stain and the cells appear as small, oval, naked nuclei, which measure between 7 and 10 μm, surrounded by neuropil (Fig. 14-38A). In response to neural tissue injury in the brain and spinal cord, there is a proliferation and hypertrophy of the resident neuroglial cells, which include the astrocyte, a supporting cell with branched cellular projections (Fig. 14-38B&C).

Oligodendrocytes

These are the myelin-forming cells of the central nervous system. In smears their nuclei are smaller (5 to 7 μm) and rounder than astrocytes and, like astrocytes, their cytoplasm is not well defined (Fig. 14-39). Due to their size and shape, oligodendrocytes can be mistaken for lymphocytes. Oligodendrocytes may surround neurons in a process called satellitosis.

Ependymal and Choroid Plexus Cells

Choroid plexus cells can be considered as specialized ependymal cells, lining the brain ventricles and the central canal of the spinal cord. These neuroepithelial cells show similar cytomorphologic features as they are usually organized in small, loose clusters and small sheets of cuboidal to columnar cells with a single, small, round, and centrally placed nucleus (Fig. 14-40).

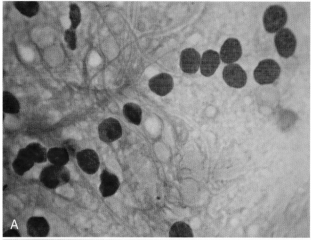

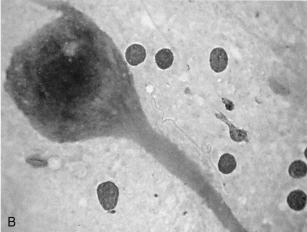

■ **FIGURE 14-37. Cerebellar cortex. Squash preparation. Dog. A, Granular cells.** Several small hyperchromatic neuron nuclei are shown from the inner granular layer of the cerebellar cortex. Note the hypercellularity and linear arrangement of the nuclei within the neuropil. Due to their small size and near absence of cytoplasm, these cells can be confused with lymphoid cells. (MGG; HP oil.) **B, Purkinje cell.** Present is a large, distinctive, flask-shaped neuron with single, central nucleus and characteristic single large, extended axon. The numerous highly branched dendrites for this cell are usually not evident with MGG stain. The cytoplasm surrounding the nucleus contains basophilic granular material known as Nissl bodies or substance. Several hyperchromatic granular cells appear in the background. (MGG; HP oil.)

Meningeal Cells

Meningeal cells are only rarely seen and recognized in brain smears. The cells are usually organized in sheets or in loose clusters showing a rather pleomorphic storiform pattern. Cell borders are poorly defined and the nuclear shape ranges from round to oval to elongate (Fig. 14-41). Occasionally, cells are organized in pseudo-acinar structures mimicking a glandular origin, which is more common in meningiomas but can also be identified in normal meningeal tissue.

Microglia

These neuroglial cells derive from bone marrow elements, likely macrophages that have specific phagocytic functions. They have small and elongated nuclei, which

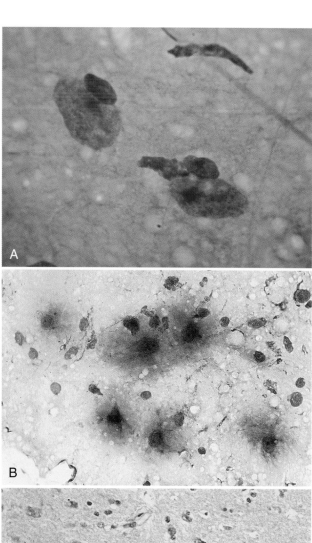

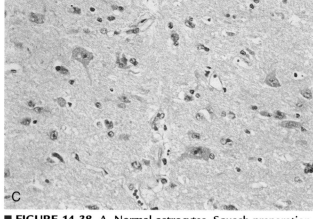

■ **FIGURE 14-38. A, Normal astrocytes. Squash preparation. Dog.** In MGG-stained samples, astrocytes appear as small, oval, naked nuclei that measure between 7 to 10 μm. Here two are surrounded by neuropil. (MGG; HP oil.) **Same case B-C. Astrocytosis. Cat. B, Brain aspirate.** Six large cells with a wispy basophilic cytoplasm are evident in this aspirate from a cat with a 14-day progression of dementia and head pressing. Nuclei are round to oval with a single small prominent nucleolus and the nuclear-to-cytoplasmic ratio is mildly increased. Cytologically, a neoplasm was suspected. (Wright-Giemsa; HP oil.) **C, Brain histology.** MRI revealed an intracranial mass. Tissue biopsy revealed normal gray matter with hypertrophied astrocytes, which is a nonspecific reaction. Although neoplastic cells were not found, adjacent neoplasia could not be ruled out. (H&E; HP oil.)

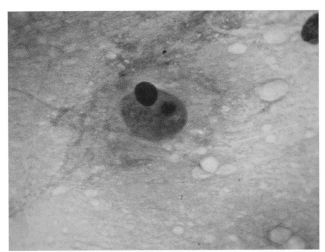

■ **FIGURE 14-39. Oligodendrocyte. Normal brain cortex. Squash preparation. Dog.** In MGG-stained smears, oligodendrocytes look like round, naked nuclei that often surround neurons in a process called satellitosis. (MGG; HP oil.)

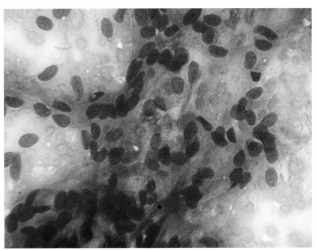

■ **FIGURE 14-41. Normal meningeal cells. Squash preparation. Dog.** The dense collection of oval nuclei is shown with associated eosinophilic streaming and whirling cytoplasm. This loose aggregate of pleomorphic meningeal cells organized in a pseudoacinar arrangement is a feature more common in meningiomas but that can be seen in samples from normal brain. (MGG; HP oil.)

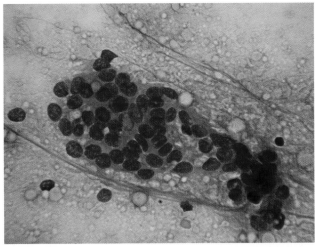

■ **FIGURE 14-40. Normal choroid cells. Squash preparation. Dog.** These lining cells arranged as small sheets of cuboidal to columnar cells have a uniform nuclear appearance and high nuclear-to-cytoplasmic ratio. The single small, round, and centrally placed nuclei are arranged occasionally in a palisade or linear arrangement. Choroid cells are cytologically indistinguishable from ependymal cells. (MGG; HP oil.)

explains their title as "rod cells." In many smears from brain cortex, microglia are localized in perivascular areas. When reactive, they show lipophagocytosis, filling the cytoplasm with well-defined vacuoles producing a foamy appearance (Fig. 14-42A&B).

Cytology of Pathologic Nervous System Tissues

Inflammatory lesions of the central nervous system can mimic neoplastic proliferation both clinically and radiographically. Cytology can be an extremely useful tool in distinguishing a true tumor from an inflammatory or reactive lesion. By using Romanowsky stain, many infectious

agents can be easily identified and recognized. In a recent report (Falzone et al., 2008), a space-occupying lesion in the temporal lobe of an adult cat was diagnosed cytologically as brain toxoplasmosis. The squash prep (Fig. 14-43) showed intense reactive gliosis surrounding round, encapsulated tissue cysts ranging from 15 μm to more than 100 μm that contained a number of elongated nucleated bradyzoites identified as *Toxoplasma* sp.

While cytologic profiles of smears of various types of human CNS tumors have been extensively described, there are very few reports in the veterinary literature that describe cytologic findings of nervous system lesions and the diagnostic accuracy of this technique.

While most describe the cytologic features from single cases or small series, Vernau et al. (2001) described the cytologic features of smears obtained from 93 primary brain tumors in dogs and cats. More recently, De Lorenzi et al. (2006) determined an accuracy value of 92.8% with a cytologic evaluation of smear samples of nervous system lesions from 42 cases in dogs and cats. In this study, once the smear considered abnormal, the specimen was designated as non-neoplastic or neoplastic. The non-neoplastic group consisted of tissues derived from inflammation, cyst, granuloma, or scar lesion, while the neoplastic group included lesions of neuroepithelial origin (neural, glial, and ependymal/choroidal proliferations) or of non-neuroepithelial origin, divided further into epithelial, mesenchymal, and round cell tumors.

The distinction between neuroepithelial and non-neuroepithelial depends to a large extent on pattern recognition and individual cell morphology. Therefore, misinterpretations may be due to different factors, such as the overlapping of morphologic features in neoplastic and non-neoplastic lesions and the primitive tumor heterogeneity.

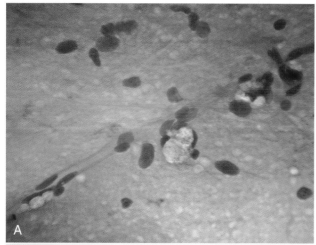

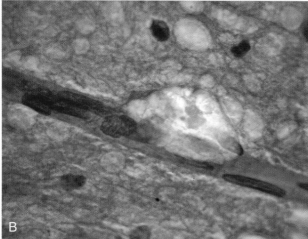

■ **FIGURE 14-42. Microglial cells. Normal brain cortex. Squash preparation. A, Dog.** Several perivascular microglial cells are shown in the center, which display an abundant foamy cytoplasm. The background contains other glial cells along with neural fibrils. (MGG; HP oil.) **B, Cat.** A single vacuolated, lipid-filled microglial cell is noted adjacent to a blood vessel. When reactive, these macrophage-derived cells undergo lipophagocytosis. (MGG; HP oil.)

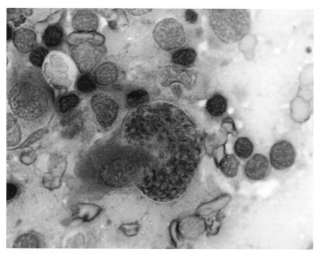

■ **FIGURE 14-43. Toxoplasmosis tissue cyst. Brain mass. Squash preparation. Cat.** A round, encapsulated structure or tissue cyst is filled with nucleated bradyzoites of *Toxoplasma* sp. (MGG; HP oil.)

Cytologic features suggesting a neuroepithelial origin include highly cellular smears related to the soft texture of the specimen, fine fibrillar background, perivascular arrangement with processes approaching the vascular lumen, round nuclei with finely stippled chromatin, and endothelial cell proliferation. Cytologic features of non-neuroepithelial lesions can vary considerably due to the extreme heterogeneous morphology of these groups. Nevertheless, the presence of cohesive cellular clusters or epithelial sheets; tightly packed spindle cells; whorls; large, round cells with prominent nucleoli and discernable cytoplasm; and numerous inflammatory cells suggests consideration of non-neuroepithelial tumors.

More specific cytologic features are described for different tumors.

Neoplasms of the Meninges and Nerve Sheaths

Non-neuroepithelial tumors that arise from the arachnoid meningeal layer are termed *meningiomas.* These are the most common intracranial tumor in dogs and cats. The tumors are derived from leptomeningocytes that associate with neural crest tissue and have both epithelial and fibro-blastic ultrastructural characteristics. As a result, these tumors have several variant forms (Montoliu et al., 2006) that are found both in cervical and lumbar regions of the spinal cord as well as intracranially and within the retro-bulbar region (Zimmerman et al., 2000). Spinal cord meningiomas are mostly extramedullary but few reports note the radiographic presentation of them as intramedullary (Hopkins et al., 1995). According to Bailey and Higgins (1986), meningiomas had the highest prevalence of pleocytosis, with a predominance of neutrophils often associated with necrosis. The meningioma was unique of all the tumors reviewed in this study, being the only tumor with CSF nucleated cell counts greater than 50/μl. Nevertheless in a more recent work (Dickinson et al., 2006) pleocytosis was detected in only 27% of 56 dogs with confirmed intracranial meningioma, and pleocytosis with a predominance of neutrophils was detected in only 19% of dogs with the conclusion that neutrophilic pleocytosis, especially with total nucleated cells count greater than 50 cells/μl, was not typical in CSF samples from dogs with intracranial meningiomas. Myelography, MRI, and CT are imaging tools used currently to identify tumors of the brain and spinal cord. Fine-needle aspirations, crush preparations (De Lorenzi et al., 2006; Moissonier et al., 2002), and incisional cutting needles (Platt et al., 2002) have been used to obtain cytologic and tissue samples for biopsy. The cytologic features of meningiomas have been discussed in several reports (Zimmerman et al., 2000; Hopkins et al., 1995).

Crush preparations from wet-fixed, rapid HE–stained meningiomas from 44 dogs and 7 cats were evaluated (Vernau et al., 2001). At low magnification, tumor cells were broken up into many clusters or cohesive cell aggregates, as well as separated into individual cells. Meningioma cells had round to slightly elongate, uniform-sized nuclei with a small, prominent nucleolus, diffusely coarse chromatin, and a well-defined nuclear border. Rarely there were intranuclear cytoplasmic evaginations, but these were plentiful in some individual tumor cells of the meningothelial subtype (Fig. 14-44A). More elongated

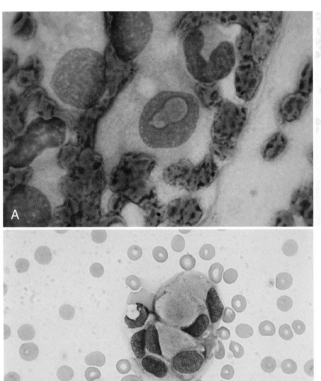

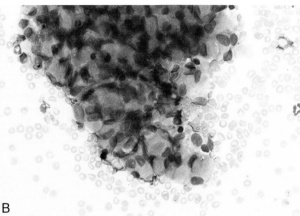

■ **FIGURE 14-44. A, Meningioma with nuclear inclusion. Squash preparation from surgical biopsy. Dog.** A single meningothelial cell contains an intranuclear inclusion that is thought to represent cytoplasmic evagination. Cytoplasmic evagination is an uncommon feature in meningioma cells but may be more commonly encountered in meningiomas of meningothelial origin. (MGG; HP oil.) **Same case B-C. Meningioma. CSF. Dog. B,** Large clump of cells in a sample taken from the cerebellomedullary cistern of a dog having a spinal cord lesion in the C1-2 region that presented with weakness. (Wright-Giemsa; HP oil.) **C,** Higher magnification of the cell clusters showing plump cells with oval to round eccentric nuclei and occasional prominent nucleoli. The cytoplasm contains an eosinophilic secretory material. Necropsy confirmed the presence of a locally extensive meningioma. (Wright-Giemsa; HP oil.)

cells sometimes had a central bar or fold through the longitudinal axis of their nucleus. There were variable amounts of eosinophilic, granular, wispy to solid cytoplasm that appeared round to elongate, often with a polar location. Mitotic figures were extremely rare. Some tumors had marked cellular anaplasia or nuclear atypia. Neutrophils were usually found in those tumors that had histologic foci of necrosis and focal accumulations.

Tumors with a sarcomatous appearance may have a disseminated nature. Two examples of spinal cord meningiomas with a meningotheliomatous appearance are shown (Figs. 14-44B&C and 14-45A&B). Meningiomas with a more common spindle cell cytologic appearance and a psammomatous histologic appearance are included (Figs. 14-46 to 14-48).

Another tumor associated with the meninges is the granular cell tumor, an uncommon tumor of animals and humans that occurs both within or outside the nervous system. The cell of origin is unclear but the morphologic appearance is thought to be the result of the accumulation of lysosomes, as demonstrated by electron microscopy (Sharkey et al., 2004), that reflect metabolic derangements in the cell. The cytologic features include large, round cells with eccentric nuclei and cytoplasm distended by many variably stained eosinophilic granules (Fig. 14-49A–C). Cells stain strongly positive for PAS as well as for the immunocytochemical stain for ubiquitin. Other staining reactions for these cells include a variably

positive reaction for S-100, a-1-antichymotrypsin, a-1-antitrypsin, and vimentin as well as a negative reaction for glial fibrillary acidic protein, pancytokeratins, and markers for subpopulations of leukocytes and macrophages (Higgins et al., 2001; Sharkey et al., 2004).

Peripheral nerve sheath tumors (PNST) may be encountered in cytologic preparations. These are most often associated with peripheral nerve roots and include those of the neural crest–derived Schwann cell that assists in myelination as well as fibroblastic connective tissue cells that surround nerve bundles. A cytologic distinction among benign PNST (Schwannoma and neurofibroma) can be difficult or impossible (Fig. 14-50). Moreover, sometimes benign Schwannomas and neurofibromas can show cytologic features of atypia so that differentiation between benign and malignant PNST becomes even more difficult.

A diagnosis of suspect PNST can be made in the presence of neoplasms associated with a peripheral nerve root, showing cytologic features of moderate to high cellularity. The cells are mainly grouped in thick fragments even if smaller clusters or single cells can be present and are characteristically spindle-shaped with elongated nuclei and inconspicuous nucleoli.

An unusual cytologic presentation of PNST from the forelimb of one cat was described (Tremblay et al., 2005). The cells revealed a pleomorphic population of individual round cells resembling histiocytes or plasma cells

Text continued on p. 358

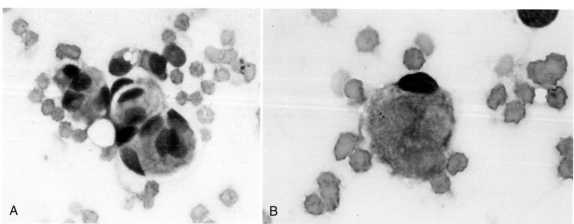

■ **FIGURE 14-45. Meningioma. Tissue imprint. Dog. Same case A-B. A,** A spinal cord mass from a dog with a 2-year history of neck pain and front leg paresis was obtained at surgery. Cytologic features demonstrate cohesive ball formation with epithelial-like appearance. (Wright; IP.) **B,** Individual meningeal cell with histiocytic appearance. The cytoplasm is abundant with eosinophilic secretory material that was positive for acid mucopolysaccharides. (Wright; HP oil.)

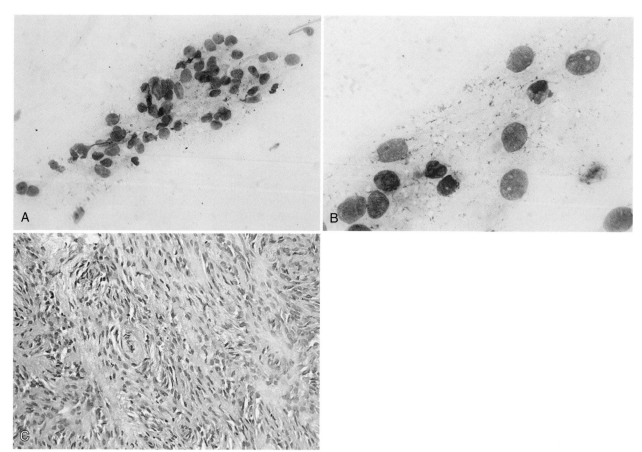

■ **FIGURE 14-46. Meningioma. Dog. Same case A-C. A-B, Tissue imprint. A,** Progressive quadriparesis was present with a circular lesion on MRI suggesting an intramedullary disease. Large cellular aggregates of mesenchymal-appearing cells are shown against a pink, finely granular background. (Wright-Giemsa; HP oil.) **B,** Higher magnification of a meningioma demonstrating the round to oval nucleus with finely granular chromatin, small nucleoli, and lightly basophilic cytoplasm that forms wispy tails. A finely granular eosinophilic material surrounds the cells and is seen within the cytoplasm as well. (Wright-Giemsa; HP oil.) **C, Tissue section.** Interweaving bundles of spindle cells are prominent with dense collagenous bands separating the cells. A small psammoma body with presumed calcified center is present (left center). (H&E; IP.)

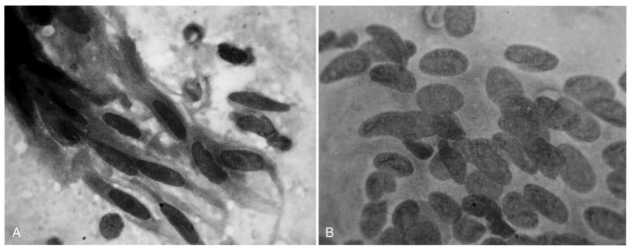

■ **FIGURE 14-47. Meningioma. Spindle pattern. Squash preparation from surgical biopsy. Dog. A,** Spindle-like tumor cells are arranged in a storiform pattern. These elongate cells with oval nuclei have a single small but prominent nucleolus. The cytoplasm is basophilic with wispy, pointed ends. (MGG; HP oil.) **B,** The tumor cells have oval or elongate uniform nuclei with moderately coarse chromatin. The cytoplasmic borders are not as defined as those in A and instead are almost nondetectable with cells appearing as an aggregate of multiple nuclei. The cytoplasm is eosinophilic. (MGG; HP oil.)

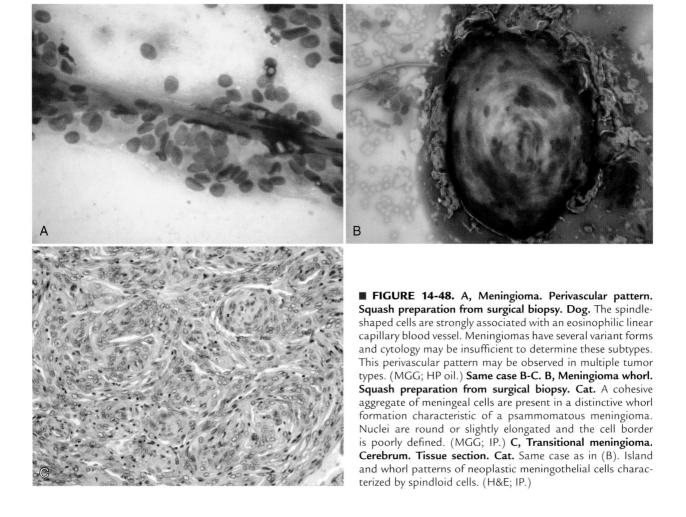

■ **FIGURE 14-48. A, Meningioma. Perivascular pattern. Squash preparation from surgical biopsy. Dog.** The spindle-shaped cells are strongly associated with an eosinophilic linear capillary blood vessel. Meningiomas have several variant forms and cytology may be insufficient to determine these subtypes. This perivascular pattern may be observed in multiple tumor types. (MGG; HP oil.) **Same case B-C. B, Meningioma whorl. Squash preparation from surgical biopsy. Cat.** A cohesive aggregate of meningeal cells are present in a distinctive whorl formation characteristic of a psammomatous meningioma. Nuclei are round or slightly elongated and the cell border is poorly defined. (MGG; IP.) **C, Transitional meningioma. Cerebrum. Tissue section. Cat.** Same case as in (B). Island and whorl patterns of neoplastic meningothelial cells characterized by spindloid cells. (H&E; IP.)

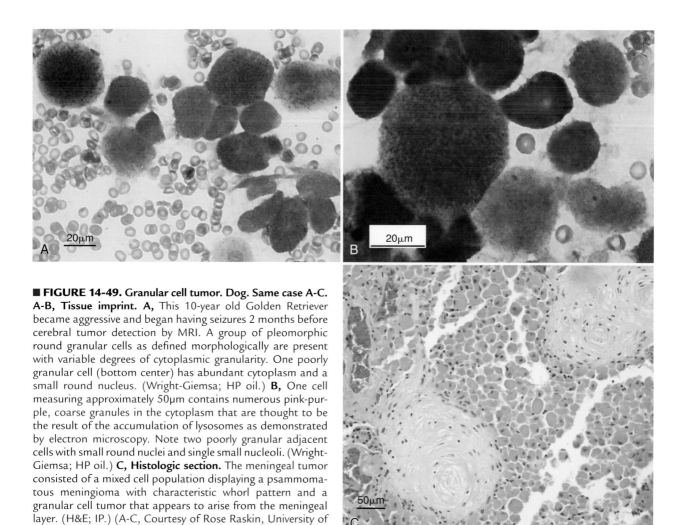

■ **FIGURE 14-49. Granular cell tumor. Dog. Same case A-C. A-B, Tissue imprint. A,** This 10-year old Golden Retriever became aggressive and began having seizures 2 months before cerebral tumor detection by MRI. A group of pleomorphic round granular cells as defined morphologically are present with variable degrees of cytoplasmic granularity. One poorly granular cell (bottom center) has abundant cytoplasm and a small round nucleus. (Wright-Giemsa; HP oil.) **B,** One cell measuring approximately 50μm contains numerous pink-purple, coarse granules in the cytoplasm that are thought to be the result of the accumulation of lysosomes as demonstrated by electron microscopy. Note two poorly granular adjacent cells with small round nuclei and single small nucleoli. (Wright-Giemsa; HP oil.) **C, Histologic section.** The meningeal tumor consisted of a mixed cell population displaying a psammomatous meningioma with characteristic whorl pattern and a granular cell tumor that appears to arise from the meningeal layer. (H&E; IP.) (A-C, Courtesy of Rose Raskin, University of Florida.)

with round, central to eccentric nuclei, basophilic cytoplasm, numerous mitotic figures, and large, multinucleated cells.

A benign nerve sheath tumor is shown (Fig. 14-51A&B). Malignant nerve sheath tumors may be locally extensive and recur more often. The histologic distinction between malignant fibroblasts and malignant Schwann cells is not readily discernible without immunohistochemistry and electron microscopy. A presumed neurofibrosarcoma is shown (Fig. 14-52A&B).

Neoplasms of Neuroepithelial Cells

Gliomas refer to neoplasms of specific neuroglial cells that include oligodendrocytes and astrocytes. Tumors from these cells most often produce a normal CSF related to their deep parenchymal location. One report of oligodendrogliomas in cats described their cytologic features as they appeared in cytospin preparations of the CSF (Dickinson et al., 2000). Cells were large with nuclei four to six times the size of red cells. Nuclei were eccentric within a densely basophilic, moderately abundant cytoplasm. An aspirate from an oligodendrogliomas presenting

as a brain mass is shown (Fig. 14-53A–C). Normally these cells are responsible for myelination of neurons in the CNS and appear as small cells with condensed chromatin. Tumors often demonstrate a unique honeycomb appearance and increased proliferation of blood vessels.

Astrocytes provide nutritional support to neurons, act as metabolic buffers or detoxifiers, and assist in repair and scar formation. They have been described as histiocytic in appearance (Fernandez et al., 1997). An example of reactive astrocytes was described previously (see Fig. 14-38A&B). Astrocytomas examined by crush preparation preserve the cytoplasmic features of an eccentrically placed nucleus within a moderately abundant basophilic cytoplasm (Fig. 14-54A–C). Glial fibrillary acidic protein (GFAP) is a marker used to distinguish astrocytes from other neuroglial and meningeal cells but may sometimes yield a positive reaction in neuroepithelial tumors, such as ependymoma and choroid plexus tumor (Fernandez et al., 1997), and meningeal tumors (Montoliu, 2006).

Neuroepithelial cells also include ependymal cells and choroid plexus cells. The ependymal cells line the

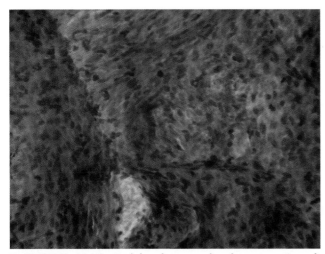

■ **FIGURE 14-50. Peripheral nerve sheath tumor. Squash preparation from surgical biopsy. Dog.** A dense collection of pleomorphic, elongated cells with oval nuclei is organized in a storiform pattern with focal palisade arrangement. Distinction between Schwannoma and neurofibroma is not possible by cytology. The diagnosis of PNST can be more easily performed if a neoplasm with these cytomorphologic features is associated with a peripheral nerve root. (MGG; IP.)

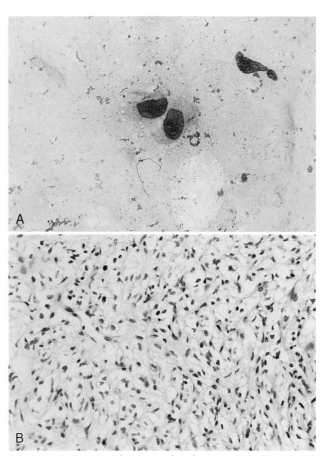

■ **FIGURE 14-51. Benign nerve sheath tumor. Dog. Same case A-B. A, Tissue imprint.** Two intact plump spindle cells demonstrate minimal anaplastic features. A compressive extradural lesion was found in the spinal canal at the nerve root region of C2-3. Clinical presentation included tetraparesis, ataxia, cervical pain, and Horner syndrome. (Wright-Giemsa; HP oil.) **B, Tissue section.** Neoplastic mesenchymal cells with eosinophilic fibrillary cell borders are arranged loosely within a fibroblastic stroma. (H&E; HP oil.)

ventricular system of the brain and central canal of the spinal cord. The ependymoma is a rare tumor (Fig. 14-55) that was reported in the cat with neoplastic cells found in the CSF with a moderately elevated protein content, mild pleocytosis, and macrophages as the predominant cell type along with evidence of chronic hemorrhage. The neoplastic cells were described as large cells having nuclear hyperchromatism, prominent nucleoli, and moderately abundant, highly basophilic agranular cytoplasm appearing singly and in clusters. An anaplastic ependymoma in a dog was diagnosed from partial positive staining with GFAP and vimentin but a negative reaction with S100, CD3, and cytokeratin (Fernandez et al., 1997). The choroid plexus cells represent a highly vascular portion of the pia mater that projects into the ventricles of the brain and is thought to secrete the CSF. Positive cytokeratin staining is expected in choroid plexus tumors. A cytologic example of a choroid plexus tumor is shown as an imprint of the tumor mass and within the CSF (Fig. 14-56A&B). The choroid plexus tumors were associated with an increased protein content and increased nucleated cell count in a study (Bailey and Higgins, 1986). These cells appear similar to mesothelial cells in the CSF, having a large, round nucleus with abundant, well-defined, deeply basophilic cytoplasm having surface projections (Fig. 14-56C). A papillary appearance with epithelial features can be seen in cytologic preparations of choroid plexus papilloma (Fig. 14-56A). Two choroid plexus carcinomas were cytologically misdiagnosed as choroid plexus papillomas (De Lorenzi et al., 2006). Both of these tumors occurred within a ventricular site and consisted of large, pedunculated, friable masses that presented cytologically as well-formed papillary structures, usually showing a fine fibrovascular core covered by uniform, cuboidal or columnar epithelium having

minimal cytologic atypia with moderate pleomorphism (Fig. 14-57A). The final histologic diagnosis of carcinoma was made based of the presence of single-cell infiltration into the fibrovascular cores, suggesting that a definitive diagnosis of choroid plexus carcinoma can be made only after thorough histologic examination of the resected specimen (Fig. 14-57B).

A potential diagnostic pitfall among tumors of different neuroectodermal and non-neuroectodermal origin can arise with ependymal or choroid plexus tumors and metastasis from well-differentiated adenocarcinomas. In fact, these two categories of neoplasms can share some analogous cytomorphologic findings such as epithelioid aspects, with cohesive glandlike fragments, round to polygonal cellular shape, and well-defined cytoplasm with distinct margins and roundish nuclei often with evident nucleoli. Additional information, such as the breed and the age of the patient, the precise location within the brain or the spinal cord, and a complete clinical history, especially the presence of a known primary tumor, may be critical in making the correct diagnosis.

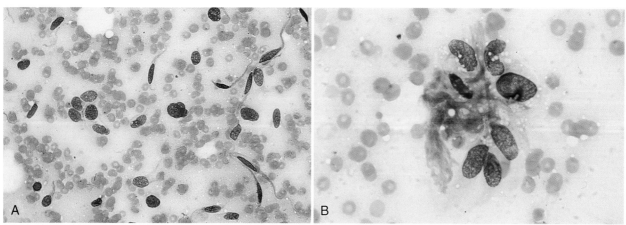

■ **FIGURE 14-52. Malignant nerve sheath tumor. Tissue imprint. Dog. Same case A-B. A,** Clinical presentation included paraparesis that progressed to tetraparesis. A mass within the spinal canal at the C2-3 nerve root was resected but recurred 2 months later. Spindle cells predominate with two populations present. Some cells have elongated fusiform nuclei and others have plump round to oval nuclei. The cytoplasm forms tails more distinct on the more elongated cells. (Wright-Giemsa; HP oil.) **B,** Aggregate of neoplastic cells with associated amorphous eosinophilic collagenous stroma. Cells have oval nuclei with coarse chromatin, small distinct nucleoli, and vacuolated scant pale blue cytoplasm. Histologic diagnosis was neurofibrosarcoma. (Wright-Giemsa; HP oil.)

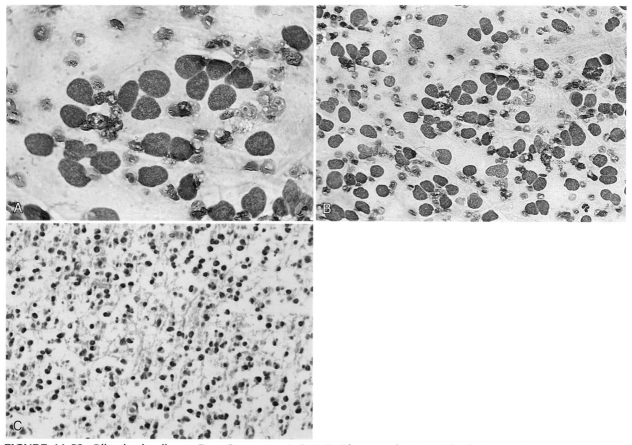

■ **FIGURE 14-53. Oligodendroglioma. Dog. Same case A-C. A-B, Tissue aspirate. A,** This brain specimen was taken from a dog with demented behavior. MRI identified a 5-cm mass in the cerebrum that extended into the lateral ventricle. Nuclei measured two to three times a red cell and appeared free with clear area present around the cell when viewed against the proteinaceous background. Nuclei are round to oval with fine chromatin and indistinct nucleoli. (Wright-Giemsa; HP oil.) **B,** A monomorphic population of large mononuclear cells arranged in loose sheets or small clusters. (Wright-Giemsa; HP oil.) **C, Tissue section.** Tissue section showing linear arrays of round hyperchromatic cells surrounded by clear spaces producing a honeycomb appearance. (H&E; HP oil.)

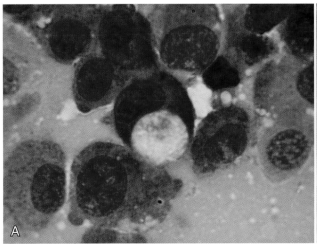

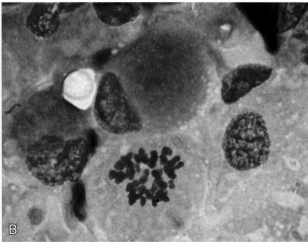

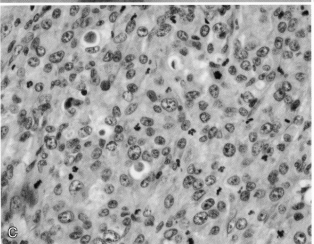

■ **FIGURE 14-54. Astrocytoma. A, Brain. Squash preparation. Dog.** Pleomorphic cells are individualized having an eccentrically placed nucleus with prominent nucleoli and moderately abundant, deeply basophilic cytoplasm. One cell appears to contain a vacuole. This appearance strongly resembles a plasma cell tumor. (MGG; HP oil.) **B, Spinal mass. Squash preparation from surgical biopsy. Cat.** This intradural spinal mass is composed of large cells with a histiocytic appearance having an eccentrically placed nucleus and abundant pink, granular cytoplasm. Also present is a normal-appearing mitotic figure. A positive immunohistochemical stain for glial fibrillary acid protein was determined, which confirmed the astrocytic origin. (MGG; HP oil.) **C, Spinal mass. Tissue section. Cat.** Medium-grade astrocytoma (anaplastic astrocytoma) with astrocytic neoplastic population characterized by high cellularity and pleomorphism, marked nuclear atypia, and numerous mitotic figures. (H&E; IP.)

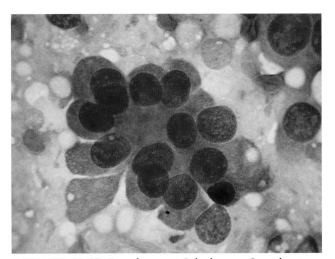

■ **FIGURE 14-55. Ependymoma. Spinal mass. Squash preparation from surgical biopsy. Dog.** These monomorphic cuboidal cells are arranged in a tight cluster with an acinar pattern. Cellular atypia is present as mild anisokaryosis and occasionally prominent nucleoli. Nuclei are round with uniform chromatin features. Cytoplasm is scant to moderately abundant and pink-blue with fine granularity. (MGG; HP oil.)

Extramedullary Tumors

Two different papers describe the cytologic features of a canine thoracolumbar spinal tumor (nephroblastoma) in two young dogs (De Lorenzi et al., 2007; Neel and Dean, 2000). In the more recent case report, a triphasic pattern, denoting the coexistence in the same smear of three different tumor cell populations, was described in analogy with human renal nephroblastoma.

THE FUTURE OF NERVOUS SYSTEM CYTOLOGY

Cerebrospinal fluid cytology and fluid analysis are likely to continue to be an important part of the investigation of neurologic disease in dogs and cats. During the last decade, there has been an increased use of sophisticated imaging techniques with increased surgical investigation and surgical and medical treatment of neurologic disease. These trends indicate there may be opportunity to expand the use of nervous system cytology to include examination of fine-needle aspirates of lesions identified within the brain or spinal cord, ventricular fluids obtained by direct aspiration or by cannula, and squash preparations of

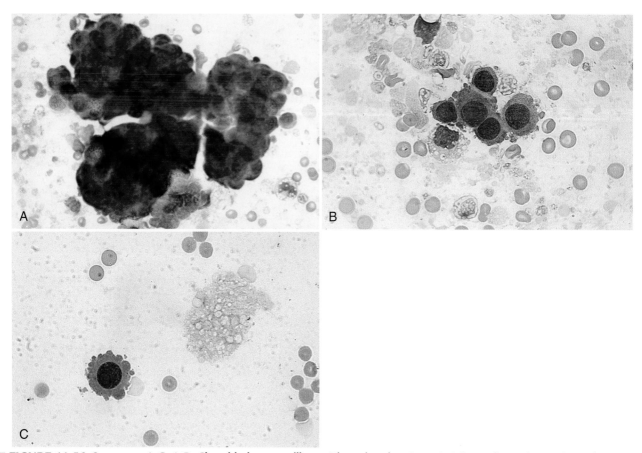

■ **FIGURE 14-56. Same case A-C. A-B, Choroid plexus papilloma. Tissue imprint. Dog. A,** Seizure, dementia, ataxia, and tetraparesis were clinical signs present in this dog in which MRI diagnosed a ventricular mass. The sample was highly cellular with large, dense,
cohesive clusters of cells having moderately abundant, deeply basophilic cytoplasm. (Wright-Giemsa; HP oil.) **B,** Higher magnification
demonstrating the tight cohesion between cells. The nuclear-to-cytoplasmic ratio is high. The nucleus is round with finely granular chromatin and large prominent nucleoli. The cytoplasmic is basophilic and finely granular. (Wright-Giemsa; HP oil.) **C, Choroid plexus
papilloma with presumed myelin fragments. CSF. Dog.** The fluid had increased protein (98 mg/dl) and a normal nucleated cell count.
One neoplastic cell was present in two cytospin preparations. The nucleus is very large and round with dispersed chromatin and a single
prominent nucleolus. The cytoplasm is dark blue with smooth surface projections. To the right of the cell is granular, gray-blue material
consistent with myelin, which suggests a degenerative process. (Wright-Giemsa; HP oil.)

small biopsy specimens or tissue fragments. All of these
techniques are currently used in cytologic evaluations of
human patients (Bigner, 1997) and to a limited extent in
veterinary medicine (De Lorenzi et al., 2006; Moissoinier
et al., 2002; Vernau et al., 2001). There may be increased
demand and/or need for development of special prepa-
rative techniques such as cell blocks and immunocytochemistry for more precise identification of primary or
metastatic tumors, inflammatory cell types, or immunophenotype of malignant or nonmalignant lymphoid proliferations. This has occurred in human medicine for the
purpose of diagnosis, prognosis, and disease monitoring.

A recent study (Tilgner et al., 2005) retrospectively
analyzed 5000 consecutive stereotactic brain biopsy
smear preparations from 4589 patients. In this huge series of cases the intraoperative, cytologic diagnosis was
correct in 90.3% of cases. The authors conclude that

intraoperative diagnosis with stereotactic biopsy has
high validity and that immediate treatment based on
smear preparations can be justified. Although in a much
smaller series of cases, similar results have been published in veterinary literature as well, with a satisfactory
cytologic diagnosis obtained in more than 90% of examined cases (De Lorenzi et al., 2006).

The future of veterinary nervous system evaluation
may include types of collection, preparation, and analysis
that differ significantly from those currently used. Even if
histopathologic and immunohistochemical evaluation of
biopsy specimens remains the cornerstone of the final
diagnosis, neurocytopathology can be considered, in experienced hands, an extremely useful tool in the workup
of patients with nervous system diseases. New approaches
using biochemical markers in the CSF (Turba et al., 2007)
may provide future areas of diagnostic tools in veterinary

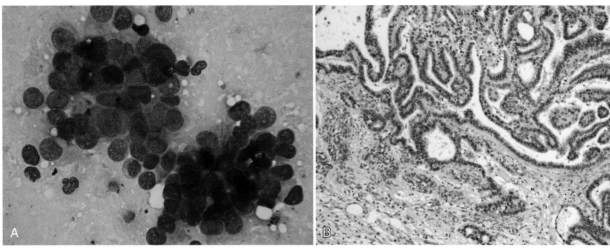

■ **FIGURE 14-57. Choroid plexus carcinoma. Dog. Same case A-B. A, Squash preparation.** Cells are grouped in tight clusters; the upper left in an acinar arrangement. Cellular atypia include moderate anisokaryosis, prominent nucleoli, coarse chromatin, and high nuclear-to-cytoplasmic ratio. These cytomorphologic features resemble metastatic carcinomas from well-differentiated tumor cells. (MGG; HP oil.) **B, Tissue section.** Papillary figures characterized by cuboidal to columnar neoplastic neuroepithelial cells of one or more layers in thickness. The adjacent subependymal brain tissue appears to be infiltrated by the tumor. (H&E; LP.)

medicine. To avoid inappropriate conclusions, diagnostic data provided by cytology should always be in accord and consistent with those derived from an accurate clinicoradiologic investigation. The combination of these approaches should significantly enhance the accuracy of smear cytology.

SUMMARY

Cerebrospinal fluid evaluation is an important part of the investigation of neurologic disease. An alteration in CSF protein content, cell counts, or cytologic findings that provides a definitive diagnosis is infrequent. However, when considered in combination with clinical signs, presentation, history, and results of other tests, a high degree of confidence can be achieved in establishing a clinical diagnosis. Knowledge of methods of collection, sites of collection, methods for analysis, and possible contaminants is an important part of establishing expertise in laboratory and cytologic evaluation of the nervous system. In the future, emerging techniques, new testing methods, and new applications of current test methods may provide information different from or complementary to existing techniques.

REFERENCES

Abate O, Bollo E, Lotti D, et al: Cytological, immunocytochemical and biochemical cerebrospinal fluid investigations in selected central nervous system disorder of dogs, *Zentralbl Veterinarmed* [B] 45:73-85, 1998.

Amude AM, Alfieri AA, Balarin MRS, et al: Cerebrospinal fluid from a 7-month-old dog with seizure-like episodes, *Vet Clin Pathol* 35:119-122, 2006.

Bailey CS, Higgins RJ: Characteristics of cerebrospinal fluid associated with canine granulomatous meningoencephalomyelitis: a retrospective study, *J Am Vet Med Assoc* 188:418-421, 1986.

Baker R, Lumsden JH: *Color atlas of cytology of the dog and cat*, St. Louis, Mosby, 2000, pp 95-115.

Baroni M, Heinold Y: A review of the clinical diagnosis of feline infectious peritonitis viral meningoencephalomyelitis, *Prog Vet Neurol* 6:88-94, 1995.

Bauer NB, Basset H, O'Neill EJ et al: Cerebrospinal fluid from a 6-year-old dog with severe neck pain, *Vet Clin Pathol* 35:123-125, 2006.

Behr S, Cauzinille L: Aseptic suppurative meningitis in juvenile boxer dogs: retrospective study of 12 cases, *J Am Anim Hosp Assoc* 42:277-282, 2006.

Behr S, Trumel C, Cauzinille L, et al: High resolution protein electrophoresis of 100 paired canine cerebrospinal fluid and serum, *J Vet Intern Med* 20:657-662, 2006.

Berthelin CF, Legendre AM, Bailey CS, et al: Cryptococcosis of the nervous system in dogs, Part 2: Diagnosis, treatment, monitoring, and prognosis, *Prog Vet Neurol* 5:136-145, 1994.

Bienzle D, Kwiecien JM, Parent JM: Extramedullary hematopoiesis in the choroid plexus of five dogs, *Vet Pathol* 32:437-440, 1995.

Bienzle D, McDonnell JJ, Stanton JB: Analysis of cerebrospinal fluid from dogs and cats after 24 and 48 hours of storage, *J Am Vet Med Assoc* 216:1761-1764, 2000.

Bigner SH: Central nervous system. In Bibbo M (ed): *Comprehensive cytopathology*, Philadelphia, WB Saunders, 1997, pp 477-492.

Boettcher IC, Steinberg T, Matiasek K: Use of anti-coronavirus antibody testing of cerebrospinal fluid for diagnosis of feline infectious peritonitis involving the central nervous system, *J Am Vet Med Assoc* 230:199-206, 2007.

Bohn AA, Willis TB, West CL, et al: Cerebrospinal fluid analysis and magnetic resonance imaging in the diagnosis of neurologic disease in dogs: a retrospective study, *Vet Clin Pathol* 35:315-320, 2006.

Bush WW, Barr C, Darrin EW, et al: Results of cerebrospinal fluid analysis, neurological examination findings, and age at the onset of seizures as predictors for results of magnetic resonance imaging of the brain in dogs examined because of seizures: 115 cases (1992-2000), *JAVMA* 220:781-784, 2002.

Carmichael N: Nervous system. In Davidson M, Else R, Lumsden J (eds): *Manual of small animal clinical pathology*, Cheltenham, UK, British Small Animal Veterinary Association, 1998, pp 235-240.

Caswell JL, Nykamp SG: Intradural vasculitis and hemorrhage in full sibling Welsh springer spaniels, *Can Vet J* 44:137-139, 2003.

Cellio BC: Collecting, processing, and preparing cerebrospinal fluid in dogs and cats, *Compend Contin Educ Pract Vet* 23:786-794, 2001.

Chamberlain MC: Comparative spine imaging in leptomeningeal metastases, *J Neuro Oncol* 23:233-238, 1995.

Chrisman CL: Special ancillary investigations. In Chrisman CL (ed): *Problems in small animal neurology*, ed 2, Philadelphia, Lea & Febiger, 1991, pp 81-117.

Chrisman CL: Cerebrospinal fluid analysis, *Vet Clin North Am Small Anim Pract* 22:781-810, 1992.

Christopher MM: Bone marrow contamination of canine cerebrospinal fluid, *Vet Clin Pathol* 21:95-98, 1992.

Cizinauskas S, Jaggy A, Tipold A: Long-term treatment of dogs with steroid-responsive meningitis-arteritis: clinical, laboratory and therapeutic results, *J Small Anim Pract* 41:295-301, 2000.

Clemmons RM: Therapeutic considerations for degenerative myelopathy of German Shepherds, New Orleans, Proceedings of the 9th ACVIM Forum, 1991, pp 773-775.

Cook JR, DeNicola DB: Cerebrospinal fluid, *Vet Clin North Am Small Anim Pract* 18:475-499, 1988.

De Lorenzi D, Bernardini M, Mandara MT. Nuove applicazioni in citologia diagnostica veterinaria: il sisterna nervoso centrale. In Proceedings of the 48th SCIVAC National Congress, Rimini, Italy, 2004, pp 136-138.

De Lorenzi D, Mandara MT, Tranquillo M et al: Squash-prep cytology in the diagnosis of canine and feline nervous system lesions: a study of 42 cases, *Vet Clin Pathol* 35:208-214, 2006.

De Lorenzi D, Baroni M, Mandara MT: A true "triphasic" pattern: thoracolumbar spinal tumor in a young dog, *Vet Clin Pathol* 36:200-203, 2007.

Desnoyers M, Bédard C, Meinkoth JH, et al: Cerebrospinal fluid analysis. In Cowell RL, Tyler RD, Meinkoth JH, DeNicola DB (eds): *Diagnostic cytology and hematology of the dog and cat*, ed 3, St. Louis, Mosby, 2008, pp 215-234.

Dickinson PJ, Keel MK, Higgins RJ, et al: Clinical and pathologic features of oligodendrogliomas in two cats, *Vet Pathol* 37:160-167, 2000.

Dickinson PJ, Sturges BK, Kass PH et al: Characteristics of cisternal cerebrospinal fluid associated with intracranial meningiomas in dogs: 56 cases (1985-2004), *J Am Vet Med Assoc* 228:564-567, 2006.

Di Stefano D, Scucchi LF, Cosentino L, et al: Intraoperative diagnosis of nervous system lesions, *Acta Cytol* 42:346-356, 1998.

Duque C, Parent J, Bienzle D: The immunophenotype of blood and cerebrospinal fluid mononuclear cells in dogs, *J Vet Intern Med* 16:714-719, 2002.

Fallin CW, Raskin RE, Harvey JW: Cytologic identification of neural tissue in the cerebrospinal fluid of two dogs, *Vet Clin Pathol* 25:127-129, 1996.

Falzone C, Baroni M, De Lorenzi D, et al: *Toxoplasma gondii* brain granuloma in a cat: diagnosis using cytology from an intraoperative sample and sequential magnetic resonance imaging, *J Small Anim Pract* 49:95-99, 2008.

Fenner WR: Diseases of the brain. In Ettinger SJ, Feldman EC (eds): *Textbook of veterinary internal medicine*, ed 5, Philadelphia, WB Saunders, 2000, pp 552-602.

Fenner WR: Central nervous system infections. In Greene CE (ed): *Infectious diseases of the dog and cat*, ed 2, Philadelphia, WB Saunders; 1998, pp 647-657.

Fernandez FR, Grindem CB, Brown TT, et al: Cytologic and histologic features of a poorly differentiated glioma in a dog, *Vet Clin Pathol* 26:182-186, 1997.

Fluhemann G, Konar M, Jaggy A, et al: Cerebral cholesterol granuloma in a cat, *J Vet Intern Med* 20:1241-1244, 2006.

Fry MM, Vernau W, Kass PH, et al: Effects of time, initial composition, and stabilizing agents on the results of canine cerebrospinal fluid analysis, *Vet Clin Pathol* 35:72-77, 2006.

Gaitero L, Anor S, Montoliu P, et al: Detection of *Neospora caninum* tachyzoites in canine cerebrospinal fluid, *J Vet Intern Med* 20:410-414, 2006.

Galloway AM, Curtis NC, Sommerlad SF, et al: Correlative imaging findings in seven dogs and one cat with spinal arachnoid cyst, *Vet Radiol Ultrasound* 40:445-452, 1999.

Gama FGV, Santana AE, de Campos Filho E, et al: Agarose gel electrophoresis of cerebrospinal fluid proteins of dogs after sample concentration using a membrane microconcentrator technique, *Vet Clin Pathol* 36:85-88, 2007.

Garma-Aviña A, Tyler JW: Large granular lymphocyte pleocytosis in the cerebrospinal fluid of a dog with necrotizing meningoencephalitis, *J Comp Pathol* 121:83-87, 1999.

Glass EN, Cornetta AM, deLahunta A, et al: Clinical and clinicopathologic features in 11 cats with *Cuterebra* larvae myiasis of the central nervous system, *J Vet Intern Med* 12:365-368, 1998.

Greenberg MJ, Schatzberg SJ, deLahunta A, et al: Intracerebral plasma cell tumor in a cat: a case report and literature review, *J Vet Intern Med* 18:581-585, 2004.

Herzberg AJ: Neurocytology. In Herzberg AJ, Raso DS, Silverman JF (eds): *Color atlas of normal cytology*, Churchill Livingstone, New York, 1999, pp 415-443.

Higgins RJ, LeCouteur RA, Vernau KM, et al: Granular cell tumor of the canine central nervous system: two cases, *Vet Pathol* 38:620-627, 2001.

Hopkins AL, Garner M, Ackerman N, et al: Spinal meningeal sarcoma in a Rottweiler puppy, *J Small Anim Pract* 36:183-186, 1995.

Hurtt AE, Smith MO: Effects of iatrogenic blood contamination of results of cerebrospinal fluid analysis in clinically normal dogs and dogs with neurologic disease, *J Am Vet Med Assoc* 211:866-867, 1997.

Johnsrude JD, Alleman AR, Schumacher J, et al: Cytologic findings in cerebrospinal fluid from two animals with GM_2-gangliosidosis, *Vet Clin Pathol* 25:80-83, 1996.

Keebler CM, Facik M: Cytopreparatory techniques. In Bibbo M, Wilbur D (eds): *Comprehensive cytopathology*, ed 3, St. Louis, Saunders, 2008, pp 977-1003.

Kipar A, Baumgartner W, Vogl C, et al: Immunohistochemical characterization of inflammatory cells in brains of dogs with granulomatous meningoencephalitis, *Vet Pathol* 35:43-52, 1998.

Lipsitz D, Levitski RE, Chauvet AE: Magnetic resonance imaging of a choroid plexus carcinoma and meningeal carcinomatosis in a dog, *Vet Radiol Ultrasound* 40:246-250, 1999.

Long SN, Anderson TJ, Long FHA, et al: Evaluation of rapid staining techniques for cytologic diagnosis of intracranial lesions, *AJVR* 3:381-386, 2002.

Mariani CL, Platt SR, Scase TJ, et al: Cerebral phaeohyphomycosis caused by *Cladosporum spp.* in two domestic shorthair cats, *J Am Anim Hosp Assoc* 38:225-230, 2002.

Mesher CI, Blue JT, Guffroy MRG, et al: Intracellular myelin in cerebrospinal fluid from a dog with myelomalacia, *Vet Clin Pathol* 25:124-126, 1996.

Messer JS, Kegge SJ, Cooper ES, et al: Meningoencephalomyelitis caused by *Pasteurella multocida* in a cat, *J Vet Intern Med* 20:1033-1036, 2006.

Mikszewski JS, Van Winkle TJ, Troxel MT: Fibrocartilagineous embolic myelopathy in five cats, *J Am Anim Hosp Assoc* 42:226-233, 2006.

Moissonnier P, Blot S, Devauchelle P, et al: Stereotactic CT-guided brain biopsy in the dog, *J Small Anim Prac* 43:115-123, 2002.

Montoliu P, Añor S, Vidal E, et al: Histological and immunohistochemical study of 30 cases of canine meningioma, *J Comp Path* 135:200-207, 2006.

Munana KR, Luttgen PJ: Prognostic factors for dogs with granulomatous meningoencephalomyelitis: 42 cases (1982-1996), *J Am Vet Med Assoc* 212:1902-1906, 1998.

Neel J, Dean GA: A mass in the spinal column of a dog (nephroblastoma), *Vet Clin Pathol* 29:87-89, 2000.

Parent JM, Rand JS: Cerebrospinal fluid collection and analysis. In August JR (ed): *Consultations in feline internal medicine*, ed 2, Philadelphia, Saunders, 1994, pp 385-392.

Platt SR, Alleman AR, Lanz OI, et al: Comparison of fine-needle aspiration and surgical-tissue biopsy in the diagnosis of canine brain tumors, *Vet Surg* 31:65-69, 2002.

Pumarola M, Balash M: Meningeal carcinomatosis in a dog, *Vet Rec* 25:523-524, 1996.

Radaelli ST, Platt SR: Bacterial meningoencephalomyelitis in dogs a retrospective study of 23 cases (1990-1999), *J Vet Intern Med* 16:159-163, 2002.

Rand JS: The analysis of cerebrospinal fluid in cats. In Bonagua JD, Kirk RW (eds): *Kirk's current veterinary therapy XII: small animal practice*, Philadelphia, Saunders, 1995, pp 1121-1126.

Rand JS, Parent J, Jacobs R, et al: Reference intervals for feline cerebrospinal fluid: cell counts and cytological features, *Am J Vet Res* 51:1044-1048, 1990.

Rand JS, Parent J, Percy D, et al: Clinical, cerebrospinal fluid and histological data from thirty-four cats with primary noninflammatory disease of the central nervous system, *Can Vet J* 35:174-181, 1994.

Ruotsala K, Poma R, da Costa RC, et al: Evaluation of the ADVIA 120 for analysis of canine cerebrospinal fluid, *Vet Clin Pathol* 37:242-248, 2008.

Shah AB, Muzumdar GA, Chitale AR, et al: Squash preparation and frozen section in intraoperative diagnosis of central nervous system tumors, *Acta Cytol* 41:1149-1154, 1998.

Sharkey LC, McDonnell JJ, Alroy J: Cytology of a mass on the meningeal surface of the left brain in a dog, *Vet Clin Pathol* 33:111-114, 2004.

Sheppard BJ, Chrisman CL, Newell SM, et al: Primary encephalic plasma cell tumor in a dog, *Vet Pathol* 34:621-627, 1997.

Simpson ST, Reed RB: Manometric values of normal cerebrospinal fluid pressure in dogs, *J Am Anim Hosp Assoc* 23:629, 1987.

Singh M, Foster DJ, Child J, et al: Inflammatory cerebrospinal fluid analysis in cats: clinical diagnosis ad outcome, *J Feline Med Surg* 7:77-93, 2005.

Skeen TM, Olby NJ, Munana KR, et al: Spinal arachnoid cysts in 17 dogs, *J Am Anim Hosp Assoc* 39:271-282, 2003.

Snyder JM, Shofer FS, Van Winkle TJ, et al: Canine intracranial primary neoplasia: 173 cases (1986-2003), *J Vet Intern Med* 20:669-765, 2006.

Sorjonen DC: Clinical and histopathological features of granulomatous meningoencephalomyelitis in dogs, *J Am Anim Hosp Assoc* 26:141-147, 1990.

Stalis IH, Chadwick B, Dayrell-Hart B, et al: Necrotizing meningoencephalitis of Maltese dogs, *Vet Pathol* 32:230-235, 1995.

Stampley AR, Swaynev DE, Prasse KW: Meningeal carcinomatosis secondary to a colonic signet-ring cell carcinoma in a dog, *J Am Anim Hosp Assoc* 23:655-658, 1986.

Thompson CA, Russell KE, Levine JM, et al: Cerebrospinal fluid from a dog with neurologic collapse, *Vet Clin Pathol* 32:143-146, 2003.

Thomson CE, Kornegay JN, Stevens JB: Analysis of cerebrospinal fluid from the cerebellomedullary and lumbar cisterns of dogs with focal neurologic disease: 145 cases (1985-1987), *J Am Vet Med Assoc* 196:1841-1844, 1990.

Tilgner J, Herr M, Ostertag C, et al: Validation of intraoperative diagnoses using smear preparations from stereotactic brain biopsies: intraoperative versus final diagnosis—influence of clinical factors, *Neurosurgery* 56:257-265, 2005.

Timmann D, Konar M, Howard J, et al: Necrotizing encephalitis in a French bulldog, *J Small Anim Pract* 48:339-342, 2007.

Tipold A, Fatzer R, Jaggy A, et al: Necrotizing encephalitis in Yorkshire terriers, *J Small Anim Pract* 34:623-628, 1993.

Tipold A, Vandevelde M, Zurbriggen A: Neuroimmunological studies in steroid-responsive meningitis-arteritis in dogs, *Res Vet Sci* 58:103-108, 1995.

Tremblay N, Lanevschi A, Doré M, et al: Of all the nerve! A subcutaneous forelimb mass in a cat, *Vet Clin Pathol* 34:417-420, 2005.

Troxel MT, Vite CH, Van Winkle TJ, et al: Feline intracranial neoplasia: review of 160 cases (1985-2001), *J Vet Intern Med* 17:850-859, 2003.

Turba ME, Forni M, Gandini G, et al: Recruited leukocytes and local synthesis account for increased matrix metalloproteinase-9 in cerebrospinal fluid of dogs with central nervous system neoplasm, *J Neurooncol* 81:123-129, 2007.

Uchida K, Hasegawa T, Ikeda M, et al: Detection of an autoantibody from pug dogs with necrotizing encephalitis (pug dog encephalitis), *Vet Pathol* 36:301-307, 1999.

Vernau KM, Higgins RJ, Bollen AW, et al: Primary canine and feline nervous system tumours: intraoperative diagnosis using the smear technique, *Vet Pathol* 38:47-57, 2001.

Zimmerman KL, Bender HS, Boon GD, et al: A comparison of the cytologic and histologic features of meningiomas in four dogs, *Vet Clin Pathol* 29:29-34, 2000.

Zimmerman K, Almy F, Carter L, et al: Cerebrospinal fluid from a 10-year-old dog with a single seizure episode, *Vet Clin Pathol* 35:127-131, 2006.

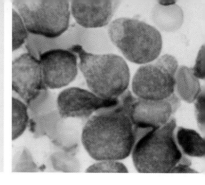

CHAPTER 15

Eyes and Adnexa

Rose E. Raskin

Cytologic examination of the eye and surrounding structures is frequently helpful in determining general categories of pathology before performing more invasive or expensive procedures. The following cytodiagnostic categories apply to the various anatomic sites of the eye. It should be noted that more than one presentation might occur in a specimen at a time.

General Cytodiagnostic Groups for Ocular Cytology
- Normal tissue
- Cystic or hyperplastic tissue
- Inflammation
- Neoplasia
- Response to tissue injury

Cytologic Biopsy Considerations

Aspiration of focal and diffuse lesions is recommended for the lesions of the eyelid, eye, and other associated structures. The thinner conjunctival tissue requires scraping with a blunt instrument such as an ophthalmic spatula or soft brush. The use of a brush was shown to reduce cellular clumping of samples and provide less cellular distortion (Willis et al., 1997). Exudate material, duct washings, and aspirate material can be used as specimens of the nasolacrimal apparatus.

EYELIDS

Normal Histology and Cytology

The dorsal and ventral eyelids are thin extensions of facial skin that meet at the lateral and medial margins, called canthi. Two to four rows of lashes are found on the upper eyelid at the free margin of the dog, while the cat has a row of cilia (Samuelson, 1999). The outermost layer resembles typical skin, with keratinized squamous epithelium and numerous hair follicles that lie in close association with sebaceous and modified sweat glands. Striated muscle fibers course through the deeper layers. The innermost layer, the palpebral conjunctiva, is lined by pseudostratified columnar epithelium containing numerous

goblet cells. Near the margins of both eyelids at the posterior end are the meibomian or tarsal glands. These large sebaceous glands lie adjacent to the palpebral conjunctiva and contribute to the lipid component of the tear film.

Inflammation

Blepharitis refers to inflammatory conditions of the eyelid. Cytologically it is characterized by the predominant cell type. Neutrophilic or purulent blepharitis most often involves bacteria such as *Staphylococcus* and *Streptococcus* sp.; however, immune-mediated disease or foreign body reactions may result in purulent inflammation. Eosinophilic inflammation should be considered for allergic reactions, some autoimmune conditions, parasitic migration (*Cuterebra* sp.), or conditions associated with collagen degeneration. Dermatophytosis or other fungal infections may be associated with granulomatous inflammation containing macrophages alone or mixed with other cell types.

Neoplasia

Diffuse neoplasms of the eyelids involve squamous cell carcinoma (especially in cats), sarcoma, mast cell tumor, and lymphoma. Focal presentations involve sebaceous gland adenoma/adenocarcinoma (canine), papilloma (canine), mast cell tumor (feline), melanoma (canine), squamous cell carcinoma (feline), cutaneous basilar epithelial neoplasm (feline), and histiocytoma (canine). Benign tumors predominate but occasionally malignant tumors such as apocrine sweat gland tumors can invade the globe and extensively damage the eye (Hirai et al., 1997).

Cyst

Chalazion, or meibomian cyst, refers to the granuloma formed from the irritating effects of ruptured sebaceous secretions or blockages caused by tumors. The leakage of meibomian cyst material incites an inflammatory response similar to a foreign body reaction. In this situation, numerous foamy macrophages, few giant cells, neutrophils, lymphocytes, amorphous debris, and sebaceous epithelium are present.

CONJUNCTIVAE

Normal Histology and Cytology

The palpebral conjunctiva is lined by a pseudostratified columnar epithelium containing goblet cells. Goblet cells appear as distended cells with an eccentric nucleus. The cytoplasm may contain clear vacuoles or red-blue granules. Mucus is common on cytologic specimens, appearing as lightly basophilic amorphous strands. The palpebral conjunctiva is continuous with the bulbar conjunctiva, which reflects onto the globe and joins the corneal epithelium. The junction of the two conjunctivae creates a sac termed the *fornix.* This blind sac is lined by stratified cuboidal epithelium containing many goblet cells. The bulbar conjunctiva consists of sheets of stratified nonkeratinized squamous epithelium, mostly intermediate and superficial with less than 1% goblet cells as detected by impression cytology (Bolzan et al., 2005). There are no significant numbers of inflammatory cells; however, mucosa-associated lymphoid tissue is located below the squamous layer of the palpebral conjunctiva near the fornix, where goblet cells are absent.

Hyperplasia

Conditions such as keratoconjunctivitis sicca, vitamin A deficiency, chronic disease, and trauma from mechanical irritants result in increased cell numbers, sometimes with evidence of metaplasia. These specimens contain many keratinized epithelial cells and goblet cells (Fig. 15-1A) (Murphy, 1988). Increased pigmentation of the epithelium may also occur such that the cytoplasm contains numerous fine, black-green melanin granules (Fig. 15-1B).

Inflammation

The predominant cell type present characterizes the conjunctivitis. Neutrophilic conjunctivitis may be associated with infectious agents such as bacteria and viruses as well as noninfectious causes. One should suspect a bacterial origin if degenerative changes are present. With viruses such as feline herpesvirus and chronic canine distemper virus, nondegenerate neutrophils predominate (Fig. 15-2A). Multinucleated epithelial cells (Fig. 15-2B) were found in approximately half of the cases with feline herpesvirus (FHV-1) infection diagnosed by culture or immunofluorescent assay (Naisse et al., 1993). Eosinophils have been associated with FHV-1 infection (Fig. 15-3A&B) (Volopich et al., 2005). Intranuclear inclusions in FHV-1 infection are occasionally encountered in conjunctival smears (Volopich et al., 2005) but are more readily seen in histologic sections. A polymerase chain reaction (PCR) test has greater sensitivity for detection of the virus than other tests (Stiles et al., 1997). Canine distemper inclusions appear pink with alcohol-based Romanowsky stains but purple with aqueous-based Wright stains.

Other infectious causes include feline chlamydiosis, which presents as variably sized discrete basophilic to bright magenta bodies in the cytoplasm of epithelium within first 2 weeks of infection. Small elementary bodies (0.3 μm) are shed that infect new cells and grow into larger (0.5 to 1.5 μm) initial bodies (Greene, 1998). The initial bodies (Fig. 15-4A&B) proliferate to become a large, membrane-bound reticulate body containing many elementary bodies (Fig. 15-5). In the Naisse et al. study (1993), visible epithelial inclusions were present in only a third of the cases positively identified by immunofluorescent assay as *Chlamydia psittaci,* currently called *Chlamydophila felis.* Besides fluorescent antibody detection, cell inoculation, enzyme-linked immunosorbent assay (ELISA), PCR procedures, or immunochemistry may be used (Volopich et al., 2005; von Bomhard et al., 2003). In one case reported, chlamydial infection in a cat was possibly transmitted from a macaw (Lipman et al., 1994).

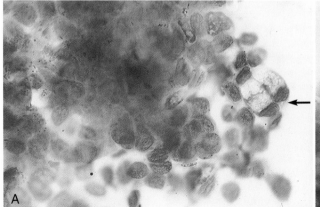
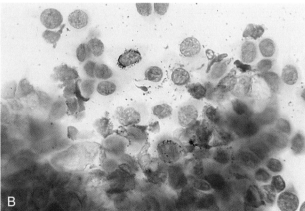

■ **FIGURE 15-1. Conjunctival scraping. Cat. Same case A-B. A, Goblet cell hyperplasia.** Chronic conjunctival disease in this animal resulted in increased numbers of goblet cells. Two are shown *(arrow)* characterized by columnar shape, eccentric nucleus, and pale foamy cytoplasm. (Wright-Giemsa; HP oil.) **B, Pigmentation and hyperplastic epithelium.** Two cells are present with abundant fine black-green cytoplasmic granules. Also note the hyperplastic epithelium with increased nuclear-to-cytoplasmic ratio. (Wright-Giemsa; HP oil.)

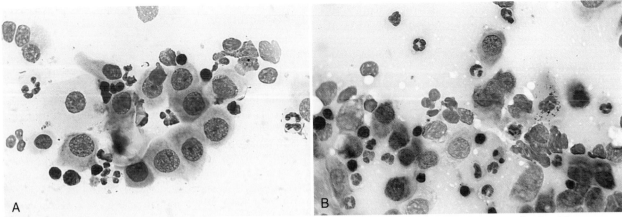

■ **FIGURE 15-2. A, Suppurative conjunctivitis. Conjunctival scraping. Cat.** The bulbar conjunctiva is hyperplastic with many nonde-generate neutrophils and few lymphocytes present in this young cat with chronic conjunctivitis. Infection with feline herpesvirus (FHV-1) was suspected. (Aqueous-based Wright; HP oil.) **B, Herpesvirus infection with suppurative conjunctivitis. Conjunctival scraping. Cat.** Many nondegenerate neutrophils are present along with reactive epithelium, including multinucleation (center). This case was confirmed previously for herpesvirus infection by polymerase chain reaction. One pigmented epithelial cell is also noted. (Wright-Giemsa; HP oil.)

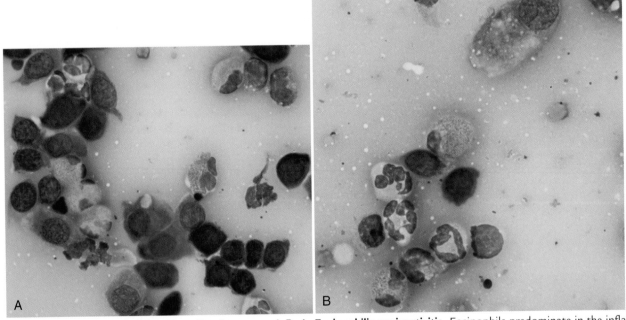

■ **FIGURE 15-3. Conjunctival brushing. Cat. Same case A-B. A, Eosinophilic conjunctivitis.** Eosinophils predominate in the inflam-matory response of this suspected herpesvirus infection with hypersensitivity in an adult cat. The small, deeply basophilic cells are the basal epithelium. Clinical signs exhibited were sneezing, tearing, blepharospasms, chemosis, and hyperemia. (Wright; HP oil.) **B, Mixed cell conjunctivitis.** In this field nondegenerate neutrophils predominate in addition to the notable increase in eosinophils. A goblet cell (upper right) is present with columnar shape and pale foamy cytoplasm. (Wright; HP oil.)

In another study, of 226 conjunctival samples, 39% were positive for non–*C. felis* chlamydial DNA, identified as *Neochlamydia hartmannellae*, in cytologic samples with eosinophilic inflammation (von Bomhard et al., 2003). Infection with feline *Mycoplasma* sp. presents as small basophilic granules similar to the elementary bod-ies of chlamydial infections with the exception that they are adherent to the surface membrane (Fig. 15-6A&B).

One study from Belgium indicated mycoplasmal infec-tion had an incidence of 25% in cats with conjunctivitis (Haesebrouck et al., 1991).

Noninfectious causes include keratoconjunctivitis sicca and allergic conditions. Eosinophilic conjunctivitis has been associated with a hypersensitivity reaction in the cat. In this situation eosinophils are seen commonly (Fig. 15-7A). Mast cell infiltrates may also be so numerous

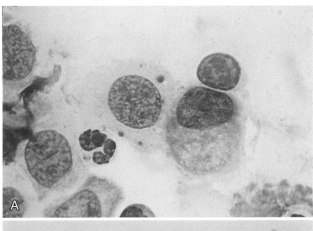

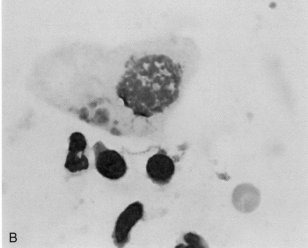

■ **FIGURE 15-4.** Chlamydiosis. Conjunctival scraping. Cat. Same case A-B. **A,** Three small basophilic initial bodies are present in the cytoplasm of one epithelial cell of this 10-month-old kitten. (Wright-Giemsa; HP oil.) **B,** Degenerating epithelial cells contain several small basophilic granular initial bodies. Another cat in the house and the owner have conjunctivitis. Nondegenerate neutrophils and small lymphocytes are also present in this sample. (Wright-Giemsa; HP oil.)

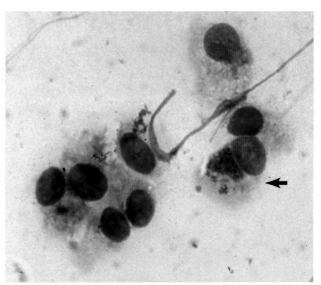

■ **FIGURE 15-5.** Chlamydiosis. Conjunctival scraping. Cat. One week earlier this cat developed pyrexia, conjunctivitis, rhinitis, and oral ulcers. The indicated cell *(arrow)* contains a perinuclear reticulate body filled with numerous elementary bodies. Diagnosis was confirmed by fluorescent antibody testing. (Wright) (Photo courtesy of John Kramer, Washington State University; presented at the 1989 ASVCP case review session.)

Miscellaneous Finding

Large amorphous basophilic inclusions within the cytoplasm of squamous epithelium have been attributed to ophthalmic ointment use, particularly those medications containing neomycin (Prasse and Winston, 1999; Young and Taylor, 2006).

NICTITATING MEMBRANE

Normal Histology and Cytology

The third eyelid, or nictitating membrane, is a large fold of conjunctiva protruding from the medial canthus. It contains a T-shaped cartilaginous plate surrounded by glandular epithelium that is serous in the cat and seromucoid in the dog (Samuelson, 1999). The palpebral and bulbar surfaces are covered by nonkeratinized stratified squamous epithelium. The free margin of the membrane is pigmented and, cytologically, fine green-black melanin granules can be found within the epithelium. Numerous variably sized lymphoid aggregates with overlying epithelium having microvilli or microfolds (M cells) on the apical surface are associated with the bulbar surface of the nictitating membrane (Giuliano et al., 2002). The stroma also contains fibrous connective tissue.

Inflammation

With follicular conjunctivitis there is a mixed population of lymphoid cells that resembles a hyperplastic lymph node (Fig. 15-8A&C). Plasma cell infiltrates (plasmacytic conjunctivitis or plasmoma) have been seen in German

that there is concern for a conjunctival mast cell tumor (Fig. 15-7B). Lymphocytes and plasma cells have been associated with allergic conditions as well as with early canine distemper infection or with chronic inflammation of the conjunctiva.

Neoplasia

Epithelium is frequently atypical and hyperplastic as a result of severe inflammation; therefore, neoplasia may be difficult to diagnose confidently. Neoplasms found associated with the conjunctival area include squamous cell carcinoma, papilloma, melanoma, lymphoma, hemangiosarcoma, and mast cell tumor. An uncommon location of transmissible venereal tumor has been the conjunctivae of the upper and lower eyelids (Boscos et al., 1998).

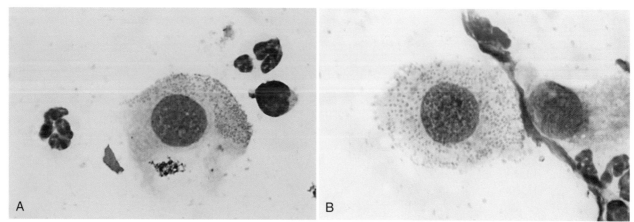

■ **FIGURE 15-6. Mycoplasmosis. Conjunctival scraping. Goat. Same case A-B. A,** This animal had keratoconjunctivitis clinically. Numerous small gray granules are associated with the cell and few organisms are found extracellularly in the background. Nondegenerate neutrophils are frequent. Stain precipitate or cellular debris is present below the cell. (Wright-Giemsa; HP oil.) **B,** Note the numerous organisms over the cytoplasm and nucleus. These granules are adherent to the surface membrane and extend into the background. (Wright-Giemsa; HP oil.)

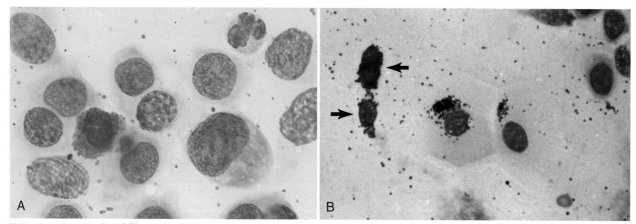

■ **FIGURE 15-7. Eosinophilic conjunctivitis. Conjunctival scraping. Cat. Same case A-B. A,** Bilateral conjunctivitis is present in this animal. An eosinophil is shown at the upper right and a mast cell is at left center. Note the mast cell granules in the background. This response occurred with a suspected hypersensitivity reaction of noninfectious causes. (Wright-Giemsa; HP oil.) **B,** Many mast cell granules are free in the background. Two mast cells *(arrows)* and two pigmented epithelial cells are present in the center. The numerous mast cells present cause concern for a mast cell tumor, but they appear fully mature and benign. (Wright-Giemsa; HP oil.)

Shepherd dogs. These thickened depigmentating lesions are composed of numerous well-differentiated plasma cells.

Neoplasia

These are similar to those seen in the conjunctivae. Adenocarcinomas, papillomas, and malignant melanomas are most common in dogs. A report of an adenocarcinoma affecting the gland of the nictitating membrane in a cat demonstrated the presence of malignant epithelial cells from impression smears of excisional biopsy material (Komaromy et al., 1997). Squamous cell carcinoma, when present on the nictitating membrane, is considered an extension from the eyelid. It appears similar to those found in the skin often with nonseptic purulent inflammation (Fig. 15-9A–E). Dogs and cats most commonly

present with hemangiosarcoma and hemangioma within the nonpigmented epithelium of the nictitating membrane compared with the conjunctivae. Exposure to ultraviolet light is suspected to be a risk factor for these endothelial neoplasms (Pirie et al., 2006; Pirie and Dubielzig, 2006).

SCLERA

Normal Histology and Cytology

The sclera is a fibrous covering of the globe that merges with the peripheral cornea and bulbar conjunctiva at the limbus, where it is pigmented. Pigment is found in all layers of the limbus except the superficial squamous cells. The underlying stroma contains dense collagen fibers, elastic fibers, fibrocytes, melanocytes, and blood vessels.

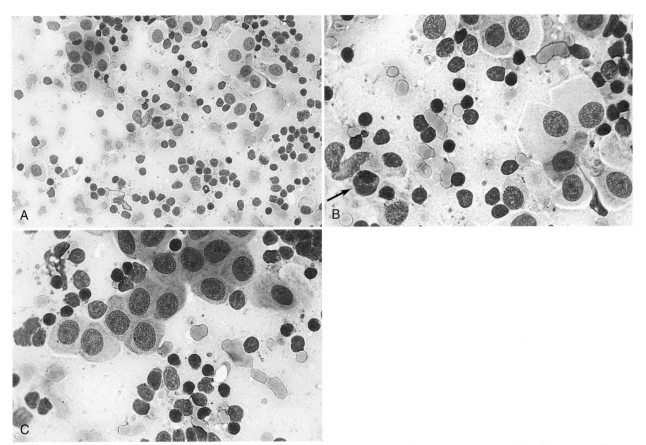

■ **FIGURE 15-8. Follicular hyperplasia. Nictitating membrane. Cat. Same case A-C. A,** Numerous small lymphocytes predominant. (Aqueous-based Wright; HP oil.) **B,** Higher magnification to demonstrate the presence of a plasma cell *(arrow)* and several intermediate lymphocytes in addition to the small lymphocytes. (Aqueous-based Wright; HP oil.) **C,** Reactive epithelium accompanies the reactive lymphoid population. (Aqueous-based Wright; HP oil.)

Aspirates may be poorly cellular, with mostly collagen present and occasional melanocytes.

Inflammation

Nodular fasciitis is a dome-shaped lesion composed of lymphoid cells, macrophages, plasma cells, fibroblasts, and few neutrophils. Melanocytes may be seen. Onchocerciasis should be a differential consideration in cases of canine episcleral nodules or periorbital swelling, particularly in dogs from the western United States. These granulomas contain the adult worm along with a variable number of eosinophils (Zarfoss et al., 2005).

Neoplasia

Neoplasms present in the sclera include melanoma, mast cell tumor, lymphoma, and sarcoma.

CORNEA

Normal Histology and Cytology

The surface of the cornea is composed of nonkeratinized stratified squamous epithelium (Fig. 15-10A). Below this surface is a thick layer of parallel bundles of collagenous stroma (Fig. 15-10B) with infrequent intermixed fibrocytes called *keratocytes.* Deeper to the stroma is a basement membrane, termed *Descemet's membrane,* composed of fine collagen fibrils. The deepest layer consists of a single layer of flattened endothelium. Cytologically, basal and intermediate squamous epithelial cells that normally lack pigmentation predominate in scrapings.

Inflammation

Infectious keratitis involves bacterial and fungal agents. Bacterial agents such as *Pseudomonas* sp., *Streptococcus* sp and *Staphylococcus* sp. produce suppurative responses with degenerative neutrophils. Fungal agents commonly isolated in mycotic keratitis are *Aspergillus* sp., *Fusarium* sp., and *Candida* sp. (Fig. 15-11). These infections produce mostly neutrophilic infiltration, but macrophages are common with occasional eosinophils. Hyphal elements are best seen with stains such as Gomori's methenamine silver. Samples should be obtained from deep within the lesion or at its edge. When used together with microbial culture, cytologic evaluation of scrapings from corneal ulcers has resulted in a maximal identification of infectious ulcerative keratitis (Massa et al., 1999).

Eosinophilic keratitis is a raised vascular lesion with white granular surface seen in cats. It is composed of

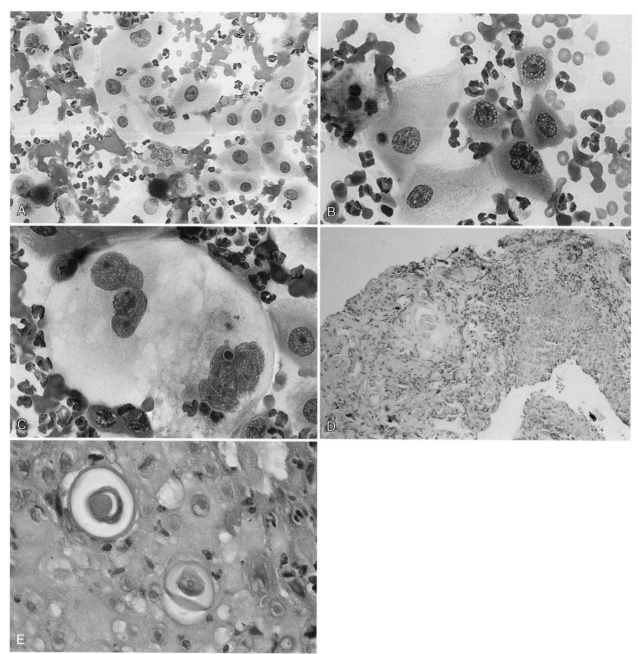

■ **FIGURE 15-9. Squamous cell carcinoma. Nictitating membrane. Cat. Same case A-E. A,** Several weeks duration of erythema and edema along with proliferative lesions on the conjunctiva and third eyelid were present in this 14-year-old cat. Sheets of epithelium appear with some features of malignancy, including anisokaryosis, multinucleation, variable nucleocytoplasmic ratio, and coarse chromatin. Many nondegenerate neutrophils are noted without evidence of sepsis. (Aqueous-based Wright; HP oil.) **B,** In addition to the previously mentioned malignant features there is perinuclear vacuolation, a feature often associated with malignant squamous epithelium. The presence of severe suppurative inflammation likely accounts for some of the dysplastic changes in the epithelium. (Aqueous-based Wright; HP oil.) **C,** Two giant epithelial cells with multiple nuclei. The presence of very bizarre morphologic changes and the absence of sepsis further supports the malignant, not dysplastic nature of the epithelium. (Aqueous-based Wright; HP oil.) **D,** This section is taken from the junction between the palpebral conjunctiva on the left and the nictitating membrane on the right. Note the marked disorganization of the mucous membrane and dermis. This tumor is thought to originate from the eyelid with extension to the nictitating membrane. (H&E; IP.) **E,** Two keratin pearls that are often associated with malignant squamous epithelium appear in the center and help to identify the neoplasm. (H&E; HP oil.)

squamous epithelium, cellular debris, including eosinophil granules, and numerous mast cells with lower numbers of intact eosinophils (Fig. 15-12A). Deeper scrapings contain predominantly eosinophils and lymphoid cells (Fig. 15-12B&C) (Prasse and Winston, 1999).

The histopathology and cytology have been well described in an article by Prasse and Winston (1996) in which they demonstrate that mast cells are most frequent in scrapings that avoid the white surface exudate. In a study involving detection of feline herpesvirus

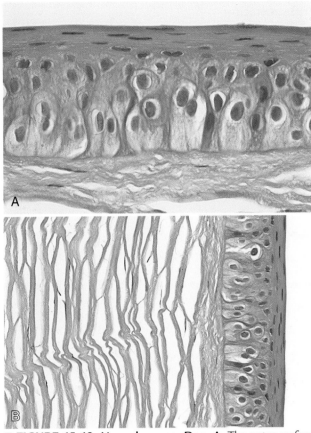

■ **FIGURE 15-10. Normal cornea. Dog. A,** The outer surface is composed of nonkeratinized stratified squamous epithelium. **B,** Below the surface epithelium is a thick layer of parallel bundles of collagenous stroma. (H&E; HP oil.)

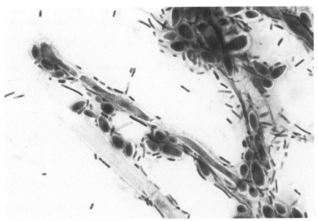

■ **FIGURE 15-11. Mycotic keratitis. Corneal scraping. Dog.** There is a 1-week history of raised white punctate masses on the cornea. Against the background of extracellular rod-shaped bacteria are hyphal elements and many spore forms. Infection with *Candida* sp. was suspected. Neutrophils were present in other fields of the specimen. (Aqueous-based Wright; HP oil.)

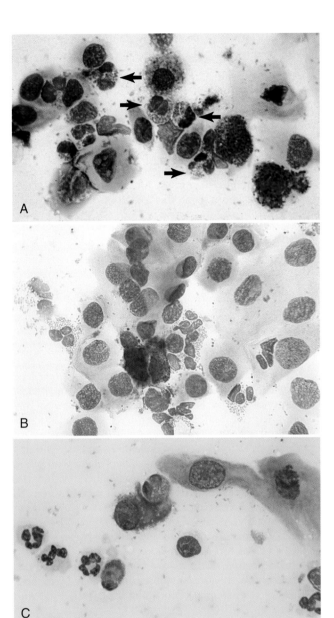

■ **FIGURE 15-12. Same case A-B. Eosinophilic keratitis. Corneal scraping. Cat. A,** There was a gritty, white proliferative mass at the lateral limbus of this animal with recurrent keratitis. Note the mixture of eosinophils *(arrows)* and many mast cells along with corneal epithelium. Surface granular material often contains high numbers of mast cells in addition to eosinophils. (Wright-Giemsa; HP oil.) **B,** This sample was likely taken from deeper into the cornea since it contains many more eosinophils than mast cells. (Wright-Giemsa; HP oil.) **C, Corneal brushing.** This sample is taken from an adult cat with a raised white proliferative lesion of two months duration. Reactive squamous epithelium is shown along with a mixed population of nondegenerate neutrophils and eosinophils. Rod-shaped eosinophil granules produce the stippled background. (Wright-Giemsa; HP oil.)

infection, there was a significant association between viral presence and epithelial keratitis (Volopich et al., 2005). In another study of eosinophilic keratitis, 76% of these cases had detectable FHV-1 DNA by PCR analysis suggesting a role for the virus in the pathogenesis of this disease (Naisse et al., 1998).

Pannus, or chronic superficial keratitis, is a common condition seen in German Shepherds that reflects a chronic progressive disease. It initially appears at the limbus as a red, vascularized lesion that progresses centrally, becoming fleshlike and later pigmented and scarred. Initially it appears cytologically as mixed inflammation with plasma cells, lymphocytes, macrophages, and neutrophils.

Response to Tissue Injury

Noninflammatory opaque corneal lesions may result from disease. Lipid corneal degeneration may be seen in old dogs with renal disease. Cytologically, only normal epithelium is seen. Another condition is mineralization, which appears as a granular plaque. On cytology, nonstaining crystalline material is found which often stains positive for calcium using the von Kossa stain.

Neoplasia

Squamous cell carcinoma, papilloma, melanoma, and sarcoma are the predominant tumor types, although tumors of the cornea are rare.

IRIS AND CILIARY BODY

Normal Histology and Cytology

The iris and ciliary body are termed the *anterior uvea.* The uvea is highly vascular and often pigmented (Fig. 15-13). The anterior border layer contains a single layer of fibroblasts with several underlying layers of melanocytes (Samuelson, 1999). These melanocytes in the dog and cat contain rod to oval brown melanin granules. The iris stroma consists of fine collagenous fibers along with blood vessels and nerves. Unstriated muscle fibers within the stroma help to dilate the iris. The posterior iridal surface is covered by pigmented epithelium that is continuous with the ciliary body. As an extension of the choroid layer, the ciliary body provides nutrients and removes wastes for the cornea and lens through formation of the aqueous humor. The main portion of the ciliary body consists of smooth muscle along with vascular sinuses and heavily pigmented epithelium at the surface containing large, round melanin granules.

Inflammation

Pyogranulomatous or granulomatous inflammation may occur with fungal infections such as coccidioidomycosis, blastomycosis, cryptococcosis, and histoplasmosis. Feline infectious peritonitis may also produce an anterior uveitis with pyogranulomatous iridocyclitis (Fig. 15-14). Other infectious conditions associated with lymphoplasmacytic uveitis include canine and feline bartonellosis, and canine monocytic ehrlichiosis (Michau et al., 2003; Ketring et al., 2004; Panciera et al., 2001; Komnenou et al., 2007). Lens-induced uveitis may produce a lymphocytic-plasmacytic infiltration consistent with immune reactivity to lens proteins.

Neoplasia

Melanomas are the most common primary intraocular tumor in the dog, with the anterior uvea most often affected. When melanoma occurs in the cat, it involves more often the iris and ciliary body. Ocular melanoma is more common than oral and dermal melanomas in the cat (Patnaik and Mooney, 1988). Ocular melanoma is also more malignant than dermal melanoma, with higher rates of mortality and metastasis. Aspiration of the neoplasm may be accomplished through the anterior chamber using a 25-gauge or smaller needle. Cytologic features of mitotic index, nuclear size and pleomorphism, and degree of pigmentation are helpful for prognostic purposes in the dog but not in the cat. The presence of anisokaryosis, variable nuclear-to-cytoplasmic ratio, and prominent nucleoli should help to distinguish malignant melanocytes from melanophages.

Ciliary neoplasms such as iridociliary adenoma and adenocarcinoma are the second most common primary intraocular tumors in the dog (Fig. 15-15). These tumors are rare in the cat. Lymphoma has been recognized as the most frequent intraocular tumor in cats (Glaze and Gelatt, 1999). It occurs as a diffuse or

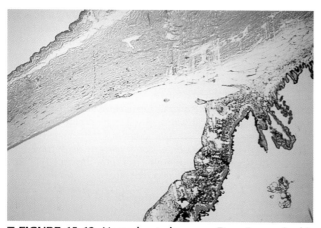

■ **FIGURE 15-13. Normal anterior uvea. Dog.** Present in this view is the cornea near the limbus where the iris and ciliary body attach at the iridocorneal angle. Portions of both the anterior and posterior chambers of the anterior humor compartment are shown. (H&E; LP.)

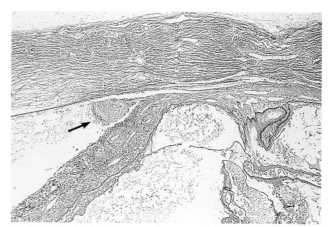

■ **FIGURE 15-14. Pyogranulomatous iridocyclitis. Cat.** Note the presence of an anterior uveitis with accumulation of inflammatory cells in the iridocorneal angle *(arrow)* and in the junction between the iris and ciliary body in this animal with confirmed feline infectious peritonitis. (H&E; LP.)

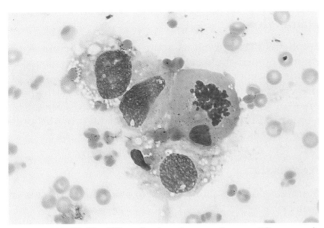

■ **FIGURE 15-15. Ciliary body adenocarcinoma. Tissue aspirate of an ocular mass extending from the iris. Dog.** Shown is a tight cluster of epithelial cells with high nuclear-to-cytoplasmic ratio, coarse chromatin, anisokaryosis, and a mitotic figure. The cytoplasm is foamy with numerous discrete vacuoles. (Wright-Giemsa; HP oil.)

nodular iris lesion. Evidence of ocular lymphoma often suggests this is metastatic from a primary site that should be found. Cytologic changes are similar to lymphoid neoplasms in other sites (Fig. 15-16A–C).

Uveal Hematopoiesis

Recent studies in six young cats with early life ocular disease (collapse of the globe, corneal perforation with protrusion of the anterior uvea) detected hematopoiesis by histomorphology in three cases. Erythroid and white cell precursors along with occasional megakaryocytes were present in the anterior and posterior uvea (Jacobi and Dubielzig, 2008). Aspirates of damaged eyes in these cases would be expected to demonstrate the extramedullary hematopoiesis.

AQUEOUS HUMOR

Normal Cytology and Collection

When aqueous humor is cloudy, cytologic evaluation of the fluid may help to diagnose the presence of infectious agents or neoplasms. Fine-needle aspiration is conducted under anesthesia using a 25-gauge or smaller needle by entering at the limbus through the bulbar conjunctiva. A small amount of fluid is removed, which is then evaluated immediately. A direct cell count using a hemocytometer is performed followed by sedimentation of the fluid for smear or cytospin preparation. Additional fluid is used to measure total protein by a microprotein technique. Normal aqueous humor in the dog has a direct cell count mean of 8.2/µl (range 0 to 37) and protein mean of 36.4 mg/dl (range 21 to 65). Normal aqueous humor in the cat has a direct cell count mean of 2.2/µl (range 0 to 15) and protein mean of 43.7 mg/dl (range 22 to 75) (Hazel et al., 1985). Cytologically, the low-protein fluid is acellular with only occasional free melanin granules or melanin-containing cells.

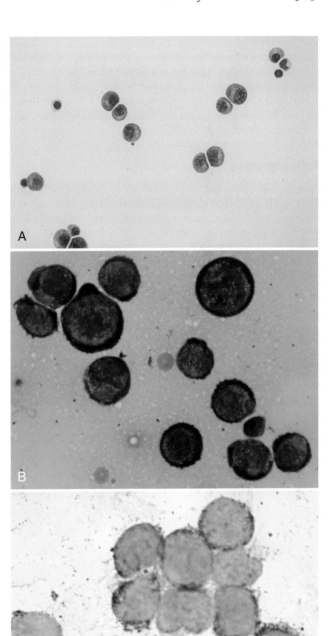

■ **FIGURE 15-16. Lymphoma. Cat. A, Iris mass aspirate.** Large, discrete, round cells with plasmacytoid features are prominent in this neoplasm. Lymphoma is the most frequent intraocular tumor in cats. (Romanowsky; HP oil.) **Same case B-C. Iris mass imprint. B,** Extremely large, deeply basophilic round cells are present. Compared with an erythrocyte and small lymphocyte (lower right), these cells measure up to 25µm in diameter. Notice the RBC size of the nucleolus in several of the cells. (Wright-Giemsa; HP oil.) **C,** Same case as in (B). Neoplastic round cell population staining positive for a B-cell marker. (anti-BLA.36; HP oil.)

This clear fluid originates from the vascular sinuses within the folds and processes of the posterior portion of the ciliary body. The humor flows from the posterior chamber of the anterior compartment through the pupil, then into the anterior chamber to the filtration angle. Excess fluid is removed at the iridocorneal angle through a vascular meshwork.

Inflammation

Anterior uveitis most often produces a neutrophilic infiltrate with infectious causes such as bacteria, *Blastomyces* sp., *Prototheca* sp., and *Leishmania* sp. Mononuclear uveitis may occur in the presence of hemorrhage. Evidence of damage to the ciliary body and/or iris can result in frequent rod to round melanin granules engulfed by macrophages (Fig. 15-17A&B).

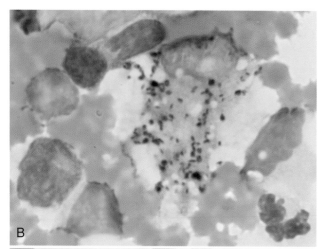
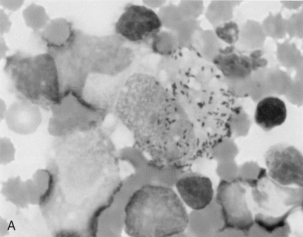

■ **FIGURE 15-17. Mixed mononuclear inflammation. Aqueous humor aspirate. Dog. Same case A-B. A,** Variably sized lymphocytes and macrophages predominate in this case with chronic anterior uveitis with secondary glaucoma. One macrophage contains numerous rod-shaped melanin granules typical of the anterior iris. (Wright-Giemsa; HP oil.) **B,** Small and intermediate lymphocytes predominate in this field. One macrophage contains both rod and round shapes of melanin granules consistent with those of the iris and ciliary body. (Wright-Giemsa; HP oil.)

Hemorrhage

Hyphema may present as acute or chronic hemorrhage. Acute hemorrhage may be indicated by the presence of erythrophagocytosis by macrophages. Platelets may be present if ongoing hemorrhage is occurring but the presence of platelets alone may indicate blood contamination only. Chronic hemorrhage is indicated by the presence of hemosiderin-laden macrophages.

Neoplasia

Metastatic tumors rarely exfoliate, with the exception of lymphoma.

RETINA

Normal Histology and Cytology

The retina is composed of 10 classical layers, which include the retinal pigment epithelium, rod and cone layer, outer limiting membrane, outer nuclear layer, outer plexiform layer, inner nuclear layer, inner plexiform layer, ganglion cell layer, nerve fiber layer, and inner limiting membrane (Fig. 15-18A). The outer nuclear layer in dogs and cats contains predominately rod nuclei, which are small, round, dense, and very distinctive in appearance (Fig. 15-18B–D). The retinal pigment epithelium is continuous with the outer layer of the ciliary body and is highly pigmented except in the region of the tapetum lucidum. Melanin within the pigmented retinal epithelial cells appear as lanceolate or elongated (Fig. 15-18E–F). External to the retina and closely adherent to the retinal pigment epithelium is the choroid, also termed the *posterior uvea,* which is mostly composed of large, round, brown to black granules (Fig. 15-18E–G).

Response to Tissue Injury

Retinal detachment may produce a subretinal cavity that contains only normal retinal cells, as was demonstrated in one feline case (Knoll, 1990).

VITREOUS BODY

Normal Cytology and Collection

Vitreocentesis may be attempted under general anesthesia using a 23-gauge or smaller needle to extract 0.2 to 0.5 mL of fluid from a region 6 to 8 mm caudal to the limbus. It is important to direct the needle caudad within the center of the globe but avoid the lens. The fluid is a transparent jellylike material that is primarily water with the remainder composed of collagen and hyaluronic acid (Samuelson, 1999). The humor is likely formed by the nonpigmented epithelium of the ciliary body. In dogs and cats the vitreous humor is dense in the center of the cavity and fluid at the periphery, unlike in primates. It is acellular except for hyalocytes, a type of histiocyte. In addition to hyalocytes, fibrocytes and glial

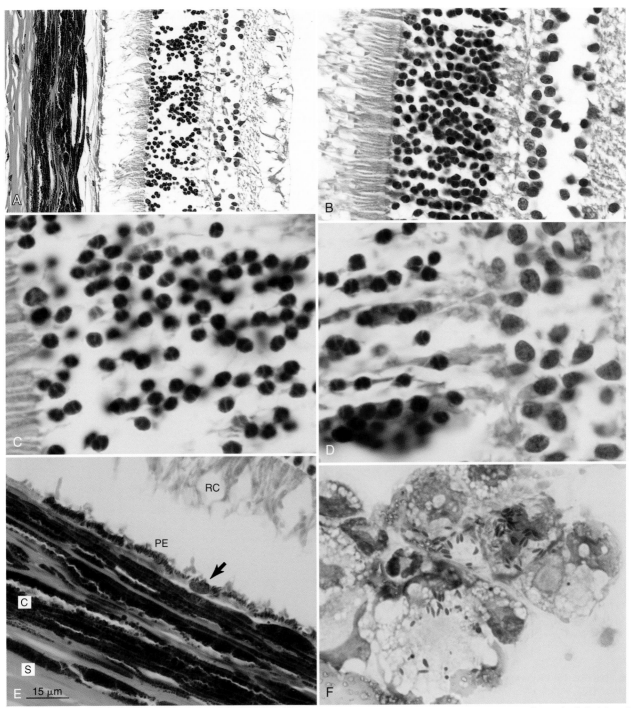

■ **FIGURE 15-18. Same case A-E, Normal retina. Dog. A,** Shown are the layers of the retina beginning externally at the left side adjacent to the pigmented choroid. They are the retinal pigment epithelium, rod and cone layer, outer limiting membrane (not visible), outer nuclear layer, outer plexiform layer, inner nuclear layer, inner plexiform layer, ganglion layer, nerve fiber layer, and inner limiting membrane. (H&E; HP oil.) **B,** Higher magnification to better demonstrate. From left to right, the rod and cone layer, outer nuclear layer, outer plexiform layer, and inner nuclear layer. (H&E; HP oil.) **C,** Portion of the rod and cone layer is shown on the left side. The outer nuclear layer in dogs and cats contains predominately rod nuclei, which are small, round, and densely stained. The nuclear appearance with its marginated chromatin is very distinctive for these cells. (H&E; HP oil.) **D,** Clusters of nuclei from the outer layer are contrasted with the large less dense nuclei of the inner nuclear layer. An outer plexiform layer lies between the two nuclear layers and the edge of the inner plexiform layer is shown at far upper right. (H&E; HP oil.) **E,** High magnification of outer retinal layers, choroid *(C)*, and external sclera *(S)*. The most external retinal layer is the pigmented epithelium *(PE)* that contains a palisading row of lanceolate melanin granules in addition to their nucleus *(arrow)*. The artifactually displaced rod and cone layer *(RC)* normally lies adjacent to the retinal pigmented epithelial layer. Notice the round brown granules of the choroid layer. (H&E; HP oil.) **F, Retinal melanin granules. Vitreous humor aspirate. Dog.** Characteristic lanceolate or caraway seed–shaped melanin granules from the pigmented retinal epithelium are present within macrophages. (Wright-Giemsa; HP oil.)

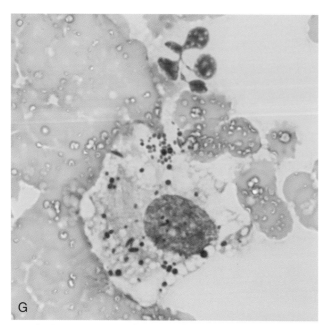

■ **FIGURE 15-18, cont'd. G, Uveal melanin granules. Vitreous humor aspirate.** Same case as in E. The choroid layer adjacent to the retina contains numerous large round brown-black granules as shown within the macrophage. Few lanceolate retinal melanin granules are also present. (Wright-Giemsa; HP oil.)

cells make up a small portion of the vitreal cells found in the fluid. Occasional lanceolate or caraway seed–shaped melanin granules may be present that are likely retinal in origin.

Inflammation

Infectious causes of endophthalmitis include bacteria, aspergillosis (Gelatt et al., 1991) (Fig 15-19A&B), blastomycosis (Fig 15-19C), cryptococcosis, histoplasmosis, and prototothecosis (Stenner et al., 2007) (Fig. 15-20).

Response to Tissue Injury

Hemorrhage (Fig. 15-21A) appears similar to that found in the aqueous humor. Lens fibers may be seen with primary lens disease or secondary to accidental puncture during sample collection. They appear as uniform amorphous basophilic strands or ribbon structures (Fig. 15-21B&C). Their degeneration may induce a neutrophilic inflammatory response. Retinal cells, when present, are usually the result of inadvertent aspiration or may reflect detachment secondary to disease e.g., uveitis or glaucoma. Photoreceptor and ganglion cells have been rarely identified on cytology; photoreceptor nuclei have marginated heterochromatin with central pale

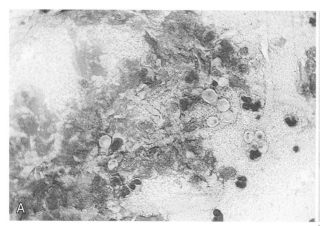

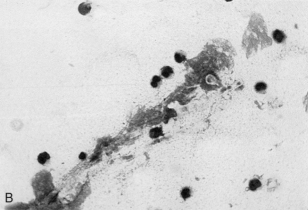

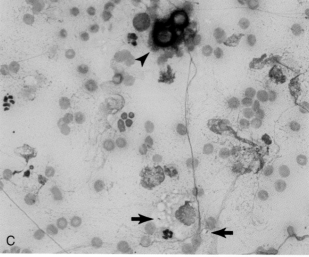

■ **FIGURE 15-19. Same case A-B, Aspergillosis. Vitreocentesis. Dog. A,** This German shepherd dog had a history of paraplegia related to discospondylitis. Bilateral uveitis was present along with other systemic signs of infection. The background is eosinophilic and granular with degenerate neutrophils. Against this proteinaceous material are the clear-staining hyphae and round spores of this fungal agent, which were cultured and identified as *Aspergillus terreus.* (Wright-Giemsa; HP oil.) **B,** Hyphae are more visible in this field. Aspergillosis is a common cause of infectious endophthalmitis. (Wright-Giemsa; HP oil.) **C, Blastomycosis. Vitreocentesis. Dog.** Two blue-stained round yeast forms *(arrowhead)* are present along with numerous degenerate neutrophils against a background of many erythrocytes and nuclear debris. One macrophage appears vacuolated and has engulfed a lanceolate retinal melanin granule *(arrow).* Another granules in noted in the background *(arrow).* (Wright; HP oil.)

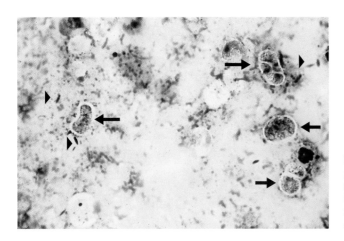

■ **FIGURE 15-20. Protothecosis. Vitreocentesis. Dog.** Shown present against the eosinophilic granular vitreal material are four sporulating forms *(arrows)* of *Prototheca zopfii*. Also present in the background are several lanceolate melanin granules typical of the retina melanocytes *(arrowheads)*. (Wright-Giemsa; HP oil.) (Photo courtesy of A. Eric Schultze, University of Tennessee.)

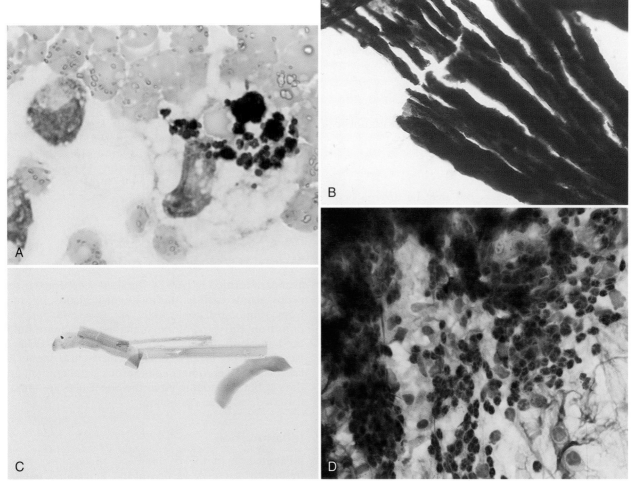

■ **FIGURE 15-21. A, Acute hemorrhage with uveal melanin granules. Vitreous humor aspirate.** Same case as in Figure 15-18E. A macrophage is shown that has engulfed an erythrocyte as well as clumps of large round brown to black melanin granules consistent with the choroid layer. (Wright-Giemsa; HP oil.) **Same case B-C. Lens fibers. Vitreocentesis. Dog. B,** Dark basophilic–staining fibers appear in parallel fashion. A mononuclear infiltrate of small lymphocytes (not shown) is present in low numbers in the vitreous humor, suggesting the presence of the lens fibers was the result of inadvertent puncture of the lens. (Wright-Giemsa; HP oil.) **C,** Isolated lightly basophilic lens fibers are recognized by the rectangular sharp outlines and ribbon-like appearance. (Wright-Giemsa; HP oil.) **Same case D-E. Retinal cells. Vitreous humor aspirate. Dog.** Cytospin preparation from patient with uveitis and secondary glaucoma. Large clusters of photoreceptor nuclei with minimal mononuclear inflammation (not shown) and erythrocytes suggest inadvertent retinal aspiration. Retinal detachment would need to be ruled out based on the clinical history. (Wright-Giemsa; HP oil.)

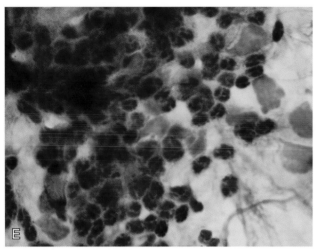

■ **FIGURE 15-21, cont'd. E,** Higher magnification of the retinal cells demonstrates the characteristic nucleus with marginated chromatin producing the appearance of nuclear segmentation. (Wright-Giemsa; HP oil.)

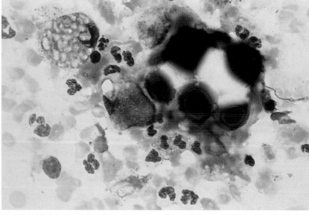

■ **FIGURE 15-22. Cryptococcosis. Tissue aspirate of periorbital mass. Dog.** This animal presented with protuberance of the frontal bone and blindness. Pyogranulomatous reaction occurred in response to the dark spherical yeast forms of *Cryptococcus neoformans*. (Wright-Giemsa; HP oil.)

euchromatin producing the appearance of a divided or segmented nucleus (Fig. 15-21D&E).

Neoplasia

This is rarely seen on cytology, but will be diagnostic when found.

ORBITAL CAVITY

The orbit has bony borders but may be approached through several sites. The most direct routes are the lateral and medial canthi by fine-needle aspiration biopsy (FNAB). Another route is the insertion of a needle behind the last upper molar into the retrobulbar space. One study compared the usefulness of FNAB in conjunction with ultrasonography in the diagnosis of clinical exophthalmos (Boydell, 1991). The procedure was diagnostic in 34 of 35 cases.

Inflammation

Bacterial infection is likely to induce a purulent response resulting in cellulitis or abscess formation. Periorbital masses may arise from fungal infections such as cryptococcosis (Fig. 15-22). Inflammation may also result from a mucocele from the zygomatic gland. The material obtained is often clear and viscid, consistent with saliva.

Neoplasia

Neoplasms involving the orbit include lymphoma, melanoma, mast cell tumor, histiocytic sarcoma squamous cell carcinoma, adenocarcinoma of the lacrimal or salivary glands (Fig. 15-23A–D), chondrosarcoma, and other sarcomas. In one case, FNAB of a suspected neoplasm posterior to the eye resulted in inadvertent aspiration of normal retinal epithelium with resultant

intraocular hemorrhage (Roth and Sisson, 1999). The classification of feline intraocular neoplasms by histochemistry and immunohistochemistry was published recently (Grahn et al., 2006). Histiocytic sarcoma must be considered in the differential diagnosis of dogs with intraocular masses, especially in Rottweilers and retriever breeds. It may be distinguished from melanoma by finding CD18-positive cells and no reactivity using Melan-A. The ocular manifestation of histiocytic sarcoma arises from the systemic form of the disease (Naranjo et al., 2007).

NASOLACRIMAL APPARATUS

Normal Histology and Cytology

Tears are formed in part by the lipid secretions of sebaceous glands such as the meibomian glands, by mucin from conjunctival goblet cells, and by seromucoid secretions from the gland of the nictitating membrane, but are predominantly formed by the aqueous fluid from the lacrimal gland located dorsolateral to the globe. The lacrimal gland is composed of serous gland epithelium in the cat but is seromucoid in the dog. Ducts are lined by flattened, cuboidal epithelium.

Inflammation

Inflammation of the lacrimal sac, or *dacryocystitis,* is frequently bacterial in origin and neutrophil exudates result obstructing the ducts.

Cyst

A cyst arising within the duct of the lacrimal gland is termed *dacryops* and contains serous or seromucoid material of low cellularity. It may be mixed with few neutrophils and macrophages (Prasse and Winston, 1999).

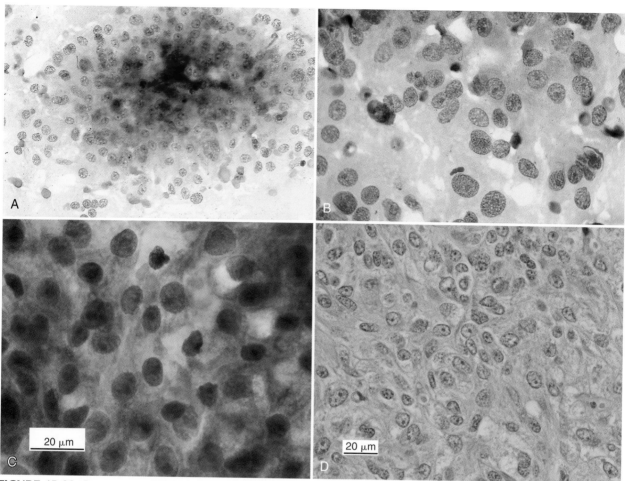

■ **FIGURE 15-23. Same case A-B. Salivary/lacrimal gland adenocarcinoma. Tissue aspirate of retrobulbar mass. Dog. A,** Dense cluster of a monomorphic population of epithelial cells having high nuclear-to-cytoplasmic ratios and anisokaryosis. The exact origin was not clear on histopathology. It produced minor degenerative changes to the retina but did not invade the globe. (Wright-Giemsa; HP oil.) **B,** Higher magnification demonstrates an acinus (upper right corner) and the foamy secretory appearance of the cytoplasm. Several nuclear features of malignancy are present, including high nuclear-to-cytoplasmic ratio, anisokaryosis, coarse chromatin, prominent nucleoli, and multinucleation. (Wright-Giemsa; HP oil.) **Same case C-D. Retrobulbar adenocarcinoma. Cat. C, Tissue aspirate.** A monomorphic cluster of small to medium epithelial cells is present that have a single round to oval nucleus set in a moderate amount of wispy, blue to grey cytoplasm with indistinct margins. The nuclei exhibit a finely stippled chromatin pattern and often contain one or two fairly prominent, round to slightly angular nucleoli. Slight anisokaryosis and anisocytosis are noted. Nuclear-to-cytoplasmic ratios are only slightly increased. The minimal anaplastic features suggest a low-grade carcinoma cytologically. (Wright; HP oil.) **D, Tissue section.** Mild to moderate anisokaryosis, moderate nuclear-to-cytoplasmic ratio, and low numbers of mitotic figures (not shown) confirm a low-grade neoplasia. Cell clusters with junctions that were confirmed by electron microscopy support the epithelial origin. The pale or foamy/vacuolar appearance of the cytoplasm suggests a secretory or glandular product. Top considerations include salivary or lacrimal origin or, less likely, nasal epithelium. (H&E; HP oil.)

REFERENCES

Bolzan AA, Brunelli ATJ, Castro MB, et al: Conjunctival impression cytology in dogs, *Vet Ophthalmol* 8: 401-405, 2005.

Boscos CM, Ververidis HN, Tondis DK, et al: Ocular involvement of transmissible venereal tumor in a dog, *Vet Ophthalmol* 1998. 1:167-170.

Boydell P: Fine needle aspiration biopsy in the diagnosis of exophthalmos, *J Sm Anim Pract* 32:542-546, 1991.

Gelatt KN, Chrisman CL, Samuelson DA, et al: Ocular and systemic aspergillosis in a dog, *J Am Anim Hosp Assoc* 27: 427-431, 1991.

Glaze MB, Gelatt KN: Feline ophthalmology. In Gelatt KN (ed): *Veterinary ophthalmology*, ed 3, Philadelphia, 1999, Lippincott Williams & Wilkins, pp 997-1052.

Grahn BH, Peiffer RL, Cullen CL, et al: Classification of feline intraocular neoplasms based on morphology, histochemical staining, and immunohistochemical labeling, *Vet Ophthalmol* 9:395-403, 2006.

Greene CE: Chlamydial infections. In Greene CE (ed): *Infectious diseases of the dog and cat*, ed 2, Philadelphia, 1998, WB Saunders, pp 172-174.

Giuliano EA, Moore CP, Phillips TE: Morphological evidence of M cells in healthy canine conjunctiva-associated lymphoid tissue, *Graefe's Arch Clin Exp Ophthalmol* 240:220-226, 2002.

Haesebrouck F, Devriese LA, van Rijssen B, et al: Incidence and significance of isolation of *Mycoplasma felis* from conjunctival swabs of cats, *Vet Microbiol* 26:95-101, 1991.

Hazel SJ, Thrall MAH, Severin GA, et al: Laboratory evaluation of aqueous humor in the healthy dog, cat, horse, and cow, *Am J Vet Res*;46:657-659, 1985.

Hirai T, Mubarak M, Kimura T, et al: Apocrine gland tumor of the eyelid in a dog, *Vet Pathol* 34:232-234,1997.

Jacobi S, Dubielzig RR: Feline early life ocular disease, *Vet Ophthalmol* 11:166-169, 2008.

Ketring KL, Zuckerman EE, Hardy WD: *Bartonella*: a new etiological agent of feline ocular disease, *J Am Anim Hosp Assoc* 40:6-12, 2004.

Knoll JS: What is your diagnosis? *Vet Clin Pathol* 19:32-34, 1990.

Komaromy AM, Ramsey DT, Render IA, et al: Primary adenocarcinoma of the gland of the nictitating membrane in a cat, *J Am Anim Hosp Assoc* 33:333-336,1997.

Komnenou AA, Mylonakis ME, Kouti V, et al: Ocular manifestations of natural canine monocytic ehrlichiosis (*Ehrlichia canis*): a retrospective study of 90 cases, *Vet Ophthalmol* 10:137-142, 2007.

Lipman NS, Yan L-L, Murphy JC: Probable transmission of *Chlamydia psittaci* from a macaw to a cat, *J Am Vet Med Assoc* 204:1479-1480, 1994.

Massa KL, Murphy CJ, Hartmann FA, et al: Usefulness of aerobic microbial culture and cytologic evaluation of corneal specimens in the diagnosis of infectious ulcerative keratitis in animals, *J Am Vet Med Assoc* 215:1671-1674, 1999.

Michau TM, Breitschwerdt EB, Gilger BC, et al: *Bartonella vinsonii* subspecies *berkhoffi* as a possible cause of anterior uveitis and choroiditis in a dog, *Vet Ophthalmol* 6:299-304, 2003.

Murphy JM: Exfoliative cytologic examination as an aid in diagnosing ocular diseases in the dog and cat, *Semin Vet Med Surg (Sm Anim)* 3:10-14, 1988.

Naisse MP, Guy JS, Stevens JB, et al: Clinical and laboratory findings in chronic conjunctivitis in cats: 91 cases (1983-1991), *J Am Vet Med Assoc* 203:834-837, 1993.

Naisse MP, Glover TL, Moore CP, et al. Detection of feline herpesvirus 1 DNA in corneas of cats with eosinophilic keratitis or corneal sequestration, *Am J Vet Res* 59: 856-858, 1998.

Naranjo C, Dubielzig RR, Friedrichs KR: Canine ocular histiocytic sarcoma, *Vet Ophthalmol* 10:179-185, 2007.

Panciera RJ, Ewing SA, Confer AW: Ocular histopathology of ehrlichial infections in the dog, *Vet Pathol* 38:43-46, 2001.

Patnaik AK, Mooney S: Feline melanoma: a comparative study of ocular, oral, and dermal neoplasms, *Vet Pathol* 25:105-112, 1988.

Pirie CG, Dubielzig RR: Feline conjunctival hemangioma and hemangiosarcoma: a retrospective evaluation of eight cases (1993-2004), *Vet Ophthalmol* 9:227-231, 2006.

Pirie CG, Knollinger AM, Thomas CB, et al: Canine conjunctival hemangioma and hemangiosarcoma: a retrospective evaluation of 108 cases (1989-2004), *Vet Ophthalmol* 9:215-226, 2006.

Prasse KW, Winston SM: Cytology and histopathology of feline eosinophilic keratitis, *Vet Comp Opthalmol* 6:74-81, 1996.

Prasse KW, Winston SM: The eyes and associated structures. In Cowell RL, Tyler RD, Meinkoth JH (eds): *Diagnostic cytology and hematology of the dog and cat*, ed 2, St Louis, 1999, Mosby, pp 68-82.

Roth L, Sisson A: Aspirate of a mass posterior to the eye. *Vet Clin Pathol* 28:89-90, 1999.

Samuelson DA: Ophthalmic anatomy. In Gelatt KN (ed): *Veterinary ophthalmology*, ed 3, Philadelphia, 1999, Lippincott Williams & Wilkins, pp 31-150.

Stenner VJ, Mackay B, King T, et al: Prototheccosis in 17 Australian dogs and a review of the canine literature, *Med Mycol* 45:249-266, 2007.

Stiles J, McDermott M, Bigsby D, et al: Use of nested polymerase chain reaction to identify feline herpesvirus in ocular tissue from clinically normal cats and cats with corneal sequestra or conjunctivitis, *Am J Vet Res* 58:338-342, 1997.

Volopich S, Benetka V, Schwendenwein I, et al: Cytologic findings, and feline herpesvirus DNA and *Chlamydophila felis* antigen detection rates in normal cats and cats with conjunctival and corneal lesions, *Vet Ophthalmol* 8:25-32, 2005.

von Bomhard W, Polkinghorne A, Lu ZH, et al: Detection of novel chlamydiae in cats with ocular disease, *Am J Vet Res* 64:1421-1428, 2003.

Willis M, Bounous DI, Hirsh S, et al: Conjunctival brush cytology: evaluation of a new cytological collection technique in dogs and cats with a comparison to conjunctival scraping, *Vet Comp Ophthalmol* 7:74-81, 1997.

Young KM, Taylor J: Laboratory medicine: Yesterday today tomorrow: Eye on the cytoplasm, *Vet Clin Pathol* 35:141, 2006.

Zarfoss MK, Dubielzig RR, Eberhard ML, et al: Canine ocular onchocerciasis in the United States: Two new cases and a review of the literature, *Vet Ophthalmol* 8:51-57, 2005.

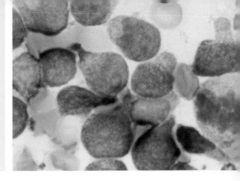

Endocrine System

A. Rick Alleman and Ul Soo Choi

The endocrine system consists of the thyroid, parathyroid, adrenal cortex, and pancreatic islet cells. These highly integrated, highly vascularized glands have sinusoids that are closely associated with secretory parenchymal cells from which hormones are produced. Also included within the endocrine system are paraganglionic cells, which are neuroendocrine cells that synthesize and secrete both catecholamines and other regulatory peptides. The neuroendocrine cells involve those of the adrenal medulla and extra-adrenal sites that are derived from neuroectoderm. The extra-adrenal paraganglionic cells include the aortic and carotid bodies, which have chemoreceptor activity in the blood gas regulation, as well as others found in the gastrointestinal tract and lung. Embryologically, neuroendocrine cells are present in gastrointestinal tissue as well as the tracheobronchial tree and liver (Hamilton et al., 1999).

Disease involving the endocrine system may involve hyperplasia, hypoplasia, inflammation, and neoplasia, with the latter condition of most interest to the cytopathologist. Endocrine system tumors are often very cellular, with the exception of aspirates from some thyroid tumors, which are often blood contaminated. Neuroendocrine neoplasms may arise from any of the endocrine glands or chemoreceptor organs giving rise to both adenomas and adenocarcinomas. Tumors arising from the neuroendocrine cells of the nasal cavity, lung, liver, skin, or gastrointestinal tract are generally termed "carcinoids." Tumors of endocrine glands and neuroendocrine cells share a characteristic cytologic feature. Slide preparations appear as naked nuclei or free nuclei embedded in a background of pale cytoplasm with few distinct cytoplasmic borders. This is an artifact of aspiration and slide preparation that results from the fragile nature of the cells from these organs. This cytologic feature should not be confused with poorly prepared samples from other tissues, where cell lysis occurs when excessive pressure is applied to the slides during sample preparation. In the later case, cell damage such as nuclear lysis and nuclear streaming will also be evident.

Although neuroendocrine tumors share common characteristics, they can often be distinguished from each other by the location of the lesion and distinctive cytologic features that may be present. Identification of the tissue of origin of the tumor is important in predicting the biologic behavior since the cytologic criteria for malignancy are not easily interpreted with these neoplasms. If criteria of malignancy are present, the tumors are likely to metastasize or locally invade surrounding structures. However, nuclei from neuroendocrine tumors often do not display anaplastic features, even when there is a likelihood of metastasis or local invasion. Thus, tumor identification and knowledge of the malignant potential of the specific neoplasms in different species is critical for prognosticating tumors of endocrine and neuroendocrine origin. This is true of all the endocrine system tumors, but is particularly important when evaluating thyroid tumors, the most commonly encountered endocrine system lesion.

THYROID TUMORS

The thyroid is composed of variably sized follicles lined by simple epithelium. Squamous to low cuboidal epithelium is present in the resting stage and cuboidal to columnar epithelium is found in the active stage (Fig. 16-1). The follicular colloid contains the thyroglobulin, from which thyroid hormone is produced. Follicles are separated by delicate fibrous septa with an abundant vascular supply. The active follicle has vacuoles adjacent to the epithelium as evidence of the endocytosis of thyroglobulin.

Thyroid tumors occur most frequently in the dog, cat, and horse (Capen, 2002). They often present clinically as a subcutaneous mass located on the neck, usually lateral to the trachea, or near the thoracic inlet. Ectopic thyroid tumors may occasionally be found in the cranial thoracic cavity, at the base of the heart, or even in the oral cavity at the base of the tongue (Lantz and Salisbury, 1989). There is marked species variation regarding the biologic behavior of thyroid tumors. Therefore, the features of

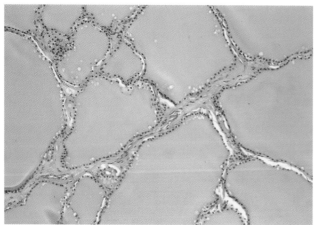

■ **FIGURE 16-1. Normal active gland. Thyroid. Cat.** Variably sized follicles that contain colloid are lined by cuboidal epithelium. Vacuoles are present adjacent to epithelium related to active endocytosis of thyroglobulin. (H&E, IP.) (Courtesy of Rose Raskin, University of Florida.)

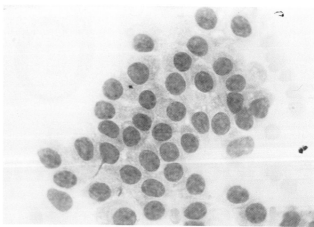

■ **FIGURE 16-2. Adenocarcinoma. Thyroid. Dog.** Tissue aspirate taken from a subcutaneous mass located on the neck. A fairly uniform cluster of cells have pale, lightly granular cytoplasm with poorly defined cytoplasmic borders, typical of an endocrine tumor. (Wright-Giemsa; HP oil.)

these lesions will be described as they relate to the dog and the cat.

Canine Thyroid Tumors

Thyroid tumors represent from 1.2% to 3.7% of all canine tumors (Harari et al., 1986). No sex predilection has been established; however, a breed predilection has been suggested for Boxers, Beagles, and Golden Retrievers (Harari et al., 1986). Approximately 50% to 70% of the thyroid tumors identified clinically in the dog are carcinomas (Bailey and Page, 2007). Aspirates from thyroid tumors, particularly carcinomas, may contain a large amount of blood contamination (Harari et al., 1986). Clusters or sheets of epithelial cells are typically seen scattered throughout the preparations. These clumps will appear as free nuclei embedded in a background of pale-blue cytoplasm, with infrequent appearance of cytoplasmic membranes or borders (Fig. 16-2). Dark-blue to black pigment is sometimes seen in the cytoplasm of epithelial cells (Fig. 16-3). Although not definitively identified as such, this pigment is thought to represent tyrosine-containing granules (Maddux and Shull, 1989). Amorphous pink material representing colloid may be associated with some clusters (Figs. 16-3 and 16-4). Colloid and/or pigmented granules, along with the naked nuclei appearance of the cells, are used to definitively identify the tissue as thyroid in origin.

The nuclei of most tumors are round to oval with minimal anaplastic features. Most thyroid tumors, even adenocarcinomas, will be composed of a fairly uniform population of cells, displaying few if any criteria of malignancy (see Figs. 16-2 to 16-4). There may be mild to moderate anisokaryosis (Fig. 16-5A) and small, indistinct nucleoli may occasionally be seen in some tumors. However, as previously mentioned, approximately 90% to 95% of the canine thyroid tumors are adenocarcinomas. Therefore, any time a canine tumor is identified as thyroid in origin it should be regarded as a probable carcinoma until histopathologic confirmation is obtained.

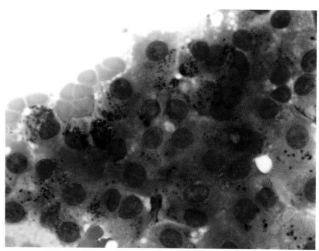

■ **FIGURE 16-3. Adenocarcinoma. Thyroid. Dog.** Tissue aspirate taken from a subcutaneous mass located on the neck. The cytoplasm of the cells has poorly defined borders and pink colloid is observed within the cluster. The dark, cytoplasmic pigment seen throughout the cluster is believed to contain tyrosine granules. The nuclei have mild anisokaryosis. (Wright-Giemsa; HP oil.)

The biologic behavior of canine thyroid tumors is well characterized. Thyroid adenocarcinomas are invasive and will metastasize if given sufficient time. The prognosis and the potential for metastasis may depend on tumor size. In one study, 14% of dogs with tumor volumes less than 20 cm³ had evidence of metastasis, whereas a metastatic rate of 75% to 100% was seen in dogs with tumor volumes between 21 and 100 cm³ (Leav et al., 1983). The earliest and most frequent site of metastasis is the lungs, resulting from invasion of tumor cells into the thyroid or jugular vein (Capen, 2002). When possible, surgical resection is the treatment of choice; however, carcinomas are rapidly invasive and may involve vital structures such as the jugular vein, carotid artery, and esophagus. In dogs, hypersecretion of

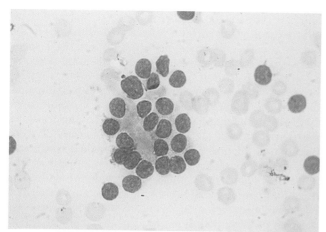

■ **FIGURE 16-4. Adenocarcinoma. Thyroid. Dog.** Tissue aspirate taken from a subcutaneous mass located on the neck. A cluster of cells has pale cytoplasm and poorly defined cytoplasmic borders. Nuclei are fairly uniform with only mild anisokaryosis. A small amount of amorphous eosinophilic material or colloid can be seen within the cluster of cells. (Wright-Giemsa; HP oil.)

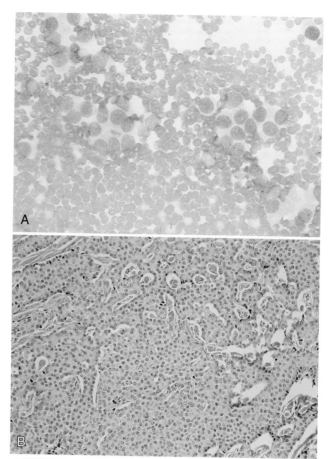

■ **FIGURE 16-5. Adenocarcinoma. Thyroid. Dog. Same case A-B. A,** This animal had an intermittent honking cough. On physical examination, a 2- to 3-cm firm, round, moveable mass was found lateral to the trachea at midneck. Present are groups of loosely adherent cells appearing as naked nuclei against a blood-contaminated background. (Wright-Giemsa; HP oil.) **B,** Variably sized compact nests and diffuse sheets of neoplastic cells efface the gland leaving normal thyroid gland with small follicles at the periphery. (H&E; IP.) (A-B, Courtesy of Rose Raskin, University of Florida.)

thyroid hormones in association with thyroid tumors may involve 10% of cases (Bailey and Page, 2007).

Feline Thyroid Tumors

Thyroid tumors in the cat are cytologically identical to those seen in the dog (Figs. 16-5 to 16-8). However, unlike in the dog, the vast majority of tumors in the cat are benign adenomas, also known as adenomatous hyperplasia. Both thyroid glands are involved in about 70% of the cases (Peterson et al., 1983). Functional adenocarcinomas occur in only 1% to 2% of cats presenting with clinical signs of hyperthyroidism (Turrel et al., 1988). In the cat, if cytologic preparations contain a very uniform population of nuclei with no criteria for malignancy, the thyroid tumor is considered most likely benign. It is not possible to cytologically differentiate between adenomas and adenocarcinomas. However, histologic evaluation of capsular or lymphatic invasion is often required to distinguish adenomas from adenocarcinomas (Capen, 2002; Turrel et al., 1988).

Unlike the canine, most thyroid adenomas in the cat actively secrete thyroid hormones. Adenomas are usually well encapsulated and the prognosis is excellent with surgical removal. If bilateral thyroidectomy is performed, the patient must be monitored for signs of hypothyroidism or hypocalcemia resulting from removal of the parathyroid glands (Bailey and Page, 2007). Adenocarcinomas are locally invasive and often metastasize to regional lymph nodes. Metastatic disease has been reported in up to 71% of cats with adenocarcinomas (Turrel et al., 1988).

Treatment may consist of antithyroid drugs, which are not cytotoxic but are used to reduce the metabolic effects of thyrotoxicosis prior to surgery. Radiotherapy with Iodine 131 (^{131}I) can alternatively be performed to reduce the neoplasm, especially for cats with hyperfunctional ectopic thyroid tissue.

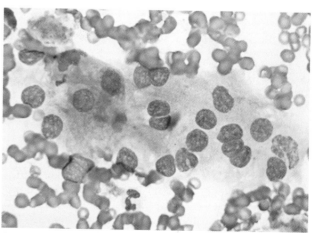

■ **FIGURE 16-6. Adenoma. Thyroid. Cat.** Tissue aspirate taken from a subcutaneous mass located on the neck. The cytoplasm of the cells has poorly defined borders, and pink colloid is observed within the cluster. The nuclei are uniform. (Wright-Giemsa; HP oil.)

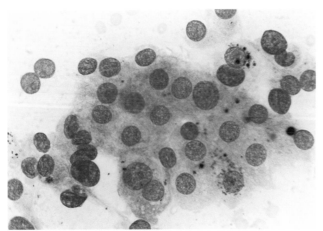

■ **FIGURE 16-7. Adenoma. Thyroid. Cat.** Tissue aspirate taken from an animal with clinical hyperthyroidism of 3 years' duration. Cat was treated 3 months earlier with radioactive iodine and now presents with reoccurrence of hyperthyroidism. Cytologically, several binucleated forms are present along with black granular cytoplasmic inclusions. Moderate degree of anisocytosis and anisokaryosis is noted that may relate to the relapse and radiation therapy. (Wright-Giemsa; HP oil.) (Courtesy of Rose Raskin, University of Florida.)

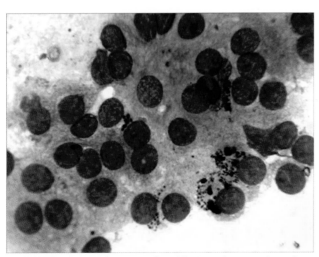

■ **FIGURE 16-8. Adenoma. Thyroid. Cat.** Tissue aspirate from a subcutaneous mass located on the neck. Cytologically, several binucleated forms appear to be present along with black granular cytoplasmic inclusions. (Wright-Giemsa; HP oil.)

PARATHYROID TUMORS

Parathyroid tumors are uncommon neoplasms in domestic animals. Most reported cases involve dogs (Berger and Feldman, 1987; DeVries et al., 1993) or cats (den Hertog et al., 1997; Kallet et al., 1991). There may be a breed predisposition in the Keeshond (Berger and Feldman, 1987). The tumors are usually recognized in older animals—for example, in dogs 7 years of age or older and cats 8 years of age or older.

The most frequently reported parathyroid tumor is the adenoma of the parathyroid chief cells. Parathyroid carcinomas are rare, but have been diagnosed in older dogs

and cats (Capen, 2002; Kallet et al., 1991; Marquez et al., 1995). Cytologic evaluation of parathyroid tumors in the dog is usually performed on surgically removed specimens since tumors are usually too small to be detected by cervical palpation. However, in one report, four of seven cats with primary hyperparathyroidism had palpable cervical masses (Kallet et al., 1991). In some cases, cytologic evaluation has been useful in making a diagnosis (den Hertog et al., 1997). Chief cells aspirated from parathyroid adenomas have a typical naked nuclei appearance on cytologic preparations. Cells appear as free nuclei in a lightly eosinophilic background of cytoplasm. In addition, some parathyroid tumors contain needle-like, eosinophilic, cytoplasmic inclusions (Fig. 16-9). The composition of these inclusions and the frequency at which they can be found in parathyroid tumors are unknown. Nuclei are round to oval and fairly uniform in size and shape. Parathyroid adenocarcinomas typically are larger than adenomas; however, they may appear similar cytologically (see Fig. 16-9). The diagnosis of adenocarcinoma is made when there is histologic or gross evidence of capsular invasion, invasion into surrounding structures, or metastasis to regional lymph or lungs (Capen, 2002).

Since parathyroid tumors, especially adenomas, are often not palpable, the presurgical diagnosis frequently relies on recognition of clinical signs and characteristic laboratory findings. The vast majority of parathyroid tumors actively secrete inappropriate amounts of parathormone, and most cases are presented for clinical signs associated with increased hormonal activity. Although some species variation may exist with regard to the frequency of observance of specific clinical signs, similarities in clinical and laboratory findings exist in all species. Commonly reported abnormalities include hypercalcemia (the most common finding), polydipsia and polyuria, muscle weakness, skeletal abnormalities, and cystic calculi (DeVries et al., 1993; Bailey and Page, 2007 Marquez et al., 1995).

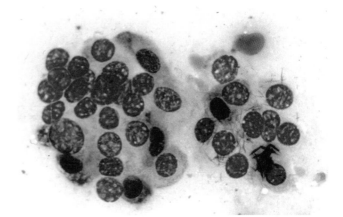

■ **FIGURE 16-9. Adenocarcinoma. Parathyroid. Dog.** Tissue imprint from a subcutaneous mass located on the neck. The animal had persistent hypercalcemia and elevated levels of parathormone. The cytoplasm of the cell cluster is pale blue with indistinct cytoplasmic borders and needle-like, eosinophilic inclusions (right). Nuclei are dense with a high nuclear-to-cytoplasmic ratio and moderate anisokaryosis. (Wright-Giemsa; HP oil.)

Surgical exploration of the cervical area is warranted if laboratory and clinical findings establish a diagnosis of primary hyperparathyroidism. Parathyroid adenomas are well encapsulated and can be surgically removed by blunt dissection. Patients must be monitored closely for the rapid development of postsurgical hypocalcemia (Bailey and Page, 2007). The long-term prognosis for patients with parathyroid adenomas is good.

TUMORS OF THE ENDOCRINE PANCREAS

The most frequently diagnosed tumor of endocrine pancreas is the insulinoma, a tumor of the beta islet cells (β-cells). These lesions have been referred to as insulinomas, insulin-producing pancreatic tumors, insulin-producing islet cell tumors, islet cell tumors, and β-cell tumors. They most commonly occur in dogs, generally large breeds over 5 years of age (Capen, 2002). Commonly affected breeds include Boxers, German Shepherds, Irish Setters, Poodles, Fox Terriers, Collies, and Labrador Retrievers. These tumors have also been identified with some frequency in the ferret and rarely in the cat (Hawks et al., 1992; Capen, 2002).

The cytologic appearance of insulinomas is typical of other endocrine tumors, with most preparations being fairly cellular containing mostly naked nuclei embedded in a background of lightly basophilic cytoplasm. In many instances, the cytoplasm of the cells contains numerous, small, punctate, clear vacuoles (Fig. 16-10). There may be a mild to moderate anisokaryosis and nuclei may contain a single prominent nucleolus, typical of some endocrine tumors. Although most β-cell tumors in the dog are carcinomas, nuclear features of malignancy are inconsistently seen, and as with other endocrine tumors, it is often difficult to predict the biologic behavior of these lesions based on the histologic or cytologic characteristics of the cells (Capen, 2002). Therefore, some

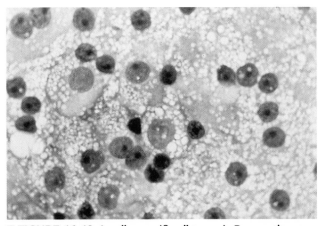

■ **FIGURE 16-10. Insulinoma (β-cell tumor). Pancreatic mass. Dog.** Tissue imprint taken from an intra-abdominal mass located in the pancreas of a hypoglycemic dog. The cytoplasmic borders of the cells are indistinct and contain numerous punctate, clear vacuoles. There is moderate anisokaryosis and a prominent, usually singular nucleolus, typical of some neuroendocrine/endocrine tumors. (Wright-Giemsa; HP oil.)

pathologists prefer to identify these lesions as islet cell tumors unless there is evidence of invasion into surrounding structures, lymphatics, or metastatic disease. If the criteria for malignancy are met, a diagnosis of adenocarcinoma can reliably be made; however, the lack of anaplastic features cannot be used to predict the biologic behavior. Even small tumors composed of well-differentiated β-cells have been known to metastasize (Capen, 2002).

The biologic behavior of these lesions is well characterized. Unlike in humans, in whom 90% of the pancreatic islet cell tumors are adenomas, most islet cell tumors in the dog are adenocarcinomas (Capen, 2002). Metastasis is via lymphatics with involvement of regional lymph nodes and liver in about 50% of the cases (Bailey and Page, 2007). Metastatic disease has been documented in other sites as well. Most tumors actively secrete inappropriate amounts of insulin, resulting in profound hypoglycemia. Because of the low blood glucose, patients often present with neuromuscular signs such as seizures, hindlimb weakness, ataxia, muscle tremors, and generalized weakness (Bailey and Page, 2007). Although not exclusively associated with insulinomas, most dogs with the disease have Whipple's triad, which consists of (1) clinical signs associated with hypoglycemia, (2) fasting blood glucose less than 40 mg/dl, and (3) alleviation of clinical signs by the administration of dextrose.

A tentative diagnosis of β-cell tumor can be made by demonstrating profound hypoglycemia and an abnormal insulin-to-glucose ratio. Confirmation can be made by exploratory celiotomy or ultrasound-guided, fine-needle aspiration if the lesion is large enough. One report suggests that once a tentative diagnosis is made, exploratory celiotomy and partial pancreatectomy are indicated in dogs since surgery significantly increases the mean survival time from 74 days (medical or dietary management) to 381 days (surgery plus medical or dietary management) (Tobin et al., 1999).

CHEMORECEPTOR TUMORS

Chemoreceptor tumors are generally referred to as *chemodectomas* or *nonchromaffin paragangliomas*. Although chemoreceptor tissue is found in several areas of the body, tumors of chemoreceptor cells are primarily found in the aortic bodies or the carotid bodies (Capen, 2002). They are uncommon tumors of the dog and have rarely been reported in cats (Tillson et al., 1994). Most dogs affected are between 10 and 15 years of age, and there is a higher incidence of these tumors in brachycephalic breeds, particularly Boxers and Boston Terriers (Capen, 2002). The majority (80% to 90%) of chemoreceptor tumors reported in animals have originated from the aortic bodies; however, there are rare reports of carotid body tumors in the dog (Obradovich et al., 1992).

The aortic body tumor or heart base tumor generally occurs as a single mass within the pericardial sac at or near the base of the heart (Capen, 2002). Presenting clinical signs are usually those associated with cardiac decompensation, particularly right heart failure resulting from significant pericardial effusion. Cytologic evaluation of the pericardial effusion rarely allows identification of tumor cells. Reactive mesothelium often associated with the fluid may be mistaken for neoplastic cells (see Chapter 6). Unlike the pericardial fluid, ultrasound-guided, fine-needle aspirates taken directly from the lesions are usually very cellular and are often diagnostically rewarding. Care must be taken when performing this procedure because of the close association of aortic body tumors with the atria and major vessels.

Cytologically, aspirates and imprints taken from these lesions are usually quite cellular. The typical naked nuclei appearance with free nuclei in a background of cytoplasm is a prominent feature (Fig. 16-11A). Nuclei are round with clumped chromatin and usually contain a single, prominent nucleolus (Fig. 11-11B) typical of neuroendocrine cell tumors. Both benign and malignant forms occur and anaplastic features of anisokaryosis and multiple, variable nucleoli are not reliable indicators of the malignant potential. Both adenomas and adenocarcinomas have scattered areas of the tumor that contain larger, more pleomorphic cells (see Fig. 16-11A) and bizarrely shaped giant cells (Capen, 2002). Carcinomas are identified by invasion into the surrounding capsule, blood vessels, lymphatics, or adjacent structures (Capen, 2002). Aortic body tumors may be difficult to distinguish from ectopic thyroid tumors, which may appear cytologically similar and may on occasion occur in the same area. The identification of colloid or pigment granules would help to identify the tissue as thyroid in origin.

Most aortic body tumors in the dog are benign adenomas (Capen, 2002). They are usually well encapsulated and are slow growing with low metastatic potential; however, they are expansive lesions and will eventually compress the atria or vena cavae. With adenomas, surgical resection is the treatment of choice; however, long-term success is limited because complete resection is difficult to achieve owing to the close association of these neoplasms with major vessels. The role of chemotherapy in the treatment of these lesions is unknown. Malignant forms or carcinomas are invasive and may spread locally to veins, lymphatics, or myocardium (Capen, 2002; Zimmerman et al., 2000). When distant metastasis occurs it is usually to the lung or the liver, but a number of organs may be involved. The prognosis for cats with chemodectomas may be worse because of the frequent invasive nature of the tumor in this species (Tillson et al., 1994).

Carotid body tumors are rare neoplasms that are located in the neck, near the angle of the jaw, at the bifurcation of the common carotid artery (Capen, 2002; Obradovich, et al., 1992). Cytologically they appear similar to aortic body tumors (Fig. 16-12A&B). The location of carotid body tumors also necessitates differentiation from thyroid tumors. Identification of colloid or pigment granules would help to identify tissue as thyroid in origin. Although case reports are limited, these tumors are more likely to be malignant than are aortic body tumors, and they are characterized by local tissue invasion and a tendency to metastasize to multiple sites in the body (Capen, 2002; Obradovich et al., 1992). Metastasis usually occurs late in the course of the disease, primarily to the liver, mediastinum, brain, heart, and lungs. Early surgical excision is the treatment of choice (Obradovich et al., 1992). The role of chemotherapy in the treatment of these tumors has not been evaluated.

ADRENAL GLAND TUMORS

Enlargement of the adrenal gland may arise from either the cortical or the medullary areas of this gland. Those enlargements originating within the cortex often result in the excessive production of corticosteroids and the clinical condition of hyperadrenocorticism. Tumors of the adrenal medulla cause the paroxysmal release of catecholamines, primarily norepinephrine.

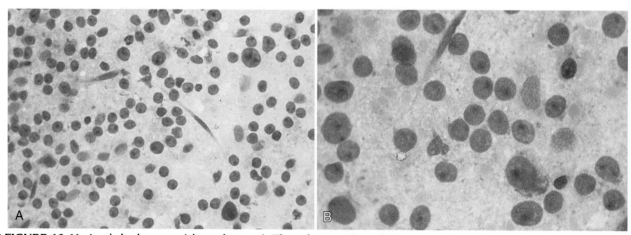

■ **FIGURE 16-11. Aortic body tumor (chemodectoma). Thoracic mass. Dog. Same case A-B. A,** Tissue aspirate taken from a mass located in the thoracic cavity, just dorsal to the base of the heart. The cells appear as naked nuclei or free nuclei within a background of lightly basophilic cytoplasm without distinct cell borders, typical of neuroendocrine tumors. There is moderate anisokaryosis and a prominent, usually singular nucleolus. (Wright-Giemsa; HP oil.) **B,** Cells display a moderate degree of anisokaryosis along with prominent, usually singular nucleoli. (Wright-Giemsa; HP oil.)

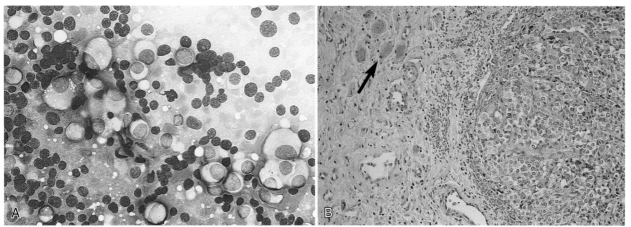

■ **FIGURE 16-12. Carotid body tumor (chemodectoma). Cervical mass. Dog. Same case A-B. A,** Surgical excision imprint from an animal that presented with a head tilt. Magnetic resonance imaging indicated the presence of the mass in the neck region near the tympanic bulla. Cytologically, there are numerous free nuclei with a small number of variably sized, intact cells. Anisocytosis and anisokaryosis are marked. (Aqueous-based Wright; HP oil.) **B,** Section contains dense sheets of neoplastic cells (right side) adjacent to fibrovascular stroma (left side) and nerve cell bodies *(arrow)*. Tumor emboli occur with blood vessels (not shown) demonstrating the invasive nature of the tumor. (H&E, IP.) (A-B, Courtesy of Rose Raskin, University of Florida.)

Tumors of the Adrenal Medulla

The most common tumor of the adrenal medulla is the pheochromocytoma, also called *chromaffin paraganglioma,* or *chromaffin cell tumor.* Rarely, other tumors, such as neuroblastomas and ganglioneuromas, may arise from the primitive neuroectodermal cells in this area (Capen, 2002). Neuroblastomas are often seen in very young animals, resulting in large intra-abdominal masses, which often metastasize to peritoneal surfaces. Ganglioneuromas are small benign tumors in the adrenal medulla.

Pheochromocytomas are tumors of the chromaffin cells of the adrenal medulla. They occur most frequently in middle-aged to older dogs with no apparent gender or breed predilection and are rarely reported in cats (Barthez et al., 1997; Patnaik et al., 1990). Clinical evidence of this tumor is usually seen on release of large amounts of catecholamines from the neoplasm. However, clinical signs are varied and vague, and in one study 57% of the cases were diagnosed as incidental findings (Barthez et al., 1997). Two cases of pheochromocytoma in dogs presented with paraparesis related to their invasion into the spinal canal (Platt et al., 1998). In addition, a large number of patients with pheochromocytomas have concurrent diseases, including other neoplasms originating from other tissues (Barthez et al., 1997; Bouayad et al., 1987). Concurrent pituitary adenomas or adrenocortical tumors resulted in some dogs with pheochromocytomas having concurrent hyperadrenocorticism. Consequently, the clinical signs may be a combination of those attributable to the release of catecholamines and those that are due to concomitant disease.

Abdominal ultrasonography is able to detect adrenal pheochromocytomas in approximately 50% of the cases (Barthez et al., 1997). In these situations, ultrasound-guided, fine-needle aspiration may be used to make a more definitive diagnosis. Care must be taken during the sampling procedure since manipulation of the affected adrenal gland could cause the paroxysmal release of catecholamines, resulting in hypertension, tachycardia, and/or arrhythmias. In addition, many of these lesions are closely associated with the caudal vena cava and, in fact, may invade this vessel.

The cytologic appearance of pheochromocytomas is typical of other neuroendocrine tumors. Much of the preparation may appear as naked nuclei against a background of cytoplasm; however, intact cells are usually identified in most carefully prepared specimens (Fig. 16-13). The cytoplasm of the cells is lightly basophilic to amphophilic with faint granules sometimes visible using Romanowsky-type stains (see Fig. 16-13). Nuclei are round to oval and a single, small nucleolus may occasionally be observed. Both benign and malignant forms of the tumor exist. Nuclear features of malignancy are unreliable in predicting the biologic behavior of the lesion since even small tumors with well-differentiated cells are known to metastasize or invade surrounding structures (Capen, 2002; Bouayad et al., 1987). The presence of nuclear criteria of malignancy would strongly suggest a high potential for local invasion or metastasis (Fig. 16-14A&B).

Pheochromocytomas may be recognized clinically on the release of large quantities of catecholamines, primarily norepinephrine, which often results in a variety of clinical signs related to the cardiovascular system and nervous system. Immunocytochemical stains (see Chapter 17) such as chromogranin A, and synaptophysin on cytologic specimens may be used to support the diagnosis of a medullary tumor. Ultrastructural studies of pheochromocytomas are helpful to demonstrate the cytoplasmic neurosecretory granules.

The prognosis for patients is guarded to poor since 50% or more of these tumors are nonresectable owing

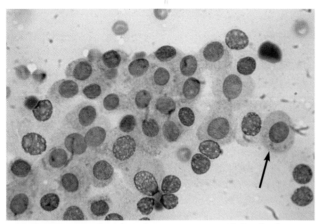

■ **FIGURE 16-13. Pheochromocytoma. Abdominal mass. Dog.** Tissue aspirate taken from an intra-abdominal mass located in the adrenal gland. The cluster of cells contains pale cytoplasm with occasional distinct cytoplasmic borders. Fine, pale, basophilic, intracytoplasmic granules can be seen in the cells *(arrow)*. There is mild anisokaryosis but no significant criteria for malignancy; however, local invasion into the caudal vena cava was detected ultrasonographically and histologically. Surgical excision resulted in complete removal of the tumor. (Wright-Giemsa; HP oil.)

to early invasion of the venous system and distant metastasis via the caudal vena cava (Barthez et al., 1997; Bouayad et al., 1987; Capen, 2002). However, with complete surgical excision long-term survival can be obtained. Several reports indicate a greater than 50% frequency of concurrent neoplasia of patients with pheochromocytomas, many of which are endocrine in origin (Barthez et al., 1997; Bouayad et al., 1987; Capen, 2002; von Dehn et al., 1995). The concurrent finding of pituitary adenoma or adrenocortical neoplasia resulted in a significant number of the dogs with pheochromocytomas having concurrent

hyperadrenocorticism (Barthez et al., 1997; von Dehn et al., 1995).

Adrenocortical Disease

Hyperadrenocorticism is a common endocrinopathy in the dog and is rarely seen in the cat. In the dog, the condition is most often the result of a pituitary tumor; however, between 10% and 20% of the cases are associated with adrenocortical neoplasia (Bailey and Page, 2007). In 89 reported cases of dogs with adrenocortical tumors, adenocarcinomas were diagnosed in 53 dogs and adenomas were found in 36 dogs (Penninck et al., 1988; Reusch and Feldman, 1991; Scavelli et al., 1986). The mean age was approximately 11 years (range 5 to 16 years). There appeared to be no significant breed or sex predilection. Both adrenocortical adenomas and adenocarcinomas have rarely been reported in the cat (Jones et al., 1992; Nelson et al., 1988).

Patients with adrenocortical tumors usually present with clinical and laboratory signs of hyperadrenocorticism. Once a diagnosis of hyperadrenocorticism is made, discriminatory tests such as the high-dose dexamethasone suppression test, measurement of endogenous adrenocorticotropic hormone (ACTH) concentrations, and abdominal ultrasonography should be used to distinguish pituitary-dependent hyperadrenocorticism (PDH) from adrenal tumors (AT). In contrast to PDH that causes bilateral adrenal enlargement, an adrenal tumor typically causes enlargement of one adrenal gland and atrophy of the contralateral adrenal gland. In one study, abdominal ultrasonography detected 18 of 25 dogs (72%) with AT (Reusch and Feldman, 1991). In this situation, an ultrasound-guided, fine-needle aspiration of the affected adrenal gland can be performed for cytologic evaluation of the lesion.

Cytologically, aspirates taken from adrenocortical adenomas contain cells resembling normal secretory cells

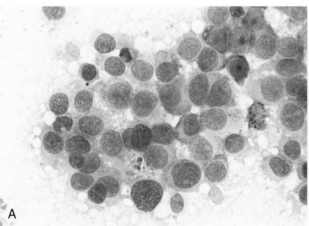

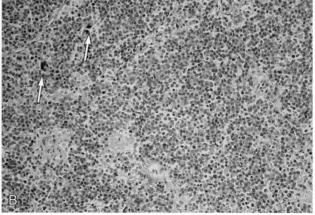

■ **FIGURE 16-14. Pheochromocytoma. Abdominal mass. Dog. Same case A-B. A,** This animal presented with cervical and thoracic pain that progressed rapidly to paraparesis. A myelogram revealed an epidural mass at Ll-2 and ultrasound examination indicated an abdominal mass. A tissue aspirate of the abdominal mass contained large, round to oval, loosely adherent cells with several criteria of malignancy including anisokaryosis, variable nuclear-to-cytoplasmic ratios, multiple prominent nucleoli, multinucleation (lower left), and coarse chromatin pattern. (Wright-Giemsa; HP oil.) **B,** The mass is composed of pleomorphic neoplastic cells arranged in a dense lobular formation separated by fibrovascular septa. Occasional multinucleate cells *(arrows)* are seen. (H&E; IP.) (A-B, Courtesy of Rose Raskin, University of Florida.)

from the zona fasciculata or zona reticularis (Capen, 2002). Preparations are typical of other endocrine tumors with most cells appearing as naked nuclei in a background of abundant cytoplasm. The cytoplasm is moderately basophilic and often contains abundant, clear, lipid vacuoles (Fig. 16-15A&C). Nuclei of adenomas are round and uniform in size. They may contain a prominent, often singular nucleolus (Fig. 16-15D). Focal areas of hematopoiesis, adipocytes, and mineral deposits may be found in some cortical adenomas (see Fig. 16-15B) (Capen, 2002). It should be noted that cells aspirated from adrenal glands that are hyperplastic, as seen in dogs with PDH, and cells from adrenal adenomas are

cytologically indistinguishable. Therefore, cytology cannot be used as a tool to distinguish between PDH and hyperadrenocorticism associated with AT.

Tumor cells from adrenocortical adenocarcinomas may be more pleomorphic compared with those from adenomas (Capen, 2002). Adenocarcinomas may display features of anaplasia, including anisokaryosis and multiple nucleoli. However, since some adenocarcinomas may contain well-differentiated cells, histologic evaluation of invasion into the capsule, adjacent structures, or vessels is the preferred method of distinction between adenomas and adenocarcinomas. Therefore, if the cytologic criteria of malignancy are fulfilled, a diagnosis of

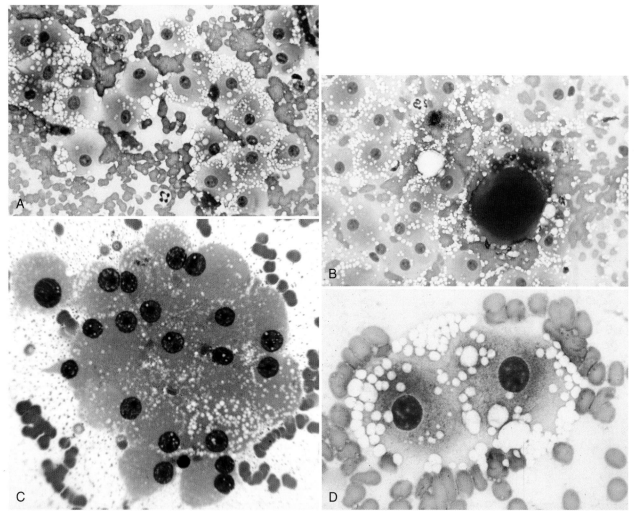

■ **FIGURE 16-15. Same case A-B&D. Adrenocortical adenoma. Adrenal mass. Aspirate. Dog. A,** Tissue aspirate taken from a single nodule off the cranial pole of the adrenal gland noted on ultrasound examination of a dog with probable hyperadrenocorticism. The cluster of uniform cells contains abundant, amphophilic cytoplasm with mostly indistinct cytoplasmic borders. The cytoplasm contains numerous clear, punctate vacuoles. (Wright-Giemsa; HP oil.) **B,** A large megakaryocyte (center) indicates the presence of extramedullary hematopoiesis, which is sometimes seen in tumors of the adrenal cortex. Evidence of chronic hemorrhage is indicated by the hemosiderin-laden macrophage (dark cell in upper center). (Wright-Giemsa; HP oil.) **C, Adrenocortical disease. Adrenal mass. Aspirate. Dog.** Sample is taken from a mass in the adrenal gland of a dog with clinical signs of hyperadrenocorticism. A cluster of adrenocortical cells with small nuclei and prominent, usually singular nucleoli are seen. There is mild to moderate anisokaryosis. The cytoplasm is lightly basophilic and contains numerous small, punctate vacuoles. (Wright-Giemsa; HP oil.) **D,** Two adrenocortical cells with small nuclei and prominent, usually singular nucleoli. The cytoplasm contains variably sized punctuate vacuoles consistent with secretory function that are present predominantly along the periphery of the cell. (Wright-Giemsa; HP oil.) (A-B, Courtesy of Peter Fernandes, University of Florida.) (D, Courtesy of Rose Raskin, University of Florida.)

adenocarcinoma can reliably be made; however, in the absence of such criteria, caution should be used in making a firm diagnosis.

Adenomas of the zona fasciculata or zona reticularis are usually small and do not metastasize. Surgical resection is treatment of choice for adenomas; however, operative and postoperative complications involving the removal of the gland are frequently seen. Approximately half of the dogs with adrenocortical adenocarcinomas have gross evidence of local invasion into the caudal vena cava or renal artery, or distant metastasis, primarily to the liver, lung, or kidney (Capen, 2002; Scavelli et al., 1986). Surgical resection of adenocarcinomas is difficult and as with adrenal adenomas, the incidence of postoperative complications is high (Scavelli et al., 1986). Treatment of adenocarcinomas with o,p-DDD (Lysodren, Bristol Laboratories, Princeton, NJ) or ketoconazole (Nizoral, Janssen Pharmaceutica, Inc., Piscataway, NJ) has had very limited success (Bailey and Page, 2007).

CARCINOIDS

Carcinoids are rare tumors arising from disseminated neuroendocrine cells in various organs. These cells are found dispersed in gastrointestinal tract, endocrine pancreas, biliary tract, respiratory tract, thymus, thyroid, urogenital tract, and skin (Klopel, 2007). These lesions were first described as *karzinoide* by Obernodorfer in 1907, referring to intestinal tumors that appeared to behave in a more indolent nature than the typical intestinal adenocarcinoma (Kulke and Mayer, 1999). Carcinoids have also been referred to as APUD (amine precursor uptake and decarboxylation) tumors, or APUDomas, because these neuroendocrine cells are able to synthesize, secrete, and metabolize biologically active amines. At present, these tumors are classified as well-differentiated neuroendocrine tumors (benign) and well-differentiated to poorly differentiated neuroendocrine carcinomas (malignant) (Klopel, 2007).

In dogs and cats, the most common location for a carcinoid is in the gastrointestinal tract. However, in dogs carcinoids have been reported to occur not only in the gastrointestinal tract (Albers et al., 1998; Christie et al., 1964; Sako et al., 2003), but also the oral cavity (Whiteley and Leininger, 1987), nasal cavity (Sako et al., 2005), pharynx (Patnaik et al., 2002), lung (Saegusa et al., 1994; Ferreira et al., 2005; Choi et al., 2008), liver (Patnaik et al., 1981; Patnaik et al., 2005a), gallbladder (Morrell et al., 2002), and skin (Konno, 1998). In the cat, carcinoid tumors have been reported in the liver and gallbladder (Patnaik et al., 2005b), stomach (Rossmeisl et al., 2002), intestines (Slawienski et al., 1997), esophagus (Patnaik et al., 1990), tracheobronchus (Rossi et al., 2007), and skin (Patnaik et al., 2001). There appears to be no apparent sex or breed predilection. Carcinoids have been reported in animals ranging from 4 month to 18 years of age, but most were reported in older animals (>7 years).

Animals with carcinoids can have a variety of clinical findings, or, in some cases, benign carcinoids have been found incidentally in the lung or intestine of clinically healthy animals during physical exam or imaging studies (Sykes and Cooper, 1982; Choi et al., 2008). Clinical signs generally reflect the anatomical location of the lesion. Gallbladder tumors can cause icterus or hematemesis (Morrell et al., 2002). In one report a cat with a 5-month history of vomiting was found with a stomach carcinoid (Rossmeisl et al., 2002).

Although neuroendocrine tumor cells may have granules containing various bioactive amines such as serotonin, histamine, substance P, kallikrein, and corticotropin, there are no known reports indicating that the release of these bioactive amines causes the development of clinical symptoms in humans or animals with benign carcinoids. However, in cases of malignant carcinoids, signs can be attributed to the release of bioactive amines. In humans, carcinoids can result in what is known as "carcinoid syndrome," a clinical syndrome consisting of diarrhea, erythema, asthenia, organomegaly, and right-sided congestive heart failure (Kulke and Mayer, 1999). These are attributed to synthesis, release, and delayed hepatic metabolism of 5-HT (hydroxytryptamine, serotonin) and tachykinins by tumors cells. In these cases measurement of serum or urine 5-HT concentration can be used as a screening test. However, unlike in humans, most dogs and cats with malignant lesions had clinical signs related to advanced stages of tumor growth and metastasis, not the release of biologically active substances. In one case, a dog with a jejunal carcinoid presented with a 4-month history of anemia, fatigue, anorexia, vomiting, intermittent diarrhea, and intestinal bleeding (Sako et al., 2003). In this animal, the concentration of serum 5-HT was approximately 10 times the reference range. There have also been rare reports of hypercortisolism in dogs with carcinoids (Churcher, 1999).

Cytologically, carcinoids as neuroendocrine tumors have a typical appearance with naked nuclei embedded in a background of cytoplasm (Fig. 16-16A). A small number of round or polygonal intact cells with a moderate to abundant amount of weakly basophilic cytoplasm may also be identified (Fig. 16-16B). The nuclei are round to polygonal with fine chromatin and occasional nucleoli. Cells from some carcinoids may contain fine, pale basophilic intracytoplasmic granules. The cytologic appearance of carcinoids is similar regardless of anatomic location. Some specific carcinoids, such as Merkel cell tumors (cutaneous carcinoids), are composed of cells that may resemble large lymphocytes with scant, basophilic cytoplasm (Orell et al., 2005). These tumors may be grossly and cytologically similar in appearance to cutaneous lymphoma and special procedures may be necessary to confirm the tissue of origin. Argentatffin and/or argyrophil stain (Grimelius, 2004). Immunohistochemistry and electron microscopy can be used to aid in the identification of carcinoid tumors. An immunohistochemical panel containing neuron specific enolase (NSE), synaptophysin, and chromogranin A antibodies can be used to histochemically identify cells of neuroendocrine origin. Electron microscopy can also be used by allowing the identification of neuroendocrine–specific, electron-dense core granules (Patnaik et al., 2005b).

As with other neuroendocrine tumors, the biologic behavior of carcinoids is difficult to predict based on cell morphology. Most of the reported neuroendocrine tumors, especially those of hepatic and intestinal origin,

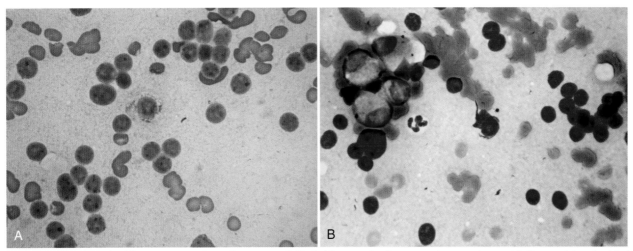

■ **FIGURE 16-16. Carcinoid. Lung mass. Dog. Same case A-B. A,** Neuroendocrine-appearing neoplasm with free nuclei embedded in lightly basophilic cytoplasmic material. Note the pale, intracytoplasmic granules in the single intact neoplastic cell (center). (Aqueous-based Wright; HP oil.) **B.** Naked nuclei are seen as a prominent feature with a low number of intact cells (upper left), which have moderate to abundant amount of light basophilic cytoplasm. (Giemsa; HP oil.)

were malignant with poor prognosis. In all of the 26 reported cases of hepatic carcinoids in dogs, the animals were either euthanized or died of the tumors because tumors were diffuse, involving all liver lobes, or had evidence of metastatic disease at the time of diagnosis (Patnaik et al., 1981; Churcher, 1999; Patnaik et al., 2005a). In cats with hepatic carcinoids, most of the animals were euthanized during or soon after surgical exploration because of either metastatic disease of diffuse involvement of all liver lobes (Patnaik et al., 2005b). In animals with gastrointestinal carcinoids—including those with lesions in the esophagus, stomach, and intestinal tract—10 of 12 canine cases and 4 of 5 feline cases had evidence of either local or distant metastasis at the time of presentation. These animals frequently presented with severe clinical signs of intestinal hemorrhage and/or vomiting. There are few reports of carcinoid tumors at sites other than liver and gastrointestinal, and in these, tumor behavior was variable. Two of 4 canine lung cases were benign and the other 2 tumors were locally invasive with severe signs of metastatic pleuritis or acute respiratory crisis (Saegusa et al., 1994; Choi et al., 2008). Two benign lung carcinoids were incidental findings and one of them was found in a patient with lymphoma. In reports of cutaneous carcinoids, one of six dogs, and one of two cats were euthanized because of local tumor recurrence or distant metastasis (Konno, 1998; Patnaik

et al., 2001). Two reports of carcinoids in the gallbladder of dogs indicated one was benign and the other malignant. Three reports of carcinoids in the nasal cavity indicated that at least one was malignant with lung metastasis. In benign tumors, surgical removal is the treatment of choice. There are no known reports of successful chemotherapeutic management of malignant carcinoids. One locally invasive, cutaneous neuroendocrine tumor was successfully treated with radiation therapy and the animal remained in complete remission for 18 months (Whiteley and Leininger, 1987).

SUMMARY

Lesions involving endocrine glands and neuroendocrine tissues are a varied group of conditions that may arise from a number of specialized organs. Even so, these lesions share cytologic features, including the appearance of naked nuclei within a background of lightly basophilic cytoplasm with indistinct borders. In addition, as a group, it is difficult to predict the biologic behavior of these lesions based solely on the presence or absence of abnormal nuclear features. Location of the lesion and distinguishing cytologic features must be used to identify the tissue of origin. The potential biologic behavior should be evaluated based on the specific tumor type and the species involved, along with histologic and/or clinical evidence of invasion.

REFERENCES

Albers TM, Alroy J, McDonnell JJ, et al: A poorly differentiated gastric carcinoid in a dog, *J Vet Diagn Invest* 10:116-118, 1998.

Bailey DB, Page RL: Tumors of the endocrine system. In Withrow SJ, Vail DM (eds): *Withrow & MacEwen's small animal clinical oncology,* ed 4, St. Louis, 2007, Saunders, pp 583-609.

Barthez PY, Marks, SL, Woo J, et al: Pheochromocytoma in dogs: 61 cases (1984-1995), *J Vet Intern Med* 11:272-278, 1997.

Berger B, Feldman EC: Primary hyperparathyroidism in dogs: 21 cases (1976-1986), *J Am Vet Med Assoc* 191:350-356, 1987.

Bouayad H, Feeney DA, Caywood DD, et al: Pheochromocytoma in dogs: 13 cases (1980-1985), *J Am Vet Med Assoc* 191:1610-1615, 1987.

Capen CC: Tumors of the endocrine glands. In Meuten DJ (ed): *Tumors in domestic animals,* ed 4, Ames, 2002, Iowa State Press, pp 607-696.

Choi US, Alleman AR, Choi J, et al: Cytologic and immunohistochemical characterization of a lung carcinoid in a dog with comparisons to human typical carcinoid, *Vet Clin Pathol* 37:249-252, 2008.

Christie GS, Jabara AG: Two cases of malignant intestinal neoplasms in dogs, *J Comp Pathol* 74:90-93, 1964.

Churcher RK: Hepatic carcinoid, hypercortisolism and hypokalaemia in a dog, *Aust Vet J* 77(10):641-645, 1999.

den Hertog E, Goossens MM, van-der-Linde-Sipman JS, et al: Primary hyperparathyroidism in two cats, *Vet Q* 19:81-84, 1997.

DeVries SE, Feldman EC, Nelson RW, et al: Primary parathyroid gland hyperplasia in dogs: six cases (1982-1991), *J Am Vet Med Assoc* 202:1132-1136, 1993.

Ferreira AJA, Peleteiro MC, Correia JHD, et al: Small-cell carcinoma of the lung resembling a brachial plexus tumour, *J Small Anim Pract* 46:286-290, 2005.

Grimelius L: Silver stains demonstrating neuroendocrine cells, *Biotech Histochem* 79(1):37-44, 2004.

Hamilton SR, Farber JL, Rubin E: Neoplasms. In Rubin E, Farber JL (eds): *Pathology*, ed 3, Philadelphia, 1999, Lippincott-Raven, pp 720-721.

Harari J, Patterson JS, Rosenthai RC: Clinical and pathologic features of thyroid tumors in 26 dogs, *J Am Vet Med Assoc* 188:1160-1164, 1986.

Hawks D, Peterson ME, Hawkins KL, et al: Insulin-secreting pancreatic (islet cell) carcinoma in a cat, *J Vet Intern Med* 6:193-196, 1992.

Jones CA, Refsal KR, Stevens BJ, et al: Adrenocortical adenocarcinoma in a cat, *J Am Anim Hosp Assoc* 28:59-62, 1992.

Kallet AJ, Richter KP, Feldman EC, et al: Primary hyperparathyroidism in cats: Seven cases (1984-1989), *J Am Vet Med Assoc* 199:1767-1771, 1991.

Klopel G: Tumour biology and histopathology of neuroendocrine tumours, *Best Pract Res Clin Endocrinol Metabol* 21(1):15-31, 2007.

Konno A, Nagata M, Nanko H: Immunohistochemical diagnosis of a Merkel cell tumor in a dog, *Vet Pathol* 35(6):538-540, 1998.

Kulke MH, Mayer RJ: Carcinoid tumors, *New Eng J Med* 340:858-868, 1999.

Lantz GC, Salisbury SK: Surgical excision of ectopic thyroid carcinoma involving the base of the tongue in dogs: three cases (1980-1987), *J Am Vet Med Assoc* 195:1606-1608, 1989.

Leav I, Schillert AL, Rijnberk A, et al: Adenomas and adenocarcinomas of the canine and feline thyroid, *Am J Pathol* 83:61-93, 1983.

Maddux JM, Shull RM: Subcutaneous glandular tissue: Mammary, salivary, thyroid, and parathyroid. In Cowell RL, Tyler RD (eds): *Diagnostic cytology of the dog and cat*, American Goleta, CA, 1989, Veterinary Publications, pp 83-92.

Marquez GA, Klausner JS, Osborne CA: Calcium oxalate urolithiasis in a cat with a functional parathyroid adenocarcinoma, *J Am Vet Med Assoc* 206:817-819, 1995.

Morrell CN, Volk MV, Mankowski JL: A carcinoid tumor in the gallbladder of a dog, *Vet Pathol* 39(6):756-758, 2002.

Nelson RW, Feldman EC, Smith MC: Hyperadrenocorticism in cats: seven cases (1978-1987), *J Am Vet Med Assoc* 193:245-250, 1988.

Obradovich JE, Withrow SJ, Powers BE, et al: Carotid body tumors in the dog: eleven cases (1978-1988), *J Vet Intern Med* 6:96-101, 1992.

Orell SR, Sterrett GF, Whitaker D: Skin and subcutis. In Orell SR, Sterrett GF, Whitaker D (eds): *Fine needle aspiration cytology*, ed 4, Oxford, 2005, Churchill Livingstone, pp 401-402.

Patnaik AK, Lieberman PH, Hurvitz AI, et al: Canine hepatic carcinoids, *Vet Pathol* 18(4):445-453, 1981.

Patnaik AK, Erlandson RA, Leiberman PH, et al: Extra-adrenal pheochromocytoma (paraganglioma) in a cat, *J Am Vet Med Assoc* 197:104-106, 1990.

Patnaik AK, Erlandson RA, Lieberman PH: Esophageal neuroendocrine carcinoma in a cat, *Vet Pathol* 27(2):128-130, 1990.

Patnaik AK, Post GS, Erlandson RA: Clinicopathologic and electron microscopic study of cutaneous neuroendocrine (Merkel cell) carcinoma in a cat with comparisons to human and canine tumors, *Vet Pathol* 38(5):553-556, 2001.

Patnaik AK, Ludwig LL, Erlandson RA: Neuroendocrine carcinoma of the nasopharynx in a dog, *Vet Pathol* 39(4):496-500, 2002.

Patnaik AK, Newman SJ, Scase T, et al: Canine hepatic neuroendocrine carcinoma: an immunohistochemical and electron microscopic study, *Vet Pathol* 42(2):140-146, 2005a.

Patnaik AK, Lieberman PH, Erlandson RA, et al: Hepatobiliary neuroendocrine carcinoma in cats: a clinicopathologic, immunohistochemical, and ultrastructural study of 17 cases, *Vet Pathol* 42(3):331-337, 2005b.

Penninck DG, Feldman EC, Nyland TG: Radiographic features of canine hyperadrenocorticism caused by autonomously functioning adrenocortical tumors: 23 cases (1978-1986), *J Am Vet Med Assoc* 192:1604-1608, 1988.

Peterson ME, Kintzer PP, Cavanagh PG, et al: Feline hyperthyroidism: pretreatment clinical and laboratory evaluations of 131 cases, *J Am Vet Med Assoc* 183:103-110, 1983.

Platt SR, Sheppard BJ, Graham J, et al: Pheochromocytoma in the vertebral canal of two dogs, *J Am Anim Hosp Assoc* 34:365-371, 1998.

Reusch CE, Feldman EC: Canine hyperadrenocorticism due to adrenocortical neoplasia, *J Vet Intern Med* 5:3-10, 1991.

Rossi G, Magi GE, Tarantino C, et al: Tracheobronchial neuroendocrine carcinoma in a cat, *J Comp Pathol* 137(2-3):165-168, 2007.

Rossmeisl JH Jr, Forrester SD, Robertson JL, et al: Chronic vomiting associated with a gastric carcinoid in a cat, *J Am Anim Hosp Assoc* 38(1):61-66, 2002.

Saegusa S, Yamamura H, Morita T, et al: Pulmonary neuroendocrine carcinoma in a four-month-old dog, *J Comp Pathol* 111(4):439-443, 1994.

Sako T, Uchida E, Okamoto M, et al: Immunohistochemical evaluation of a malignant intestinal carcinoid in a dog, *Vet Pathol* 40(2):212-215, 2003.

Sako T, Shimoyama Y, Akihara Y, et al: Neuroendocrine carcinoma in the nasal cavity of ten dogs, *J Comp Pathol* 133:155-163, 2005.

Scavelli TD, Peterson ME, Matthiesen DT: Results of surgical treatment of hyperadrenocorticism caused by adrenocortical neoplasia in the dog: 25 cases (1980-1984), *J Am Vet Med Assoc* 189:1360-1364, 1986.

Slawienski MJ, Mauldin GE, Mauldin GN, et al: Malignant colonic neoplasia in cats: 46 cases (1990-1996), *J Am Vet Med Assoc* 211(7):878-881, 1997.

Sykes GP, Cooper BJ: Canine intestinal carcinoids, *Vet Pathol* 19(2):120-131, 1982.

Tillson DM, Fingland RB, Andrews GA: Chemodectoma in a cat, *J Am Anim Hosp Assoc* 30:586-590, 1994.

Tobin RL, Nelson RW, Lucroy MD, et al: Outcome of surgical versus medical treatment of dogs with beta cell neoplasia: 39 cases (1990-1997), *J Am Vet Med Assoc* 215:226-230, 1999.

Turrel JM, Feldman EC, Nelson RW, et al: Thyroid carcinoma causing hyperthyroidism in cats: 14 cases (1981-1986), *J Am Vet Med Assoc* 193:359-364, 1988.

von Dehn BJ, Nelson RW, Feldman EC, et al: Pheochromocytoma and hyperadrenocorticism in dogs: six cases (1982-1992), *J Am Vet Med Assoc* 207:322-324, 1995.

Whiteley LO, Leininger JR: Neuroendocrine (Merkel) cell tumors of the canine oral cavity, *Vet Pathol* 24:570-572, 1987.

Zimmerman KL, Rossmeisl JH, Thorn CE, et al: Mediastinal mass in a dog with syncope and abdominal distension, *Vet Clin Pathol* 29:19-21, 2000.

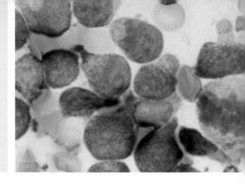

17

Advanced Diagnostic Techniques

José A. Ramos-Vara, Anne C. Avery, and Paul R. Avery

Cytopathology is a highly useful, noninvasive method for diagnosis of malignant vs. benign conditions and identification of infectious agents. However, a number of problems confront the cytopathologist on a daily basis because of limitations of conventional cytologic features. Adjunct techniques can be utilized to give additional information, which allows one to reach a definitive diagnosis. These techniques must be used in parallel with conventional cytologic features and include immunodiagnostics for cellular origin, electron microscopy for presence of subcellular structures, special histochemical stains for demonstration of chemical constituents, flow cytometry and image analysis for a quantitative evaluation of cellular markers, and molecular diagnostics for clonality or chromosomal abnormalities. In this chapter, we discuss adjunct diagnostic techniques and focus on both their applications in cytopathology and histopathology.

IMMUNODIAGNOSIS

The detection of antigens by immunologic and chemical reactions in tissue sections (immunohistochemistry-IHC-), or cytologic preparations (immunocytochemistry-ICC-) has become one of the most commonly used ancillary morphologic techniques in diagnostic pathology (Barr and Wu, 2006). The advantages of IHC and ICC are: 1) They do not require the use of expensive equipment. 2) Both prospective and retrospective studies can be done on a variety of samples. 3) Antigen detection can be correlated with morphologic changes (IHC) and its cellular location (ICC). 4) Stained slides can be stored for many months. 5) Routine processing of samples is usually acceptable for these techniques. Both IHC and ICC are practical in the characterization of poorly differentiated neoplasms, differentiation of primary from metastatic tumors, and determination of sites of origin of metastatic lesions and prognostic assessments (DeLellis and Hoda, 2006). The general consensus is that IHC/ICC methods, if properly applied and interpreted, increase diagnostic accuracy in pathology. Technical aspects of IHC and ICC, interpretation of results, and pitfalls will be reviewed. An

algorithmic approach to the diagnosis of tumors, the diagnosis of metastatic disease, and the use of antibodies as prognostic markers will be presented. This review will not include detailed IHC or ICC procedures. For this purpose, the reader is referred to other published material (Polak and Van Noorden, 2003; Ramos-Vara and Saeteele, 2007).

Immunohistochemistry

Antibodies

Immunohistochemistry (IHC) demonstrates antigens in tissue sections by incubating the sections with specific antibodies and demonstrating the immunologic reaction with a histochemical (enzyme-substrate) reaction to produce a colored (visible) reaction (Ramos-Vara, 2005). Polyclonal or monoclonal antibodies can be used. In general, *polyclonal antibodies* are usually raised in rabbits and have higher affinity but lower specificity than monoclonal antibodies. Cross-reactivity (defined as recognition of unrelated antigens) is more common with polyclonal antibodies. Key in the use of polyclonal antibodies in diagnostic IHC/ICC is their degree of purification (examples of commercially available antibodies include whole serum antibodies, antibodies purified by precipitation of immunoglobulins, and immunoglobulins purified by affinity chromatography). *Monoclonal antibodies,* produced in mice using the hybridoma technology, recognize a single epitope (a 4-8 amino acid chain in a protein) and therefore are highly specific and have constant characteristics among different batches of antibody. Rabbit monoclonal antibodies are increasingly being used in human diagnostic IHC, but despite their reported advantages over mouse monoclonal antibodies (e.g., higher affinity, no need for antigen retrieval, use on mouse tissues), some of them neither react on animal tissues nor perform better than mouse monoclonal antibodies (Reid et al., 2007; Vilches-Moure and Ramos-Vara, 2005). Selection of a particular antibody will be determined by published information or the experience of other laboratories. There are no guarantees that an antibody that recognizes an antigen in one species will do so in another species; only testing will determine if this is the case. Needless to say, the large number of species from which samples can be obtained is one of the biggest challenges that a veterinary pathologist must face in immunodiagnostics.

Fixation

The universal fixative for histopathology and diagnostic IHC is buffered formalin. Attempts to replace formalin fixative in diagnostic IHC have failed, although for specific situations the use of nonformaldehyde fixatives, particularly glyoxal-based, has been reported (Yaziji and Barry, 2006). Fixation is necessary for preservation of cellular components, to prevent autolysis and displacement of cell constituents, to stabilize cellular materials (antigens), and to facilitate conventional staining and immunostaining (Ramos-Vara, 2005). The use of formalin is not without problems. First, the quality of formalin solutions varies widely in regard to concentration of formaldehyde, pH, and presence of preservatives. Second, formalin fixation, by producing methylene bridges between amino groups and other functional groups, alters the tertiary and quaternary structure of proteins and forms cross-links between soluble tissues and proteins. These chemical reactions may modify the targeted epitope. Amino acids that are especially sensitive to formalin fixation include lysine, glycine, tyrosine, arginine, histidine, and serine. Despite the fact that formalin fixation may impair immunohistochemical detection, good fixation is paramount to detect antigens with IHC. Underfixation is as bad as or worse than overfixation, and is a fairly common problem due to reduced turnaround times in diagnostic laboratories. With the advent of heat-induced epitope retrieval (HIER), overfixation or variable fixation time among samples is less critical in the detection antigens targeted in human diagnostic IHC (Webster et al., 2009). The same will probably be true with common antigens demonstrated in animal samples. Autolysis is a common problem in diagnostic pathology. Studies addressing the effects of autolysis in IHC have shown that most antigens are still detectable despite decomposition; however, caution in the interpretation of autolyzed material is necessary due to the loss of detection of some antigens (Maleszewski et al., 2007). Necrotic tissue tends to produce more background than normal tissue; however, IHC of necrotic tissue can provide valuable information when no other tissue is available, particularly for cytokeratins and CD45. Decalcification of formalin-fixed tissues generally does not reduce the immunoreactivity of most antigens, particularly when using weak acids; some loss of reactivity is apparent when using strong acids for decalcification, but it does not affect all antigens.

Sample Processing

Processing of samples for diagnostic IHC is the same as for routine histopathology. Antigens have been successfully detected in formalin-fixed, paraffin-embedded (FFPE) tissues stored for several decades (Litlekalsoy et al., 2007). Autolyzed samples or those with biopsy artifacts should be avoided. For IHC and ICC, samples are mounted onto silanized slides, poly-L-lysine-coated slides, or charged slides to allow a strong bond between the slide and the tissue section. Pooling of reagents under the tissue section or tissue loss can occur when using noncharged slides or slides without special coatings. Complete deparaffination is critical to achieve optimal immunostaining. Deparaffination is somewhat cumbersome and there are commercial products to perform deparaffination and antigen retrieval simultaneously although results may not be completely satisfactory. A simple approach to deparaffination and antigen retrieval with heat has recently been published (Boenisch, 2007).

Antigen Retrieval

As previously mentioned, formalin fixation modifies the tertiary structure of proteins, often rendering antigens undetectable by specific antibodies. A factor in the binding of antibodies to antigens is their conformational fit, which may be modified during fixation. Antigen retrieval (AR) is intended to reverse the changes produced during fixation. In addition to conformational changes in the structure of proteins, fixation produces major changes in the electrostatic charge of proteins (antigens), which is critical for the initial attraction between antigens and antibodies. Therefore, recovery of the electrostatic charges lost during formalin fixation has been proposed as another mechanism of antigen retrieval for many (but not all) proteins. In other words, it appears that more than one mechanism may be involved in the lack of recognition of antigens by antibodies after fixation in cross-linking fixatives. The two more common AR procedures include proteolytic enzymes (e.g., pronase, trypsin, proteinase K) and immersion of slides in buffer at high temperature. Each antibody may react differently to antigen retrieval and therefore it is necessary to test several methods when optimizing the IHC procedure although some HIER procedures appear to produce optimal results in a wide variety of antibodies. With the variety of AR methods available, standardization of IHC methods among laboratories and comparison of results is very challenging at best.

Protocols

For technical aspects of IHC and detailed protocols, the reader is referred to a more recent review (Ramos-Vara and Saeteele, 2007). Table 17-1 includes the antibodies used by the Animal Disease Diagnostic Laboratory at Purdue University for infectious and neoplastic diseases of dogs and cats. Immunohistochemical protocols can be divided into three stages: 1) Pretreatment procedures; 2) Incubation of the primary antibody, secondary, and tertiary reagents; 3) Visualization of the immunologic reaction.

Pretreatment Procedures

These procedures include blocking of endogenous activities, blocking of nonspecific binding, and antigen retrieval (the lattermost already discussed). *Endogenous peroxidase* (for immunoperoxidase procedures) is common in numerous tissues although formalin fixation destroys most of it. *Endogenous alkaline phosphatase* (for alkaline

TABLE 17-1 List of Selected Antigen Markers, Sources, Tissue Controls, and Uses for Selected Antibodies Used in Dogs and Cats

Antigen	Species*	Clone/ Catalog #	Vendor	Tissue Control	Use
Actin muscle	Dog	HHF35	Dako	Skeletal muscle/heart	Muscle neoplasms
Actin sarcomeric	Dog	Alpha-Sr-1	Dako	Skeletal muscle/heart	Striated muscle tumors
Actin smooth muscle	Dog	1A4	Dako	Stomach/Intestine	Smooth muscle tumors
Adenovirus (blend)	Dog	20/11 and 2/6	Chemicon	Infected tissue	Infection
Amylin (IAPP)	Cat, Dog	R10/99	AbD Serotec	Pancreas	Pancreatic islet amyloid
Bcl-2 oncoprotein	Cat only	NCL-bcl-2	Novocastra	Lymphoid tissue	Lymphoid tumors
B-lymphocyte antigen (BLA.36)	Cat, Dog	A27-42	Dako	Lymph node, spleen	B-cell, histiocytic tumors
CD1c (ICC)	Dog only	CA13.9H11	UCD	Lymphoid tissue	Dendritic cell tumors
CD3 (ICC)	Dog only	CA17.2A12	AbD Serotec	Lymph node, spleen	T-cell lymphoma
CD3 epsilon (IHC)	Cat, Dog	CD3-12	AbD Serotec	Lymph node, spleen	T-cell lymphoma
CD10 (CALLA antigen)	Dog	56C6	Vector	Kidney,	Renal, stromal tumors
CD11d (IHC)	Dog only	CA18.3C6	UCD	Spleen	Lymphoid, histiocytic tumors
CD11d (ICC)	Cat, Dog	CA16.3D3	UCD	Spleen	Lymphoid, histiocytic tumors
CD18	Cat only	FE3.9F2	UCD	Spleen	Leukocytic tumors
CD18	Dog only	CA16.3C10	UCD	Spleen, lymph node	Leukocytic tumors
CD20	Cat, Dog	RB-9013	LabVision	Spleen, lymph node	B-cell tumors
CD31	Dog	JC/70A	Dako	Skin, other	Vascular endothelial and megakaryocytic tumors
CD45	Dog only	CA12.10C12	UCD	Spleen, lymph node	Leukocytic tumors
CD45RA	Dog only	CA21.4B3	UCD	Lymphoid tissue	Lymphoid tumors
CD79a	Cat, Dog	HM57	Dako	Lymph node, spleen	B-cell lymphoma
CD117 (*c-Kit* protein)	Dog	A4502	Dako	Mast cell tumor	Mast cell tumor
Calcitonin	Cat, Dog	A0576	Dako	Thyroid	C-cell tumors
Calponin	Dog	CALP, h-CP	Dako, Sigma	Small intestine, stomach	Smooth muscle and myoepithelial tumors
Calretinin	Cat, Dog	18-0211	Zymed	Kidney	Renal tubules, nerve tissue, adrenocortical tumors, mesothelioma
Canine distemper virus	Dog	CDV-NP	VMRD	Infected tissue	Infection
Carcinoembryonic antigen	Dog	A0115	Dako	Intestine	Epithelial tumors
Caspase-3	Dog	CASP3ACTabr	Research Diagnostics	Lymph node	Apoptotic cells
Chromogranins A+B	Dog	PRO11422	Research Diagnostics	Pancreas	Neuroendocrine marker
Coronavirus	Cat, Dog	FIPV3-70	CMI	Infected tissue	Infection
COX-1	Dog	160108	Cayman Chemical	Normal urinary bladder	Normal urothelium, endothelium
COX-2	Cat, Dog	PG 27 B	Oxford Biomedical	Transitional cell carcinoma	Carcinomas
Cytokeratin 5	Dog	XM26	Vector	Mammary gland, skin	Myoepithelium, basal cells
Cytokeratin 7	Dog	OV-TL 12/30	Dako	Skin, urinary bladder	Glandular epithelium
Cytokeratins 8/18	Dog	5D3	Novocastra	Liver, stomach	Glandular epithelium
Cytokeratins AE1-AE3	Cat, Dog	AE1 and AE3	Dako	Skin	General epithelium marker
Cytokeratins Pan	Dog	MNF116	Dako	Glandular/squamous epithelium	General epithelium marker
Cytokeratins HMW	Dog	34βE12	Dako	Skin	Squamous epithelium, mesothelium, hepatocytes
Desmin	Dog	D33	Dako	Skin, stomach, intestine	Muscle tumors
E-Cadherin	Dog	36	BD Transduction	Skin	Langerhan's cells, epithelium, histiocytoma, meningiomas
Estrogen receptor alpha	Cat, Dog	CC4-5	Novocastra	Uterus	Estrogen receptor tumors

Continued

TABLE 17-1 List of Selected Antigen Markers, Sources, Tissue Controls, and Uses for Selected Antibodies Used in Dogs and Cats—cont'd

Antigen	Species*	Clone/ Catalog #	Vendor	Tissue Control	Use
Factor VIII–related antigen	Dog	A0082	Dako	Skin, other	Vascular endothelial and megakaryocytic tumors
Feline calicivirus	Cat	S1-9	CMI	Infected tissue	Infection
Feline herpesvirus 1	Cat	FHV5	CMI	Infected tissue	Infection
Feline leukemia virus	Cat	C11D8-2C1	CMI	Infected tissue	Infection
Glial fibrillary acidic protein	Dog	Z0334	Dako	Brain	Neural (glial) tumors
Glucagon	Cat, Dog	A0565	Dako	Pancreas	Glucagon-producing tumors
Glut 1	Dog	A3536	Dako	Peripheral nerve	Peripheral nerves, stromal cells, kidney
Hepatocyte marker-1 (Hep Par 1)	Dog	OCH1E5	Dako	Liver	Hepatocellular tumors
Ig kappa chains	Dog	A0191	Dako	Lymph node	Plasmacytomas
Ig lambda chains	Dog	A0193	Dako	Lymph node	Plasmacytomas
Immunoglobulin M	Cat, Dog	CM7	CMI	Lymph node	Lymphoid tumors
Inhibin-alpha	Dog	R1	Serotec	Testicle, Sertoli cell tumor	Sex cord–stromal and adrenal cortical tumors
Insulin	Dog	Z006	Zymed	Pancreas	Insulin-producing tumors
Ki-67	Dog	7B11	Zymed	Lymphoma	Cell proliferation marker
Laminin	Cat, Dog	Z0097	Dako	Skin/Kidney	Perivascular wall tumors and basement membrane
Leptospira	Dog	–	NVSL	Infected tissue	Infection
Lysozyme	Dog	A0099	Dako	Liver, spleen	Histiocytes
Melan A	Cat, Dog	A103	Dako	Melanoma	Melanomas, steroid-producing tumors
MHC II	Dog	TAL.1B5	Dako	Histiocytoma, LN	Antigen presenting cells, lymphocytes
Microphthalmia transcription factor	Dog	C5	abcam	Melanoma	Melanomas
MUM 1 protein	Dog	MUM1p	Dako	Plasmacytoma	Plasmacytomas, myelomas, some B-cell tumors
Myeloid/histiocytic antigen	Dog	MAC 387	Dako	Spleen, liver	Macrophages, myeloid cells
Myoglobin	Dog	A324	Dako	Skeletal muscle, heart	Skeletal muscle tumors
Neospora caninum	Dog	210-70-NC	VMRD	Infected tissue	Infection
Nerve growth factor receptor	Dog	NGFR5	LabVision	Nerve	Nerves
Neurofilament-2	Dog	SMI-31	Covance	Brain	Neuron neurofilaments
Neuron specific enolase	Dog	BBS/NC/ VI-H14	Dako	Pancreas	Neuroendocrine marker
OCT3/4	Dog	C-10	Santa Cruz	Mast cell tumor	Germ cell and mast cell tumors
p63	Dog	4A4	Santa Cruz	Skin, mammary gland	Myoepithelium, basal cells
Papilloma virus	Dog	B0580	Dako	Infected tissue	Infection
Parathyroid hormone	Dog only	M7070	Dako	Parathyroid	Normal and neoplastic parathyroid
Parvovirus	Dog	A3B10	VMRD	Infected tissue	Infection
Progesterone receptor	Dog	SP21	LabVision	Uterus	Progesterone receptor tumors
Proliferating Cell Nuclear Antigen	Dog	PC10	Dako	Lymphoma, lymph node	Proliferation marker
Protein Gene Product 9.5	Cat, Dog	Z5116	Dako	Adrenal gland	Neuroendocrine marker
S-100 protein	Cat, Dog	Z0311	Dako	Nerve, brain	Neural marker, neuroendocrine tumors
Somatostatin	Dog	A0566	Dako	Pancreas	Pancreatic islet tumors, some carcinoids
Synaptophysin	Dog	SP11	LabVision	Pancreas	Neuroendocrine marker

TABLE 17-1 List of Selected Antigen Markers, Sources, Tissue Controls, and Uses for Selected Antibodies Used in Dogs and Cats—cont'd

Antigen	Species*	Clone/ Catalog #	Vendor	Tissue Control	Use
Thyroglobulin	Cat, Dog	492020	ShandonImmunon	Thyroid	Thyroglobulin-producing tumors
Thyroid transcription factor-1	Dog	8G7/G3/1	Dako	Lung, thyroid	Lung and thyroid neoplasms
Toxoplasma gondii	Cat	MAB802	Chemicon	Infected tissue	Infection
Tryptase	Dog only	AA1	Dako	Mast cell tumor	Mast cell tumors
Uroplakin III	Dog only	AU1	Res. Diagnostics	Urinary bladder	Urothelial neoplasms
Vimentin	Dog	SP20	LabVision	Skin, stomach	Mesenchymal tumor marker

* Known species reactivity is listed; Dog or Cat only - indicates both species were tested but only one is reactive

CMI, Custom Monoclonals International; *HMW*, high molecular weight; *NVSL*, National Veterinary Services Laboratories (Ames, IA); *UCD*, University of California-Davis (P. Moore)

phosphatase detection methods) is blocked in procedures using this enzyme. Mammalian tissues have two alkaline phosphatase isoenzymes; the nonintestinal form is easily blocked with levamisole; the intestinal isoform unfortunately requires acetic acid to be blocked, a chemical that can damage some antigens. Numerous tissues have *endogenous avidin-biotin activity* that must be blocked before adding biotinylated reagents in avidin-biotin detection systems. *Nonspecific binding of immunoglobulins* to tissue is blocked by incubating tissue sections with bovine serum albumin or serum from the same species as the secondary reagent before the incubation with the primary antibody. There are commercially available reagents to block endogenous activities and nonspecific immunoglobulin binding.

Immunohistochemical Reaction

The immunohistochemical reaction can be divided into an immunologic (antigen-antibody) reaction followed by its demonstration with a histochemical (colored) reaction. The sensitivity of the immunohistochemical reaction is mostly the result of the detection method used (Ramos-Vara, 2005); progress in this regard has been dramatic in the last decade. Two main enzymes are used in IHC: peroxidase and alkaline phosphatase. Peroxidase is probably the enzyme most commonly used, but in some occasions, particularly with heavily pigmented samples or samples rich in endogenous peroxidase, alkaline phosphatase is an excellent alternative. Current IHC methods can be divided into avidin-biotin or non–avidin-biotin systems. After incubation with the primary antibody, a secondary antibody specific for the primary antibody (secondary reagent) is added. For avidin-biotin systems the secondary reagent is biotinylated. For avidin-biotin methods, a tertiary reagent labeled with avidin molecules and an enzyme (peroxidase or alkaline phosphatase) is needed. The most common non–avidin-biotin method is based on polymer technology. The polymers contain many molecules of secondary antibodies and enzyme. Polymer methods are usually two-step methods, whereas avidin-biotin methods are usually three-step methods.

Polymer-based methods have fewer steps, do not have endogenous avidin-biotin background problems, and are usually more sensitive, but are beyond the scope of this review (Vosse et al., 2007). Detection of multiple antigens in the same tissue section is also possible. Issues to keep in mind in double or multiple immunostaining is the compatibility of AR among antigens to be detected, the type of primary antibodies (polyclonal or monoclonal), cellular localization of antigens, and the color of chromogens used.

Visualization of the Immunologic Reaction

The addition of a substrate for the enzyme used plus a chromogen will produce a colored reaction if there is binding of antibodies to tissue antigens. For immunoperoxidase methods, the most common chromogen is diaminobenzidine (DAB), which produces a brown deposit. Another common chromogen is aminoethylcarbazole (AEC). For alkaline phosphatase, Fast Blue and Fast Red are common chromogens. The use of a chromogen needs to be coordinated with the counterstaining and coverslipping methods.

Standardization and Validation of an IHC Test

Like any other ancillary technique, IHC needs to be standardized and validated. *Optimization* (standardization) of a new antibody/test is the process of serially testing and modifying components of the procedure (e.g., fixation, antigen retrieval, antibody dilution, detection system, incubation time, etc.) with the aim of producing a consistent, high-quality assay. The reader is advised to standardize every antibody used in his/her laboratory despite the existence of published protocols, to ensure optimal results. Standardization includes adequate tissue fixation. Tissues should be fixed in 10% neutral buffered formalin for a minimum of 8 hours. Every new antibody is tested following a standard protocol that includes three pretreatments: no antigen retrieval, AR with a proteolytic enzyme (e.g., proteinase K), and HIER (e.g., citrate buffer, pH 6.0); and four, two-fold dilutions of the primary antibody (Ramos-Vara and Beissenherz, 2000). With this standard protocol, the total of slides initially processed for each antibody is 15, including a negative reagent control for each pretreatment. The positive control section used in standardization (and later in a diagnostic setting) is one in which the antigen in question has been detected with a different method (e.g., virus isolation) and its cellular location is known. A negative control section (containing cells known by independent methods to lack the antigen in question) also should be included. Usually, the same tissue block used for the positive control can be used for the negative control.

Incubation of the primary antibody is done at room temperature; duration varies from 30 minutes to 2 hours. Overnight incubations (usually at 4 °C) may be beneficial, but disrupt the automation of the IHC procedure. Based on the results of this initial procedure, the optimal AR method and dilution of the primary antibody is selected as the slide with the best signal (specific staining)–to–noise (background staining) ratio. If staining is nonspecific or suboptimal, other AR methods and dilutions should be tested. Keep in mind that some antibodies raised against human antigens may not be reactive in animal tissues. For standardization, tissue samples are processed in the same way as the diagnostic samples that eventually will be tested.

Test validation in IHC follows standardization; however, because it is time consuming and expensive, it is seldom done in veterinary medicine. Validation of a test examines technical aspects such as the effects of prolonged fixation, but focuses more on the ability of the antibody to be used as a marker of a specific cell, tumor, or infectious agent. Antibodies used as tumor markers need to be tested against tumors that may be difficult to distinguish from the one in question (tumors with similar phenotype, e.g., round cell tumors) with routine stains and tumors present in the same location/organ (Ramos-Vara et al., 2007). Validation should also include evaluation of staining differences among different tumors, staining differences within tumors—particularly when different phenotypes are present (e.g., spindle and epithelioid melanomas staining differences with Melan-A)—and differences between primary and metastatic tumors. Validation is critical given the relative immunologic promiscuity (recognition of more than one cell type or tumor) of most antibodies. Finally, and due to the proven variation of antibody reactivity among different species, standardization and validation of an immunochemical procedure must be done in each species examined.

Immunocytochemistry

Processing of Cytologic Samples

Immunocytochemistry can be performed on most types of cytologic samples including cytospins, cell smears, cell blocks, and liquid-based monolayer preparations (Fetsch and Abati, 2004). Cytospins and cell smears are used when the sample volume is small. The advantage of cytospins is better preservation of cytomorphology. However, ICC on cytospins, cell smears, and liquid-based monolayer preparations (ThinPrep) tends to produce more background staining (Barr and Wu, 2006). Cell blocks of FFPE thrombin clots are the method of choice when

there are abundant cells (e.g., effusions). The advantage of cell blocks is the similarity of processing to surgical pathology specimens (and therefore comparable results), the possibility of preparing multiple sections of the same block (e.g., for testing multiple markers), and ease of storage. Cell blocks may present some disadvantages such as loss of cytomorphology and loss of antigenicity due to formaldehyde fixation (Brown, 2001). Cell blocks are preferred for nuclear antigens (e.g., Ki-67, p53, PCNA), whereas air-dried cytospins are preferred for the detection of surface antigens (e.g., leukocytic antigens). Thin-Preps are less suitable than cell blocks for detection of nuclear antigens (Gong et al., 2003).

ICC may be performed on previously stained Romanowsky or Papanicolau slides when that is the only available specimen and produces similar results to that of unstained slides. The ICC staining can be done with or without previous destaining (with acid alcohol) of the routine stain (Abendroth and Dabbs, 1995; Barr and Wu, 2006; Miller and Kubier, 2002). However, there are some technical drawbacks to using previously stained slides: loss of cells from the slide, cell disruption (affecting mostly ICC of membranous and cytoplasmic markers), and signal reduction for some markers (e.g., S100) due to repeated passage of the sample through graded alcohols. In cases in which only a slide is available and the area containing cells is large, multiple markers can be tested simultaneously. Alternatively, the sample can be divided following tissue-transfer techniques (Sherman et al., 1994).

Fixation

Cytology slides are either wet-fixed or air-dried and fixed immediately before performing ICC (Dabbs, 2002). When wet-fixed preparations were compared with air-dried samples, there were no significant changes in terms of cytologic preservation or ICC staining. However, air-dried preparations may lose fewer cells than wet-fixed samples. Air-dried preparations can be stored at 2 to 8 °C for up to 2 weeks before immunostain without loss of antigenicity (Fetsch and Abati, 2004). Samples are put in a plastic microscope slide box, then in a ziplock plastic bag containing desiccant. Samples should equilibrate to room temperature before the bag is opened to avoid cell rupture. Storage for several weeks can be done at −70 °C (Suthipintawong et al., 1996).

One of the main problems in comparing the quality of immunostaining in cytology preparations is the wide range of fixatives and fixation protocols used in different laboratories. This issue is very different from diagnostic IHC, in which a universal fixative, 10% buffered formaldehyde is used in most instances. Here we are giving general rules, but each laboratory should standardize and validate their protocols to obtain consistent results. Fixation is necessary to preserve cell integrity during multistep immunostaining procedures. Fixation should be performed immediately before immunostaining; theoretically, the type of fixative is selected on an antibody-by-antibody basis. In general, for lymphoid and melanoma markers, samples should be fixed for 5 to 10 minutes at room temperature in acetone; for epithelial markers, 5 minutes at room temperature in alcohol (95% ethanol or a 1:1 mixture of methanol and 100% ethanol); for nuclear antigens, 3.7% buffered formalin for 15 minutes (Fetsch and Abati, 2004). Some authors favor formal saline as a universal fixative suitable for most antigens (Leong et al., 1999). S100 protein, gross cystic disease fluid protein-15, and hormone receptors are not well demonstrated in ethanol-fixed samples due to cytoplasmic antigen leakage (Dabbs, 2002).

Method

Immunocytochemical methods parallel those of immunohistochemistry. There are several steps previous to the incubation of the primary antibody (e.g., endogenous peroxidase block, nonspecific binding block, avidin-biotin block, antigen retrieval). After the primary antibody incubation, a secondary, and sometimes a tertiary, reagent is necessary to demonstrate the immune reaction. The peroxidase block is necessary when using immunoperoxidase techniques; the usual method is with 3% H_2O_2 in deionized water. The peroxidase blocking step can be omitted in acetone-fixed specimens. Antigen retrieval is necessary in numerous occasions. Unfortunately, there is no rule to determine *a priori* whether antigen retrieval is needed or which method is optimal. The approach to standardize ICC is similar to that for IHC. A comprehensive list of antibodies used in ICC at the National Cancer Institute including antibody sources, dilution of the primary antibody, and fixation and antigen retrieval methods is available (Fetsch and Abati, 2004).

Interpretation of ICC and IHC

Immunohistochemistry is an ancillary method and therefore needs to be interpreted in conjunction with clinicopathologic data, including cytologic and surgical biopsy findings, if available. In very few cases is IHC considered a standalone technique in human or veterinary pathology. Specific knowledge of the right staining pattern of a given marker is extremely important to determine whether the staining is significant or not. Interpretation of ICC is more challenging than that of IHC because of the difficulty in obtaining positive and negative control samples treated in a similar way to the test sample and the additional difficulty of distinguishing normal from neoplastic cells. As stressed in the upcoming section on immunohistochemical diagnosis of metastatic tumors, there are very few, if any, antibodies that are truly specific for a single cell type. The interpretation of an IHC reaction is based on the expected "antibody personality profile" (see below) and the infidelity of tumor-specific markers (e.g., reactivity in T-cells with B-cell markers) (Yaziji and Barry, 2006). Simultaneous presence of an antigen in more than one cellular compartment is possible in neoplastic cells, but usually results from diffusion of proteins due to cellular damage during processing. Detection of an antigen in an unusual location should be interpreted with caution and indicated in the immunohistochemical report. Generally speaking, antibodies used in IHC can be used in ICC. In addition, some antibodies that are nonreactive in surgical biopsy specimens are suitable for cytologic preparations.

The interpretation of an immunohistochemical reaction requires a definition of positive or negative staining. This is a controversial issue so only guidelines will be given. Some markers are expected to be present in most cells in a tumor (e.g., cytokeratins in a carcinoma), whereas the detection of other markers (e.g., uroplakin III in transitional cell carcinoma) in only a small group of cells is considered a positive result. Perhaps, as recommended recently in human pathology (Goldstein et al., 2007), a statement in the IHC report indicating the intensity of the staining and the percentage of positive tumor cells would be more informative than merely a positive or negative result as provided in a recent veterinary study (Höinghaus et al., 2008). The lack of expression of a particular antigen may be as significant as its presence in prognostication (e.g., absence of expression of progesterone receptor is linked to poor outcome in human breast cancer; lack of bcl-6 expression combined with MUM1 expression in cutaneous large B-cell lymphoma is linked to short survival) (Bardou et al., 2003; Sundram et al., 2005). In human pathology IHC antibodies are classified as Class I devices by the FDA, meaning that antibodies are considered special stains as adjuncts to conventional histopathologic diagnostic examination (Rhodes, 2005). In other words, with some exceptions, IHC is not a standalone technique and results must be interpreted by the pathologist in the context of the disease. Some IHC tests (e.g., assays for ER, PR, HER2/neu) are considered class II devices with potential predictive or prognostic value. Similarly in veterinary medicine, immunohistochemical results are part of the pathology report and need to be interpreted by the pathologist (Ramos-Vara et al., 2008).

Limitations of Immunohistochemistry

Although IHC has largely displaced electron microscopy as the ancillary technique of choice in diagnostic pathology, it has some limitations (Fisher, 2006). One of the main problems is the lack of standardization and quality control among laboratories, particularly in regard to antigen retrieval. This interlaboratory lack of reproducibility is significant when dealing with prognostic markers (Mengel et al., 2002). Interpretation of immunostaining is also subjective (wide range of interobserver interpretations) and a degree of knowledge of IHC and the antibodies used is required to interpret results correctly. What constitutes a positive result (percentage of positive cells needed, intensity of the reaction) is still controversial, but a critical issue for therapeutic decisions in oncology. Some tumors do not express specific markers beyond the generic ones, which makes testing with multiple markers expensive and unrewarding. Neoplastic cells up- and downregulate gene expression, resulting in the lack of expression of expected antigens or the expression of new antigens. All these issues are perhaps more serious in veterinary medicine, where the degree of sophistication and use of IHC techniques is not as advanced as in human pathology, and are exacerbated by interspecies differences in antigen expression and detection.

Troubleshooting

General Lack of Staining

The most common cause of lack of staining in the test and control samples is improper procedure (from fixation to immunocytochemical procedure including antigen retrieval, antibody concentration, and an improper counterstain) (Dabbs, 2002). A systematic approach to the entire IHC procedure is necessary to determine the cause of staining failure.

Weak Staining

In this context, weak staining applies to both the positive (tissue) control and the test sample and is the result of too much buffer left after a rinsing step, excessive antibody dilution, insufficient incubation time, or improper storage of reagents including buffers, antibodies, and substrates (Fetsch and Abati, 2004). If weak staining only affects the test sample it might be the result of loss of epitopes in the tissue or overfixation.

Background Staining and False-Positive Staining

There are multiple causes of background staining. A common one is inadequate blocking of serum proteins. Blocking is usually done with normal serum or protein (Brown, 2001). Bovine serum albumin has been used extensively in the past as a blocking reagent of nonspecific reactions. However, there is recent evidence that adding albumin to antibody and diluent solutions increases the background of immunohistochemical reactions (Mittelbronn et al., 2006). Other causes of false-positive staining are necrotic tissue, crushed cells, improper fixation, incomplete blocking of endogenous peroxidase or endogenous biotin, and high concentration of the primary antibody (Dabbs, 2002). Samples that are too thick tend to trap reagents and produce background staining. Carcinoma cells in fluids often express vimentin and lose their immunoreactivity for cytokeratins; antigens shed into effusion fluid can be absorbed onto the surfaces of other cells present in the same fluid. Some antigens in cytologic samples such as factor VIII-rAg and immunoglobulins tend to diffuse into the surrounding tissue contributing to incorrect interpretation of immunostaining (Barr and Wu, 2006). To avoid overstaining due to the concentration of the primary antibody, retitration of primary antibodies on cytologic preparations is recommended. Other causes of background staining are included elsewhere (Ramos-Vara, 2005). When using detection kits that recognize primary antibodies made in goats, extensive background in both the positive and negative controls is observed if using tissue sections from the same or related species (ruminants) due to the presence of endogenous immunoglobulins recognized by the secondary antibody (anti–goat IgG). A similar problem is observed with rabbit monoclonal antibodies tested on rabbit tissues or mouse monoclonal antibodies tested on mouse tissues. Special detection procedures are commercially available to avoid this background staining. Although not an example of nonspecific background staining, it is very important in immunocytochemistry to distinguish positive staining in normal or reactive cells from that of neoplastic cells. This distinction can be challenging when the number of reactive cells is higher than that of the neoplastic cells (e.g., T-cell–rich B-cell lymphoma). Fig. 17-1 and Fig. 17-2 show examples of background and nonspecific staining.

The Use of Controls

The same type of controls described under IHC is used for ICC (tissue and reagent controls). Ideally, the control tissue sample should contain the antigen of interest and be fixed and processed in an identical way to the test sample. The ideal positive control should demonstrate immunoreactivity that is weak in some places and strong in others. A negative reagent control is also necessary for each antibody tested (see Fig. 17-2). For the negative reagent control, either an irrelevant antibody or nonimmune serum from the same species as the primary antibody (and ideally the same Ig isotype for monoclonal antibodies) replaces the primary antibody (Fetsch and Abati, 2004). The slide with the negative reagent control should be processed in an identical manner as the slide with the primary antibody. The negative control slide is used to assess nonspecific staining that is not the result of specific antigen-antibody binding (background staining). If only one slide is available, it may be used divided into test and negative reagent control by circling the areas of interest with a diamond or wax pen or using the cell transfer technique already mentioned (DeLellis and Hoda, 2006). In some instances, a slide negative for one marker can be used to test a second marker.

Panel Markers for Diagnostic Immunohistochemistry of Tumors

The goal of diagnostic IHC is to maximize sensitivity without compromising specificity of results. A typical approach is to cover the main tumor types with antibody panels that include cytokeratins (carcinoma), vimentin (sarcoma), S-100 (melanomas or peripheral nerve sheath tumors), and CD45 (leukocytic neoplasms). To achieve maximum sensitivity, the use of "redundant" antibodies for a given antigen is recommended: in other words, the use of several antibodies that should label the same cell type. Table 17-2 lists cell markers and their use in the immunochemical diagnosis of tumors, with emphasis on organ system. In human pathology, the following expanded panel has been proposed: Pan-cytokeratin (carcinomas), CD45 and CD43 (lymphomas), S-100 and Melan-A or gp 100 (melanomas), vimentin and collagen IV (sarcoma) (Yaziji and Barry, 2006). Some of these markers are not available or not reactive in animal tissues, so alternatives need to be found. Once other clinicopathologic data has been examined judicious use of antibodies is the best approach: it will reduce both the cost of testing and the need to explain unexpected reactions to the client. Once a particular tumor group has been identified (e.g., sarcoma), more specific markers to determine the type of tumor are used. This approach is based on

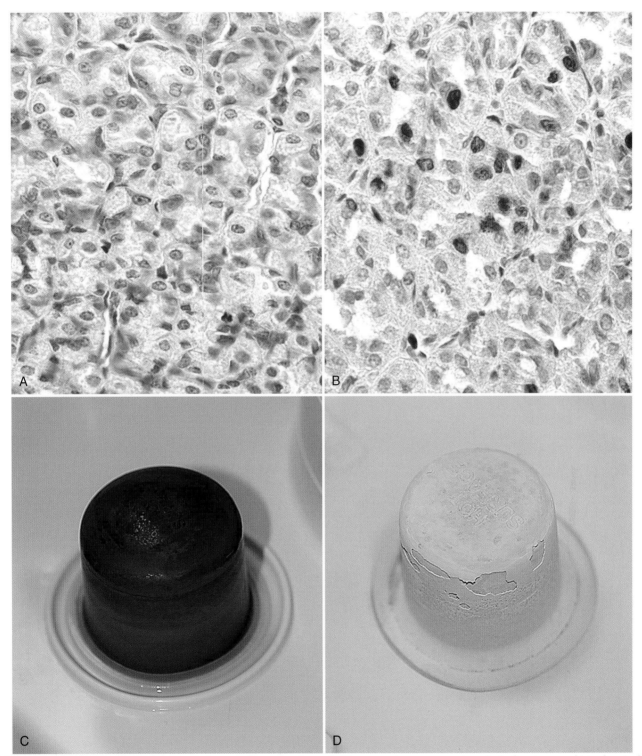

■ **FIGURE 17-1. A–P, Troubleshooting in immunohistochemistry. A,** Tissue section cut several weeks before immunohistochemical testing shows no staining for Ki67 as a result of tissue section aging. **B,** Compare the same tissue section when cut fresh and immunohistochemistry is performed that shows anti-Ki67 nuclear staining in several cells. **C,** A clean heating unit is shown, which helps avoid fluctuations in the incubation temperature. **D,** Note the buildup of salt deposits when using a steamer.

Continued

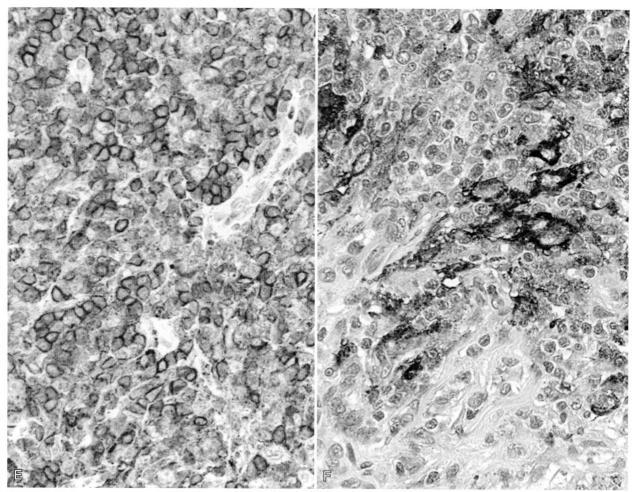

■ **FIGURE 17-1, cont'd. E,** Antigen retrieval (HIER with citrate) demonstrates MHC II-positive cells that include lymphocytes and histiocytes in a case of regressing canine cutaneous histiocytoma. **F,** Note only dendritic (Langerhans) cells are demonstrated when not using antigen retrieval.

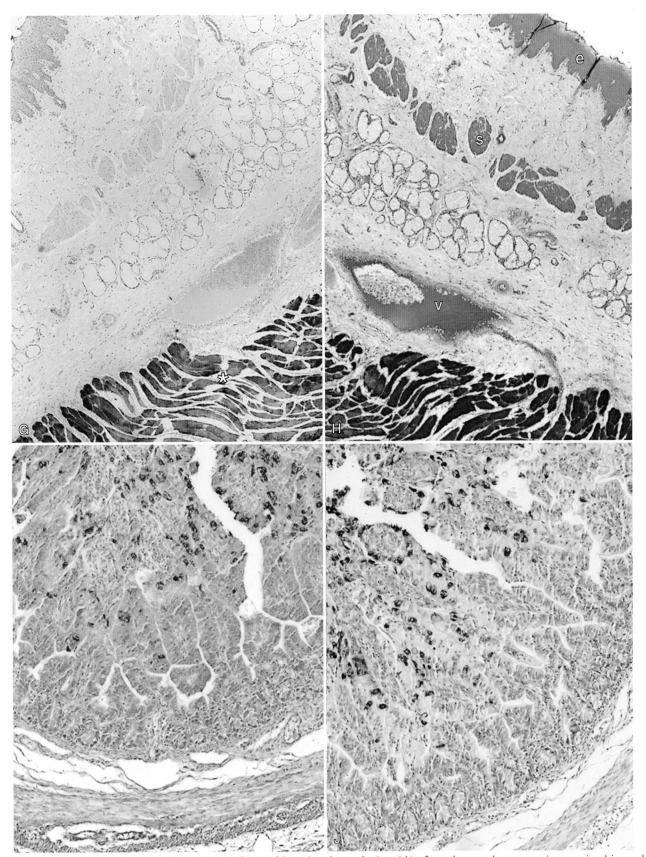

■ **FIGURE 17-1, cont'd. G,** Myoglobin is only detected in striated muscle *(asterisk)* of esophagus when no antigen retrieval is used. **H,** Nonspecific staining due to antigen retrieval with proteinase K in blood vessels *(v)*, smooth muscle *(s)*, and mucosal epithelium *(e)*. **I,** The primary antibody is too concentrated and nonspecifically reacts with many cells. **J,** Optimal dilution of the primary antibody showing reactivity for anti-Rotavirus A only in infected cells of this section of small intestine.

Continued

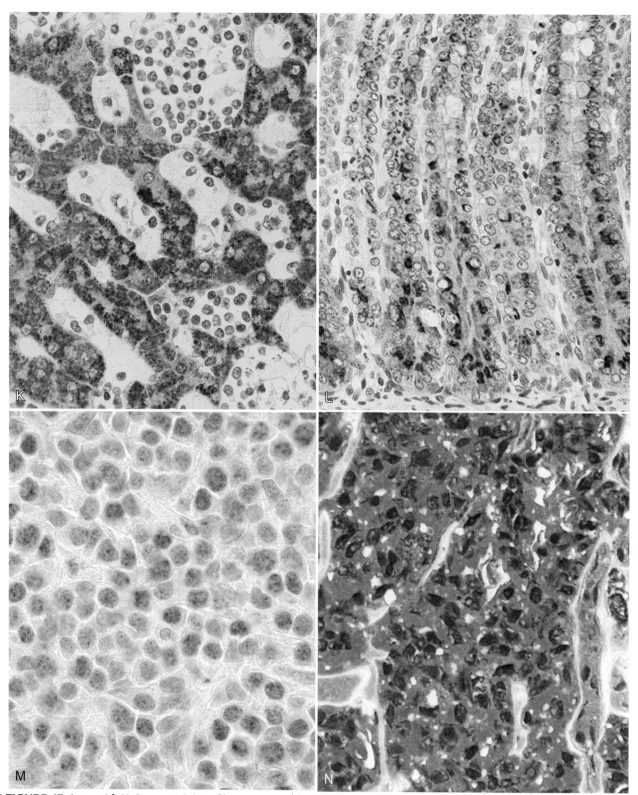

■ **FIGURE 17-1, cont'd. K,** Strong staining of hepatocytes with antibody to CD79a, a B-cell marker. **L,** The majority of epithelial cells in this section of small intestine have strong supranuclear staining with antibody to rotavirus A, which was considered nonspecific. Similar staining (supranuclear) has been observed in different mucosal epithelia with other monoclonal antibodies targeting infectious agents. **M,** CD79a antibody sometimes produces strong nuclear staining in lymphocytes without demonstrable cytoplasmic staining. This pattern of staining is considered nondiagnostic. **N,** Autolyzed tissues may show abnormal location of some proteins. Parathyroid gland showing strong nuclear and cytoplasmic staining for CKs.

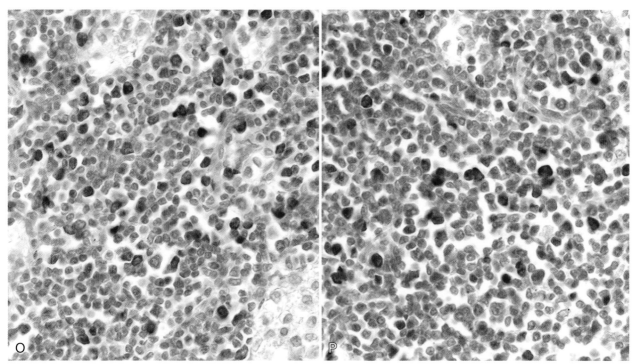

■ **FIGURE 17-1, cont'd. O,** Use of negative reagent control section to demonstrate positive nonspecific staining by numerous plasma cells in this section of lymph node with a primary antibody for natural killer cells. **P,** A similar tissue section with the primary antibody replaced with nonimmune serum. The staining is almost identical. These results are interpreted as binding of the secondary antibody to immunoglobulin-producing cells (plasma cells). (A-B, Courtesy of Dr. Kim Maratea, Purdue University.)

algorithms. Fig. 17-3 shows a basic algorithm to characterize tumors frequently found in domestic species. This algorithmic approach is borrowed from the human experience; unfortunately many markers currently used in human pathology are not reactive in animal tissues or their reactivity is different (in other words, when dealing with IHC, not all animal species and antibodies are created equal). This problem is compounded because the extensive testing (validation) of antibodies used in human diagnostic IHC is almost nonexistent in veterinary medicine. The lack of predictive behavior (percentage of positive cases of a tumor with a particular antibody) is one of the most difficult barriers to overcome in veterinary diagnostic IHC. The use of a particular marker will be also determined by its availability in the laboratory. Many antibodies with diagnostic or prognostic significance in human pathology await validation in similar tumors of animals (Capurro et al., 2003). A similar algorithmic approach can be used in immunocytochemistry.

Antibody personality profile (APF) is a new concept introduced by Yaziji and Barry (2006). An APF is defined by 1) location of expected signal (e.g., cytokeratins are exclusively cytoplasmic; S-100 protein and calretinin are cytoplasmic and nuclear; CD45, CD11 are in the cell membrane; laminin, collagen IV are found only in the interstitium); 2) antibody pattern (S-100 produces a homogeneous signal; cytokeratins, a filamentous signal; chromogranin A and Melan-A, a granular signal); 3) antibody-characteristic pattern across tissues and tumors (thyroid transcription

factor-1 [TTF-1] stains most neoplastic cells in a pulmonary carcinoma; uroplakin III stains only a small percentage of tumor cells). Knowledge of the profile facilitates accurate interpretation of immunohistochemical results. Keep in mind that the APF may vary among animal species (Ramos-Vara et al., 2000, 2002b).

Immunochemical Diagnosis of Anaplastic or Metastatic Tumors

The number of antibodies available for diagnostic purposes has increased exponentially in the last few years. This gives the diagnostician more opportunities to make a definitive diagnosis. Keep in mind that regardless of the number of markers used to characterize a particular tumor, the gold standard before attempting IHC should be HE. A careful examination of HE-stained slides will reduce the number of markers needed to arrive to a definitive diagnosis. Even after that, it is uncommon to make a definitive diagnosis with only one marker because expression (or lack of thereof) of proteins in tumor cells may differ from that in the normal cell counterpart. Upregulation and downregulation of gene expression and the proteins codified by such genes is common in neoplastic cells. The use of tumor marker panels in the diagnosis of metastatic disease is key to improving our chances of arriving at a definitive diagnosis. Considering the relatively low cost of IHC and the expenses of treating some tumors, clinicians are keen to get a definitive

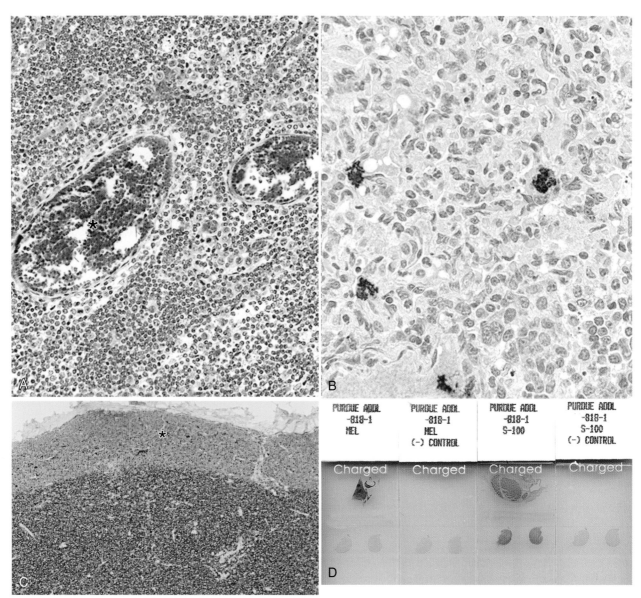

■ FIGURE 17-2. A–F, Troubleshooting in immunohistochemistry. A, This section of lymphoid tissue was not pretreated with hydrogen peroxide to remove endogenous peroxidase activity. Red blood cells *(asterisk)* contain abundant endogenous peroxidase activity. **B,** Nonspecific DAB precipitate can mimic true staining. **C,** The border of the section *(asterisk)* is less stained than the center due to loss (evaporation) of reagents during prolonged incubation, in this case of lymphoma stained for CD3. **D,** Four slides show the results for the two markers Melan-A and S100. Each marker has two tissue sections on two slides; one slide incubated with the primary antibody (slides labeled as MEL and S-100) and one slide in which the primary antibody has been replaced with nonimmune serum or immunoglobulins [slides labeled as (-) CONTROL]. It is advisable to add a known positive control to the same slide that contains the test tissue section (in this case, the positive control is the brown-stained tissue in the upper half of the slides). This case was positive for S100 and negative for Melan-A (test tissues are in the lower half of the slides).

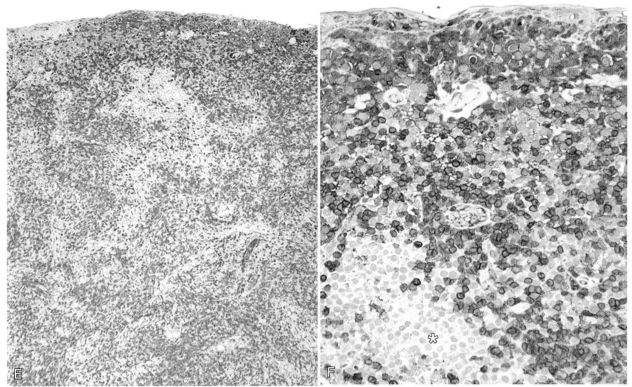

■ **FIGURE 17-2, cont'd. E,** Low magnification of a case of regressing cutaneous histiocytoma demonstrating the more abundant reactive CD3-positive lymphocytes than neoplastic Langerhans cells. **F,** Higher magnification of E showing Langerhans cells which are unstained with antibody to CD3 *(asterisk)*.

TABLE 17-2   Markers Used for the Differential Diagnosis of Major Tumor Categories

Tumor Tissue	Markers
Adrenal	Cortex: Melan-A, inhibin-alpha, calretinin
	Medulla: PGP 9.5, chromogranins, synaptophysin
Endocrine tumors (generic)	Chromogranin A, synaptophysin, PGP 9.5, neuron specific enolase (NSE), S100
Epithelial vs. mesenchymal	Cytokeratins (epithelial), vimentin (mesenchymal), E-cadherin (epithelium), p63 (basal cells, myoepithelium)
Leukocytic	CD45 (panleukocytic), CD18 (with emphasis in histiocytic), CD11d (dendritic cells), E-cadherin (Langerhan's cells), lysozyme (histiocytes), myeloid histiocytic marker (histiocytes, myeloid cells)
Liver	Hep Par 1 (hepatocytes), cytokeratin 7 (bile duct epithelium)
Lymphoid	CD3 (T-cell), CD79a and CD20 (B-cell), CD45 and CD18 (panleukocytic), MUM1 (plasma cells)
Mast cell tumors	CD117, tryptase, OCT3/4
Melanocytic tumors	Melan A, S100, NSE
Muscle differentiation	Actin muscle (all muscle), smooth muscle actin (smooth muscle), myoglobin (skeletal muscle), actin sarcomeric (striated muscle), desmin (all muscle), calponin (smooth muscle, myofibroblast, myoepithelium)
Neurogenic tumors	S100 (neurons, glial cells), neurofilament (neurons), GFAP (glial cells), glut1, nerve growth factor receptor (perineural cells)
Pancreas (endocrine)	Insulin, glucagon, somatostatin, synaptophysin, PGP 9.5, chromogranin A
Squamous vs. adenocarcinoma	Squamous cell carcinoma (CK5, p63); adenocarcinoma (CK7)
Testis and ovary	Sex cord–stromal tumors (inhibin-α, NSE); germ-cell tumors (calretinin, KIT, PGP 9.5)
Thyroid	Thyroglobulin (follicular cells), calcitonin (medulla, C-cells), TTF1 (follicles and medulla)
Urinary tumors	Uroplakin III, cytokeratin 7, COX-2, COX-1
Vascular tumors (endothelium)	Factor VIII–related antigen, CD31

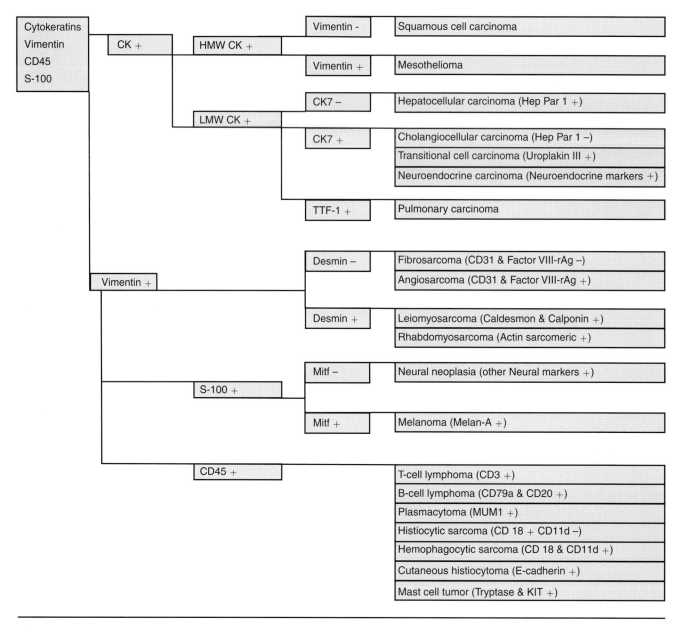

This algorithm is intended for dogs. Antibody reactivity may be similar or different in other species

+	Most tumors are positive for this marker
+/–	Variable number of cases positive for this marker
–	Tumors generally negative for this marker
CK	Cytokeratins
LMW CK	Low molecular weight cytokeratins
HMW CK	High molecular weight cytokeratins
TTF-1	Thyroid transcription factor-1
Mitf	Microphthalmia-associated transcription factor

■ **FIGURE 17-3. Simplified algorithmic approach for canine tumor diagnosis using immunochemistry.** Cytokeratins, vimentin, CD45, and S-100 provide the starting point to help distinguish several carcinomas, sarcomas, neural tumors, and hematopoietic neoplasms from each other.

answer from the pathologist. A treatment tailored to a specific tumor will more likely improve the quality of life of the animal.

The proposed series of steps to characterize a meta-static tumor has been modified from Dabbs (2006) and include: 1) Determine the cell line of differentiation using major lineage markers. 2) Determine the cytokeratin type for carcinomas and possible coexpression of vimentin. 3) Determine if there is expression of cell-specific products, cell-specific structures, or transcription factors unique to specific cell types. The main difference with the algorithmic approach for a metastatic tumor is that without knowing the location of the primary tumor, the differential diagnosis includes more tumor types and the tumor marker panel therefore includes more antibodies.

Determine the Cell Line of Differentiation

Markers should include keratins as well as lymphoid, melanoma, and sarcoma markers (Chijiwa et al., 2004; Höinghaus et al., 2008). A basic panel of markers for small animals is: pancytokeratins (clones AE1/AE3 or MNF 116), CD45 (panleukocytic marker), Melan-A or S100 (melanocytic differentiation), and vimentin (mesenchymal differentiation).

Determine the Cytokeratin Type for Carcinomas and Coexpression of Vimentin

Cytokeratins comprise approximately 20 polypeptides with different molecular weight, numbered 1 through 20. They are separated by charge into acidic (type I) and basic (type II) keratins. Cytokeratins are paired together as acidic and basic types. Most low–molecular weight keratins (e.g., CK 7, 8, 18, 20) are present in all epithelia except squamous epithelium, whereas high–molecular weight keratins (e.g., CK 1, 2, 3, 4, 9, 10) are typically present in squamous epithelium. Almost all mesotheliomas and carcinomas, except squamous cell carcinomas, have CK 8 and 18. The coordinate expression of CK 7 and CK 20 is one criterion to classify carcinomas in human pathology. This approach has proven very useful in metastatic carcinomas of undetermined origin. There is only one paper published regarding domestic animals that examines a wide range of carcinomas in dogs and cats for expression of CK 7 and CK 20 (Espinosa de los Monteros et al., 1999). Results for CK 7 were similar to those in humans, but major differences were observed for CK 20 among both animal species. CK 5 is a useful marker of myoepithelial differentiation in glandular tumors as well as for squamous epithelium and mesothelial cells. Although cytokeratins are the typical marker of epithelial differentiation, they can be detected in mesenchymal tumors (melanoma, leiomyosarcoma, gastrointestinal stromal tumors, liposarcoma, meningioma, and angiosarcoma), although usually in only a few cells, as opposed to the diffuse and strong staining of carcinomas and sarcomatoid carcinomas (Dabbs, 2006). Coexpression of intermediate filaments has been reported in certain human fetal and adult tissues.

Some carcinomas frequently express vimentin, particularly endometrial carcinoma, renal cell carcinoma, salivary gland carcinoma, spindle cell carcinoma, and thyroid follicular carcinoma. In a few cases, coexpression of CKs and vimentin is observed in colorectal, mammary, prostatic, and ovarian carcinomas.

Expression of Cell-Specific Products

This group of markers includes proteins or glycoproteins produced by a few cell types. The exact function of some of these proteins is unknown.

Neuroendocrine Markers.

Within the generic neuroendocrine markers, synaptophysin and chromogranin A are the most commonly used and specific for this group of tumors. Antibodies for these markers work well in most animal species. Keep in mind that synaptophysin, in addition to staining the majority of pheochromocytomas of the adrenal gland, may stain a significant number of adrenal cortical tumors as well. Neuron specific enolase (NSE) is another classic generic neuroendocrine marker. Unfortunately, this marker is less specific than its name claims and stains other nonendocrine cell types, making its use in diagnostic IHC questionable. A recently used neuroendocrine marker in veterinary pathology, protein gene product (PGP) 9.5, a ubiquitin hydrolase, labels many neuroendocrine cells but also labels unrelated tumors (Ramos-Vara and Miller, 2007). Antibodies to peptide hormones (e.g., thyroglobulin, calcitonin, glucagon, insulin) usually cross-react among different animal species and demonstrate specific endocrine cell types.

Specific Markers.

Every year, numerous scientific papers report the characterization of "novel" markers (antibodies) that are extremely specific for particular human cells or tumors. Most eventually will be relegated to use in combination with other antibodies (as part of a tumor panel). In this section are presented some markers that are useful in the characterization of specific animal tumors. **Thyroid transcription factor-1 (TTF1),** a nuclear transcription factor, is frequently expressed in thyroid tumors (more common in follicular, but also present in medullary, tumors) and pulmonary tumors (Ramos-Vara et al., 2002a, 2005). Other tumors, including mesotheliomas, are usually negative. **Hep Par 1 (hepatocyte paraffin 1)** is consistently detected in hepatocytes and their tumors with no staining of biliary epithelium, which makes it a good choice to distinguish these tumors, particularly when used in conjunction with CK 7 (Ramos-Vara et al., 2001a). However, some intestinal, and probably pancreatic, tumors can be positive (Ramos-Vara and Miller, 2002). **Melan-A** is one of the best specific and sensitive markers of melanomas in dogs (less sensitive in feline melanomas) and certainly more specific than other classic markers such as S100 and NSE (Ramos-Vara et al., 2000, 2002b). It should be noted that many steroid-producing tumors from the adrenal cortex, testis, and ovary show strong reactivity for Melan-A (Ramos-Vara et al., 2001b). **Uroplakin III,** a major component of the asymmetric unit of transitional epithelium, is expressed in most canine transitional cell carcinomas and, in conjunction with CK 7, the number of transitional cell carcinomas detected approaches 100% (Ramos-Vara et al., 2003). Uroplakin III has not been detected in nonurothelial normal or neoplastic tissues of dogs which makes this marker the exception to the rule (coexpression of the same marker in different cell types).

A marker widely used in human pathology to discriminate mesothelioma from carcinoma is calretinin. However, attempts to use it in canine mesotheliomas with a variety of antibodies have been unrewarding. There is a report of calretinin staining in equine mesothelioma (Stoica et al., 2004). The differential diagnosis of mesothelioma and pulmonary carcinoma is challenging in human pathology and numerous antibodies have been tested. A recent study indicates that the combination of D2-40 and calretinin (both positive in mesothelioma and negative in lung carcinoma) and CEA and TTF-1 (both negative in mesothelioma and positive in pulmonary carcinoma) antibodies is an economic way to distinguish these two types of tumors (Mimura et al., 2007). Desmin is detected in reactive mesothelial cells but not in mesothelioma or carcinoma in cytologic preparations (Afify et al., 2002). As previously mentioned, TTF-1 is a specific and sensitive marker of canine pulmonary and thyroid carcinomas. The use of CEA on animal tumors is very limited. We are not aware of D2-40 staining of mesotheliomas in animal species. The use of both cytokeratins and vimentin (usually coexpressed in mesotheliomas) is probably the best approach to distinguish mesothelioma from pulmonary carcinoma in animals (Geninet et al., 2003; Morini et al., 2006; Sato et al., 2005; Vural et al., 2007).

A smooth muscle–specific protein, calponin, has been evaluated in canine mammary tumors (Espinosa de los Monteros et al., 2002). In addition, Webster et al. (2007b) studied the expression of the embryonic transcription factor OCT4 in canine neoplasms.

Antibodies as Prognostic Markers in Veterinary Oncology

IHC in oncology is useful as a tool to determine tumor prognosis or disease outcome. This is a topic of intense investigation in human pathology, and not without controversy. Prognostic markers are currently under investigation for some animal tumors. Briefly discussed below are proliferation markers, telomerase activity, KIT stem cell factor, and immunophenotypic changes during cancer progression.

Proliferation/Cell Cycle Markers

This group includes Ki67, PCNA and cyclins, and in general indicates the proportion of proliferating/cycling cells in a given tumor; these markers correlate well with mitotic index. Malignant tumors generally have more proliferating cells than benign tumors, with some exceptions. Lymphomas, mammary tumors, melanocytic tumors, and mast cell tumors are probably the tumors in domestic species in which these markers have been studied most extensively (Ishikawa et al., 2006; Kiupel et al., 1999; Madewell, 2001; Sakai et al., 2002). In mast cell tumors, there is good correlation between decreased survival time and Ki67 index and between the histochemical detection of nuclear organizing regions (AgNORs), which determine the rate of cellular proliferation (generation time) and decreased disease-free interval (Webster et al., 2007a). In a different study (Scase et al., 2006), both AgNORs and Ki67 scores were considered useful prognostic markers for canine mast cell tumors, with Ki67 score used to divide Patnaik grade 2 mast cell tumor into 2 groups showing markedly different actual survival times. PCNA score did not correlate with differences in survival times of several types of tumors (Roels et al., 1999; Scase et al., 2006; Webster et al., 2007a). The prognostic significance of detection of cyclins in animal tumors has not been fully evaluated (Murakami et al., 2001).

Telomerase

Telomeres are portions of repetitive DNA that protect chromosomes from degradation and loss of essential genes (Cadile et al., 2007). With each cell division, telomeres progressively shorten in all somatic cells until cells undergo replicative senescence or apoptosis. Telomerase is a ribonucleoprotein enzyme complex that synthesizes telomere DNA. In normal cells telomerase is detected in male germ cells, activated lymphocytes, lens tissue, and stem cell populations but not in somatic cells. In human cancer, telomerase activity is detected in 85% to 90% of cases and in dogs more than 90% of tumors examined express telomerase activity (Kow et al., 2006). Telomerase expression in dogs is significantly associated with tumor proliferation (Ki67 labeling index) and/or tumor grade (Long et al., 2006). Immunohistochemical detection of telomerase could be useful as a prognostic marker and tool to determine the therapeutic approach to cancer (Argyle and Nasir, 2003).

KIT

The KIT protein, a tyrosine kinase receptor product of the *c-kit* proto-oncogene, is expressed in numerous tissues and cells including mast cells and mast cell tumors. Immunohistochemical staining patterns of KIT in canine mast cell tumors have been used as a prognostic tool (Kiupel et al., 2004). In a normal mast cell, KIT is localized in the cell membrane; localization within the cytoplasm in mast cell tumors has been linked to increased rate of local recurrence, decreased survival rate, or increased tumor grade (Reguera et al., 2000).

Epithelial-Mesenchymal Transition (EMT)

Observed in some human cancers is the loss or redistribution of epithelial markers and gain of mesenchymal markers. EMT is usually associated with one or more of the following tumor features: increased tumor cell motility, invasive potential, tumor grade or tumor stage (Baumgart et al., 2007). The most common proteins affected in EMT are epithelial markers (E-cadherin, beta-catenin, and plakoglobin) and mesenchymal markers (N-cadherin and vimentin). Although it is likely to occur, there is no published evidence of EMT or its prognostic significance in cancer of domestic animals.

ELECTRON MICROSCOPY

The ultrastructural examination of tissues and cells is one of the most common ancillary methods used in diagnostic cytology and pathology (Dardick et al., 1996). If the markers of immunohistochemistry are structural or secretory proteins specific for a cell or tissue, then the markers of electron microscopy (EM) are subcellular structures such as organelles or matrix constituents. Electron microscopy has contributed in great measure to an understanding of the structural features of normal and pathologic tissues. Although the use of EM has declined in the last decade and been partially replaced by other techniques (e.g., immunohistochemistry), EM is still a very valuable tool to reach a definitive diagnosis in some difficult cases, particularly in peripheral nerve sheath tumors, some synovial sarcomas, pleomorphic sarcomas, and mesotheliomas (Dardick and Herrera, 1998; Mackay, 2007). EM and IHC should be used in a complementary fashion based on the type of diagnostic problem (Fisher, 2006). As an ancillary technique, EM raises the level of confidence in diagnoses based on light microscopy. Of the three main types of ancillary techniques currently used in veterinary pathology (EM, IHC, PCR), EM is the most mature technique, meaning that it has gone through the usual stages of development, evaluation and, stabilization as opposed to the other two techniques that are still in development or evaluation stages. As the saying goes, embrace the new techniques if they are worthy and keep the proven old ones.

Pros and Cons of Electron Microscopy

Advantages of EM

- It is the only method to examine the fine detail of tissues and cells (organelles, inclusions, pigments, extracellular matrix).
- There is a wealth of information on ultrastructural pathology in the literature of the last 40-plus years.
- Although not optimal, formalin-fixed (and even paraffin-embedded) tissues can be used.
- It can identify infectious agents not previously reported (and therefore without specific antibodies or genetic probes).
- Many microorganisms are more resistant to autolysis than eukaryotic cells (and therefore warrant ultra-structural examination in suboptimally preserved tissues) (Figs. 17-4 to 17-7).
- For some tumors, it is the most reliable method for diagnosis (Fig. 17-8).
- For certain lesions (e.g., glomerular disease) EM is still the gold standard method (Fig. 17-9).
- Immunologic assays can be performed on EM samples.
- EM complements immunohistochemistry.
- Cellular structures are nearly identical among animal species at the ultrastructural level (in IHC, in contrast, it is not unusual to be unable to demonstrate a particular antigen in a new species due to lack of interspecies cross-reactivity).

Disadvantages of EM

- Sample preparation is rather tedious.
- Optimal preparation is only achieved with special fixation.
- Pathologic changes are sometimes difficult to distinguish from autolysis or processing artifacts.
- Sampling may not be representative due to small sample size (an important limiting factor for heterogeneous lesions); pitfalls include the presence of necrotic, normal, or stromal tissue.
- Overall, it is more expensive than immunohistochemistry.
- It requires expensive equipment and highly skilled technicians.

- Examination of samples is very tedious.
- Pathologists with extensive experience and interest in ultrastructural pathology are an endangered species.

Basics of Electron Microscopy

Fundamentals

The principle on which the transmission electron microscope operates is similar to that of the light microscope—i.e., lenses are used to magnify images. The main difference used to produce images is in the type of radiation, which for EM is electrons, and the means to focus, which for EM is electromagnetic lenses. The resolving power of an electron microscope is around 0.2 nm or less, much higher than that obtained with a photonic microscope (200 nm) or with a fluorescence microscope (100 nm). Processing a sample for EM is basically similar to that for light microscopy, paraffin-embedded samples, but the reagents used are different.

Fixation

The speed of fixation is critical in EM to avoid changes due to autolysis. As previously mentioned, the fixative of choice for light microscopy is formaldehyde. For routine electron microscopy glutaraldehyde is the gold standard, with secondary fixation in osmium tetroxide. These two fixatives are complementary: glutaraldehyde stabilizes proteins and osmium tetroxide stabilizes lipids. Glutaraldehyde has a slower diffusion rate than formaldehyde and very small samples (around 1 mm^3) are required for optimal fixation. Formaldehyde is not an optimal fixative but in diagnostic pathology is the most commonly used primary fixative for EM, particularly when ultrastructural studies are not considered initially in the diagnostic workup. Due to the impurities of commercially available formaldehyde solutions (e.g., formic acid, methanol), ultrastructural preservation is compromised. Tissues fixed in paraformaldehyde (an aldehyde from which formaldehyde is produced) are more amenable to immunoelectron microscopy than those fixed in glutaraldehyde.

Processing of Fixed Samples

Fixed samples are dehydrated and embedded in a liquid resin that polymerizes to produce a hard block that is cut using special glass or diamond knives in an ultramicrotome. Epoxy resins are the standard embedding material, but for special procedures (e.g., immunoelectron microscopy) acrylic resins such as Lowicryl and LR White resins are preferred (Bancroft and Gamble, 2007). For cell suspensions (fine-needle aspirates, cytology samples), samples are pre-embedded in a protein medium (e.g., agar, bovine serum albumin). Semi-thin sections (0.5 to 1.0 μm) are first cut to localize the most appropriate portion of the sample to section at an approximate thickness of 60 to 90 nm (silver to straw-colored ultrathin sections). Routine sections are usually stained with uranyl acetate and lead citrate (osmium fixative will also stain membranes and lipid vacuoles). FFPE tissues can be used when no other sample is available. Keep in mind that the degree of preservation of organelles and membranes in FFPE samples may be severely compromised.

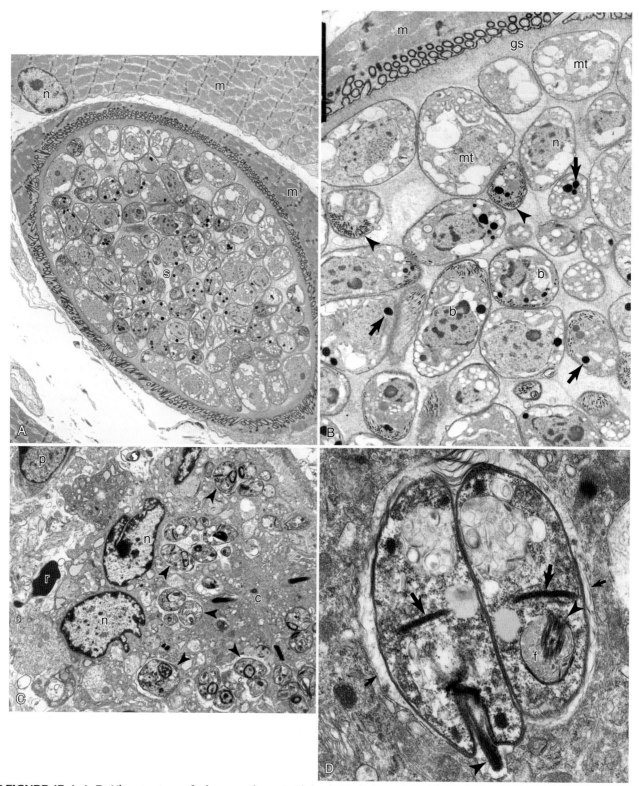

■ **FIGURE 17-4. A–D, Ultrastructure of microorganisms. A,** Skeletal muscle in a mink with *Sarcocystis* cyst *(s)* within a skeletal muscle cell *(m)* with its nucleus *(n)*. **B,** Higher magnification of the *Sarcocystis* cyst reveals metrocytes *(mt)*, bradyzoites *(b)*, and ground substance *(gs)* surrounded by the cyst wall *(cw in white lettering)*. Typical structures of coccidian parasites are micronemes *(arrowheads)* and rhoptries *(arrows)*. Skeletal muscle *(m)* contains the cyst. Note the nucleus *(n)* of a bradyzoite. **C,** The dermis of a horse with *Leishmania* amastigotes *(arrowheads)* within a multinucleate giant cell. Note the nucleus *(n)* and cytoplasm *(c)* of multinucleate giant cell. A red blood cell *(r)* and plasma cell nucleus *(p)* are partially visible. **D,** Higher magnification of two *Leishmania* amastigotes showing the kinetoplast *(thick arrows)*, flagellum *(arrowhead)*, and flagellar pocket *(f)* within the parasitophorous vacuole *(thin arrows)*.

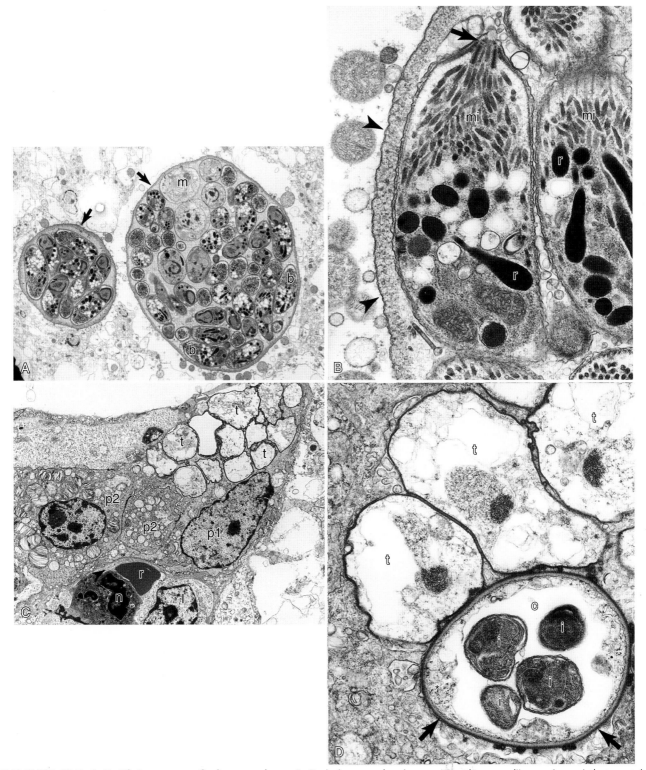

■ **FIGURE 17-5. A–D, Ultrastructure of microorganisms. A,** Brain in a cat showing two *Toxoplasma gondii* cysts *(arrows)* that contain numerous bradyzoites *(b in white lettering)* and fewer immature merozoites *(m)*. **B,** *Toxoplasma* bradyzoites with conoid *(arrow)*, micronemes *(mi)*, and rhoptries *(r)* surrounded by a cyst wall *(arrowheads)*. **C,** Lung of a pig with numerous *Pneumocystis carinii* trophozoites *(t)* on the alveolar surface. Note the type one *(p1)* and type 2 *(p2)* pneumocytes, red blood cell *(r)*, neutrophil *(n)*, and lymphocyte *(l)*. **D,** Three trophozoites *(t)* and one cyst *(c)* form. Note the cyst has a thick cell wall *(arrows)*, a rudimentary cytoplasm *(asterisk)*, and four intracystic bodies *(i)*.

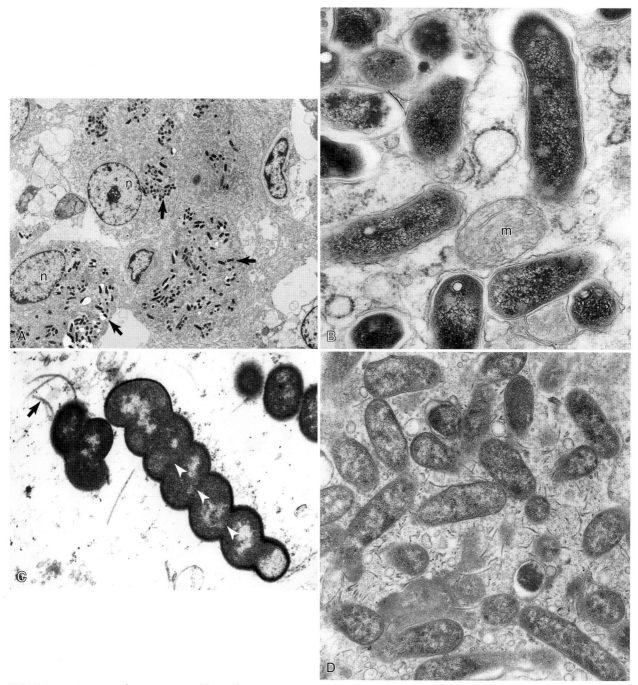

■ **FIGURE 17-6. A–D, Ultrastructure of bacteria. A,** Goat intestine with *Mycobacterium avium* subsp. *paratuberculosis (arrows)* within epithelioid macrophages. Note the nucleus *(n)* of the macrophages. **B,** Higher magnification of mycobacterial organisms indicating a mitochondrion *(m)*. **C,** Pig stomach with *Helicobacter* sp. Note flagella *(arrow)* and periplasmic filaments *(arrowheads in white)*. **D,** Dog stomach with *Campylobacter*-like organisms. Numerous flagella are observed in this field.

Approach to Diagnostic Ultrastructural Pathology

Sample selection and interpretation of electron micrographs is heavily biased by the clinical history and light microscopy findings. After examination of FFPE tissues under the light microscope, differential diagnoses are made and additional ancillary techniques (e.g., EM, IHC) are requested for further characterization of that lesion.

After examining a lesion by light microscopy, the pathologist will determine which features to seek at the ultrastructural level. During the ultrastructural examination, a good observer may find additional, unexpected features that prompt reconsideration of the original diagnosis. Formalin fixation or delayed fixation will probably create artifacts that may render the sample unsuitable for thorough ultrastructural evaluation but still adequate to detect specific features (e.g., viral particles, parasites,

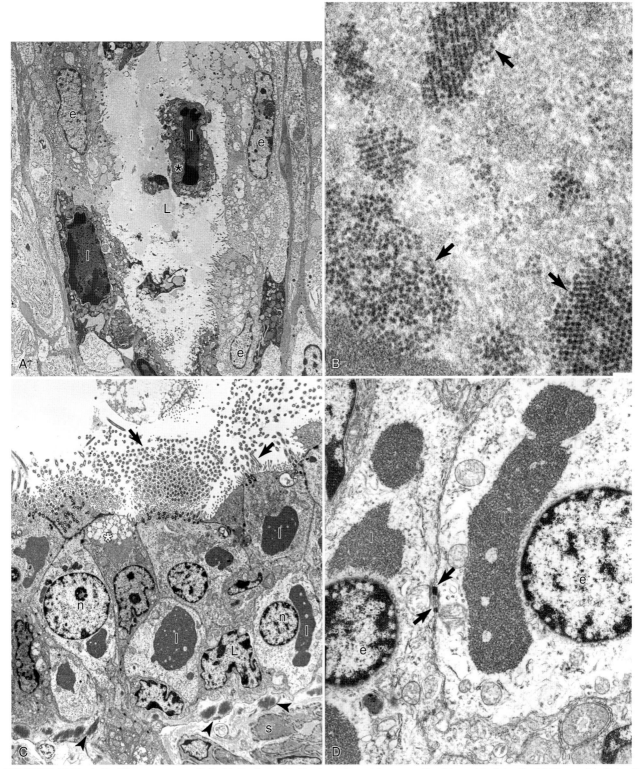

■ **FIGURE 17-7. A–D, Ultrastructure of viral infections. A,** Cat intestine with a crypt lined by epithelial cells *(e)*. Two epithelial cells, one free *(asterisk in white)* in the crypt lumen *(L)*, have pyknotic nuclei and intranuclear feline panleukopenia viral inclusions *(I in white lettering)*. **B,** Higher magnification of feline panleukopenia viral particles forming distinct arrays *(arrows)*. **C,** Mink bronchiole with numerous ciliated cells that contain intracytoplasmic distemper viral inclusions *(I in white lettering)*. Note the nucleus *(n)* of a ciliated epithelial cell with many cilia *(arrows)*, mucus cell *(asterisk)*, basement membrane with collagen bundles *(arrowheads)*, and smooth muscle cell *(s)*. **D,** Higher magnification of bronchiole demonstrating distemper viral inclusions *(I in white lettering)*. Note the intercellular junctions *(arrows)* between two infected epithelial cells and the nuclei of the two epithelial cells *(e)*.

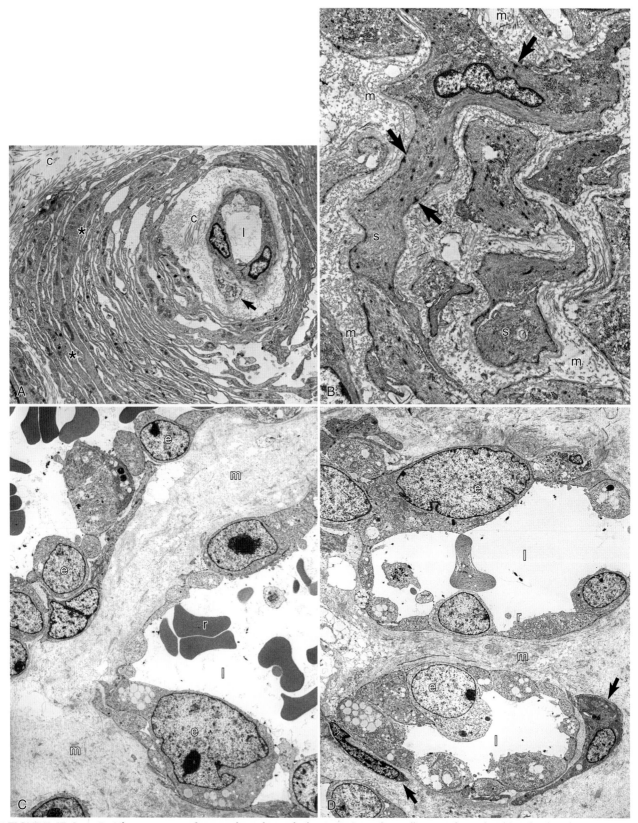

■ **FIGURE 17-8. A–D, Ultrastructure of mesenchymal neoplasia. A,** Perivascular wall tumor from the skin of a dog demonstrating a capillary vessel lumen *(l)* that is lined by endothelial cells *(e)*, a pericyte *(arrow)*, and collagen fibers *(c)*. Neoplastic pericytes *(asterisks in white)* form multiple layers around the vessel. **B,** Leiomyosarcoma in the intestine of a dog with spindloid neoplastic cells *(s)* that have characteristic subplasmalemmal and cytoplasmic densities *(arrows)* of smooth muscle cells. Note the extracellular matrix *(m)*. **C,** Low magnification and **(D)** higher magnification. of a canine case of hemangiosarcoma in the skin. The neoplastic capillary vessel lumens *(l)* are lined by atypical endothelial cells *(e)* that have a large nucleus with abundant euchromatin and a prominent nucleolus. Also present are red blood cells *(r)*, extracellular matrix *(m)*, and pericytes *(arrows)*.

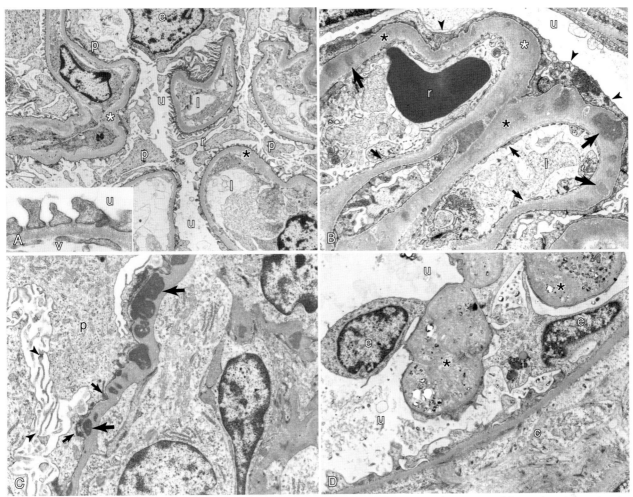

■ **FIGURE 17-9. A–D, Ultrastructure of normal kidney and glomerular disease. A,** Normal structure of the equine glomerulus showing the urinary space *(u)* with basement membrane *(asterisks)* lined by podocyte processes *(p)*. Note that foot processes of podocytes are distributed evenly over the surface of the basement membrane. Lumen of capillary *(l)* is shown. Inset: Higher magnification of the filtration unit of the glomerulus showing the urinary side *(u)* versus the vascular side *(v)*. **B,** Membranous glomerulonephritis in a cat reveals irregular thickening of the basement membrane *(asterisks)* of the glomerulus. The basement membrane has multiple immune-complex electron-dense deposits *(long arrows)*. Note the fused foot processes of podocytes *(arrowheads)*. Lumen of capillary vessel *(l)* is surrounded by a fenestrated lining *(short arrows)*. Also shown is a red blood cell *(r)* and the urinary space *(u)*. **C,** Membranous glomerulonephritis in a dog demonstrates irregular thickening of basement membrane that contains multiple immune-complex electron-dense deposits *(long arrows)*, some in a subepithelial location *(short arrows)*. Note microvilli *(arrowheads)* on the surface of a podocyte *(p)*. **D,** Canine glomerulocystic kidney disease has parietal epithelium *(e)* that is hypertrophic and distorted, containing abundant, mildly electron-dense material *(asterisks)*. The associated Bowman's capsule *(c)* is expanded by extracellular matrix and surrounds the urinary space *(u)*.

inclusions, crystals). Buffered formaldehyde (approximately pH 7.4) will reduce the loss of cellular components and tissue shrinkage.

A sequential (orderly) approach to the ultrastructural study of tumors involves: topographic cellular relationships → external lamina → cell contours → intercellular junctions → cytoplasmic granules → cytoplasmic filaments; cytoplasmic vacuoles and vesicles → type and distribution of organelles → nuclear and nucleolar morphology → stroma.

In case of a conflict of interpretation between light microscopy and electron microscopy, re-evaluation of findings is mandatory. As a rule, if discrepancies still persist, light microscopy findings should prevail due to the far greater amount of tissue examined. However,

the current specialization of pathology makes the use of multiple ancillary techniques (EM, IHC, PCR) common in difficult cases and careful evaluation of all results needs to be made before establishing a final diagnosis. Malignancy cannot be determined on ultrastructural grounds. Establishment of a malignant phenotype is in the realm of light microscopy and tumor biologic behavior, supported in very specific cases by immunohistochemical and molecular tests. Tables 17-3 and 17-4 are intended to give the reader a general approach to the ultrastructural characterization of common tumors.

There are excellent atlases on ultrastructural pathology (Dickersin, 2000; Dvorak and Monahan-Earley, 1992; Erlandson, 1994; Eyden, 1996; Ghadially, 1998).

TABLE 17-3 Organelle Approach to Tumor Diagnosis

Organelle	Features	Tumor
Basal lamina	50- to 100-nm–thick, moderately dense layer following the contours of the cell membrane	Epithelium, mesothelium, meningothelium, granulosa cell, Sertoli cell, muscle, nerve sheath, adipose, and endothelial tumors. (Not present in: hematopoietic cells, fibroblasts, neurons, chondrocytes, osteoblasts, myofibroblasts)
Extracellular matrix	*Collagen:* Cross-striated periodicity of 50 nm, 50- to 100-nm-thick. *Elastin:* Amorphous, moderately dense component and 10- to 12-nm tubular filaments in different arrangements. *Proteoglycans:* Poorly stained, amorphous with occasional granular to filamentous structures.	Numerous epithelial and mesenchymal tumors. Chondrosarcoma. Variable in mesenchymal tumors.
Fibronexus	Cell-to-matrix structure composed of fibronectin filaments in the extracellular space and subplasmalemmal plaques with intracellular smooth muscle myofilaments. Difficult to observe in formalin-fixed tissues.	Myofibroblastic tumors. (Not present in smooth muscle tumors and fibrosarcomas)
Filaments, intermediate	About 10 nm thick. Located in cytoplasmic matrix. *Noncytokeratin:* vimentin, desmin, neurofilaments, glial filaments. Impossible to distinguish them by EM. Variable amounts; between organelles, forming bands of spheroidal masses. *Cytokeratins:* tonofibril (bundles of cytokeratin filaments). Loosely organized (nonsquamous epithelium e.g., mesothelium) or high electron density (squamous and basal cell epithelium).	Carcinomas, neuroendocrine tumors, melanomas, sarcomas. Squamous, basal cell, mesothelioma, endocrine, ameloblastoma, synovial, and epithelioid sarcomas. Myoepithelium (along with myofilaments).
Filament, smooth muscle	5- to 7-nm (actin) and 15-nm (myosin) thick with dense bodies and attachment plaques.	Leiomyosarcoma, hemangiopericytoma, myoepithelium, myofibroblast.
Filaments, striated muscle	Variable degree of differentiation (organization) of sarcomeric myofilaments (actin, myosin).	Rhabdomyosarcoma, rhabdomyoma.
Glycogen	Small, pale to dense particles (30 nm) or rosettes (100-200 nm). Empty areas of cytoplasm due to extraction during processing.	Muscle and liver tumors. Variable amount in many carcinomas and sarcomas.
Golgi apparatus	Packaging and biochemically altering proteins produced in RER. Stacks of membranes.	No specific tumor types.
Intercellular junctions	**Desmosomes:** uniform width of 20-30 nm with intermediate linear density, subcytoplasmic membrane plaques and tonofilaments. **Gap junctions:** Closely apposed membranes (2-nm space) without associated filaments or dense material.	Many epithelial and mesenchymal tumors.
Lipid	Not membrane-bound with amorphous to lamellar, variably dense matrix. Membrane-bound if in lysosomes.	Abundant in steroidogenic tumors, adipose tumors, sebaceous carcinoma, renal cell carcinoma.
Melanosomes	Rod-shaped or elliptical, 200-600 nm, single membrane granules.	Melanoma, melanocytic schwannoma.
Melanosome, compound	Aggregates of melanomes within secondary lysosomes. Variable stages of digestion.	Keratinocytes, macrophages, fibroblasts.
Microtubules	Long, cytoplasmic, 25-nm diameter tubules.	Abundant in neuronal and neuroendocrine tumors.
Mitochondria	Rounded, ovoid, rod-shaped, elongated, branched, annular (1000-nm width). Two limiting membranes and intermediate clear space. Cristae represent infoldings of inner membrane. Tubular or tubulovesicular cristae in cells with lipid and SER indicate steroidogenic phenotype (liver, adrenal cortex, Leydig, and ovarian cells).	Abundant in oncocytomas, hepatocellular tumors, renal cell carcinoma, steroid and muscle tumors.
Mucin granules	Single limiting membrane granules with flocculent, filamentous, reticulate, or homogeneous matrix with no halo.	Mucinous carcinomas.
Neuroendocrine granules	Location: below plasma membrane, within basal cytoplasm and cell processes. Size: Typical 200-400 nm, with range from 60 to 1000 nm. Center: very dense matrix (core) separated from the membrane by clear halo.	Neuroendocrine, paraneuronal, neuronal tumors.
	Small granules (80-150 nm)	Retinoblastoma, neuroblastoma, Merkel cell tumor
	Large granules (1000 nm)	Pituitary gland tumors
	Norepinephrine granules: eccentric cores	Pheochromocytomas, paragangliomas
	Biphasic (rounded and rod-shaped profiles) granules	Abdominal and urogenital neuroendocrine tumors
	Crystal-like granules and sometimes multiple cores	Insulinoma

TABLE 17-3   Organelle Approach to Tumor Diagnosis—cont'd

Organelle	Features	Tumor
Nucleus	Nuclear irregularities are common in neoplastic cells. Artifact of sectioning with contained portions of cytoplasm (pseudoinclusions or nuclear pockets). Multilobation: multiple nuclear profiles connected by thin bridges. Multinuclearity: Nuclear profiles not joined.	Multiple tumor types. Nonspecific feature. Osteoclast-like giant cell tumors. Myeloid leukemia, large B-cell lymphoma.
Primary lysosomes	Small (100-300 nm), rounded, or oval, single-membrane–bound granules. Dense, homogeneous, granular matrix. Crystalline core in eosinophil granules.	Myeloid sarcomas, histiocytic sarcomas, follicular thyroid carcinoma. Endocrine and steroidogenic tumors, granular cell tumors.
RER	Common; active protein synthesis (immunoglobulins, matrix, neuroendocrine, lysosomes).	Fibrosarcoma, plasmacytoma, osteosarcoma.
SER	Common in cells rich in lipid, glycogen, or steroid metabolism.	Sex cord–stromal tumors, hepatocellular tumors.
Secondary lysosomes	Variably sized, single-membrane–bound organelles with remnants of digested material.	Granular cell tumor. Myeloid leukemias, histiocytic sarcoma, prostatic and neuroendocrine tumors.
Serous/zymogen granules	Large (up to 1000 nm), single membrane–bound with a dense to pale matrix and no halo.	Serous carcinomas (e.g., salivary, pancreatic)
Synaptic vesicles	40- to 80-nm, membrane-bound structures with clear interior	Differentiated neuronal tumors

RER, Rough endoplasmic reticulum.
SER, Smooth endoplasmic reticulum.

SPECIAL HISTOCHEMICAL STAINS

The term "special stains" groups most of the histochemical stains used in histopathology and arbitrarily separates them from the standard hematoxylin-eosin. Special stains have been and still are important techniques in the characterization of numerous lesions and tissues. Before the advent of immunohistochemistry and molecular techniques, special stains were the main tool to characterize lesions beyond an HE. The majority of laboratories are capable of doing special stains with the same equipment available for routine histopathology.

Advantages of Special Stains

• They are easy and usually quick to produce.
• Most have standard and very reproducible protocols.
• Currently, numerous special stains can be purchased as kits and used in automatic stainers.
• They have been extensively validated and numerous variations to original protocols have been produced to improve their quality.
• They are fairly inexpensive.
• They detect substances to which there are no commercial antibodies to be detected by IHC.

Disadvantages of Special Stains

• Some stains are somewhat unpredictable.
• Due to the nature of the histochemical reaction, large chemical groups rather than a small number of amino acids encompassing an epitope of an antigen (immunohistochemistry) or short sequences of nucleic acids (molecular techniques) are detected; in other words, they are less specific than IHC or molecular techniques.

Staining Principles

Numerous factors contribute to dye-tissue affinities including: 1) Solvent-solvent interactions (e.g., hydrophobic bonding between enzymes and their substrates); 2) Stain-stain interactions (e.g., metachromatic staining with basic dyes, silver impregnation); 3) Reagent-tissue interactions of Coulombic attractions (e.g., acid and basic dyes); Van der Waal's forces (e.g., detection of large molecules such as elastic fibers); hydrogen bonding (e.g., staining of polysaccharides by carminic acid from nonaqueous solutions); or covalent bonding (e.g., nuclear detection by the Feulgen reaction, PAS stain) (Bancroft and Gamble, 2007).

Special stains are used mainly to demonstrate specific chemical groups characteristic of a substance (e.g., glycogen, myelin) (Fig. 17-10 and Table 17-5) and to demonstrate the general morphology of microorganisms (e.g., fungi, bacteria) (Fig. 17-11 and Table 17-6). There are excellent books regarding special stains and other aspects of histotechnology (Bancroft and Gamble, 2007; Carson, 1997; Prophet, 1992).

FLOW CYTOMETRY

While cytomorphology alone is often sufficient for cell identification, there are many instances where more objective or detailed identification is needed to provide diagnostic or prognostic information. Flow cytometry is a valuable and readily available tool that allows the analysis of individual cells as they pass in front of a laser as a single cell suspension. The light absorbance and scatter properties of the cells can provide information about cell size and internal complexity/granularity respectively, and the use of specific antibodies allows the quantification of both intracellular and surface-expressed components.

TABLE 17-4   Common Ultrastructural Features of Tumors

Tumor Type	Cellular Features	Extracellular Matrix
Adenocarcinoma	Microvilli. Lumens. Junctional complexes. Secretory granules. Golgi apparatus. Endoplasmic reticulum. Cilia (+/−).	Basal lamina
Carcinoid/islet cell tumors	Insular arrangement of cells. Intercellular junctions (e.g., desmosomes). Numerous dense-core granules (variable size and morphology depending of tumor type). Variable intermediate filaments.	Basal lamina surrounding cell clusters Collagen
C-cell carcinoma of thyroid	Dense-core granules. Variable number of organelles (Golgi apparatus, RER, mitochondria).	Basal lamina surrounding cell clusters Collagen
Chondrosarcoma	Scalloped or villous-like cell surface. Abundant and dilated RER. Large Golgi apparatus. Abundant glycogen. Variable intermediate filaments.	Variable. Collagen, glycoprotein, glycos-aminoglycans
Fibrosarcoma	Abundant rough endoplasmic reticulum. Cytoplasmic filaments. Golgi apparatus. Filopodia (+/−).	No basal lamina. Abundant collagen.
Gastrointestinal stromal tumor	Lack of distinct nuclear/cytoplasmic features or morphology similar to smooth, fibroblastic or nerve cells.	Basal lamina (+/−). Collagen.
Glomus tumor	Epithelioid cells. Many mitochondria. Thin filaments. Dense bodies. Pinocytotic vesicles.	Basal lamina. Collagen.
Granular cell tumor	Tightly apposed cells. Numerous cytoplasmic, membrane-bound, variable electron-dense granules (secondary lysosomes).	Basal lamina around groups of cells.
Hemangiopericytoma	Palisading arrangement around capillaries. Focal attachments and intercellular junctions. Pinocytotic vesicles. Intermediate filaments. Variable number of mitochondria, RER.	Abundant basal lamina and matrix.
Hemangiosarcoma	Prominent junctional complexes. Villous-like projections on the luminal aspect. Pinocytotic vesicles. Intermediate cytoplasmic filaments. Free ribosomes. Some mitochondria and RER.	Basal lamina.
Histiocytic sarcoma	Variably sized and shaped nuclei. Numerous cytoplasmic organelles (lysosomes, mitochondria, Golgi apparatus, lipid droplets [+/−]). Phagocytosed red blood cells or leukocytes (+/−).	No basal lamina.
Langerhans histiocytosis	Large, irregularly shaped nucleus. Numerous organelles (mitochondria, free ribosomes, rough endoplasmic reticulum, primary lysosomes). Filopodia. Absence of secondary lysosomes.	No basal lamina.
Leiomyosarcoma	Thin (6-nm) filaments and dense bodies among filaments within cytoplasm and subjacent to plasmalemma. Pinocytotic vesicles. Little RER. Round-ended nuclei. Contraction indentations of nuclei.	Basal lamina.
Leydig cell tumor	Lipid droplets. Abundant SER. Mitochondria with tubular cristae. Microvilli on cell surface. Canalicular-like spaces between cells.	Partial basal lamina.
Liposarcoma	Lipid droplets. Pinocytotic vesicles. Glycogen (+/−). Intermediate filaments. Mitochondria (+/−), Golgi apparatus (+/−), SER and RER (+/−).	Basal lamina.
Lymphoma	Many free ribosomes or polyribosomes. No intercellular junctions. Smooth, indented or convoluted nuclear membrane	No basal lamina.
Mast cell tumor	Round, indented nucleus. Numerous membrane-bound cytoplasmic granules of variable density. Filopodia	No basal lamina. Collagen.
Meningioma	Long, interdigitating cellular processes. Numerous intermediate filaments. Numerous intercellular junctions (e.g. desmosomes). Variable number of organelles. Glycogen (+/−).	Basal lamina (−/+).
Mesothelioma	Numerous long microvilli. Intercellular junctions. Filaments. Tonofibrils. Glycogen. Intracytoplasmic lumens. Lack of mucinous granules and glycocalix	Basal lamina.
Myofibroblastic sarcoma	Spindle shape. Prominent RER. Some thin (6-nm) and peripherally located filaments with focal densities. Fibronexus junction (+/−).	No basal lamina. Abundant matrix with collagen, proteoglycans, and glycos-aminoglycans. Fibronectin.
Osteosarcoma	Scalloped or villus-like cell surface. Abundant and dilated RER. Large Golgi apparatus. Abundant glycogen.	Hydroxyapatite deposits on collagen fibers (osteoid) (+/−).

TABLE 17-4 Common Ultrastructural Features of Tumors—cont'd

Tumor Type	Cellular Features	Extracellular Matrix
Paraganglioma	Clusters of cells. Round, dense-core granules. Prominent Golgi apparatus. Interweaving cytoplasmic processes. Paranuclear filaments (+/−). Sustentacular (Schwann-like) cells with filaments at the periphery of cell clusters.	Basal lamina surrounding cell clusters.
Parathyroid carcinoma	Islands of cells. Intercellular junctions. Interdigitation of lateral membranes. Dense-core secretory granules. Variable glycogen and cell organelles (RER, SLE, mitochondria, Golgi). Occasional clusters of oncocytic cells.	Basal lamina surrounding cell clusters.
Perineuroma	Whorls of slender cells with bipolar cytoplasmic processes. Pinocytotic vesicles. Scant organelles.	Discontinuous basal lamina. Collagen.
Pheochromocytoma	Clusters of polygonal cells. Large, pleomorphic, dense-core granules (sometimes clear or partially filled). Prominent Golgi apparatus. No significant number of sustentacular cells.	Basal lamina surrounding cell clusters. Many small blood vessels.
Plasmacytoma	Abundant rough endoplasmic reticulum. Membrane-bound dense bodies (+/−). Intercellular junctions (+/−). Eccentric nucleus. Paranuclear area with Golgi apparatus, centriole, mitochondria.	No basal lamina. Amyloid (+/−).
Rhabdomyosarcoma	Thick (15-nm) myosin filaments. Z-band formations. Sarcomeres. Thin (6-nm) filaments. Glycogen. Mitochondria (+/−).	Incomplete basal lamina. Collagen.
Schwannoma	Long intertwining processes. Variable number of mitochondria, RER, lysosomes. Intermediate filaments.	Basal lamina. Collagen in matrix.
Seminoma	Close, appositioned, round to polygonal cells. Intercellular junctions. Large, euchromatic nucleus. Prominent nucleoli. Abundant glycogen. Variable number of organelles; mainly free ribosomes.	Basal lamina (+/−).
Sertoli cell tumor	Polygonal cells. Intercellular junctions. Indented nuclei. Junctional complexes. Interdigitating lateral cell membranes. Abundant SER. Lipid droplets. Mitochondria with tubular cristae. Secondary lysosomes.	Basal lamina. Collagenous matrix.
Squamous cell carcinoma	Desmosomes. Keratohyalin granules. Tonofibrils.	Basal lamina.

(+/−) = Feature not present in all tumors or cells.
(−/+) = Feature rarely observed.

The most widely used clinical application involves incubating cells with fluorescently labeled antibodies directed at surface antigens to allow the determination of both the frequency of cells that express the given molecule as well as the relative expression levels on individual cells. Because antibodies can be labeled with a variety of fluorochromes that have different excitation and emission wavelengths, the expression of several surface molecules can be detected simultaneously. The major advantage of flow cytometry is that it allows the rapid and objective identification of large numbers of cells. Clinically, flow cytometry is generally used for the analysis of hematopoietic cells, in order to characterize lymphoma and leukemia, and to quantify cells in cases of suspected immunologic disorders.

Methodology

Sample Collection

To analyze a sample with flow cytometry the cells must be in suspension and free of any clumping or debris. Anticoagulated whole blood or cavity effusions can generally be submitted directly to a flow cytometry facility for analysis. Aspirates from solid tissue can be resuspended in media with serum. In university or laboratory settings, tissue culture media such as RPMI or DMEM, buffered with HEPES and supplemented with 5% to 10% fetal bovine serum is ideal. However in the clinic setting, 0.9% saline can be used, and 10% serum from the patient can be added. Serum from another patient of the same species may also be used. Because a minimum of 10,000 cells are needed for each antibody combination, several tissue aspirates are needed for a complete analysis. If samples are to be shipped, they must be shipped overnight with a cold pack.

Laboratory Preparation of Sample

The preparation of cells for flow cytometry varies widely between laboratories (Lana et al., 2006a; Ruslander et al., 1997; Vernau and Moore, 1999; Villiers et al., 2006; Wilkerson et al., 2005), and at present there is no consensus about the best method. Most commonly, the first step in cell preparation is to remove the red blood cells by lysis in a hypotonic solution. An alternative method is to prepare the cells by differential density centrifugation through a solution such as Histopaque. Neutrophils, red blood cells, and platelets will pass through the solution, whereas mononuclear cells will remain on top of the

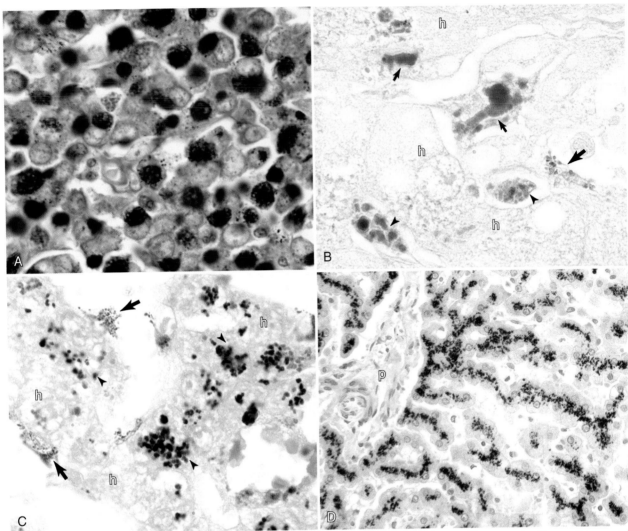

■ **FIGURE 17-10.** A–D, Detection of granules and pigments by special histochemical stains. **A, Giemsa stain. Mast cell tumor. Skin. Dog.** Cells are filled with numerous dense metachromatic granules (purple) characteristic of mast cells. **B, Hall's stain. Liver. Dog.** The green pigment present within bile canaliculi *(thin arrows)* and Kupffer cells *(arrowheads)* is bile. Hemosiderin *(thick arrow)* is not stained but apparent due to its refractile nature. Hepatocytes *(h)* are noted. **C, Rubeanic acid stain. Liver. Dog.** This stain reveals copper granules *(arrowheads)* within hepatocytes *(h)*. Kupffer cells with hemosiderin granules *(arrows)* are shown. **D, Perl's stain for iron. Liver. Dog.** Iron pigment appears blue within hepatocytes. The portal area *(p)* is shown.

Histopaque layer. While this technique concentrates the mononuclear cells considerably, it is possible that cells of interest may pass through the density gradient and be lost from the analysis.

For analysis of antigens expressed on the cells' surface, such as CD4 and CD8, cells are incubated with antibodies to cell surface markers. Primary antibodies are either unlabeled or have been directly conjugated to a fluorescent molecule called a fluorochrome. The directly conjugated antibodies can be visualized immediately after staining and they greatly facilitate the use of multiple markers simultaneously. Cells stained with unlabeled antibodies must be subjected to a second staining reaction using a labeled antibody that will recognize the immunoglobulin portion of the primary antibody. In general, only a single unconjugated antibody can be used in a staining reaction, preventing the simultaneous quantification of

multiple markers on individual cells. It is important to include control reactions for each sample. Controls consist of the same cells left unstained and cells stained with an antibody of the same isotype that should not specifically bind to any antigens on the cells of interest. The unstained cells allow the operator to correct for autofluorescence, and the fluorescent intensity of the irrelevant antibody reaction can be used to determine the level of background staining.

Laboratories use a variety of different antibodies in different combinations for immunophenotyping. Table 17-7 lists a suggested panel for dogs and cats, although most laboratories (including our own) use a more extensive array of antibodies. The largest supplier of directly conjugated antibodies for use in routine veterinary flow cytometry is Abd Serotec *(www.ab-direct.com),* and the clones listed in Table 17-7 are all available through this

TABLE 17-5 Special Histochemical Stains for Intracellular and Extracellular Substances

Stain	Substance or Structure	Color
Acid phosphatase	Prostate	Black
Alcian Blue	Sialomucins, hyaluronic acid, sulfated mucosubstances	Blue
Alizarin red S	Calcium	Orange-red
Best's Carmine	Glycogen	Deep red
Bielschowsky's silver stain	Axons	Black
Congo red	Amyloid	Orange-red*
Cresyl Violet	Nissl substance	Violet
Dunn-Thompson	Hemoglobin	Emerald green
Feulgen	DNA	Red-purple
Fontana-Masson	Melanin	Black
Gordon and Sweets Reticulin Fiber	Reticulin fibers	Black
Grimelius	Argyrophilic granules	Black
Hall's	Bile/biliverdin	Green
Jone's Methenamine	Basement membranes	Black
Kinyoun's (modified Ziehl-Neelsen)	Lipofuscin	Red
Luxol Fast Blue	Myelin	Blue
Mallory's PTAH	Muscle, fibrin, glial processes	Dark blue
Masson's Trichrome	Muscle, collagen	Muscle: Red
		Collagen: Blue
Mayer's Mucicarmine	Mucin, hyaluronic acid, chondroitin sulfate	Rose to red
Methyl Green Pyronin	Nucleic acids	DNA: Green-blue
		RNA: Red
Oil Red O	Fat	Orange–bright red
Periodic acid-Schiff (PAS)	Glycogen, mucin	Red
Prussian Blue	Iron	Blue
Rubeanic Acid	Copper	Green
Schmorl's Reaction	Melanin, lipofuscin	Dark blue
Sudan Black B	Fat	Black
Tolouidine Blue	Mast cells	Purple
Verhoeff	Elastic fibers	Black
Von Kossa	Calcium	Black

* Apple green birefringency with polarized light

company. Other suppliers, such as R&D Systems *(www.rndsystems.com),* B-D Biosciences *(www.bdbiosciences.com),* and Southern Biotech *(www.southernbiotech.com,* cats only) have fewer antibodies.

The cells are washed after the final staining reaction, and then can either be fixed in paraformaldehyde for later analysis or analyzed immediately without fixation. If cells are analyzed immediately, they can be additionally stained with propidium iodide, which will label cells with a disrupted cell membrane and can therefore be used to exclude dead cells from the analysis. This technique is extremely useful because dead cells tend to nonspecifically bind antibodies.

In addition to surface molecules, several useful antigens are located within the cell cytoplasm. For example, most human T-cell acute lymphoblastic leukemia (ALL) lack surface expression of CD3, but have cytoplasmic expression of CD3 (Szczepanski et al., 2006). The CD3 reagent commonly used for IHC in dogs can also be used for flow cytometry (Wilkerson et al., 2005) and could be included in a panel used to phenotype acute leukemia. The monocyte/granulocyte lineage markers myeloperoxidase (MPO) and MAC387 are also cytoplasmic and can be useful for analyzing acute myeloid origin leukemia (Villiers et al., 2006). In order to expose these cytoplasmic molecules,

cell membranes must be permeabilized using commercially available permeabilization reagents before staining.

Data Analysis

The most important aspect of flow cytometry is data analysis, which begins with the examination of the light scatter properties of the cells. As cells pass in front of the laser, they scatter the light, and detectors record the amount of forward-scattered and side-scattered light. The total amount of forward-scattered light detected depends on cell surface area or size, whereas the amount of side-scattered light indicates cellular complexity or granularity. Figure 17-12 demonstrates a typical scatter plot from canine peripheral blood, where each dot represents an individual cell placed relative to the amount of forward and side scatter recorded as it passes in front of the laser. Typical scatter properties allow the identification of lymphocyte, monocyte, and neutrophil populations.

Although there is no consensus on analysis methods in veterinary medicine, in general the first step of an analysis is to "gate" different populations of cells based on their scatter properties. As shown in Figure 17-12, lymphocytes have lower forward and side scatter, whereas neutrophils have higher forward and side scatter, with monocytes falling in between.

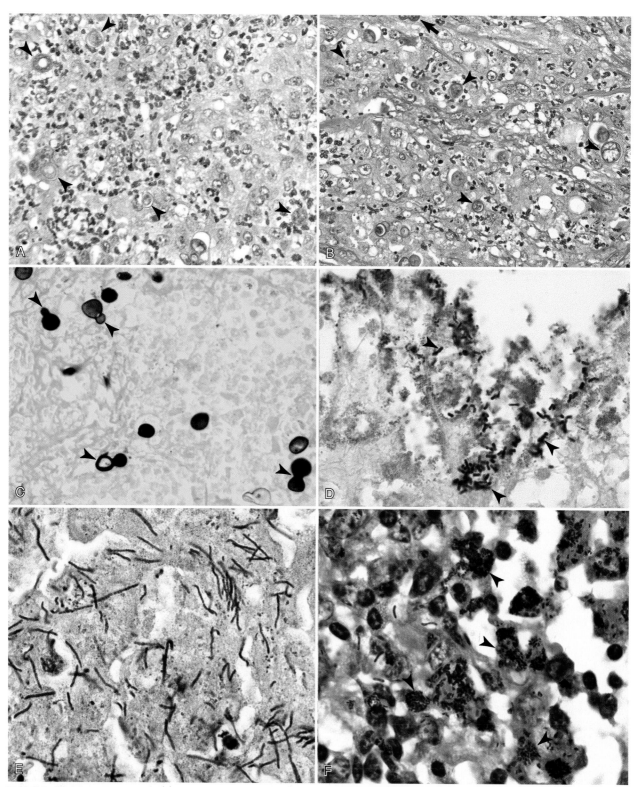

■ **FIGURE 17-11. A–F, Detection of microorganisms by special histochemical stains. Pyogranulomatous dermatitis. Skin. Dog. Blastomycosis. Same case A-C. A,** With routine hematoxylin-eosin stain, cellular detail of the inflammatory reaction is excellent, but detection of yeasts *(arrowheads)* is difficult. **B,** PAS stain improves the detection of yeasts due to staining cell walls magenta *(arrowheads)*. Note the broad-based budding formation *(arrow)*. **C,** Grocott methenamine silver stain demonstrates excellent yeast morphology but detail of the inflammatory process is poor. Numerous broad-based budding yeasts are observed *(arrowheads)*. **D,** Canine intestine with Gram stain depicts many gram-positive bacterial rods *(arrowheads)*. **E, Warthin-Starry stain. Liver. Horse.** *Clostridium piliformis.* This staining method is excellent to detect microorganisms due to the high contrast with the background. **F, Ziehl-Neelsen stain. Skin. Dog,** mycobacterial dermatitis. Acid-fast organisms *(arrowheads)* are strongly stained bright red. Note the presence of unstained bacilli *(arrows in white)*.

TABLE 17-6   Special Histochemical Stains for Microorganisms

Stain	Microorganism
Giemsa	Metachromatic granules. Good stain for protozoa and some bacteria.
Gram	Standard staining for bacteria.
Grocott methenamine silver	Fungi, *Pneumocystis*
Jimenez	Chlamydiae
Macchiavello	Chlamydiae
Mucicarmine	Capsule of *Cryptococcus*
Periodic acid-Schiff	Fungi
Steiner and Steiner silver	Numerous bacteria including *Helicobacter* (good contrast between the black staining of the bacteria and the background)
Toluidine blue	Metachromatic granules.
Wade-Fite	Acid-fast bacteria including mycobacteria, *Nocardia*
Warthin-Starry	Similar uses to Steiner stain.
Ziehl-Neelsen	Acid fast bacteria. *Nocardia* is difficult to detect.

TABLE 17-7   Antibody Panels for Characterization of Canine and Feline Leukocytes by Flow Cytometry

Cell Type	Antigen	Clone(s)	Species Antibody Produced Against
Dog Panel			
Dendritic cells/monocytes	CD1c	CA13.9H11	Dog
T cells	CD3	CA17.2A12	Dog
T cell subset/neutrophils	CD4	YKIX302.9/CA13.1E4	Dog
T cells	CD5	YKIX322.3	Dog
T cell subset	CD8α	YCATE55.9/CA9.JD3	Dog
Macrophages, some T-cells	CD11d	CA16.3D3	Dog
Monocytes/Neutrophils*	CD14	TUK4/UCHM1	Human
B cells	CD21	CA2.1D6/LB21	Dog/human
Precursors	CD34	1H6	Dog
B cells	CD79a	HM57	Human
All leukocytes	CD45	YKIX716.13/CA12.10C12	Dog
Cat Panel			
T cells	CD3ε	CD3-12	Human
T cell subset	CD4	vpg39	Cat
T cells	CD5	FE1.1B11	Cat
T cell subset	CD8α/β	vpg9	Cat
Monocytes	CD14	TUK4*	Cat
B cells	CD21	CA2.1D6/LB21	Dog/human
B cells	CD79a	HM57	Human

*TUK4 does not appear to stain neutrophils, but UCHM1 does.

The next step is to determine the percentage of cells within each population that expresses the markers of interest by looking at the fluorescence profile of each population. The fluorochromes used to label antibodies are excited by the laser and emit a particular peak emission wavelength, which can be detected by the flow cytometer. Different fluorochromes have distinct peak emission wavelengths so antibodies conjugated to two different fluorochromes can be used simultaneously in one staining reaction. The amount of fluorescent signal detected is proportional to the number of fluorochrome molecules on the cell. The data can then be displayed as a single parameter in the form of a histogram, or two parameters can be displayed simultaneously as a dot plot (Fig. 17-13). Two-parameter dot plots allow individual events/cells to be displayed so that the relative fluorescence for two individual markers can be displayed.

Electronic gating of different populations allows the user to determine the percentage of cells in each population that are positive for a given molecule (see Fig. 17-13). The percentage of positive cells is usually determined by first analyzing the isotype control and setting gates based on this control. The percentage of positive cells is determined by the number of cells that fall above the gate set by the negative control (see Fig. 17-13). While the isotype control is used as a guideline, it is generally accepted that there is some flexibility in the placement of gates to include logical populations of cells.

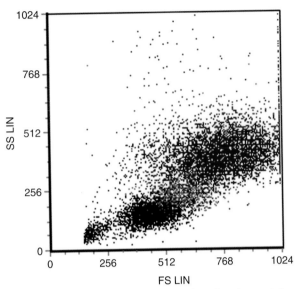

■ FIGURE 17-12. Light scatter properties of canine peripheral blood by flow cytometry. Forward (x axis) and side scatter (y axis) of peripheral blood showing individual neutrophils *(blue)*, monocytes *(red)* and lymphocytes *(black)*.

Reporting Flow Cytometry Data

All laboratories report flow cytometry data differently. In peripheral blood analysis, the most useful information is the absolute number of a lymphocyte subset in peripheral blood per microliter. When only percentages are reported, it may be difficult to distinguish loss of one population from expansion of another population. Although normal values have been published (Byrne et al., 2000), preparation methods differ so widely between laboratories that each lab should generate their own normal values.

For other samples, percentages of lymphocyte subsets are reported usually after gating on the relevant population by size. For example, in lymph node aspirates from dogs with lymphoma, the neoplastic lymphocytes are usually large. Therefore, the percentage of each lymphocyte subset will be determined after gating on the large cells. In addition to the percentage of cells expressing different markers, cells with an abnormal phenotype, such as loss of an antigen or aberrant expression of an antigen, should also be described or quantified.

Uses for Flow Cytometry

Reactive vs. Neoplastic Lymphocytosis

Routine immunophenotyping of circulating lymphocytes is becoming more prevalent in veterinary medicine as more cross-reactive and species-specific antibodies become available. A number of studies have described the immunophenotypic markers of canine lymphoma and leukemia (Appelbaum et al., 1984; Day, 1995; Caniatti et al., 1996; Ruslander et al., 1997; Grindem et al., 1998; McDonough and Moore, 2000; Modiano et al., 1998; Ponce et al., 2003). Distinguishing a reactive from a neoplastic process is often the first task faced by the clinician. Finding of a phenotypically homogeneous population of lymphocytes suggests a neoplastic, rather than a reactive, process. For example, canine chronic lymphocytic leukemia (CLL) most commonly involves an expansion of CD8+ T cells, and less frequently B cells (Vernau and Moore, 1999; Workman and Vernau, 2003). CD8 T cells usually comprise 25% to 35% of canine peripheral blood, and B cells usually comprise 5% to 20% (Byrne et al., 2000; Greeley et al., 2001). Leukemia would be the primary differential diagnosis in a dog with persistent lymphocytosis when a majority of peripheral blood lymphocytes are CD8+ T or B cells, although no criteria have been established in veterinary medicine for making this distinction. A rare exception to such an interpretation in dogs would be lymphocytosis in *Ehrlichia canis* infection, which can be associated with the selective expansion of CD8+ T cells (Heeb et al., 2003; McDonough and Moore, 2000; Weiser et al., 1991). To our knowledge, there are no such examples in cats. Studies of the predictive value of an expanded lymphocyte population and the absolute lymphocyte counts that can be used to define leukemia would be important and clinically useful, but at present no such reports are available in the veterinary literature.

Aberrant expression of surface molecules can provide a definitive diagnosis of leukemia or lymphoma (Rezuke et al., 1997) as reactive lymphocytes will generally retain expression of their normal constellation of antigens. Human T-cell leukemias are characterized by their tendency to lose expression of normal T-cell antigens, or to express aberrant combinations of antigens (Jennings and Foon, 1997). For example in one study of 87 human malignant T-cell disorders, complete loss of any T-cell antigen (CD2, CD5, CD7) or the panleukocyte antigen CD45 was diagnostic for malignancy (Gorczyca et al., 2002). In order to detect aberrant antigen expression it is useful to examine a large panel of antigens using multicolor fluorescence protocols. In our experience, loss of the panleukocyte marker CD45 is the most common form of aberrant antigen expression in T-cell leukemia while smaller numbers of cases have been documented that have lost expression of CD4 and CD8 (Vernau and Moore, 1999). Despite the utility in helping to diagnose T-cell leukemia, decreased expression of CD45 does not appear to be associated with prognosis (Williams et al., 2008).

Prognostic Significance of Immunophenotype

Lymphoma.

Studies of canine multicentric lymphoma have consistently demonstrated that immunophenotype (B versus T) provides prognostically useful information in conjunction with clinical stage (Ruslander et al., 1997; Teske et al., 1994). T-cell lymphomas typically have a worse prognosis than B-cell lymphomas. It is important to note, however, that there are histologic subtypes of T cell lymphoma (Ponce et al., 2004) that have a good prognosis, and histologic subtypes of B-cell lymphoma that have a poor prognosis (Raskin and Fox, 2003). In human medicine, surface markers have been identified to help distinguish between some histologic subtypes of lymphoma via flow cytometry but, because we have not yet reached that point in veterinary medicine, immunophenotype should ideally be combined with histologic subtyping.

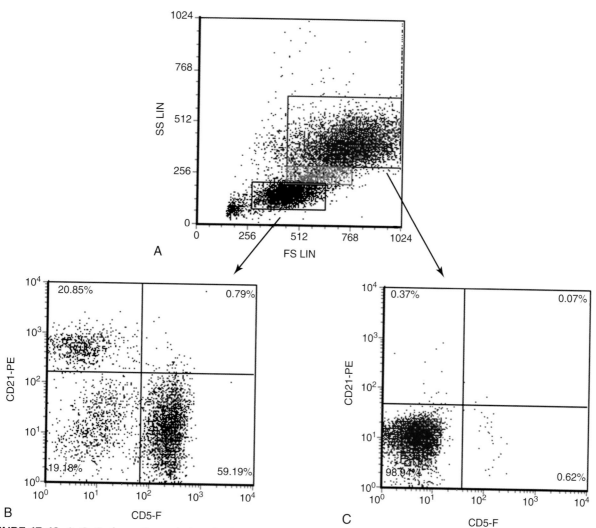

■ **FIGURE 17-13. A–C, Gating cell populations by flow cytometry. A,** Forward and side scatter histogram used to gate different leukocyte populations. **B,** Expression of CD5 (x axis, FITC fluorochrome) and CD21 (y axis, PE fluorochrome) on the lymphocyte population showing that 60% of the cells express CD5, and 20% of the cells express CD21. The quadrants were drawn so that in the isotype control, 95% of the cells were in the lower left quadrant (not shown). **C,** Expression of CD5 and CD21 on the neutrophil population, demonstrating that these cells do not express either marker.

Peripheral Lymphocytosis.

Willliams et al. (2008) have examined the immunophenotype of canine lymphoproliferative disorders involving peripheral lymphocytosis (without distinguishing lymphoma from leukemia) and its prognostic significance. Analyzing peripheral blood samples, immunophenotype, plus one additional clinical or cellular feature allowed dogs with circulating neoplastic lymphocytes to be placed in good and poor prognostic categories. In B-cell disorders, the size of the circulating lymphocytes was prognostic (larger B cells were associated with shorter survival), and in CD8 T-cell disorders, the lymphocyte count was prognostic (cases with >30,000 lymphocytes/μl had shorter survival times) (Williams et al., 2008).

Classification of Acute Leukemia

Acute leukemia, diagnosed by cellular morphology, has long been known to have a poor prognosis. The use of anti–canine CD34, a marker generally found on precursor lymphocytes, is useful in objectively identifying cases of acute leukemia. CD34 is most likely expressed on both ALL and AML (Villiers et al., 2006; Workman and Vernau, 2003), but there are presently no published studies examining the distribution of CD34 on different leukemic subtypes. In addition, because the traditional classification scheme for acute leukemia has relied on cellular morphology alone, the correlation between blast morphology and CD34 expression has not been established. Despite this fact, recent work has documented a significantly shortened survival time in dogs with increased numbers of circulating CD34+ cells (Williams et al., 2008).

Often when blasts are identified in the peripheral blood or bone marrow it is difficult to assign a cell lineage, and flow cytometry can be extremely useful in these cases although again, few reports have been published correlating morphologic characteristics with immunophenotype. Cytoplasmic staining of acute leukemias may be more useful than surface staining, because human T-cell ALL express CD3 only in their cytoplasm

(Szczepanski et al., 2006), and the B cell marker CD79a is located in the cytoplasm. Leukemias staining with either of these markers can generally be classified as lymphoid. Cells staining with surface markers such as CD14 or CD11b are classified as myeloid. Intracellular staining with an antibody to myeloperoxidase or using the antibody MAC387 may provide further confirmation of the myeloid origin of these cells. There is an excellent study correlating AML subclassification (AML-M1, M4 and M5) with immunophenotype using a variety of markers (Villiers et al., 2006), but similar studies are not available for ALL.

Diagnosis of Mediastinal Masses

A particularly useful application of flow cytometry involves distinguishing lymphoma from thymoma in cases of lymphocyte-rich mediastinal masses (Lana et al., 2006a). Thymic lymphocytes coexpress the markers CD4 and CD8 whereas all other T cells express either CD4 or CD8. A proportion of the lymphocytes associated with the neoplastic epithelial tissue in a thymoma will coexpress CD4 and CD8 so that this phenotype, together with the small size of the cells, is diagnostic for thymoma (Fig. 17-14). Lymphomas involving the mediastinum are generally T cell, but express only one or neither of the subset markers CD4 or CD8. Since making the distinction between lymphoma and thymoma determines whether a patient will have chemotherapy or surgery, this is a particularly important use for this assay.

IMAGE ANALYSIS

Complementary to flow cytometry is image analysis. Image analysis is the measuring and counting of microscopic images in order to obtain information of diagnostic importance. Although image analysis has existed for some time, the advent of computer-assisted analysis has led to a more rapid, sensitive, and quantitative

method of evaluation (Meijer et al., 1997). Typically, a television camera receives images from a light microscope. These signals are converted into digits by an interfaced computer, creating digitized cell images that can be displayed on a monitor.

Image analysis can be divided into three different areas: for example, cellular morphometry, counting cellular components, and cytometry. Morphometry is the quantitative description of geometric features of cellular structures of any dimension. The counting of cellular components or object counting is usually applied to the assessment of cell kinetics by evaluating proliferative markers in tumors. This allows for the quantitation of the proliferative fraction or number of mitoses in a cell population, which has been shown to be useful for evaluation of the biologic behavior of tumors. Proliferation markers include bromodeoxyuridine (BrdU), proliferating cell nuclear antigen (PCNA), Ki67, and AgNOR method.

DNA cytometry is the measurement of DNA content in tumor cells and is used as a marker of malignancy in oncology. Image cytometry is used to measure the amount of ICC or IHC stained proteins in cells.

Laser scanning cytometry is a newer technology that scans cells on a slide, which are evaluated by flow cytometry type analysis (Darzynkiewicz et al., 1999). Laser cytometry permits the observer to view cells and correlate flow cytometry data directly with cells measured and classify those cells by standard morphologic criteria.

PCR FOR ANTIGEN RECEPTOR REARRANGEMENTS (PARR)

In human medicine, determination of clonality by detecting clonally rearranged antigen receptor genes is often the test of choice if routine cytology, histology and immunophenotyping are not able to provide a definitive diagnosis of lymphoid malignancy (Swerdlow, 2003).

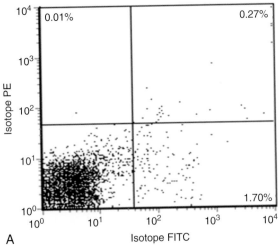
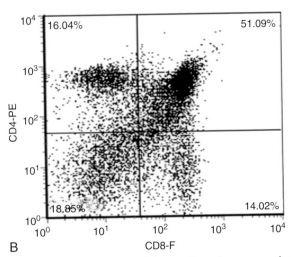

■ **FIGURE 17-14. A&B, Detection of thymoma by flow cytometry.** Both panels show fluorescence of the small lymphocyte population, gated based on forward and side scatter (not shown). **A,** Isotype control showing placement of quadrants. **B,** CD4 and CD8 fluorescence, showing that 51% of the cells coexpress CD4 and CD8 (upper right quadrant). Note the presence of cells that express only CD4 or CD8. These cells represent the stage of thymic differentiation following the double positive (CD4+CD8+) stage, when one or the other of the two markers have been downregulated.

Clonality testing is based on the observation that lymphocytes mount a diverse response to antigens, whether they are derived from the environment (such as allergens), from pathogens, or from self (autoantigens). By contrast, malignant lymphocytes are homogeneous, arising from a single transformed cell. Normal lymphocyte differentiation depends on the process of antigen receptor rearrangement; therefore, all mature lymphocytes have antigen receptor genes that have undergone V-J or V-D-J rearrangement. Immunoglobulin genes are rearranged in B lymphocytes, and T-cell receptor genes α/β and/or γ/δ in T lymphocytes (Jung and Alt, 2004). During this process (Fig. 17-15) nucleotides are trimmed or added between genes as they recombine, resulting in significant length and sequence heterogeneity, particularly within the complementarity determining region 3 (CDR3). Further diversity within B-cell immunoglobulin genes is created by somatic hypermutation during antigen-driven B cell activation. The end result of this differentiation is a diverse population of lymphocytes with virtually limitless antigen specificity and a large variety of CDR3 sequences and lengths. Lymphocytes derived from the same clone will have CDR3 regions of the same length and sequence. The term PARR is used to distinguish it from other types of PCR assays and from other methods of determining clonality. Additional means of determining clonality in human medicine would include the amplification of BCL1-IGH and BCL2-IGH genes, because the chromosomal translocation that brings the BCL and IGH loci together is relatively common in human B cell lymphomas (van Dongen et al., 2003).

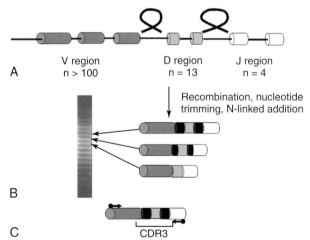

■ **FIGURE 17-15. A–C, Immunoglobulin gene recombination.** **A,** One V region gene (of more than 100 in the human genome) recombines with a randomly selected D region gene and a J region gene, looping out the intervening DNA. **B,** During this process, nucleotides are added *(black bars)* between genes, which generate length and sequence diversity in the complementarity determining region 3 (CDR3). Differentially sized DNA can be separated on a polyacrylamide gel and will appear as a ladder representing different populations of B cells (shown at left). **C,** Primers with homology to the conserved framework regions of V and J regions *(arrows)* will amplify PCR products of different sizes when the DNA is derived from different lymphocytes. Primers are located outside the hypervariable CDR3.

Methodology

Sample Collection

The principle behind this assay has been described more detail (Avery, 2004; Workman and Vernau, 2003). The steps to carry out a clonality assay begin with DNA extraction from tissue. Virtually any type of tissue can be used as a source of DNA, including blood, cavity fluids, aspirates, CSF, stained or unstained cytology preps, and tissue in paraffin blocks. The latter is the least desirable because formalin fixation degrades DNA and can result in both more false negatives and false positives.

DNA Amplification

Primers that hybridized to the conserved portions of V and J region genes of immunoglobulin and T-cell receptor genes are then used to amplify DNA in a PCR reaction. Although T-cell receptors can either be α/β or γ/δ, primers recognizing TCRγ are used. Since there are fewer TCRγ genes, fewer primers are needed to detect the majority of malignancies, and TCRγ is rearranged before TCRβ, so will be clonal even if the malignancy ultimately expresses TCRα/β. In human medicine, primers recognizing TCRγ, TCRβ, TCRδ, as well V-J, D-J and BCL-IgH rearrangements, are used to detect clonality (van Dongen et al., 2003).

Data Analysis

Analysis of these PCR products can be carried out using a variety of methods designed to evaluate the size of the products, and in some cases the sequence heterogeneity. Polyacrylamide gel electrophoresis separates the PCR products by size. The presence of a dominant, single-sized product indicates the presence of a group of lymphocytes that share an identically sized CDR3 region (e.g., clonally expanded). The presence of a variably sized products suggests a polyclonal population of lymphocytes. For gel electrophoresis to be used, the gels must have the ability to resolve products that are three base pairs different in size (thus agarose gels cannot be used). Alternative methods include heteroduplex analysis (Moore et al., 2005), which resolves products by both size and sequence heterogeneity (and thus may provide more resolving power), capillary gel electrophoresis, which separates products by size but is less time consuming, and melt curve analysis (Xu et al., 2002), which uses Syber Green technology and also relies on both size and sequence heterogeneity.

Data Interpretation

Figure 17-16 shows PCR products separated by size using polyacrylamide gel electrophoresis (Burnett et al, 2003). Each case has a positive control (lane 1) to confirm the presence of DNA. The positive control DNA is amplified with any primers that will give a single product, thereby confirming the relative quantity and quality of the extracted DNA. Two sets of primers are used to amplify immunoglobulin genes in separate reactions (lanes 2 and 3), and two sets of primers are used to

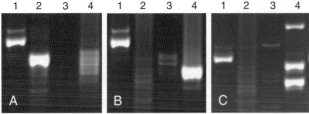

■ **FIGURE 17-16.** A–C, PARR assay analyzed by polyacrylamide gel electrophoresis. Each panel represents four reactions from a different dog. Lane 1: Positive control indicating the presence of DNA. Primers are specific for Cmu, but could be for any gene. Lanes 2 and 3: Two different sets of primers for immunoglobulin genes. Lane 4: Primers for T-cell receptor genes. **A,** Dog with B-cell lymphoma with a single band in lane 2 of greater strength than the positive control. Note the other lanes show no products of a smear. **B,** Dog with T-cell lymphoma with a single band in lane 4. **C,** Dog with T-cell lymphoma and several discrete clonal PCR products.

amplify TCRγ (lane 4) in the same reaction (there are technical reasons for this arrangement).

Amplification can result in no product (for example lane 3 in panel A), a smear (lane 4 in panel A), a single-sized PCR product (lane 2 panel A), or multiple discrete products (lane 4 panel C). A smear or no product is interpreted as a negative result (no evidence of clonality), while one or more prominent, discrete products is considered a positive result (indicating the presence of a clonally expanded population[s]). In Figure 17-16, the dog in panel A had a clonal B cell population and the dogs in panels B and C had clonal T cell populations.

The most common positive result is one or two PCR products. Two PCR products is most likely the result of rearrangements of both chromosomes in the tumor. However it is not unusual to see multiple rearrangements (Kisseberth et al., 2007). The reason for more than two discrete PCR products is not clear. It may also be possible that a derivative of the original neoplastic clone underwent additional recombination events. These questions may be resolved by sequencing individual PCR products, but this has not yet been done.

It is important that as laboratories develop this assay, they provide sensitivity and specificity numbers for their assay—published results from one laboratory do not translate to another because of the wide variation in the way the assay is carried out. In the authors' laboratory, the sensitivity of the assay on canine cases of histologically or cytologically confirmed lymphomas or leukemias is 80%. The reasons for false negative results may be: 1) it is not possible to generate primers that detect all V or J region genes, and the malignancy uses a gene to which the primers do not hybridize; 2) the malignancy has lost the chromosome carrying the antigen receptor genes; 3) somatic hypermutation in cases of B-cell lymphoma or leukemia has altered the sequence to which the primers hybridize; 4) the malignancy is NK in origin and therefore does not contain a rearranged antigen receptor gene.

The presence of a clonal population is 94% specific for malignancy. The 6% of cases in which there is a clonal population of B or T cells, but no lymphoproliferative

disease, have included single cases of Lyme disease, Rocky Mountain Spotted Fever, *Bartonella* infection, and several cases of *Ehrlichia canis* infection. There are likely additional reasons for detecting a clonal lymphocyte population in non-neoplastic conditions, which need to be determined.

Applications

Diagnosis of Lymphoma and Leukemia

Clonality testing is now available for dogs and cats on a routine basis. The first large-scale study of this technique was reported by Burnett et al. (2003) following earlier studies that demonstrated the presence of clonally rearranged T-cell receptor genes in canine malignancy (Dreitz et al., 1999; Fivenson et al., 1994; Vernau and Moore, 1999).

The most common application of this technique is in cases where cytology or histology is ambiguous. Because the assay can detect between 1:100 and 1:1000 neoplastic cells within a population of normal cells (Burnett et al., 2003), it can be useful in early cases of lymphoma or leukemia. Stained or unstained cytology slides or cells freshly aspirated into EDTA tubes are the best samples for this purpose. Interpretation of the results will vary depending on the sensitivity and specificity of the assay in each laboratory offering the test.

Staging Lymphoma and Monitoring Disease

Since the PARR assay is more sensitive than visual examination of cells, it can detect neoplastic cells in the peripheral blood when they are not detected by cytology (Keller et al., 2004). Approximately 75% of stage III lymphomas, which have no visually detectable circulating neoplastic cells, will have a PARR+ result in the peripheral blood (Lana et al., 2006b). The presence of these cells does not appear to correlate with a worse outcome; however, clinical staging remains the most useful predictor of prognosis. It may be possible to use PARR to monitor the progression of disease following chemotherapy and to predict relapse before it is clinically evident, but this application has not yet been explored.

Clonal Relationships between Tumors

The sequence of the CDR3 region that is amplified during the PCR process is unique to each lymphocyte clone. Therefore this sequence can be used to establish the relationship between neoplastic cells that arise in different places in the body, arise at different times, or have a dramatically different morphologic appearance. For example, the relationship between *Helicobacter pylori* infection and human gastric lymphoma was established by showing that the B-cell lymphoma in a patient with a history of *Helicobacter* infection had the same CDR3 sequence as clones found in reactive gastritis biopsy specimens obtained several years earlier (Zucca et al., 1998).

The unique CDR3 sequence can be used to determine if two tumors with morphologically different phenotypes are related. Brauninger et al. (1999) described two human patients with two distinct forms of lymphoma occurring simultaneously. Both patients had classic

Hodgkin's lymphoma while one also had a follicular lymphoma and the other had a T cell–rich B-cell lymphoma. The CDR3 sequence of the immunoglobulin gene in the Reed-Sternberg cells of the Hodgkin's lymphoma was identical to the CDR3 sequence of the other form of B-cell lymphoma in both patients. This finding indicates that a single clone can evolve into dramatically different morphologic phenotypes. Burnett et al. (2004) carried out a similar study in a dog treated for classical non-Hodgkin's B-cell lymphoma which then developed multiple myeloma. By sequencing the CDR3 regions of both tumors, it was shown that the B cells from the lymphoma and the plasma cells from the multiple myeloma had the same clonal origin

Clonality Assays in Cats

The sequences of TCRγ and immunoglobulin genes from cats have been published and used for clonality assays in cases of visceral B-cell lymphoma and intestinal T-cell lymphoma (Moore et al., 2005; Werner et al., 2005). In a study using these primers in cases of feline intestinal lymphoma, the sensitivity of the T cell primers was 89%, and the sensitivity of the B cell primers was 68%. In our laboratory, when applied to all forms of feline lymphoma and leukemia, these primers currently can detect approximately 60% of all confirmed feline lymphomas and leukemias. Additional primers are being developed in an attempt to increase sensitivity. This assay will be particularly useful for distinguishing inflammatory bowel disease from lymphoma in cats, a distinction that is often difficult to make histologically.

DETECTION OF CHROMOSOMAL ABNORMALITIES

Lymphoma and leukemia are frequently associated with translocations because the process of recombining antigen receptor genes leaves lymphocytes susceptible to mistakes in recombination. Most translocations found in human leukemia and lymphoma involve the immunoglobulin heavy chain gene locus. For example, the t(11;14) translocation juxtaposes the locus encoding cyclin D1 on chromosome 11 to an immunoglobulin-enhancer sequence on chromosome 14. This translocation, which results in the overexpression of cyclin D1,

is found in virtually all cases of mantle cell lymphoma (Campo, 2003). Detection of the translocation by PCR or the overexpressed protein by immunohistochemistry can be used to confirm the diagnosis of mantle cell lymphoma in histologically ambiguous cases. Recently, a consortium of European researchers found that the combined use of clonality determination through antigen receptor rearrangements together with detection of this and other translocations by PCR resulted in detection of a clonal population in 95% of cases of confirmed lymphoid malignancies (van Krieken et al., 2003).

Chromosomal aberrations have been detected in dogs by conventional karyotyping (Hahn et al., 1994) and by comparative genome hybridization (Thomas et al., 2003). Aberrations include the gain or loss of portions of chromosomes, as well as balanced translocations between different chromosomes. The assays used to detect these chromosomal changes are not yet amenable to routine diagnostic testing, and may not be sufficiently sensitive for detecting early malignancy or a small number of malignant cells within a population of reactive cells. Despite this fact, studies of this sort will almost certainly lead to the discovery of targeted PCR and immunohistochemistry or flow cytometry–based assays that can be used for detecting malignant lymphocytes in ambiguous cases.

CHOOSING ANCILLARY TESTS FOR SUSPECTED LYMPHOID NEOPLASIA

The primary utility of the PARR assay is to help establish the presence of lymphoma or leukemia in cases where more routine diagnostic tests are ambiguous. Some examples of situations where PARR is useful include: lymph node aspirates where lymphoma is suggested but cannot be concluded (e.g., a predominance of small to intermediate-sized lymphocytes or the mild expansion of intermediate-sized to large lymphocytes), lymphocyte-rich, nonchylous effusions, or increased plasma cell numbers in the marrow. Flow cytometry is the first test of choice for animals with peripheral lymphocytosis. In cases of cytologically or histologically confirmed lymphoma, flow cytometry, immunohistochemistry, or immunocytochemistry are the best methods for immunophenotyping. Table 17-8 lists common

TABLE 17-8   Ancillary Diagnostic Testing in Lymphoma and Leukemia

Presenting Complaint	Best Site to Test	Best Test(s) to Use
Lymphoma, confirmed, need phenotype	Lymph node	Flow cytometry, IHC, ICC
Lymphoma, suspect, equivocal cytology/histology	Lymph node or involved organ	PARR
Lymphocytosis or leukemia	Peripheral blood	Flow cytometry, ICC
Rare suspicious cells in the peripheral blood, no lymphocytosis	Peripheral blood	PARR
Splenomegaly, equivocal cytology/histology	Spleen	PARR
Mass or aspirate with cells of unclear origin	Mass	IHC, ICC, Flow cytometry if cellular; PARR if not
Lymphocyte rich effusion	Effusion fluid	Flow cytometry, IHC, ICC

IHC, Immunohistochemistry; *ICC*, immunocytochemistry; *PARR*, PCR for antigen receptor rearrangements.

diagnostic dilemmas involving lymphoproliferative disorders, and the type of test that is most useful in each. Note that while this list applies to both dogs and cats, both flow cytometry and PARR are less rewarding in cats. There are fewer antibodies for flow cytometry in this species, resulting in less complete characterization of lymphoproliferative diseases, and the PARR assay is currently less sensitive in cats.

REFERENCES

Abendroth CS, Dabbs DJ: Immunocytochemical staining of unstained versus previously stained cytologic preparations, *Acta Cytol* 39:379-386, 1995.

Appelbaum FR, Sale GE, Storb R, et al: Phenotyping of canine lymphoma with monoclonal antibodies directed at cell surface antigens: Classification, morphology, clinical presentation and response to chemotherapy, *Hematol Oncol* 2:151-168, 1984.

Afifiy AM, Al-Khafaji BM, Paulino AFG, et al: Diagnostic use of muscle markers in the cytologic evaluation of serous fluids, *Appl Immunohistochem Mol Morphol* 10:178-182, 2002.

Argyle DJ, Nasir L: Telomerase: a potential diagnostic and therapeutic tool in canine oncology, *Vet Pathol* 40:1-7, 2003.

Avery PR, Avery AC: Molecular methods to distinguish reactive and neoplastic lymphocyte expansions and their importance in transitional neoplastic states, *Vet Clin Pathol* 33:196-207, 2004.

Bancroft JD, Gamble M (eds): *Theory and practice of histological techniques*, ed 6, Edinburgh, 2007, Churchill Livingstone.

Bardou VJ, Arpino G, Elledge RM, et al: Progesterone receptor status significantly improves outcome prediction over estrogen receptor status alone for adjuvant endocrine therapy in two large breast cancer databases, *J Clin Oncol* 21:1973-1979, 2003.

Barr NJ, Wu NCY: Cytopathology/FNA. In Taylor CR, Cote RJ (eds): *Immunomicroscopy: a diagnostic tool for the surgical pathologist*, ed 3, Philadelphia, 2006, Saunders, pp 397-416.

Baumgart E, Cohen MS, Neto BS, et al: Identification and prognostic significance of an epithelial-mesenchymal transition expression profile in human bladder tumors, *Clin Cancer Res* 13:1685-1694, 2007.

Boenisch T: Pretreatment for immunohistochemical staining simplified, *Appl Immunohistochem Mol Morphol* 15:208-212, 2007.

Bräuninger A, Hansmann M-L, Strickler JG, et al: Identification of common germinal-center B-cell precursors in two patients with both Hodgkin's disease and non-Hodgkin's lymphoma, *N Engl J Med* 340:1239-1247, 1999.

Brown RW: Immunocytochemistry. In Ramzy I (ed): *Clinical cytopathology and aspiration biopsy: fundamental principles and practice*, New York, 2001, McGraw-Hill, pp. 535-548.

Burnett RC, Blake MK, Thompson LJ, et al: Evolution of a B-Cell lymphoma to multiple myeloma after chemotherapy, *J Vet Intern Med* 18:768-771, 2004.

Burnett RC, Vernau W, Modiano JF, et al: Diagnosis of canine lymphoid neoplasia using clonal rearrangements of antigen receptor genes, *Vet Pathol* 40:32-41, 2003.

Byrne KM, Kim HW, Chew BP, et al: A standardized gating technique for the generation of flow cytometry data for normal canine and normal feline blood lymphocytes, *Vet Immunol Immunopath* 73:167-182, 2000.

Cadile CD, Kitchell BE, Newman RG, et al: Telomere length in normal and neoplastic canine tissues, *Am J Vet Res* 68:1386-1391, 2007.

Campo E: Genetic and molecular genetic studies in the diagnosis of B-cell lymphomas I: mantle cell lymphoma, follicular lymphoma, and Burkitt's lymphoma, *Hum Pathol* 34:330-335, 2003.

Caniatti M, Roccabianca P, Scanziani E, et al: Canine lymphoma: immunocytochemical analysis of fine-needle aspiration biopsy, *Vet Pathol* 33:204-212, 1996.

Capurro M, Wanless IR, Sherman M, et al: Glypican-3: a novel serum and histochemical marker for hepatocellular carcinoma, *Gastroenterology* 125:89-97, 2003.

Carson FL: *Histotechnology: a self-instructional text*, ed 2, 1997, American Society for Clinical Pathology.

Chijiwa K, Uchida K, Tateyama S: Immunohistochemical evaluation of canine peripheral nerve sheath tumors and other soft tissue sarcomas, *Vet Pathol* 41:307-318, 2004.

Dabbs DJ: Immunocytology. In Dabbs DJ (ed): *Diagnostic immunohistochemistry*, New York, 2002, Churchill Livingstone, pp 625-639.

Dabbs DJ: Immunohistology of metastatic carcinoma of unknown primary. In Dabbs DJ (ed): *Diagnostic immunohistochemistry*, ed 2, New York, 2006, Churchill Livingstone.

Dardick I, Herrera GA: Diagnostic electron microscopy of neoplasms, *Hum Pathol* 29:1335-1338, 1998.

Dardick I, Eyden B, Federman M, et al (eds.): *Handbook of diagnostic electron microscopy for pathologists-in-training*, New York, 1996, Igaku-Shoin.

Darzynkiewica Z, Bedner E, Li X, et al: Laser-scanning cytometry: a new instrumentation with many applications, *Exp Cell Res* 249:1-12, 1999.

Day MJ: Immunophenotypic characterization of cutaneous lymphoid neoplasia in the dog and cat, *J Comp Pathol* 112:79-96, 1995.

DeLellis RA, Hoda RS: Immunohistochemistry and molecular biology in cytological diagnosis. In Koss LG, Melamed MR (eds): *Koss' diagnostic cytology and its histopathologic basis*, Philadelphia, 2006, Lippincott Williams & Wilkins, pp 1635-1680.

Dickersin GR (ed): *Diagnostic electron microscopy: a text/atlas*, ed 2, New York, 2000, Springer.

Dreitz MJ, Ogilvie G, Sim GK: Rearranged T lymphocyte antigen receptor genes as markers of malignant T cells, *Vet Immunol Immunopath* 69:113-119, 1999.

Dvorak AM, Monahan-Earley RA (eds.): *Diagnostic ultrastructural pathology I*, Boca Raton, 1992, CRC Press.

Erlandson RA (ed.): *Diagnostic transmission electron microscopy of tumors*, New York, 1994, Raven Press.

Espinosa de los Monteros A, Fernández A, Millán MY et al: Coordinate expression of cytokeratins 7 and 20 in feline and canine carcinomas, *Vet Pathol* 36:179-190, 1999.

Espinosa de los Monteros A, Millán MY, Ordás J, et al: Immunolocalization of the smooth muscle-specific protein calponin in complex and mixed tumors of the mammary gland of the dog: assessment of the morphogenetic role of the myoepithelium, *Vet Pathol* 39:247-256, 2002.

Eyden B (ed): *Organelles in tumor diagnosis: an ultrastructural atlas*, New York, 1996, Igaku-Shoin.

Fetsch PA, Abati A: Ancillary techniques in cytopathology. In Atkinson BF (ed), *Atlas of diagnostic cytopathology*, ed 2, Philadelphia, 2004, Saunders, pp 747-775.

Fisher C: The comparative roles of electron microscopy and immunohistochemistry in the diagnosis of soft tissue tumors, *Histopathology* 48:32-41, 2006.

Fivenson DP, Saed GM, Beck ER, et al: T-cell receptor gene rearrangement in canine mycosis fungoides: further support for a canine model of cutaneous T cell lymphoma, *J Invest Derm* 102:227-230, 1994.

Geninet C, Bernex F, Rakotovao F, et al: Sclerosing peritoneal mesothelioma in a dog: a case report, *J Vet Med A* 50:402-405, 2003.

Ghadially FN (ed): *Diagnostic ultrastructural pathology: a self-evaluation and self-teaching manual*, ed 2, Boston, 1998, Butterworth-Heinemann.

Goldstein NS, Hewitt SM, Taylor CR, et al: Recommendations for improved standardization of immunohistochemistry, *Appl Immunohistochem Mol Morphol* 15:124-133, 2007.

Gong Y, Sun X, Michael CW, et al: Immunocytochemistry of serous effusion specimens: a comparison of ThinPrep vs. cell block, *Diagn Cytopathol* 28:1-5, 2003.

Gorczyca W, Weisberger J, Liu Z, et al: An approach to diagnosis of T-cell lymphoproliferative disorders by flow cytometry, *Cytometry* 50:177-190, 2002.

Greeley EH, Ballam JM, Harrison JM, et al: The influence of age and gender on the immune system: a longitudinal study in Labrador Retriever dogs, *Vet Immunol Immunopath* 82:57-71, 2001.

Grindem CB, Page RL, Ammerman BE, et al: Immunophenotypic comparison of blood and lymph node from dogs with lymphoma, *Vet Clin Pathol* 27:16-20, 1998.

Hahn KA, Richardson RC, Hahn EA, et al: Diagnostic and prognostic importance of chromosomal aberrations identified in 61 dogs with lymphosarcoma, *Vet Pathol* 31:528-540, 1994.

Heeb HL, Wilkerson MJ, Chun R, et al: Large granular lymphocytosis, lymphocyte subset inversion, thrombocytopenia, dysproteinemia, and positive Ehrlichia serology in a dog, *J Am Anim Hosp Assoc* 39:379-384, 2003.

Höinghaus R, Hewicker-Trautwei M, Mischke R: Immunocytochemical differentiation of canine mesenchymal tumors in cytologic imprint preparations, *Vet Clin Pathol* 37:104-111, 2008.

Ishikawa K, Sakai H, Hosoi M, et al: Evaluation of cell proliferation in canine tumors by the bromodeoxyuridine labeling method, immunostaining of Ki-67 antigen and proliferating cell nuclear antigen, *J Toxicol Pathol* 19:123-127, 2006.

Jennings CD, Foon KA: Recent advances in flow cytometry: application to the diagnosis of hematologic malignancy, *Blood* 90:2863-2892, 1997.

Jung D, Alt FW: Unraveling V(D)J recombination; insights into gene regulation, *Cell* 116:299-311, 2004.

Keller RL, Avery AC, Burnett RC, et al: Detection of neoplastic lymphocytes in peripheral blood of dogs with lymphoma by polymerase chain reaction for antigen receptor gene rearrangement, *Vet Clin Pathol* 33:145-149, 2004.

Kisseberth WC, Nadella WV, Breen M, et al: A novel canine lymphoma cell line: a translational and comparative model for lymphoma research, *Leuk Res* 31:1709-1720, 2007.

Kiupel M, Teske E, Bostock D: Prognostic factors for treated canine malignant lymphoma, *Vet Pathol* 36:292-300, 1999.

Kiupel M, Webster JD, Kaneene JB, et al: The use of KIT and tryptase expression patterns as prognostic tools for canine cutaneous mast cell tumors, *Vet Pathol* 41:371-377, 2004.

Kow K, Bailey SM, Williams ES, et al: Telomerase activity in canine osteosarcoma, *Vet Comp Oncol* 4:184-187, 2006.

Lana S, Plaza S, Hampe K, et al: Diagnosis of mediastinal masses in dogs by flow cytometry, *J Vet Intern Med* 20:1161-1165, 2006a.

Lana SE, Jackson TL, Burnett RC, et al: Utility of polymerase chain reaction for analysis of antigen receptor rearrangement in staging and predicting prognosis in dogs with lymphoma, *J Vet Intern Med* 20:329-334, 2006b.

Leong ASY, Suthipintawong C, Vinyuvat S: Immunostaining of cytologic preparations: a review of technical problems, *Appl Immunohistochem Mol Morphol* 7:214-220, 1999.

Litlekalsoy J, Vatne V, Hostmark JG, et al: Immunohistochemical markers in urinary bladder carcinomas from paraffin-embedded archival tissue after storage for 5-70 years, *BJU Int* 99:1013-1019, 2007.

Long S, Argyle DJ, Nixon C, et al: Telomerase reverse transcriptase (TERT) expression and proliferation in canine brain tumors, *Neuropathol Appl Neurobiol* 32:662-673, 2006.

Mackay B: Electron microscopy in tumor diagnosis. In Fletcher CDM (ed): *Diagnostic histopathology of tumors*, ed 3, New York, 2007, Churchill Livingstone, pp 1831-1859.

Madewell BR: Cellular proliferation in tumors: a review of methods, interpretation, and clinical applications, *J Vet Intern Med* 15:334-340, 2001.

Maleszewski J, Lu J, Fox-Talbot K, et al: Robust immunohistochemical staining of several classes of proteins in tissues subjected to autolysis, *J Histochem Cytochem* 55:597-606, 2007.

McDonough SP, Moore PF: Clinical, hematologic, and immunophenotypic characterization of canine large granular lymphocytosis, *Vet Pathol* 37:637-646, 2000.

Meijer GA, Belien JAM, van Diest PJ, et al: Image analysis in clinical pathology, *J Clin Pathol* 50:365-370, 1997.

Mengel M, Wasielewski R, Wiese B, et al: Inter-laboratory and inter-observer reproducibility of immunohistochemical assessment of the Ki-67 labelling index in a large multi-centre trial, *J Pathol* 198:292-299, 2002.

Miller RT, Kubier P: Immunohistochemistry on cytologic specimens and previously stained slides (when no paraffin block is available), *J Histotechnol* 25:251-257, 2002.

Mimura T, Ito A, Sakuma T, et al: Novel marker D2-40, combined with calretinin, CEA, and TTF-1: an optimal set of immunodiagnostic markers for pleural mesothelioma, *Cancer* 109:933-938, 2007.

Mittelbronn M, Dietz K, Simon P, et al: Albumin in immunohistochemistry: foe and friend, *Appl Immunohistochem Mol Morphol* 14:441-444, 2006.

Modiano JF, Smith R, Wojcieszyn J, et al: The use of cytochemistry, immunophenotyping, flow cytometry, and in vitro differentiation to determine the ontogeny of a canine monoblastic leukemia, *Vet Clin Pathol* 27:40-49, 1998.

Moore PF, Woo JC, Vernau W, et al: Characterization of feline T cell receptor gamma (TCRG) variable region genes for the molecular diagnosis of feline intestinal T cell lymphoma, *Vet Immunol Immunopath* 106:167-178, 2005.

Morini M, Bettini G, Morandi F, et al: Deciduoid peritoneal mesothelioma in a dog, *Vet Pathol* 43:198-201, 2006.

Murakami Y, Tateyawa S, Uchida K, et al: Immunohistochemical analysis of cyclins in canine normal testes and testicular tumors, *J Vet Med Sci* 63:909-912, 2001.

Polak JM, Van Noorden S: *Introduction to immunocytochemistry*, ed 3, Oxford, 2003, Garland Science/BIOS Scientific Publishers.

Ponce F, Magnol JP, Marchal T, et al: High-grade canine T cell lymphoma/leukemia with plasmacytoid morphology: a clinical pathological study of nine cases, *J Vet Diagn Invest* 15:330-337, 2003.

Ponce F, Magnol JP, Ledieu D, et al: Prognostic significance of morphological subtypes in canine malignant lymphomas during chemotherapy, *Vet J* 167:158-166, 2004.

Prophet EB (ed): *AFIP laboratory methods in histotechnology*, Washington DC, 1992, American Registry of Pathology.

Ramos-Vara JA: Technical aspects of immunohistochemistry, *Vet Pathol* 42:405-426, 2005.

Ramos-Vara JA, Beissenherz ME: Optimization of immunohistochemical methods using two different antigen retrieval methods on formalin-fixed, paraffin-embedded tissues: experience with 63 markers, *J Vet Diagn Invest* 12:307-311, 2000.

Ramos-Vara JA, Miller MA: Immunohistochemical characterization of canine intestinal epithelial and mesenchymal tumors with a monoclonal antibody to hepatocyte paraffin 1 (Hep Par 1), *Histochem J* 34:397-401, 2002.

Ramos-Vara JA, Miller MA: Immunohistochemical detection of protein gene product 9.5 (PGP 9.5) in canine epitheliotropic T-cell lymphoma (mycosis fungoides), *Vet Pathol* 44:74-79, 2007.

Ramos-Vara JA, Saeteele J: Immunohistochemistry. In Howard GC, Kaser MR (eds), *Making and using antibodies: a practical handbook*, Boca Raton, 2007, CRC Press, pp 273-314.

Ramos-Vara JA, Beissenherz ME, Miller MA, et al: Retrospective study of 338 canine oral melanomas with clinical, histologic, and immunohistochemical review of 129 cases, *Vet Pathol* 37:597-608, 2000.

Ramos-Vara JA, Miller MA, Johnson GC: Immunohistochemical characterization of canine hyperplastic hepatic lesions and hepatocellular and biliary neoplasms with monoclonal antibody hepatocyte paraffin 1 and a monoclonal antibody to cytokeratin 7, *Vet Pathol* 38:636-643, 2001a.

Ramos-Vara JA, Beissenherz ME, Miller MA, et al: Immunoreactivity of A103, an antibody to Melan-A, in canine steroid-producing tissues and their tumors, *J Vet Diagn Invest* 13:328-332, 2001b.

Ramos-Vara JA, Miller MA, Johnson GC, et al: Immunohistochemical detection of thyroid transcription factor-1, thyroglobulin, and calcitonin in canine normal, hyperplastic, and neoplastic thyroid gland, *Vet Pathol* 39:480-487, 2002a.

Ramos-Vara JA, Miller MA, Johnson GC, et al: Melan A and S100 protein immunohistochemistry in feline melanomas: 48 cases, *Vet Pathol* 39:127-132, 2002b.

Ramos-Vara JA, Miller MA, Boucher M, et al: Immunohistochemical detection of uroplakin III, cytokeratin 7, and cytokeratin 20 in canine urothelial tumors, *Vet Pathol* 40:55-62, 2003.

Ramos-Vara JA, Miller MA, Johnson GC: Usefulness of thyroid transcription factor-1 immunohistochemical staining in the differential diagnosis of primary pulmonary tumors of dogs, *Vet Pathol* 42:315-320, 2005.

Ramos-Vara JA, Miller MA, Valli VEO: Immunohistochemical detection of multiple myeloma 1/interferon regulatory factor 4 (MUM1/IRF-4) in canine plasmacytoma: comparison with CD79a and CD20, *Vet Pathol* 44:875-884, 2007.

Ramos-Vara JA, Kiupel M, Baszler T, et al: Suggested guidelines for immunohistochemical techniques in veterinary diagnostic laboratories, *J Vet Diagn Invest* 20:393-413, 2008.

Raskin RE, Fox LE: Clinical relevance of the World Health Organization classification of lymphoid neoplasms in dogs (Abst), *Vet Pathol* 40:593, 2003.

Reguera MJ, Rabanal RM, Puigdemont A, et al: Canine mast cell tumors express stem cell factor receptor, *Am J Dermatopathol* 22:49-54, 2000.

Reid V, Doherty J, McIntosh G, et al: The first quantitative comparison of immunohistochemical rabbit and mouse monoclonal antibody affinities using Biacore analysis, *J Histotechnol* 30:177-182, 2007.

Rezuke WN, Abernathy EC, Tsongalis GJ: Molecular diagnosis of B- and T-cell lymphomas: fundamental principles and clinical applications, *Clin Chem* 43:1814-1823, 1997.

Rhodes A: Quality assurance of immunocytochemistry and molecular morphology. In Hacker GW, Tubbs RR (eds): *Molecular morphology in human tissues: techniques and applications*, Boca Raton, 2005, CRC Press, pp 275-293.

Roels S, Tilmant K, Ducatelle R: PCNA and Ki67 proliferation markers as criteria for prediction of clinical behavior

of melanocytic tumors in cats and dogs, *J Comp Pathol* 121: 13-24, 1999.

Ruslander DA, Gebhard DH, Tompkins MB, et al: Immunophenotypic characterization of canine lymphoproliferative disorders, *In vivo* 11:169-172, 1997.

Sakai H, Noda A, Shirai N, et al: Proliferative activity of canine mast cell tumors evaluated by bromodeoxyuridine incorporation and Ki-67 expression, *J Comp Pathol* 127:233-238, 2002.

Sato T, Miyoshi T, Shibuya H, et al: Peritoneal biphasic mesothelioma in a dog, *J Vet Med A* 52:22-25, 2005.

Scase TJ, Edwards D, Miller J, et al: Canine mast cell tumors: correlation of apoptosis and proliferation markers with prognosis, *J Vet Intern Med* 20:151-158, 2006.

Sherman ME, Jimenez-Joseph D, Gangi MD, et al: Immunostaining of small cytologic specimens: facilitation with cell transfer, *Acta Cytol* 38:18-22, 1994.

Stoica G, Cohen N, Mendes O, et al: Use of immunohistochemical marker calretinin in the diagnosis of a diffuse malignant metastatic mesothelioma in an equine, *J Vet Diagn Invest* 16:240-243, 2004.

Sundram U, Kim Y, Mraz-Gernhard S, et al: Expression of the bcl-6 and MUM1/IRF4 proteins correlate with overall and disease-specific survival in patients with primary cutaneous large B-cell lymphoma: a tissue microarray study, *J Clin Pathol* 32:227-234, 2005.

Suthipintawong C, Leong ASY, Vinyuvat S: Immunostaining of cell preparations: a comparative evaluation of common fixatives and protocols, *Diagn Cytopathol* 15:167-174, 1996.

Swerdlow SH: Genetic and molecular genetic studies in the diagnosis of atypical lymphoid hyperplasias versus lymphoma, *Hum Pathol* 34:346-351, 2003.

Szczepanski T, van der Velden VH, Van Dongen JJ: Flow-cytometric immunophenotyping of normal and malignant lymphocytes, *Clin Chem Lab Med* 44:775-796, 2006.

Teske E, van Heerde P, Rutteman GR, et al: Prognostic factors for treatment of malignant lymphoma in dogs, *J Am Vet Med Assoc* 205:1722-1728, 1994.

Thomas R, Smith KC, Ostrander EA, et al: Chromosome aberrations in canine multicentric lymphomas detected with comparative genomic hybridisation and a panel of single locus probes, *Br J Cancer* 89:1530-1537, 2003.

van Dongen JJ, Langerak AW, Bruggemann M, et al: Design and standardization of PCR primers and protocols for detection of clonal immunoglobulin and T-cell receptor gene recombinations in suspect lymphoproliferations: report of the BIOMED-2 Concerted Action BMH4-CT98-3936, *Leukemia* 17:2257-2317, 2003.

van Krieken JH, Langerak AW, San Miguel JF, et al: Clonality analysis for antigen receptor genes: preliminary results from the Biomed-2 concerted action PL 96-3936, *Hum Pathol* 34:359-361, 2003.

Vernau W, Moore PF: An immunophenotypic study of canine leukemias and preliminary assessment of clonality by polymerase chain reaction, *Vet Immunol Immunopath* 69:145-164, 1999.

Vilches-Moure JG, Ramos-Vara JA: Comparison of rabbit monoclonal and mouse monoclonal antibodies in immunohistochemistry in canine tissues, *J Vet Diagn Invest* 17:346-350, 2005.

Villiers E, Baines S, Law AM, et al: Identification of acute myeloid leukemia in dogs using flow cytometry with myeloperoxidase, MAC387, and a canine neutrophil-specific antibody, *Vet Clin Pathol* 35:55-71, 2006.

Vosse BAH, Seelentag W, Bachmann A, et al: Background staining of visualization systems in immunohistochemistry. Comparison of the avidin-biotin complex system and the EnVision+ system, *Appl Immunohistochem Mol Morphol* 15:103-107, 2007.

Vural SA, Ozyldilz Z, Ozsoy SY: Pleural mesothelioma in a nine-month-old dog, *Irish Vet J* 60:30-33, 2007.

Webster JD, Yuzbasiyan-Gurkan V, Miller RA, et al: Cellular proliferation in canine cutaneous mast cell tumors: associations with *c-KIT* and its role in prognostication, *Vet Pathol* 44:298-308, 2007a.

Webster JD, Yuzbasiyan-Gurkan V, Trosko JE, et al: Expression of the embryonic transcription factor OCT4 in canine neoplasms: a potential marker for stem cell subpopulations in neoplasia, *Vet Pathol* 44:893-900, 2007b.

Webster JD, Miller MA, DuSold D, et al: Effects of prolonged formalin-fixation on diagnostic immunohistochemistry in domestic animals, *J Histochem Cytochem*. Available at *http://www.jhc.org/cgi/content/abstract/jhc.2009.953877v1*. Accessed April 30, 2009.

Weiser MG, Thrall MA, Fulton R, et al: Granular lymphocytosis and hyperproteinemia in dogs with chronic ehrlichiosis, *J Am Anim Hosp Assoc* 27:84-88, 1991.

Werner JA, Woo JC, Vernau W, et al: Characterization of feline immunoglobulin heavy chain variable region genes for the molecular diagnosis of B-cell neoplasia, *Vet Pathol* 42:596-607, 2005.

Wilkerson MJ, Dolce K, Koopman T, et al: Lineage differentiation of canine lymphoma/leukemias and aberrant expression of CD molecules, *Vet Immunol Immunopath* 106:179-196, 2005.

Williams MJ, Avery, AC, Lana, SE, et al: Canine lymphoproliferative disease characterized by lymphocytosis: immunophenotypic markers of prognosis, *J Vet Intern Med* 22:596-601, 2008.

Workman HC, Vernau W: Chronic lymphocytic leukemia in dogs and cats: the veterinary perspective, *Vet Clin North Am Small Anim Pract* 33:1379-1399, 2003.

Xu D, Du J, Schultz C, et al: Rapid and accurate detection of monoclonal immunoglobulin heavy chain gene rearrangement by DNA melting curve analysis in the LightCycler system, *J Mol Diag* 4:216-222, 2002.

Yaziji H, Barry T: Diagnostic immunohistochemistry: what can go wrong? *Adv Anat Pathol* 13:238-246, 2006.

Zucca E, Bertoni F, Roggero E, et al: Molecular analysis of the progression from Helicobacter pylori-associated chronic gastritis to mucosa-associated lymphoid-tissue lymphoma of the stomach, *N Eng J Med* 338:804-810, 1998.

Index

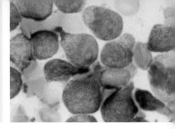

Page numbers followed by f indicate figures; t, tables; b, boxes.

439